PATHOLOGIC FEATURES

GROSS FINDINGS

Cribriform hyperplasia is not recognizable grossly.

MICROSCOPIC FINDINGS

This lesion is characterized by a crowded cribriform and complex papillary proliferation of epithelial cells (Fig. 1-22A). The nuclei are small, bland, and without prominent nucleoli. Frequently, the cribriform glands have clear cytoplasm and uniform, round lumina (Fig. 1-22B). On low power, the lesion typically has a nodular appearance. Around many of the glands is a strikingly prominent basal cell layer consisting of a row of cuboidal, darkly stained cells beneath the clear cells (Fig. 1-22C).

ANCILLARY STUDIES

IMMUNOHISTOCHEMISTRY

Immunostains for HMWCK can highlight the basal cell layer (Fig. 1-23), although this usually is unnecessary.

DIFFERENTIAL DIAGNOSIS

Cribriform clear cell hyperplasia can be confused with both high-grade PIN and cribriform adenocarcinoma. The distinction of cribriform hyperplasia from cribri-

form carcinoma is based on the nodularity, presence of basal cells, and lack of significant cytologic atypia. In contrast to high-grade PIN, cells in cribriform hyperplasia do not exhibit nuclear atypia, and there is a prominent basal cell layer around some of the glands.

PROGNOSIS AND THERAPY

Clear cell cribriform hyperplasia is a benign lesion and requires no treatment.

BASAL CELL HYPERPLASIA

BCH is typically seen as part of the spectrum of benign prostatic hyperplasia, usually in samples from the TZ. However, it can be found in the PZ of the prostate, associated with inflammation. BCH is, in association with atrophy, a common reactive response in the setting of antiandrogen therapy.

CLINICAL FEATURES

BCH is uncommon, with an incidence of 3% to 15%. It is usually identified in TURP specimens but may be

---

CRIBRIFORM CLEAR CELL HYPERPLASIA—PATHOLOGIC FEATURES

Gross Findings
► Nonrecognizable

Microscopic Findings
► Glands contain cribriform and complex papillary proliferation of epithelial cells
► Clear cytoplasm and uniform, round lumina
► Small, bland nuclei without prominent nucleoli
► Nodular appearance at low power
► Strikingly prominent basal cell layer focally present

Immunohistochemical Features
Basal cell positive for HMWCK

Differential Diagnosis
► High-grade PIN
► Cribriform adenocarcinoma of the prostate
► Central zone epithelium

BASAL CELL HYPERPLASIA—FACT SHEET

Definition
► Nodular and diffuse expansion of uniform round and occasional cribriform glands associated with acellular stroma, as part of the spectrum of benign prostatic hyperplasia

Incidence and Location
► Uncommon: incidence 3-15%
► Most common in transition zone; can be found in peripheral zone associated with inflammation

Morbidity and Mortality
► Incidental histologic finding

Gender, Race, and Age Distribution
► Men 60-80 years

Clinical Features
► Patients present with symptoms of prostatism
► Common reactive response in the setting of antiandrogen therapy

Prognosis and Treatment
► Benign lesion
► Conservative treatment

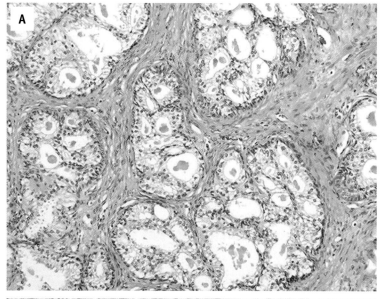

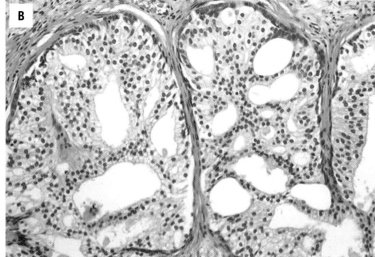

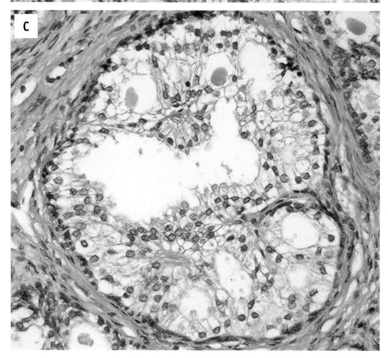

FIGURE 1-22

A, At low power, the lesion of cribriform clear cell hyperplasia is characterized by crowded cribriform and complex papillary proliferation of epithelial cells. **B,** Frequently, the cribriform glands have clear cytoplasm and uniform, round lumina. **C,** At high power, the nuclei are small, bland, and without prominent nucleoli. A strikingly prominent basal cell layer is present around many of the glands.

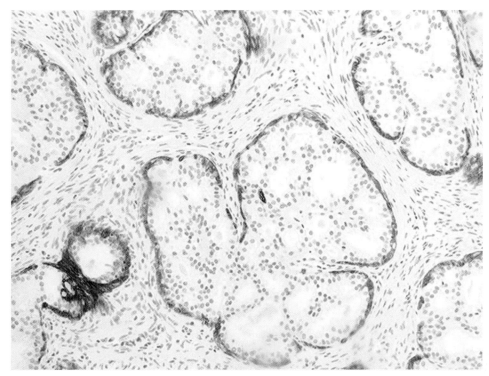

FIGURE 1-23
Immunostains for high-molecular-weight cytokeratin (HMWCK) can highlight the basal cell layer in cribriform clear cell hyperplasia.

encountered in needle biopsies. Patients typically are 60 to 80 years of age and present with symptoms of prostatism.

prostatic entities that contain well-formed lamellar calcifications in up to half of the cases (Fig. 1-24C). Another unique feature is the presence of intra-cytoplasmic eosinophilic globules.

PATHOLOGIC FEATURES

GROSS FINDINGS

BCH is not recognizable grossly.

MICROSCOPIC FINDINGS

BCH is usually characterized by nodular expansion of uniform, round glands associated with normal-appearing stroma (Fig. 1-24A). It may be divided into complete or incomplete forms, usual and "atypical" types. The complete form is characterized by solid nests of dark, blue cells with lack of luminal cell differentiation. The incomplete form is characterized by residual small lumina lined by secretory cells with clear cytoplasm, surrounded by multiple layers of basal cells (Fig. 1-24B). In both types, the basal cells are dark with scant cytoplasm and display round to oval, or spindled, hyperchromatic nuclei. Nucleoli are often indistinct. In some cases, nucleoli are prominent; this initially was termed "atypical basal cell hyperplasia" but is currently referred to as "basal cell hyperplasia with prominent nucleoli," so as to not cause unnecessary concern for patients and clinicians. BCH is also one of the few

---

BASAL CELL HYPERPLASIA—PATHOLOGIC FEATURES

Gross Findings
▶ Nonrecognizable

Microscopic Findings
▶ *Complete:* solid nests of dark, blue cells with lack of luminal differentiation
▶ *Incomplete:* residual small lumina lined by secretory cells with clear cytoplasm, surrounded by multiple layers of basal cells
▶ Basal cells are dark with scant cytoplasm and display round to oval, or spindled, hyperchromatic nuclei
▶ Nucleoli are indistinct but may be more prominent ("basal cell hyperplasia with prominent nucleoli")
▶ Well-formed lamellar calcifications (half of cases)
▶ Intracytoplasmic eosinophilic globules

Immunohistochemical Features
▶ Strong positivity for HMWCK, p63
▶ Weak and focal positivity for PSA and PSAP

Differential Diagnosis
▶ Prostatic adenocarcinoma
▶ High-grade PIN

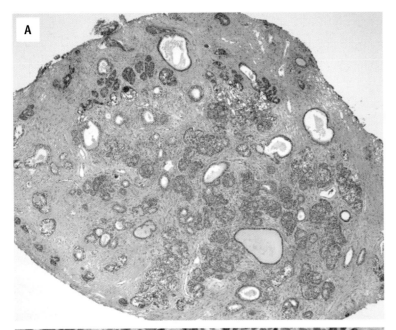

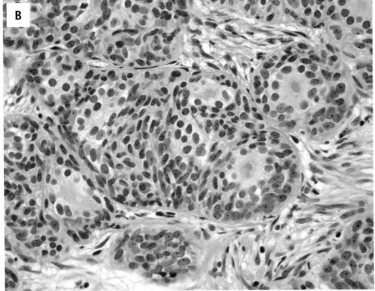

FIGURE 1-24

A, At low power basal cell hyperplasia is characterized by a nodular expansion of uniform, round glands associated with normal-appearing stroma. **B,** The incomplete form is characterized by residual small lumina lined by secretory cells with clear cytoplasm, surrounded by multiple layers of basal cells. **C,** At high power, the basal cells are dark, with scant cytoplasm and round-to-oval hyperchromatic nuclei. Nucleoli are often indistinct. Well-formed lamellar calcifications *(center)* are noted in up to half of the cases.

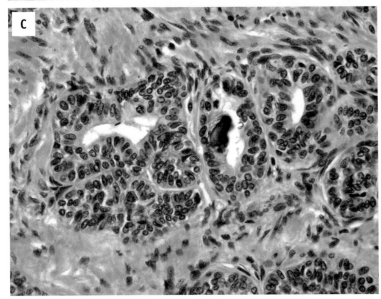

ANCILLARY STUDIES

IMMUNOHISTOCHEMISTRY

Special histochemical stains have shown acid and neutral mucin in BCH, whereas immunoperoxidase stains demonstrate a phenotype similar to that of normal basal cells: strong positivity for HMWCK and p63, and weaker and focal positivity for PSA and PSAP.

DIFFERENTIAL DIAGNOSIS

BCH with prominent nucleoli can be difficult to distinguish from high-grade PIN. Differentiating features within BCH include rounder nuclei, atrophic luminal cytoplasm, occasional presence of atypical cells beneath benign-appearing secretory cells, in some cases solid nests, and immunohistochemical demonstration of multiple layers of basal cells. BCH with nucleoli is distinguished from adenocarcinoma by the multilayering of nuclei, the presence of solid nests, atrophic cytoplasm, and the presence of basal cells.

PROGNOSIS AND THERAPY

There is no known association between BCH showing prominent nucleoli and either acinar adenocarcinoma or basaloid carcinoma of the prostate.

NEPHROGENIC ADENOMA OR METAPLASIA

Nephrogenic metaplasia (nephrogenic adenoma) is a benign proliferation of gland-like structures that most commonly involve the urinary bladder. Despite its earlier designation as nephrogenic adenoma, this lesion is thought to arise from metaplasia of the underlying urothelium. The lesion has been associated with radiation, surgery, stones, instrumentation, intravesical thiotepa and bacille Calmette-Guérin (BCG), and renal transplantation.

CLINICAL FEATURES

The largest series of nephrogenic metaplasia reported 80 cases. The majority of lesions occur in the bladder; the prostatic urethra and ureter are less frequently involved.

PATHOLOGIC FEATURES

GROSS FINDINGS

Nephrogenic metaplasia is usually a small, solitary, incidental lesion, but tumors up to 4.0 cm in diameter have been reported. It may appear as papillary, polypoid,

---

NEPHROGENIC ADENOMA OR METAPLASIA—FACT SHEET

Definition
- Benign proliferation of gland-like structures that most commonly involve the urinary bladder

Incidence and Location
- Rare (80 cases reported in largest series of nephrogenic metaplasia)
- Most common in bladder and prostatic urethra; ureter less frequently involved

Morbidity and Mortality
- Benign metaplastic proliferation
- Multifocal in 18% of cases

Clinical Features
- Associated with radiation, surgery, stones, instrumentation, intravesical thiotepa, BCG, renal transplantation

Prognosis and Treatment
- Can rarely recur

NEPHROGENIC ADENOMA OR METAPLASIA—PATHOLOGIC FEATURES

Gross Findings
- Small, solitary, incidental lesion
- Papillary, polypoid, hyperplastic, fungating, friable, or velvety lesion

Microscopic Findings
- Four patterns: tubular, cystic, polypoid-papillary, and diffuse
- Small, solid to hollow tubules lined by low columnar or cuboidal epithelial cells
- Eosinophilic (occasionally clear cell) cytoplasm
- Minimal cytologic atypia
- Mitotic figures are absent to very rare
- Occasionally cells exhibit a hobnail configuration
- Thickened hyaline sheath around some tubules
- Occasional eosinophilic secretions
- May extend into underlying smooth muscle

Immunohistochemical Features
- Frequently positive for HMWCK
- Focal positive tubular secretions for PSA and PSAP
- Strong cytoplasmic positivity for AMACR in up to 58% of cases

Differential Diagnosis
- Well-differentiated prostatic adenocarcinoma

hyperplastic, fungating, friable, or velvety lesions. In approximately 18% of cases, multiple lesions are identified.

MICROSCOPIC FINDINGS

Three main histologic patterns have been described: tubular, cystic, diffuse and polypoid-papillary (Fig. 1-25A). The majority of the cases consist of small hollow tubules lined by low columnar or cuboidal epithelial cells with eosinophilic to clear cell cytoplasm and minimal cytologic atypia. Mitotic figures are absent to very rare. Occasionally, cells exhibit a hobnail configuration. A distinguishing feature of nephrogenic adenoma is the presence of a thickened hyaline sheath around some of the tubules, which may enhance with

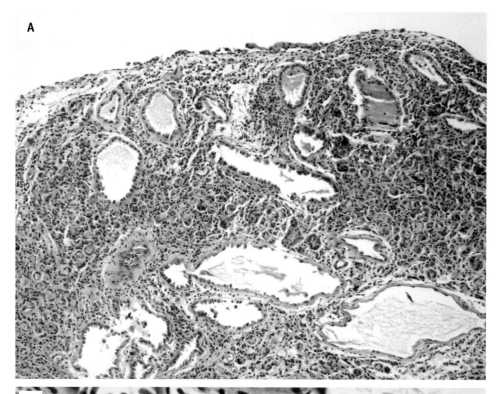

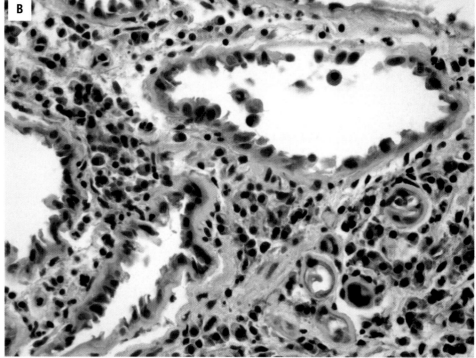

FIGURE 1-25

A, Low-power view of tubulocystic nephrogenic adenoma. **B,** At high power, a distinguishing feature is the presence of a thickened hyaline sheath around some of the tubules *(right lower corner)*. Hobnail cells with reactive atypia line the cystic spaces *(center)*.

PAS stains. Cystic tubules may contain colloid-like eosinophilic secretions. Some tubules are lined by hobnail cells with reactive atypia, resembling vessels. Inflammation is almost always present (Fig. 1-25B).

ANCILLARY STUDIES

IMMUNOHISTOCHEMISTRY

Cytoplasmic staining for HMWCK is found in more than half of cases of nephrogenic adenoma. Focal cytoplasmic staining and/or positive tubular secretions for PSA and PSAP may be seen in almost half of the cases. Strong cytoplasmic positivity for AMACR, ranging from patchy to diffuse, has been reported in up to 58% of nephrogenic adenomas.

DIFFERENTIAL DIAGNOSIS

The presence in a TURP specimen of small glands with occasionally prominent nucleoli within smooth muscle bundles can closely mimic prostate cancer. The small size of the acini, atrophic cytoplasm, cystic dilatation, hyaline rim of connective tissue around some of the glands, inflamed stroma, and distinctive patterns (papillary, tubules with colloid secretions, tubules resembling vessels) separate nephrogenic adenoma arising from the prostatic urethra from adenocarcinoma of the prostate.

PROGNOSIS AND THERAPY

Nephrogenic adenoma is a benign lesion and may rarely recur. According to a recent study, in those cases arising in renal transplantation patients this entity is neither metaplastic nor neoplastic in nature. Molecular studies in this setting suggest that nephrogenic adenoma is thoroughly nephrogenic in origin and results from the implantation of renal tubular cells at sites of prior urothelial injury, with subsequent proliferation of epithelial elements. Whether this is the universal mechanism or more than one etiology is possible is unknown.

MESONEPHRIC REMNANT HYPERPLASIA

Mesonephric remnant hyperplasia is well documented in the female genital tract but is an uncommon incidental histologic finding in the prostate and periprostatic tissue, with 16 cases reported. In a series of almost 700 transurethral resections, 0.6% contained mesonephric remnants. Mesonephric ducts give rise to the ejaculatory ducts and the primordial ureters; remnants may persist in the bladder neck and trigone region.

CLINICAL FEATURES

The mean age of the patients is 70 years (range, 50 to 85 years). Most patients present with prostatism and undergo TURP.

PATHOLOGIC FEATURES

GROSS FINDINGS

Mesonephric remnant hyperplasia is not recognizable grossly.

MICROSCOPIC FINDINGS

The lesion is characterized by a vaguely lobular or infiltrative proliferation of crowded, small tubules lined by a single layer of cuboidal epithelial cells (Fig. 1-26A). Two histologic patterns have been described: One consists of small atrophic acini that contain colloid-like secretion (Fig. 1-26B); the second pattern consists of small atrophic acini with occasional papillary buds with empty lumina, reminiscent of nephrogenic metaplasia. Cytologically, the lining cells are bland, usually with no evidence of nuclear enlargement or prominent nucleoli (Fig. 1-26C).

MESONEPHRIC REMNANT HYPERPLASIA—FACT SHEET

Definition
▶ Benign proliferation of mesonephric remnant

Incidence and Location
▶ Uncommon: 16 cases reported
▶ Incidence in TURP: 0.6%

Morbidity and Mortality
▶ Benign incidental finding

Gender, Race, and Age Distribution
▶ Men; mean age, 70 years (range 50-85 years)

Clinical Features
▶ Patients present with prostatism and undergo TURP

Prognosis and Treatment
▶ Benign proliferation
▶ No treatment needed

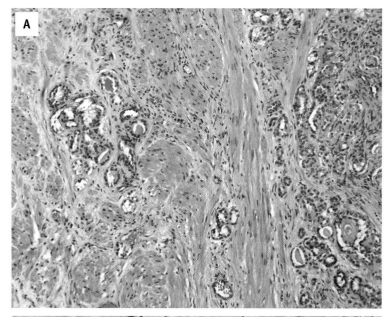

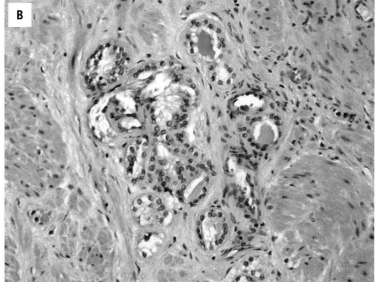

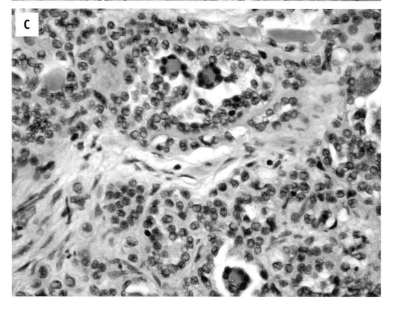

FIGURE 1-26

A, At low power the lesion of mesonephric remnant hyperplasia shows a vaguely lobular or infiltrative proliferation of crowded, small tubules. **B,** Small atrophic acini containing colloid-like secretion. **C,** At high power, the lining cells are bland, with no evidence of nuclear enlargement or prominent nucleoli.

MESONEPHRIC REMNANT HYPERPLASIA—PATHOLOGIC FEATURES

Gross Findings
► Nonrecognizable

Microscopic Findings
► Vaguely lobular or infiltrative proliferation of crowded, small tubules lined by a single layer of cuboidal epithelial cells with scant cytoplasm
► Small acini that contain colloid-like secretion
► Small acini or solid nests with empty lumen
► Lining cells are bland, usually with no evidence of nuclear enlargement or prominent nucleoli

Immunohistochemical Features
► Secretion is positive for PAS and Alcian blue
► Variable staining for HMWCK
► Negative PSA and PSAP immunostains

Differential Diagnosis
► Prostatic adenocarcinoma
► Nephrogenic metaplasia

ANCILLARY STUDIES

IMMUNOHISTOCHEMISTRY

Histochemically, the secretions in the acini are positive for PAS and Alcian blue. Immunohistochemically, mesonephric hyperplasia displays variable immunoreactivity for HMWCK but lacks staining for PSA and PSAP.

DIFFERENTIAL DIAGNOSIS

Because of the infiltrative appearance and the apparent infiltration of the stroma, perineural spaces, and extraprostatic extension, mesonephric remnant hyperplasia should be differentiated from infiltrating PCa. Immunophenotype, the presence of dense eosinophilic luminal substance, in contrast to the loose granular eosinophilic material typically seen in acinar carcinoma, atrophic cytoplasm, and papillary features are helpful tools in the differential diagnosis. Nephrogenic metaplasia closely resembles mesonephric hyperplasia, but this process tends to be periurethral.

PROGNOSIS AND THERAPY

Mesonephric remnant hyperplasia is not a risk factor for malignancy.

PROSTATIC URETHRAL POLYP

Prostatic urethral polyps are benign, single, polypoid to papillary structures that grow into the prostatic urethra in and around the verumontanum. They are most likely hyperplastic and represent an exaggerated proliferation of urethral mucosa.

CLINICAL FEATURES

About 200 cases have been reported. The lesion may occur in a wide age range, from 13 to 84 years of age, although younger adults (27 to 41 years) are most often affected. In addition to the prostatic urethra, the lesion occurs within the bladder, usually around the trigone, where they are termed *ectopic prostatic polyps*. These lesions typically manifest with gross and microscopic hematuria and frequently with hemospermia, dysuria, and frequency.

PATHOLOGIC FEATURES

GROSS FINDINGS

The lesion is grossly characterized as small, papillary or frond-like exophytic tissue or as a polyp.

PROSTATIC URETHRAL POLYP—FACT SHEET

Definition
► Benign, single, polypoid to papillary growth of prostatic tissue

Incidence and Location
► About 200 cases have been reported
► Prostatic urethra around the verumontanum
► Most common location is within the bladder, usually around the trigone

Morbidity and Mortality
► Recurrence is uncommon

Gender, Race, and Age Distribution
► Occur in a wide age range, 13-84 years
► Younger adults, aged 27-41 years, are often affected

Clinical Features
► Gross and microscopic hematuria
► Frequently hemospermia, dysuria, and frequency

Prognosis and Treatment
► Benign lesion
► Cystoscopic excision and fulguration

PROSTATIC URETHRAL POLYP—PATHOLOGIC FEATURES

Gross Findings

▶ Small, papillary or frond-like exophytic tissue or polyp

Microscopic Findings

▶ Papillae lined by benign columnar prostatic and/or transitional epithelium
▶ Fibrovascular cores with benign prostatic acini
▶ Secretory cells are bland without nuclear atypia
▶ No mitotic activity

Immunohistochemical Features

▶ Positive for PSA and PSAP

Differential Diagnosis

▶ Ductal adenocarcinoma of the prostate
▶ Papillary urothelial neoplasms
▶ Villous adenomas

MICROSCOPIC FINDINGS

The lesion consists of a papillary to polypoid growth of fibrovascular cores lined by benign columnar prostatic and/or transitional epithelium. The submucosal component of the polyp is composed of stroma and normal-appearing prostatic acini (Fig. 1-27). In some areas, the acini may be closely packed and cystically dilated. The acini have a typical secretory cell layer with underlying basal cells. The secretory cells are bland without nuclear atypia. No mitotic activity is noted.

ANCILLARY STUDIES

IMMUNOHISTOCHEMISTRY

Immunohistochemically, the surface glandular columnar cells and acini are positive for PSA and PSAP.

DIFFERENTIAL DIAGNOSIS

The differential diagnosis is with ductal adenocarcinoma of the prostate, papillary urothelial neoplasms, and villous adenomas. In contrast to these entities, the cells lining prostatic urethral polyps are indistinguishable from normal prostatic glandular epithelium.

PROGNOSIS AND THERAPY

Prostatic urethral polyps are totally benign lesions. They are treated by cystoscopic excision and fulguration. Recurrence is uncommon.

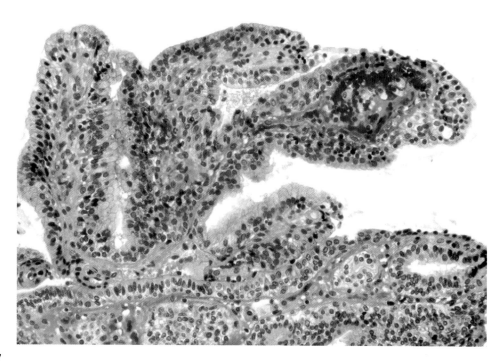

FIGURE 1-27
Prostatic urethral polyp is a polypoid growth of fibrovascular cores lined by benign columnar prostatic epithelium. The submucosal component of the polyp is composed of stroma and normal-appearing prostatic acini.

VERUMONTANUM MUCOSAL GLAND HYPERPLASIA

Verumontanum mucosal gland hyperplasia (VMGH) is a benign, small acinar proliferation that occurs exclusively in the verumontanum and adjacent posterior prostatic urethra, where the utricle and the ejaculatory ducts merge with the prostatic urethra.

CLINICAL FEATURES

VMGH is an uncommon lesion in prostate needle biopsies and is almost never sampled in TURP because of the sparing of the verumontanum by this procedure. The lesion is invariably small, less than 1 mm, and often multicentric. VMGH is identified as an incidental histologic finding in 14% of radical prostatectomy specimens in men 47 to 87 years of age. The small size and the crowded nature of VMGH may simulate low-grade PCa.

PATHOLOGIC FEATURES

GROSS FINDINGS

VMGH is not recognizable grossly.

VERUMONTANUM MUCOSAL GLAND HYPERPLASIA—FACT SHEET

Definition
▶ Benign, small acinar proliferation

Incidence and Location
▶ Uncommon
▶ Incidental finding in 14% of radical prostatectomy specimens
▶ Occurs in the verumontanum and adjacent to the posterior prostatic urethra

Morbidity and Mortality
▶ Benign lesion

Gender, Race, and Age Distribution
▶ Men, 47-87 years of age

Clinical Features
▶ The lesion is invariably small, <1 mm

Prognosis and Treatment
▶ Associated with the presence of adenosis
▶ Not a risk factor for malignancy
▶ No treatment necessary

VERUMONTANUM MUCOSAL GLAND HYPERPLASIA— PATHOLOGIC FEATURES

Gross Findings
▶ Nonrecognizable

Microscopic Findings
▶ Uniform, closely packed, round small acini
▶ Intact basal cell layer
▶ Small, uniform nuclei and inconspicuous nucleoli
▶ Found adjacent to and often contiguous with urothelium
▶ Intraluminal corpora amylacea and distinctive brown-orange concretions
▶ Lipofuscin pigment may be present

Immunohistochemical Features
▶ Mucosal glands stain positively with PSA
▶ Basal cells stain with HMWCK and are S-100 protein negative

Differential Diagnosis
▶ Low-grade adenocarcinoma of the prostate

MICROSCOPIC FINDINGS

The lesion is characterized by relatively uniform, closely packed, round, small acini, with an intact basal cell layer, small uniform nuclei, and inconspicuous nucleoli (Fig. 1-28). VMGH is characteristically identified adjacent to and often contiguous with urothelium. Intraluminal corpora amylacea and distinctive brown-orange concretions are frequent (Fig. 1-28). Lipofuscin pigment may be present within the cytoplasm of the glandular cells.

ANCILLARY STUDIES

IMMUNOHISTOCHEMISTRY

Immunophenotypically, verumontanum mucosal glands are similar to prostatic acini: the secretory cells of these mucosal glands stain positively with antibodies to PSA, whereas the basal cells stain with antibodies to HMWCK and are S-100 protein negative.

DIFFERENTIAL DIAGNOSIS

The main entity to exclude in the differential diagnosis is low-grade PCa. The glands of VMGH lack the infiltrative and haphazard arrangement of the glands typically found in adenocarcinoma. The distinctive intraluminal concretions and basal cell layer further distinguish this entity from prostate cancer.

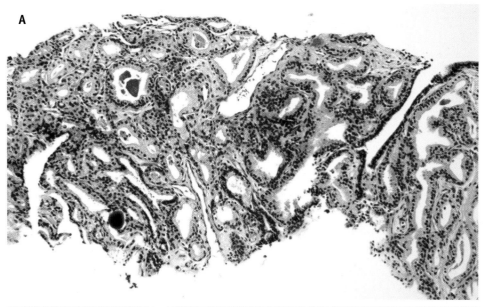

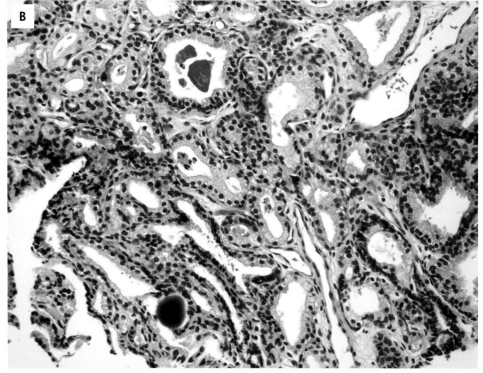

FIGURE 1-28
A, At low power, verumontanum mucosal gland hyperplasia (VMGH) is a proliferation of relatively uniform, closely packed, round, small acini. **B,** At high power, the luminal cells have small uniform nuclei and inconspicuous nucleoli. An intact basal cell layer is present. Intraluminal distinctive brown-orange concretions are frequent.

PROGNOSIS AND THERAPY

VMGH has been associated with the presence of adenosis, but it is not a risk factor for malignancy.

NORMAL NONPROSTATIC TISSUE IN PROSTATE SPECIMENS

Seminal vesicles, ejaculatory duct apparatus, Cowper's gland, paraganglia, skeletal muscle within prostate gland, and nerves with involvement by benign prostate glands are normal anatomic structures that are readily recognized and easily separated from malignancy. However, they may in some situations present a diagnostic problem, particularly with limited sampling.

SEMINAL VESICLES AND EJACULATORY DUCT APPARATUS

Occasionally, seminal vesicle tissue or ejaculatory duct apparatus, or both, are present in specimens obtained by transurethral resection or needle biopsy of the prostate.

Due to the limited amount of tissue, it may sometimes be difficult to recognize the characteristic architectural pattern; moreover, the cytologic atypia can also be a source of overdiagnosis of PCa. The recognition of seminal vesicle tissue or ejaculatory duct apparatus rests on appreciating their architectural as well as cytologic features.

PATHOLOGIC FEATURES

GROSS FINDINGS

The seminal vesicles are paired, coiled and tubular male sex accessory glands bounded by the prostate distally, the base of the bladder anteriorly, and Denonvillier's fascia and the rectum posteriorly. In adults, they measure approximately 6 cm in length and 2 cm in width, although marked variation has been reported. The duct originating from each seminal vesicle joins the ampulla of the vasa deferentia to form the paired ejaculatory ducts, which are located medially to the seminal vesicles and run through the base of the prostate to the urethra.

MICROSCOPIC FINDINGS

Seminal vesicles are characterized by large, dilated lumina with numerous small glands clustered around the periphery. Often, the glands appear to bud off from the central lumen. A common finding on needle biopsy

is the dilated irregular lumen of the seminal vesicle seen at the edge of the tissue core, where the core is fragmented as it enters the seminal vesicle lumen. At higher magnification, the epithelium lining the lumina and small glands is characterized by cells showing nuclear hyperchromasia and pleomorphism that is at times striking (Fig. 1-29). The nucleoli are markedly enlarged, with bizarre shapes, and often obscure the nuclear details. Despite the pleomorphic features of the nuclei, mitoses are not identified. The atypia appears degenerative in nature, similar to what is seen in association with radiation. Small nuclear pseudoinclusions are commonly seen. Prominent golden-brown lipofuscin granules are typically identified. Morphologically, ejaculatory duct apparatus epithelium is similar to that of seminal vesicles, but, in contrast to the latter, the ducts are surrounded by a band of loose fibrovascular connective tissue and lack a well-formed muscular wall (Fig. 1-30).

ANCILLARY STUDIES

IMMUNOHISTOCHEMISTRY

Negative immunostaining for PSA and PSAP and positive staining for HMWCK and p63 are helpful in excluding the diagnosis of carcinoma. Caution must be used with immunohistochemistry involving polyclonal antibodies to PSA, because they can label seminal vesicle tissue. Monoclonal antibodies to PSA do not exhibit this cross-reactivity.

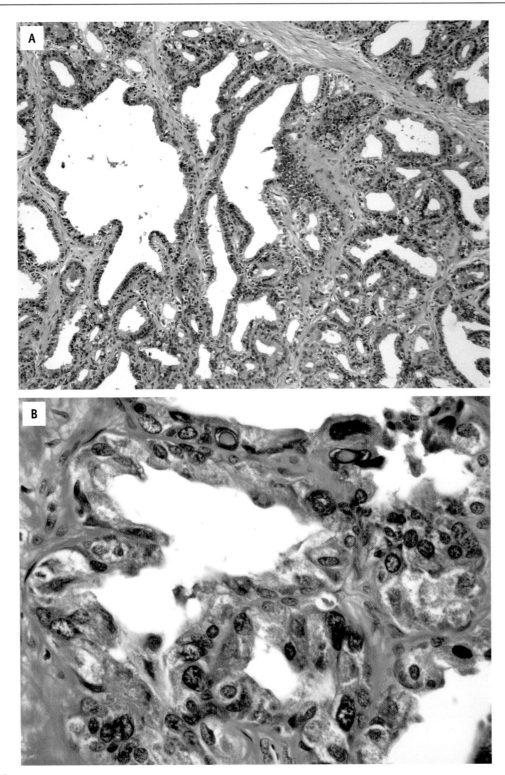

FIGURE 1-29
A, At low power, seminal vesicle tissue consists of large, dilated lumina with numerous small glands clustered around the periphery. **B,** At higher magnification, the epithelium lining the lumina and small glands shows nuclear hyperchromasia and pleomorphism. Nuclear pseudoinclusions are commonly seen. Prominent golden-brown lipofuscin granules are typically identified.

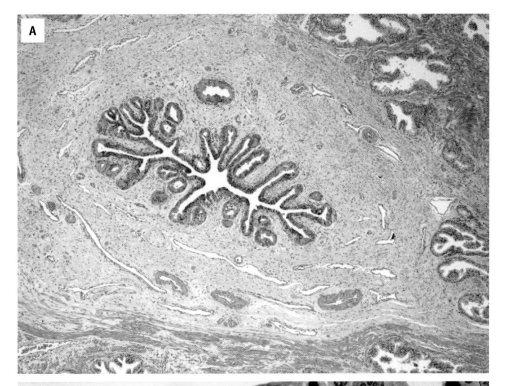

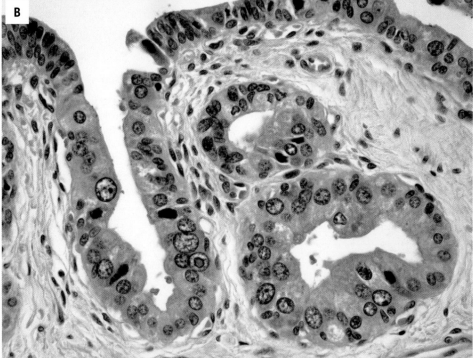

FIGURE 1-30
A, At low power, the ejaculatory ducts are surrounded by a band of loose fibrovascular connective tissue and lack a well-formed muscular wall.
B, At high power, the ejaculatory duct epithelium is similar to that of the seminal vesicles.

DIFFERENTIAL DIAGNOSIS

Seminal vesicle tissue and ejaculatory duct apparatus can be confused with PCa in limited biopsy specimens. When the epithelial atypia and the presence of pigment are not prominent, the diagnosis can be challenging. Even in poorly differentiated prostatic carcinoma lacking glandular differentiation, one rarely sees the severe atypia present within seminal vesicle cells. Benign prostate tissue, high-grade PIN, and, rarely, carcinoma contain lipofuscin; however, the pigment differs in that the granules are smaller and more red-orange or blue. The distinction between seminal vesicles and ejaculatory duct apparatus, although difficult, is of practical importance, because the presence of prostatic carcinoma in ejaculatory duct tissue does not indicate extraprostatic extension, whereas seminal vesicle involvement indicates high-stage disease.

PROGNOSIS AND THERAPY

Seminal vesicles and ejaculatory duct apparatus are normal anatomic structures.

COWPER'S GLANDS

Cowper's glands, also referred to as bulbourethral glands, are paired pea-shaped glands extrinsic to the prostate that are located in the urogenital diaphragm lateral to the membranous urethra near the prostatic apex. Cowper's glands are rarely sampled in prostatic specimens.

CLINICAL FEATURES

Cowper's glands can be seen in specimens obtained by transurethral resection or needle biopsy. The incidental sampling in needle biopsy is a rare event, with an incidence of 0.006%.

PATHOLOGIC FEATURES

GROSS FINDINGS

These small glands measure, on average, 1.0 cm in diameter in adult men.

MICROSCOPIC FINDINGS

Cowper's glands are composed of a circumscribed lobule of small, uniformly sized acini lined by mucus-containing cells with a central duct. The glands may be located within skeletal muscle. Bland cytologic features, including small nuclei and inconspicuous nucleoli, are a characteristic feature (Fig. 1-31).

ANCILLARY STUDIES

IMMUNOHISTOCHEMISTRY

Cowper's glands are mucicarmine, PAS-D (Fig. 1-32), Alcian blue, and cytokeratin positive; they are typically negative for S-100, PSAP, and HMWCK. Staining for

---

COWPER'S GLANDS—FACT SHEET

Definition
► Normal, paired, pea-shaped mucous glands

Incidence and Location
► Extrinsic to the prostate
► Located in urogenital diaphragm lateral to the membranous urethra, near the prostatic apex
► Incidental sampling in needle biopsy is a rare event with an incidence of 0.006%

Gender, Race, and Age Distribution
► Normal finding in all men

Clinical Features
► Seen in TURP or on needle biopsy specimens

Prognosis and Treatment
► Normal anatomic structures

COWPER'S GLANDS—PATHOLOGIC FEATURES

Gross Findings
► Small glands, 1.0 cm in diameter in adult men

Microscopic Findings
► Circumscribed lobule of small, uniformly sized acini
► Lined by mucus-containing cells with a central duct
► Typically located within skeletal muscle
► Bland cytologic features, including small nuclei and inconspicuous nucleoli

Immunohistochemical Features
► Mucicarmine, PAS-D, and Alcian blue positive
► Typically negative for S-100, PSAP
► Staining for PSA is variable
► Basal cells show SMA reactivity
► The ductal cells exhibit HMWCK staining

Differential Diagnosis
► Low-grade prostatic adenocarcinoma
► Foamy gland carcinoma
► Mucinous metaplasia

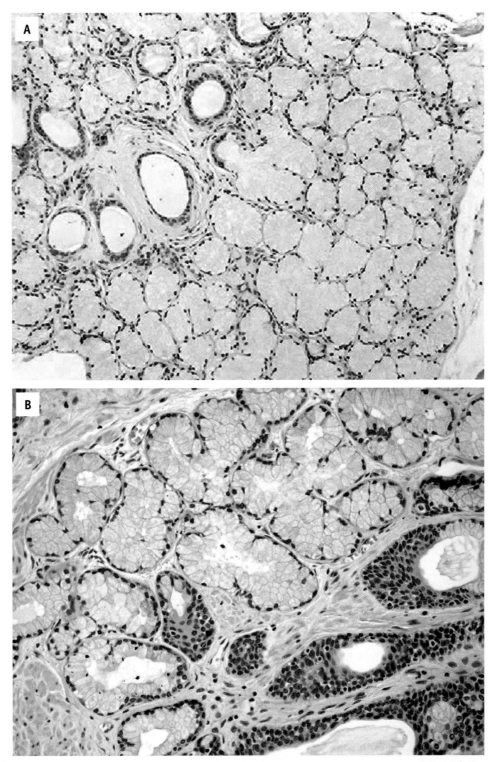

FIGURE 1-31
A and **B,** Cowper's glands are composed of a circumscribed lobule of small, uniform acini lined by mucus-containing cells with a central duct. Bland cytologic features, including small nuclei and inconspicuous nucleoli, are typical features.

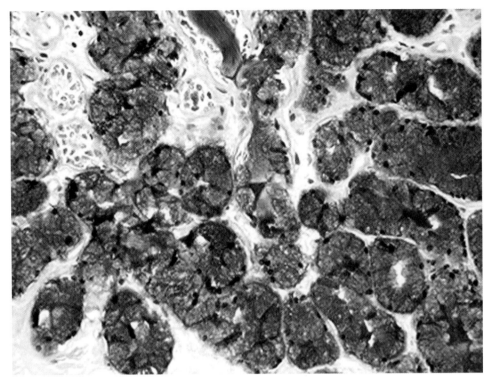

FIGURE 1-32
Cowper's glands are periodic acid-Schiff-positive after diastase digestion (PAS-D).

PSA is variable. Smooth muscle actin (SMA) reactivity has been reported in the basal cells at the periphery of the acini. The ductal cells exhibit HMWCK staining.

DIFFERENTIAL DIAGNOSIS

Cowper's glands may resemble low-grade adenocarcinoma, foamy gland carcinoma, or mucinous metaplasia. The presence of glands in skeletal muscle may further mimic cancer. Cowper's glands can be separated from adenocarcinoma by its lobular architecture, bland cytologic features, and abundant mucus-filled cytoplasm. Although prostate cancer cytoplasm may contain neutral mucinous secretions, in prostate cancers one does not see abundant mucinous cytoplasm to the extent that the lumina are almost occluded. Foamy gland carcinomas have almost as abundant cytoplasm, yet in foamy gland cancer the glands are larger and the mucin stains are negative. The separation between Cowper's glands and mucinous metaplasia is based chiefly on whether the process is intraprostatic or exterior to the gland.

PARAGANGLIA

Paraganglia are located in or adjacent to the lateral neurovascular bundle and can occasionally be identified within prostatic stroma or in the bladder neck smooth muscle. They are situated in smooth muscle but are not admixed with benign prostate glands.

CLINICAL FEATURES

Paraganglia has been identified in 8% of radical prostatectomy specimens. Rarely, paraganglia may be seen in TURP or needle biopsy specimens, where they can be misdiagnosed as high-grade PCa. A more common issue is the misinterpretation of extraprostatic paraganglial tissue in radical prostatectomy specimens as cancer, potentially leading to overstaging.

PATHOLOGIC FEATURES

GROSS FINDINGS

Paraganglia are not recognizable grossly.

MICROSCOPIC FINDINGS

Paraganglia consist of small, solid nests of cells with clear or, more commonly, amphophilic, finely granular cytoplasm, often with a "zellballen" arrangement. A prominent vascular pattern, often intimately related to nerves, is present. The nuclei are often hyperchromatic, but nucleoli are inconspicuous to small (Fig. 1-33).

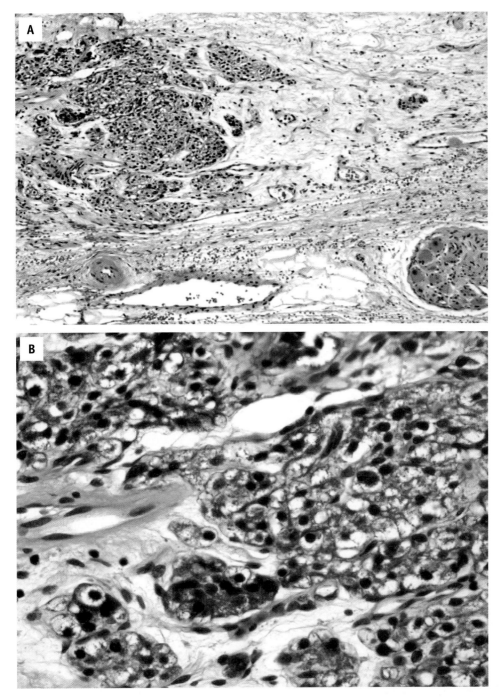

FIGURE 1-33

A, At low power, paraganglia consist of small, solid nests of cells separated by a delicate vascular network. **B,** At high power, the cells have amphophilic, finely granular cytoplasm. The nuclei are often hyperchromatic, but nucleoli are inconspicuous to small.

ANCILLARY STUDIES

IMMUNOHISTOCHEMISTRY

The cells are chromogranin, neuron-specific enolase (NSE), S-100, and synaptophysin positive; they are PSAP and PSA negative.

DIFFERENTIAL DIAGNOSIS

Although paraganglia closely mimic high-grade PCa, the highly vascular setting and the characteristic granular, typically amphophilic cytoplasm are clues to prevent a misdiagnosis. Verification of the diagnosis can be accomplished with immunohistochemistry.

SKELETAL MUSCLE WITHIN PROSTATE GLAND

Skeletal muscle of the urogenital diaphragm not uncommonly extends into the periphery of the prostate gland, especially in the apical and anterior portion. Recognition of this finding is important, because non-neoplastic prostate glands may occasionally be seen admixed with skeletal muscle fibers and should not be diagnosed as prostate carcinoma (Fig. 1-34). Moreover, the presence of prostatic adenocarcinoma glands between skeletal muscle fibers is not diagnostic of extraprostatic extension by carcinoma.

BENIGN GLANDS IN PERINEURAL SPACE

Benign prostatic glands can, on occasion, indent peripheral nerves and can even be found, in extremely rare cases, within nerves. Perineural indentation by benign glands must be distinguished from perineural invasion by cancer. The bland cytology, the benign architecture (i.e., papillary infolding), and the recognition that the glands do not circumferentially surround the nerves are helpful findings in diagnosing perineural indentation by benign glands (Fig. 1-35).

BENIGN STROMAL LESIONS OF THE PROSTATE

BLUE NEVUS

Melanotic lesions of the prostate can be subdivided according to the distribution of the pigment. *Blue nevus* is a term used to describe melanin deposition in spindle stromal cells. The presence of melanin in glandular epithelium, with or without associated stromal melanocytes, is called *melanosis.*

CLINICAL FEATURES

About 22 cases of prostatic blue nevus have been reported. Prostatic blue nevus is an incidental histologic finding, most commonly seen in patients who undergo prosta-

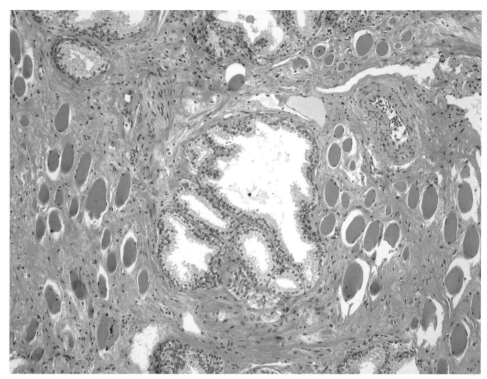

FIGURE 1-34
Non-neoplastic prostate glands may occasionally be seen admixed with skeletal muscle fibers, especially apically and anteriorly.

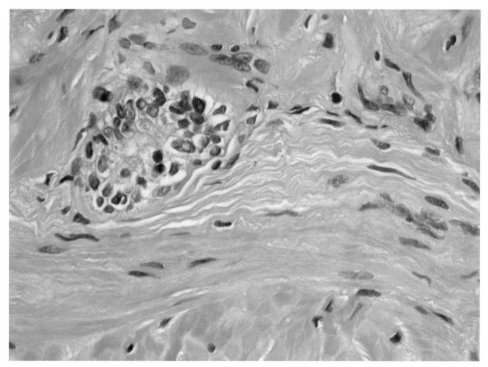

FIGURE 1-35
Benign prostatic glands can on occasion indent peripheral nerves.

BLUE NEVUS—FACT SHEET

Definition
▶ Melanin deposition in spindle stromal cells

Incidence and Location
▶ Rare; about 22 cases reported
▶ Incidence ranges from 0.03% to 4%

Morbidity and Mortality
▶ Benign lesion

Gender, Race, and Age Distribution
▶ The average age at detection is 66 years (range, 50-80 years)

Clinical Features
▶ Incidental histologic finding in patients who underwent prostatectomy for BPH symptoms

Prognosis and Treatment
▶ Not a risk factor for the development of malignancy

tectomy for BPH symptoms. The incidence is 0.03% to 4% of prostatic tissue samples. The average age at detection is 66 years, with a range from 50 to 80 years.

PATHOLOGIC FEATURES

GROSS FINDINGS

Brown to black streaks or areas 0.1 to 2.0 cm in diameter can be appreciated in some cases.

BLUE NEVUS—PATHOLOGIC FEATURES

Gross Findings
▶ Brown to black streaks or areas 0.1 to 2.0 cm in diameter

Microscopic Findings
▶ Deeply pigmented, melanin-filled spindle cells within the fibromuscular stroma
▶ The stromal cells containing the pigment are haphazardly dispersed

Immunohistochemical Features
▶ Pigment stains black with Fontana-Masson and disappears after bleaching with potassium permanganate
▶ Iron and lipofuscin (Luxol fast blue) stains are negative
▶ Pigmented cells stain for S-100 protein
▶ PSA, PSAP, and CEA are negative
▶ HMB-45 can be negative

Differential Diagnosis
▶ Malignant melanoma of the prostate
▶ Hemosiderin-laden stromal macrophages

MICROSCOPIC FINDINGS

Blue nevi are characterized by deeply pigmented, melanin-filled spindle cells within the fibromuscular stroma. The stromal cells containing the pigment are haphazardly dispersed. In two cases, in addition to glandular and stromal melanosis, melanin was also seen in adjacent glands of adenocarcinoma.

ANCILLARY STUDIES

IMMUNOHISTOCHEMISTRY

Histochemically, the pigment stains black with Fontana-Masson and disappears after bleaching with potassium permanganate (Fig. 1-36). Iron and lipofuscin (Luxol fast blue) stains are negative. The pigmented cells stain for S-100 protein, whereas PSA, PSAP, and carcinoembryonic antigen (CEA) immunostains are negative. HMB-45 has been negative in two cases.

DIFFERENTIAL DIAGNOSIS

Blue nevus should be distinguished from malignant melanoma of the prostate and from hemosiderin-laden stromal macrophages. Blue nevus and prostatic melanosis lack the destructive growth and cytologic atypia of melanoma. Hemosiderin is characterized by clumps of golden-yellow pigment, whereas melanin is brown-black and more uniformly and finely granular.

PROGNOSIS AND THERAPY

Prostatic blue nevus is not a risk factor for the development of malignancy, including malignant melanoma.

ENDOMETRIOSIS

A case of endometriosis occurring in a 78-year-old man with a long course of estrogen therapy has been reported. The lesion arose in a small, red-tan raised mass proximal to the internal urethral orifice. The patient was treated with estrogen therapy for prostatic carcinoma. This case and similar lesions reported in the male bladder were invariably associated with hematuria and chlorotrianisene therapy for PCa.

Ductal adenocarcinoma of the prostate is in the differential diagnosis, but, unlike endometriosis, ductal carcinoma displays cytologic atypia, is PSA immunoreactive, and lacks endometrial stroma.

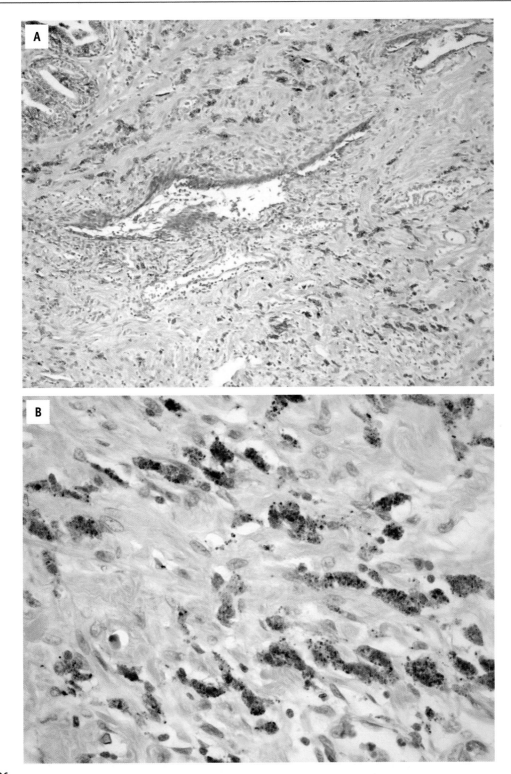

FIGURE 1-36
A, At low power, blue nevi are characterized by deeply pigmented, melanin-filled spindle cells within the fibromuscular stroma. **B,** The stromal cells containing the pigment are haphazardly dispersed (Fontana-Masson stain).

ELASTOSIS

Elastosis of the prostate may be seen in needle biopsy and radical prostatectomy specimens, but its signifi-cance is unknown. The presence of elastosis correlates with age, prostatic atrophy, local and generalized arteriosclerosis, nodular prostatic hyperplasia, and acute inflammation. Elastosis was detected in 65 of 100 consecutive autopsy specimens.

SUGGESTED READINGS

Bostwick DG, Eble JN: Urologic Surgical Pathology. Philadelphia, Mosby, 1997.

Epstein JI, Yang XJ: Prostate Biopsy Interpretation, 3rd ed. Philadelphia, Lippincott, 2002.

Humphrey PA: Prostate Pathology. Chicago, AJCP Press, 2003.

Srigley JR: Benign mimickers of prostatic adenocarcinoma. Mod Pathol 2004;17:328–348.

Benign Prostatic Hyperplasia

Littlejohn JO Jr, Ghafar MA, Kang YM, Kaplan SA: Transurethral resection of the prostate: The new old standard. Curr Opin Urol 2002;12:19–23.

McNeal J: Pathology of benign prostatic hyperplasia: Insight into etiology. Urol Clin North Am 1990;17:477–486.

Walsh PC: Benign prostatic hyperplasia. In Walsh, PC, Retik AB, Stammey TA, et al (eds): Campbell's Urology, 6th ed. Philadelphia, WB Saunders, 1992.

Xia Z, Roberts RO, Schottenfeld D, et al: Trends in prostatectomy for benign prostatic hyperplasia among black and white men in the United States: 1980 to 1994. Urology 1999;53:1154–1159.

Nonspecific Granulomatous Prostatitis

Garcia Solano J, Sanchez Sanchez C, Montalban Romero S, Perez-Guillermo M: Diagnostic dilemmas in the interpretation of fine-needle aspirates of granulomatous prostatitis. Diagn Cytopathol 1998;18:215–221.

Miralles TG, Gosalbez F, Menendez P, et al: Fine needle aspiration cytology of granulomatous prostatitis. Acta Cytol 1990;34:57–62.

Mondal A., Mukherjee B, Ghosh E: Transrectal fine needle aspiration cytology of granulomatous prostatitis. Indian J Pathol Microbiol 1994;37:275–279.

Oppenheimer JR, Kahane H, Epstein JI: Granulomatous prostatitis on needle biopsy. Arch Pathol Lab Med 1997;121:724–729.

Stanley MW, Horwitz CA, Sharer W, et al: Granulomatous prostatitis: A spectrum including nonspecific, infectious, and spindle cell lesions. Diagn Cytopathol 1991;7:508–512.

Stillwell TJ, Engen DE, Farrow GM: The clinical spectrum of granulomatous prostatitis: A report of 200 cases. J Urol 1987;138:320–323.

Acute and Chronic Prostatitis

Collins MM, Stafford RS, O'Leary MP, Barry MJ: How common is prostatitis? A national survey of physician visits. J Urol 1998;159:1224–1228.

Palapattu GS, Sutcliffe S, Bastian PJ, et al: Prostate carcinogenesis and inflammation: Emerging insights. Carcinogenesis 2005;26:1170–1181.

Platz EA, De Marzo AM: Epidemiology of inflammation and prostate cancer. J Urol 2004;171:S36–S40.

Roberts RO, Bergstralh EJ, Bass SE, et al: Prostatitis as a risk factor for prostate cancer. Epidemiology 2004;15:93–99.

Roberts RO, Lieber MM, Bostwick DG, Jacobsen SJ: A review of clinical and pathological prostatitis syndromes. Urology 1997;49:809–821.

Schaeffer AJ: NIDDK-sponsored Chronic Prostatitis Collaborative Research Network (CPCRN): 5-year data and treatment guidelines for bacterial prostatitis. Int J Antimicrob Agents 2004;24(Suppl 1):S49–S52.

Postbiopsy Granuloma

Epstein JI, Hutchins GM: Granulomatous prostatitis: Distinction among allergic, nonspecific, and post-transurethral resection lesions. Hum Pathol 1984;15:818–825.

Henry L, Wagner B, Faulkner MK, et al: Metal deposition in post-surgical granulomas of the urinary tract. Histopathology 1993;22:457–465.

Mies C, Balogh K, Stadecker M: Palisading prostate granulomas following surgery. Am J Surg Pathol 1984;8: 217–221.

Xanthoma

Nelson RS, Epstein JI: Prostatic carcinoma with abundant xanthomatous cytoplasm: Foamy gland carcinoma. Am J Surg Pathol 1996;20:419–426.

Sebo TJ, Bostwick DG, Farrow GM, Eble JN: Prostatic xanthoma: A mimic of prostatic adenocarcinoma. Hum Pathol 1994;25:386–389.

Malakoplakia

Agostinho AD, Correa LA, Amaro JL, et al: Malakoplakia or prostate cancer? Similarities and differences. Urol Int 1998;61:47–49.

Repassy DL, Ivanyi A, Csata S, Tamas G: Combined occurrence of prostate carcinoma and malakoplakia. Pathol Oncol Res 2002;8:202–203.

Sarma HN, Ramesh K, al Fituri O, et al: Malakoplakia of the prostate gland: Report of two cases and review of the literature. Scand J Urol Nephrol 1996;30:155–157.

Atrophy

De Marzo AM, Platz EA, Epstein JI, et al. A working group classification of focal prostate atrophy lesions. Am J Surg Pathol (in press).

De Marzo AM, Marchi VL, Epstein JI, Nelson WG: Proliferative inflammatory atrophy of the prostate: Implications for prostatic carcinogenesis. Am J Pathol 1999;155:1985–1992.

De Marzo AM, Meeker AK, Zha S, et al: Human prostate cancer precursors and pathobiology. Urology 2003;62:55–62.

Ruska KM, Sauvageot J, Epstein JI: Histology and cellular kinetics of prostatic atrophy. Am J Surg Pathol 1998;22:1073–1077.

Adenosis (Atypical Adenomatous Hyperplasia)

Cheng L, Shan A, Cheville JC, et al: Atypical adenomatous hyperplasia of the prostate: A premalignant lesion? Cancer Res 1998;58:389–391.

Grignon DJ, Sakr WA: Atypical adenomatous hyperplasia of the prostate: A critical review. Eur Urol 1996;30:206–211.

Yang XJ, Wu CL, Woda BA, et al: Expression of alpha-methylacyl-CoA racemase (P504S) in atypical adenomatous hyperplasia of the prostate. Am J Surg Pathol 2002;26:921–925.

Sclerosing Adenosis

Grignon DJ, Ro JY, Srigley JR, et al: Sclerosing adenosis of the prostate gland: A lesion showing myoepithelial differentiation. Am J Surg Pathol 1992;16:383–391.

Jones EC, Clement PB, Young RH: Sclerosing adenosis of the prostate gland: A clinicopathological and immunohistochemical study of 11 cases. Am J Surg Pathol 1991;15:1171–1180.

Luque RJ, Lopez-Beltran A, Perez-Seoane C, Suzigan S: Sclerosing adenosis of the prostate: Histologic features in needle biopsy specimens. Arch Pathol Lab Med 2003;127:e14–e16.

Cribriform Clear Cell Hyperplasia

Frauenhoffer EE, Ro JY, el-Naggar AK, et al: Clear cell cribriform hyperplasia of the prostate: Immunohistochemical and DNA flow cytometric study. Am J Clin Pathol 1991;95:446–453.

Montironi R, Diamanti L: Morphologic changes in benign prostatic hyperplasia following chronic treatment with the 5-alpha-reductase inhibitor finasteride. J Urol Pathol 1996;4:123–135.

Basal Cell Hyperplasia

Amin MB, Schultz DS, Zarbo RJ: Analysis of cribriform morphology in prostatic neoplasia using antibody to high-molecular-weight cytokeratins. Arch Pathol Lab Med 1994;118:260–264.

Bullock MJ, Srigley JR, Klotz LH, Goldenberg SL: Pathologic effects of neoadjuvant cyproterone acetate on nonneoplastic prostate, prostatic intraepithelial neoplasia, and adenocarcinoma: A detailed analysis of radical prostatectomy specimens from a randomized trial. Am J Surg Pathol 2002;26:1400–1413.

Civantos F, Marcial MA, Banks ER, et al: Pathology of androgen deprivation therapy in prostate carcinoma: A comparative study of 173 patients. Cancer 1995;75:1634–1641.

Rioux-Leclercq NC, Epstein JI: Unusual morphologic patterns of basal cell hyperplasia of the prostate. Am J Surg Pathol 2002;26:237–243.

Thorson P, Swanson PE, Vollmer RT, Humphrey PA: Basal cell hyperplasia in the peripheral zone of the prostate. Mod Pathol 2003;16:598–606.

Nephrogenic Adenoma or Metaplasia

Allan CH, Epstein JI: Nephrogenic adenoma of the prostatic urethra: A mimicker of prostate adenocarcinoma. Am J Surg Pathol 2001;25:802–808.

Gupta AMW, Hanlin L, Policarpio-Nicolas, ML, et al: Expression of alpha-methylacyl-coenzyme A racemase in nephrogenic adenoma. Am J Surg Pathol 2004;28:1224–1229.

Mazal PR, Schaufler R, Altenhuber-Muller R, et al: Derivation of nephrogenic adenomas from renal tubular cells in kidney-transplant recipients. N Engl J Med 2002;347:653–659.

Oliva E, Young RH: Nephrogenic adenoma of the urinary tract: A review of the microscopic appearance of 80 cases with emphasis on unusual features. Mod Pathol 1995;8:722–730.

Skinnider BF, Oliva E, Young RH, Amin MB: Expression of alpha-methylacyl-CoA racemase (P504S) in nephrogenic adenoma: A significant immunohistochemical pitfall compounding the differential diagnosis with prostatic adenocarcinoma. Am J Surg Pathol 2004;28:701–705.

Mesonephric Remnant Hyperplasia

Bostwick DG, Qian J, Ma J, Muir TE: Mesonephric remnants of the prostate: incidence and histologic spectrum. Mod Pathol 2003;16:630–635.

Gikas PW, Del Buono EA, Epstein JI: Florid hyperplasia of mesonephric remnants involving prostate and periprostatic tissue: Possible confusion with adenocarcinoma. Am J Surg Pathol 1993;17:454–460.

Prostatic Urethral Polyp

Anjum MI, Ahmed M, Shrotri N, et al: Benign polyps with prostatic-type epithelium of the urethra and the urinary bladder. Int Urol Nephrol 1997;29:313–317.

Butterick JD, Schnitzer B, Abell MR: Ectopic prostatic tissue in urethra: A clinicopathological entity and a significant cause of hematuria. J Urol 1971;105:97–104.

Remick DG Jr, Kumar NB: Benign polyps with prostatic-type epithelium of the urethra and the urinary bladder: A suggestion of histogenesis based on histologic and immunohistochemical studies. Am J Surg Pathol 1984;8:833–839.

Verumontanum Mucosal Gland Hyperplasia

Gagucas RJ, Brown RW, Wheeler TM: Verumontanum mucosal gland hyperplasia. Am J Surg Pathol 1995;19:30–36.

Gaudin PB, Wheeler TM, Epstein JI: Verumontanum mucosal gland hyperplasia in prostatic needle biopsy specimens: A mimic of low grade prostatic adenocarcinoma. Am J Clin Pathol 1995;104:620–626.

Muezzinoglu B, Erdamar S, Chakraborty S, Wheeler TM: Verumontanum mucosal glands hyperplasia is associated with atypical adenomatous hyperplasia of the prostate. Arch Pathol Lab Med 2001;125:358–360.

Seminal Vesicles and Ejaculatory Duct Apparatus

De Marzo AM, Yang X, Nelson WG, et al: Distinguishing seminal vesicles (SV) from prostate cancer using immunohistochemistry (IHC). Mod Pathol 1999;12:93A.

Cowper's Glands

Cina SJ, Silberman MA, Kahane H, Epstein JI: Diagnosis of Cowper's glands on prostate needle biopsy. Am J Surg Pathol 1997;21:550–555.

Saboorian MH, Huffman H, Ashfaq R, et al: Distinguishing Cowper's glands from neoplastic and pseudoneoplastic lesions of prostate: Immunohistochemical and ultrastructural studies. Am J Surg Pathol 1997;21:1069–1074.

Paraganglia

Denford A, Vaughan M, Mayall F: Paraganglia as an unusual mimic of carcinoma in the prostate. Br J Urol 1997;80:677–678.

Gaudin PB, Reuter VE: Benign mimics of prostatic adenocarcinoma on needle biopsy. Anat Pathol 1997;2:111–134.

Kawabata K: Paraganglion of the prostate in a needle biopsy: A potential diagnostic pitfall. Arch Pathol Lab Med 1997;121:515–516.

Ostrowski ML, Wheeler TM: Paraganglia of the prostate: Location, frequency, and differentiation from prostatic adenocarcinoma. Am J Surg Pathol 1994;18:412–420.

Skeletal Muscle within Prostate Gland

Kost LV, Evans GW: Occurrence and significance of striated muscle within the prostate. J Urol 1964;92:703–704.

Manley CJ: The striated muscle of the prostate. J Urol 1966;95:234–240.

Benign Glands in Perineural Space

Carstens P: Perineural glands in normal hyperplastic prostate. J Urol 1980;123:686–688.

Cramer S: Benign glandular inclusion in prostatic nerves. Am J Clin Pathol 1981;75:854–855.

McIntire TL, Franzini DA: The presence of benign prostatic glands in perineural spaces. J Urol 1986;135:507–509.

Blue Nevus

Jao W, Fretzin DF, Christ ML, Prinz LM: Blue nevus of the prostate gland. Arch Pathol 1971;91:187–191.

Martinez Martinez CJ, Garcia Gonzalez R, Castaneda Casanova AL: Blue nevus of the prostate: Report of two new cases with immunohistochemical and electronmicroscopy studies. Eur Urol 1992;22:339–342.

Ro JY, Grignon DJ, Ayala AG, et al: Blue nevus and melanosis of the prostate: Electron-microscopic and immunohistochemical studies. Am J Clin Pathol 1988;90:530–535.

Endometriosis

Beckman EN, Pintado SO, Leonard GL, Sternberg WH: Endometriosis of the prostate. Am J Surg Pathol 1985;9:374–379.

Borda A, Petrucci MD, Berger N: Miscellaneous benign lesions of the bladder and urinary tract. Ann Pathol 2004;24:18–30.

Elastosis

Billis A, Magna LA: Prostate elastosis: A microscopic feature useful for the diagnosis of postatrophic hyperplasia. Arch Pathol Lab Med 2000;124:1306–1309.

2 Neoplasms of the Prostate and Seminal Vesicles

Ming Zhou • Cristina Magi-Galluzzi • Jonathan I. Epstein

PROSTATIC INTRAEPITHELIAL NEOPLASIA

CLINICAL FEATURES

Prostatic intraepithelial neoplasia (PIN) is an atypical epithelial proliferation within the pre-existing prostatic acini and ducts, i.e., a PIN gland has a benign architecture, but is lined with cytologically atypical cells. It is divided into low-grade (LGPIN) and high-grade (HGPIN) types, based on the degree of cytologic atypia. There is no proven association between LGPIN and prostate carcinoma. HGPIN, on the other hand, is strongly associated with prostate carcinoma and is accepted as a precursor lesion to prostate carcinoma.

HIGH-GRADE PROSTATIC INTRAEPITHELIAL NEOPLASIA (HGPIN)— FACT SHEET

Definition
▶ Secretory epithelial proliferation that displays severe cytologic atypia within the preexisting prostatic acini and ducts

Prevalence, Race, and Age Distribution
▶ Prevalence increases with age
▶ Higher prevalence and more extensive HGPIN in African Americans compared with Caucasian Americans (7%, 26%, 46%, 72%, 75%, and 91% in African American versus 8%, 23%, 29%, 49%, 53%, and 67% in Caucasian between the third and eighth decades)

Clinical Features
▶ Does not result in abnormal DRE or elevated PSA
▶ Diagnosed only by histological examination

Radiologic Features
▶ May appear as a hypoechoic lesion, indistinguishable from prostate carcinoma

Prognosis and Treatment
▶ Presumptive premalignant lesion
▶ HGPIN in needle biopsy denotes a 20–25% risk of finding prostate carcinoma in subsequent rebiopsy. Consider rebiopsy in 0 to 6 months
▶ No treatment for HGPIN as an isolated finding in needle biopsy

---

AGE AND RACE DISTRIBUTION

The prevalence of HGPIN increases with age. In addition, higher prevalence and more extensive HGPIN are observed in African Americans as compared with Caucasian Americans. An autopsy study identified HGPIN in 7%, 26%, 46%, 72%, 75% and 91% of African Americans between the third and eighth decade, compared with 8%, 23%, 29%, 49%, 53%, and 67% in Caucasians.

PREVALENCE OF HGPIN IN SURGICAL PROSTATE SPECIMENS

The prevalence of HGPIN ranges from 4% to 16% in prostate needle biopsy specimens and from 2% to 3% in specimens obtained by transurethral resection of the prostate (TURP). HGPIN is found in 85% to 100% of radical prostatectomies performed for prostate carcinoma, reflecting a strong association between the two.

MOLECULAR AND GENETIC ASPECTS OF HGPIN

The incidence of aneuploidy in HGPIN is 50% to 70%, slightly lower than or similar to that in invasive prostate carcinoma. Genetic changes tend to be very similar to those in prostate carcinoma. The most common change involves chromosome 8, including loss of 8p and gain of 8q. Other common changes include gains of chromosomes 10, 7, 12, and Y and loss of 10q, 16q, and 18q. HGPIN has decreased expression of NKX3.1, a prostate-specific, homeodomain transcription factor, and p27, a cell cycle regulatory protein. *TP53* gene mutation and protein accumulation, and *c-myc (MYC)* gene amplification are identified in some HGPIN. *GSTP1*, a gene involved in detoxification of genotoxins, is inactivated by promoter hypermethylation in 70% of HGPIN. Overexpression of α-methylacyl-coenzyme A racemase (AMACR) is seen in the majority of HGPIN specimens.

CLINICAL SIGNS AND SYMPTOMS

PIN does not result in abnormality on digital rectal examination (DRE), nor does it lead to elevation of serum prostate-specific antigen (PSA). It can only be diagnosed by histological examination of the prostate tissue.

RADIOLOGIC FEATURES

HGPIN may appear as a hypoechoic lesion, indistinguishable from prostate carcinoma, on ultrasonography.

PATHOLOGIC FEATURES

GROSS FINDINGS

PIN is not grossly visible.

MICROSCOPIC FINDINGS

The histologic diagnosis is based on architectural and cytologic features. PIN, at low scanning power, appears darker than normal prostatic glands due to higher nuclear density and increased cytoplasmic eosinophilia or amphophilia (Fig. 2-1A). LGPIN shows crowding of luminal secretory cells, irregular nuclear spacing, and stratification. Nuclei are enlarged and vary in size, although the chromatin appears normal and nucleolar prominence is rare or absent (Fig. 2-1B). The basal cell layer is intact. It is difficult to reproducibly distinguish LGPIN from normal or hyperplastic epithelium; therefore, a diagnosis of LGPIN is not recommended.

HGPIN also shows intraluminal epithelial proliferation, with a variety of architectural patterns. Cytologically, individual cells are more uniformly enlarged, with nuclear variation less than that observed in LGPIN. Many cells show large and prominent nucleoli, as well as hyperchromatic and clumpy chromatin (Fig. 2-2), similar to that seen in prostate carcinoma. The basal cell layer is often discontinuous and occasionally is absent.

Four major architectural patterns of HGPIN—tufting, micropapillary, flat, and cribriform—have been described, although these patterns are important only for diagnostic consideration and in general have no clinical significance. Tufting pattern is most common and has cells piling up to form undulating mounds of nuclei (Fig. 2-2A). Micropapillary pattern is the second most common pattern and has columns of atypical cells without fibrovascular cores (Fig. 2-2B). Flat pattern has no significant architectural changes (Fig. 2-2C). Cribriform pattern, the least common type, has more complex architecture, with Roman bridges and cribriform formations (Fig. 2-2D). Other rare patterns include solid and inverted variants. The inverted type is characterized by polarization of enlarged nuclei toward the glandular lumen of HGPIN (Fig. 2-2E), usually of tufting or micropapillary type. HGPIN may partially involve a prostatic gland (Fig. 2-3), and different patterns may exist in the same gland.

HGPIN glands are composed of dysplastic cells that are morphologically similar or identical to prostate carcinoma. Histologic variants that correspond to virtually all the morphologic variants of prostate carcinoma have been described, including signet-ring, mucinous, foamy gland, and small cell neuroendocrine variants (Fig. 2-2F).

HIGH-GRADE PROSTATIC INTRAEPITHELIAL NEOPLASIA (HGPIN)— PATHOLOGIC FEATURES

Gross Findings
▶ Not visible grossly

Microscopic Findings
▶ Luminal cell crowding, irregular spacing, "piling-up" with chromatin hyperchromasia, clumping and prominent nucleoli
▶ Architectural patterns: flat, tufting, micropapillary, and cribriform
▶ Histologic variants: signet-ring, mucinous, inverted, and small cell neuroendocrine

Immunohistochemical Features
▶ Secretory cells + for pancytokeratins and low-molecular-weight cytokeratin; + but often reduced expression of PSA and PSAP; 60% to 80% + for AMACR (P504S)
▶ HMWCK (34βE12) and p63 demonstrate complete or discontinuous basal cell layers

Differential Diagnosis
▶ Prostatic central zone glands
▶ Seminal vesicle/ejaculatory duct epithelium
▶ Reactive atypia due to inflammation, infarction, or radiation
▶ Metaplasia (transitional cell, squamous cell)
▶ Hyperplasia (clear cell cribriform hyperplasia, basal cell hyperplasia)
▶ Prostate carcinoma with cribriform pattern
▶ Ductal adenocarcinoma
▶ Urothelial carcinoma

ANCILLARY STUDIES

IMMUNOHISTOCHEMISTRY

HGPIN is positive for pancytokeratins (AE1/3 and Cam5.2) and prostate-specific markers (PSA and prostate-specific acid phosphatase [PSAP]). Stains for basal cells (high-molecular-weight cytokeratin [HMWCK] and p63) demonstrate complete or discontinuous, occasionally absent, basal cell layers (Fig. 2-4A,B). Expression of AMACR is detected in the majority of HGPIN samples (Fig. 2-4C).

DIFFERENTIAL DIAGNOSIS

Normal central zone glands have architectural complexity, with eosinophilic cytoplasm and nuclear stratification, but lack the nuclear atypia that characterizes HGPIN. Seminal vesicle or ejaculatory duct epithelium does not show the characteristic nuclear changes of HGPIN, in particular the prominent nucleoli. It often has pleomorphic, hyperchromatic nuclei of degenerative nature scattered among normal-appearing nuclei. Nuclear pseudoinclusions are frequent. Golden-brown lipofuscin

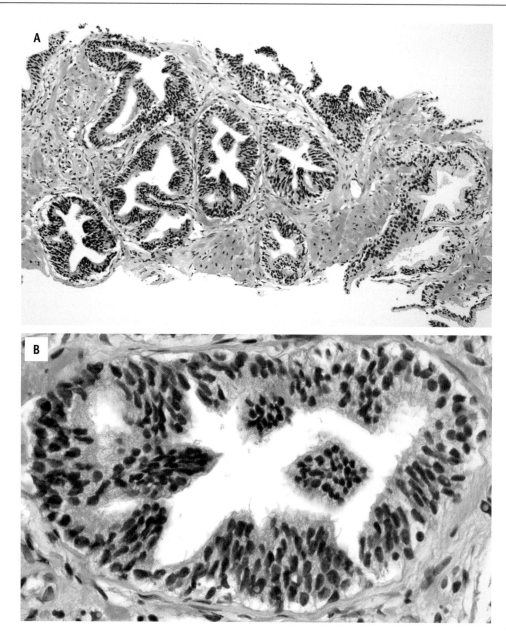

FIGURE 2-1

(**A**) At low magnification, low-grade prostatic intraepithelial neoplasia (LGPIN) glands (*left*) have an architecture similar to normal glands (*right*), but they appear darker than the latter. Secretory cells show focal nuclear crowding and stratification. Nuclei are enlarged with size variation; however, there are no conspicuous nucleoli (**B**).

pigment is almost invariably present, although similar pigment can occasionally be found in HGPIN.

Prostate glands and ducts adjacent to inflammation or infarction may show nuclear atypia, including prominent nucleoli, but they do not have the prominent architectural changes of HGPIN. Benign glands after irradiation often show basal cell prominence and multi-layering and streaming of cells. Squamous metaplasia is also common. Although usually pronounced, the nuclear atypia appears degenerative and varies from gland to gland.

Transitional cell metaplasia is usually multilayered. However, the nuclei are frequently oval to slightly elon-gated with nuclear grooves. Nuclear atypia, including prominent nucleoli, is absent.

Basal cell hyperplasia often appears as small and solid nests, although some may retain lumina, in con-trast to the medium- to large-caliber glands affected by HGPIN. "Atypical basal cell hyperplasia" is a term applied to basal cell hyperplasia with prominent nucleoli. However, the nucleoli are in the basal cells rather than in secretory cells. One can often find secretory cells on top of the hyperplastic basal cells. Immunostains for basal cell markers (p63 or HMWCK) can sometimes aid in establishing a definitive diagnosis: basal cell hyper-plasia is positive for these markers, whereas in HGPIN,

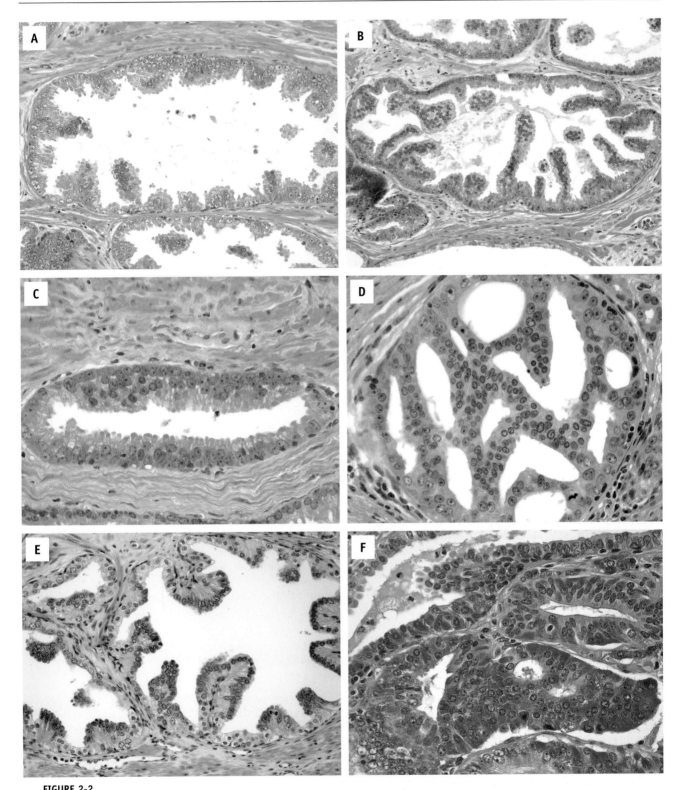

FIGURE 2-2

Secretory cells of high-grade prostatic intraepithelial neoplasia (HGPIN) show prominent nucleoli and are hyperchromatic with clumpy chromatin. Cells may form undulating mounds (tufting pattern, **A**) or cellular columns without fibrovascular cores (micropapillary pattern, **B**). Flat pattern has no significant architectural changes (**C**). Cribriform pattern has complex architecture with Roman bridges and cribriform formations (**D**). Inverted HGPIN is characterized by polarization of enlarged nuclei toward the glandular lumen (**E**). Neuroendocrine HGPIN contains red cytoplasmic granules (F).

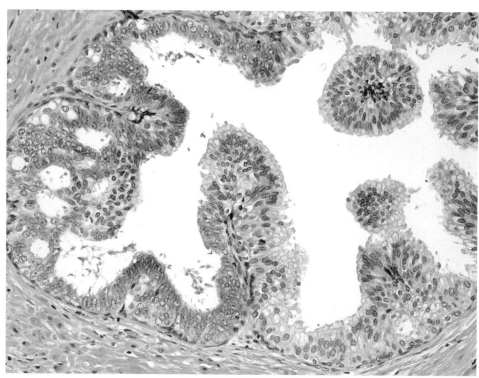

FIGURE 2-3

High-grade prostatic intraepithelial neoplasia (HGPIN), showing partial involvement of a prostatic gland.

the apical secretory cells are negative and only residual basal cells are highlighted by such stains.

Clear cell cribriform hyperplasia is a benign condition that is most commonly found in transition zone. It has cribriform architecture at low magnification. Cytologic atypia is absent. In addition, the basal cells are often prominent and form a collarette around the gland.

It is more problematic to differentiate HGPIN from invasive cribriform prostate carcinoma and intraductal carcinoma, a recently described yet controversial entity. All three entities consist of atypical cells spanning the entire diameter of the involved prostatic glands. Figure 2-5 provides an algorithm for working up atypical cribriform lesions in prostate needle biopsy. The most salient histologic feature that distinguishes intraductal carcinoma from HGPIN is the presence of multiple cribriform glands with prominent nuclear atypia and comedonecrosis. When a diagnosis of intraductal carcinoma is made, a note should be included in the diagnosis to indicate that it is invariably associated with an invasive prostate carcinoma component.

Ductal adenocarcinoma usually involves the prostatic urethra and verumontanum and extends into periurethral ducts, sites that are uncommonly affected by HGPIN. However, ductal adenocarcinoma may occasionally arise in the peripheral zone, or ordinary acinar prostate carcinoma may focally have ductal adenocarcinoma features. In addition, ductal adenocarcinoma usually retains basal cell layers. However, the papillae in ductal adenocarcinoma have true fibrovascular cores,

and cells may show significant nuclear atypia with a high mitotic rate and extensive necrosis, features uncommon in HGPIN.

Urothelial carcinoma that involves prostatic ducts and acini replaces the ductal-acinar epithelium with predominantly solid, highly atypical, and mitotically active neoplastic cells. The cytoplasm of these cells is dense or "hard" and may show squamous differentiation, compared with the granular cytoplasm of HGPIN.

PROGNOSIS AND TREATMENT

HGPIN in prostate needle biopsy is a risk factor for detection of prostate carcinoma in subsequent biopsies, whereas LGPIN is not. The incidence of detecting invasive cancer on rebiopsy ranges from 36% in patients who were diagnosed of HGPIN in the early 1990s, to 21% in patients who were diagnosed after 2000. The cancer risk is 18% after a LGPIN diagnosis, and 20% after a diagnosis of benign prostatic tissue. Between 80% and 90% of prostate carcinomas are detected on the first rebiopsy after a HGPIN diagnosis, and rebiopsy may detect persistent HGPIN in 5% to 43% of cases. The current recommendation is that patients with a HGPIN diagnosis should undergo rebiopsy in 0 to 6 months regardless of their serum PSA level and DRE findings. Rebiopsy should sample the entire gland, because HGPIN confers an increased risk for cancer

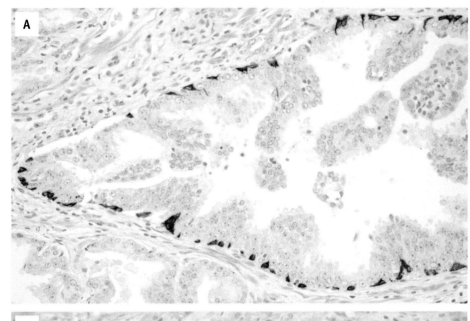

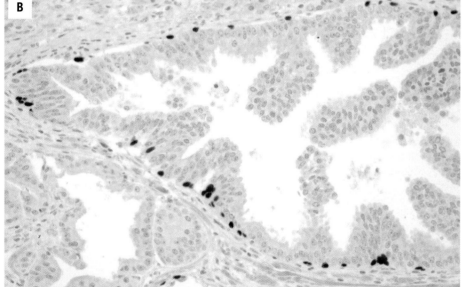

FIGURE 2-4

High-grade prostatic intraepithelial neoplasia (HGPIN) gland has discontinuous basal cell layer, as demonstrated by high-molecular-weight cytokeratin (HMWCK) (**A**) and p63 (**B**) immunostains. In contrast, basal cells are absent in cancer glands *(left lower corner)*. HGPIN also has weak expression of α-methylacyl-coenzyme A racemase (AMACR) (**C**), although weaker than the adjacent cancer glands.

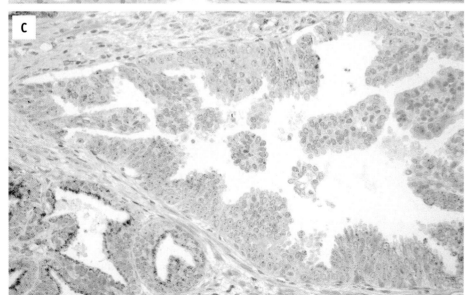

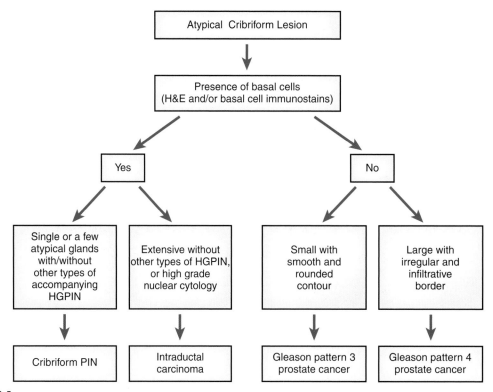

FIGURE 2-5

Differential diagnosis of atypical cribriform lesions on prostate needle biopsies.

throughout the gland. No therapy is indicated for HGPIN as an isolated finding. Because the risk of cancer after a biopsy diagnosis of HGPIN in more recent studies is decreasing, the current recommendation for repeat biopsy may change in the near future.

Atypical glands adjacent to HGPIN (PINATYP) may represent a microinvasive prostate cancer budding off the HGPIN gland, or tangential sectioning of the HGPIN gland (Fig. 2-6). PINATYP seems to confer a higher risk for subsequent detection of cancer than does HGPIN alone, with a risk of 53%. All patients with PINATYP therefore should undergo rebiopsy.

PROSTATE CARCINOMA

CLINICAL FEATURES

PREVALENCE

Prostate carcinoma is the most common noncutaneous malignancy in American men and the third most common cancer in men worldwide, with 230,000 new cases in the United States in 2004. The incidence and mortality have increased in the last several decades, due in part to the introduction of newer diagnostic tests, such as PSA screening. However, prostate carcinoma is a less prominent cause of cancer death, accounting for 10% of all cancer deaths in men in the United States. The incidence varies greatly with geographic location, ethnic background, and age. The highest incidence is seen in the United States, Australia, and Scandinavian countries, whereas prostate carcinoma is relatively uncommon in countries of the Far East. In the United States, blacks have a much higher incidence and mortality than whites. The incidence rises dramatically with age. The clinical disease is uncommon before the age of 50 years. The hazard of detection is 40 times greater for men older than 65 years, compared with younger men. One autopsy study showed 83% prevalence among patients 90 years of age and older.

ETIOLOGY

Multiple genetic and environmental factors are involved in prostate carcinogenesis. Age, family history, and race are definitive risk factors. A family history of prostate carcinoma confers a higher risk. The degree of risk is related to the age and number of affected relatives, with the greatest risk conferred by a father or brother with onset before 40 years of age. These observations strongly support a genetic basis for prostate carcinoma. Many susceptibility loci and several candidate genes have been identified for hereditary prostate cancer. Racial background, with American blacks having higher incidence, higher grade, and more extensive cancer, may be related to various genetic and environmental factors.

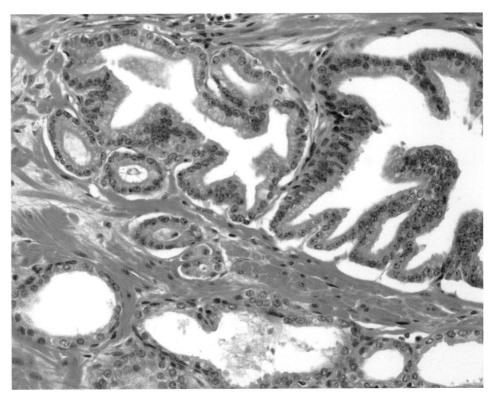

FIGURE 2-6

Adjacent to a high-grade prostatic intraepithelial neoplasia (HGPIN) gland are several small, atypical glands suspicious for cancer. They may represent a minute focus of invasive prostate carcinoma or tangential sectioning of the HGPIN gland.

Dietary fat and sex hormone levels are probable risk factors for prostate carcinoma. High fat intake, especially from red meat, is strongly associated with development of prostate carcinoma. On the other hand, fruit and vegetable consumption may protect against prostate carcinoma.

Sex hormones play an important role in the development and growth of prostate carcinoma. Testosterone is converted to more potent dihydrotestosterone (DHT) by the enzyme 5-α-reductase. Testosterone and DHT then bind to the androgen receptor (AR), which is a transcription factor that regulates androgen-dependent cell growth. Genetic polymorphisms in 5-α-reductase and AR genes affect the enzyme and receptor activities.

Other potential risk factors include increased plasma insulin-like growth factor I expression, exposure to herbicides, exposure to cadmium, and low levels of vitamin D, vitamin E, and selenium.

MOLECULAR BIOLOGY

Linkage analysis has identified at least seven candidate loci for hereditary prostate cancer. Of them, three genes have been cloned: *RNASEL* on 1q24-25, *HPC2* on 17p, and *MSR1* on 8p22-23. These three genes do not account for all the hereditary prostate cancer, and more than 10 other genes also have been implicated. Of particular importance to the inherited susceptibility for prostate carcinoma are the common polymorphisms in a number of low-penetrance genes, or genetic modifiers.

It is hypothesized that specific combinations of these variants, in the proper environmental setting, can profoundly affect the risk of development of prostate carcinoma.

Mutations in any of the classic oncogenes and tumor suppressor genes are detected only infrequently in sporadic prostate carcinomas. They harbor nonrandom somatic genomic alterations. The most common chromosomal alterations include losses at 1p, 6q, 8p, 10q, 13q, 16q, and 18q and gains at 1q, 2p, 7, 8q, 18q, and Xq. Many genes have been implicated in prostate carcinogenesis and progression, including *GSTP1*; *NKX3-1*, a homeobox gene involved in the prostate carcinoma progression; and *PTEN*, a tyrosine phosphatase with tumor suppressor function. Other genes include p27 and E-cadherin. Another very common somatic genomic alteration is telomere shortening, which leads to genomic instability in prostate carcinoma and other epithelial cancers.

CLINICAL SIGNS AND SYMPTOMS

Most prostate carcinoma is asymptomatic. About three-fourths of prostate carcinomas arise in the peripheral zone, and some can result in abnormal findings on DRE. Rarely, prostate carcinoma can lead to urinary obstruction when a large tumor mass arises in the transition zone or extends into the transition zone from the peripheral zone, or invades the bladder neck. Locally aggressive prostate carcinoma that involves the bladder

---

PROSTATE ADENOCARCINOMA—FACT SHEET

Definition
► Invasive carcinoma with prostatic secretory cell differentiation

Incidence and Location
► Most common noncutaneous malignancy in United States
► 230,000 new cases in 2004
► 70% to 75% in peripheral zone, 15% to 20% in transition zone, 10% in central zone

Gender, Race, and Age Distribution
► Incidence rises dramatically with age; uncommon before 50 years of age
► Highest incidence in United States, Australia, and Scandinavian countries; relatively uncommon in Far East countries
► Blacks have much higher incidence and mortality than whites in United States

Clinical Features
► Most asymptomatic
► Some with abnormal DRE
► Occasionally obstructive urinary symptoms
► Rarely symptoms and signs related to metastasis to bone, brain, and other sites
► 70% to 75% has PSA >4 ng/mL

Prognosis and Treatment
► Expectant management—localized prostate carcinoma with life expectancy <10 years
► Radical prostatectomy/radiation therapy—localized prostate carcinoma
► Hormonal ablation + radiation—locally advanced prostate carcinoma
► Hormonal ablation—metastatic prostate carcinoma
► Prognosis highly variable and depends on host, tumor, and treatment parameters

---

and rectum can cause hematuria, rectal bleeding, or obstruction.

Rarely, patients present with symptoms and signs that are related to prostate carcinoma metastatic to different anatomic sites, most commonly bone, regional lymph nodes, lung, and brain.

Currently, most prostate carcinomas are clinically detected by serum PSA screening and by DRE, not by clinical symptoms.

DIAGNOSIS

Prostate-specific Antigen

PSA is a serine protease secreted by the epithelial cells of prostatic ducts and acini to liquefy the seminal coagulum. Benign and malignant prostatic tissue produces PSA. Only a small percentage of PSA in serum is free; the majority is complexed with α-1-antichymotrypsin and α-2-macroglobulin.

Patients with prostate carcinoma in general have higher serum PSA than those without the disease. A serum PSA level greater than 4 ng/mL is considered abnormal. However, serum PSA lacks sensitivity and specificity for prostate carcinoma. Approximately 70% to 75% of prostate carcinomas have serum PSA values greater than 4 ng/mL. The positive predictive value of serum PSA is higher when the concentration is greater than 10 ng/mL, or when accompanied by abnormal DRE findings. However, some nonmalignant conditions, including benign prostatic hyperplasia (BPH), inflammation, infarction, instrumentation, and ejaculation, also increase the serum PSA level.

Total serum PSA correlates well with advancing age. To improve the specificity, the following age-specific normal PSA reference ranges are proposed: 2.5 ng/mL for men 40 to 49 years of age, 3.5 ng/mL for those age 50 to 59 years, 4.5 ng/mL for age 60 to 69 years, and 6.5 ng/mL for 70 to 79 years of age.

Other modifications of PSA testing have been introduced to improve the test's specificity, including the ratio of free to total PSA, which is decreased in prostate carcinoma; the PSA density, which is the ratio of total PSA to prostate glandular volume as measured by transrectal ultrasound (TRUS) and is higher in prostate carcinoma; and the PSA velocity, or the rate of PSA change over time, which is increased in prostate carcinoma.

PSA testing has significantly affected the clinical and pathologic attributes of detected prostate carcinoma. Most prostate carcinomas detected by PSA screening are of intermediate grade and confined to the prostate. In addition, 5% to 27% of prostate carcinomas are considered potentially clinically insignificant.

Preoperative PSA is often used in combination with Gleason grade in needle biopsy and clinical stage to predict pathologic stage, including the probability for organ-confined disease, extraprostatic extension, seminal vesicle invasion, and lymph node metastasis and the likelihood of disease recurrence after therapy. These probability estimates are helpful in discussions with patients about risks versus benefits when choosing treatment options.

PSA levels may also be used to monitor the response to various treatments. After radical prostatectomy, the serum PSA should drop to an undetectable level; elevated PSA levels signal recurrence or residual disease. After radiation therapy, three consecutive increases in PSA level after it initially reaches a nadir indicate a biochemical failure.

Prostate Needle Biopsy

The standard method for detection of prostate carcinoma is by TRUS-guided sextant core biopsies that systematically sample the parasagittal midlobe regions of apex, middle, and base. Several modifications of the sextant protocol have been made. More recently, the standard has been to sample the gland with approximately 10 to 12 cores, in particular from the more lateral aspect of the peripheral zone, where the majority of prostate carcinomas arise. In cases with high suspicion for cancer despite negative biopsies, "saturation biopsy" may be performed, collecting 10 to 15 biopsies from each side of the prostate. The addition of a transition zone biopsy is also used typically only when the initial biopsy is negative and the clinical suspicion for cancer is high. More needle cores may also be taken for larger prostates.

Information concerning the anatomic locations of needle biopsies should be preserved by either embedding the samples in separate blocks or inking in different colors. This information is critical for the prognostication and therapy-planning. It is also important when a diagnosis of "atypical glands suspicious for prostate carcinoma" is made. Rebiopsy strategy entails concentration in the initial atypical region in addition to sampling of the rest of the prostate. At least three levels of the biopsy core should be cut for hematoxylin and eosin (H&E) staining. An option is for one or two intervening sections to be cut on positive charged slides for potential immunohistochemical studies.

Transurethral Resection of the Prostate

TURP mainly detects transition zone prostate carcinoma and bulky peripheral zone prostate carcinoma that extends into the transition zone. Initially, eight cassettes should be submitted in random fashion. In younger patients (< 65 years of age), submission of all the tissue is justified to identify all T1a lesions (i.e., those in which tumor occupies < 5 % of the total specimen). If T1b disease (in which tumor occupies > 5 % of the total specimen) is found on the initial eight slides, it is not necessary to submit additional tissue. However, if T1a prostate carcinoma is found on the initial eight slides, the remaining tissue should be submitted for review.

Transrectal Ultrasound

The sonographic appearance of prostate carcinoma is not specific, with 70 % to 75 % prostate carcinomas being hypoechoic and the remaining isoechoic and indistinguishable from surrounding tissue. Many significant prostate carcinomas are missed by TRUS. It remains as a means of guidance for prostate needle biopsies.

Computed Tomography and Magnetic Resonance Imaging

Both computed tomography and magnetic resonance imaging are of limited use because of low sensitivity to detect and stage prostate carcinoma.

Radioimmunoscintigraphy

A bone scan provides the most sensitive method to detect bony metastasis. ProstaScint (capromab pendetide), a radioisotope-labeled monoclonal antibody against prostate-specific membrane antigen (PSMA), may detect microscopic metastasis. The sensitivity can be improved by using it in combination with PSA, biopsy Gleason grade, and clinical stage data.

PATHOLOGIC FEATURES

GROSS FINDINGS

Gross examination of TURP specimens is of little significance, because benign processes can mimic prostate carcinoma. On radical prostatectomies, grossly identifiable prostate carcinoma is typically of higher grade and stage and larger diameter. In contrast to the adjacent normal benign prostate tissue, which appears tan and spongy, grossly evident prostate carcinoma is firm and solid and ranges in color from white-grey to yellow-orange (Fig. 2-7). Prostate carcinomas discovered by PSA screening are less visible grossly; these cancers are often small (< 5 mm) and of lower grade and stage.

Patterns of Spread and Metastasis

Local extraprostatic extension typically occurs anteriorly for transition zone cancer and posteriorly and posterolaterally for peripheral zone cancer. Prostate carcinoma can also spread superiorly into the bladder neck. Rarely, it can penetrate Denonvillier's fascia posteriorly to involve the rectum. Metastatic prostate carcinoma most commonly involves regional lymph nodes and bones of the pelvis and axial skeleton, where a characteristic osteoblastic response is often elicited.

MICROSCOPIC FINDINGS

Prostate carcinoma has a constellation of architectural, cytoplasmic, nuclear, and intraluminal features.

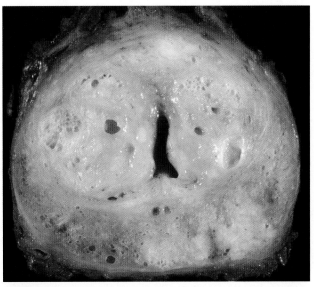

FIGURE 2-7

Prostate carcinoma, manifesting as firm, solid areas ranging from white-grey to yellow-orange with involvement of the left posterolateral and anterior zones. In contrast, benign prostate tissue appears tan and spongy. Also note that the transition zones are expanded by benign prostatic hyperplasia.

PROSTATE CARCINOMA—PATHOLOGIC FEATURES

Gross Findings

▶ Firm, solid, white-grey to yellow-orange, in contrast to tan, spongy benign prostatic tissue
▶ PSA-detected cancer often not grossly visible

Microscopic Findings

▶ Architectural features: haphazard glandular arrangement; infiltrative growth; less differentiated glands with cribriform, fused glands, cords, sheets, or single tumor cells
▶ Typically small glands with straight luminal border
▶ Cytologic features: pale to amphophilic cytoplasm; no lipofuscin pigment
▶ Nuclear features: enlargement, hyperchromasia, variably prominent nucleoli; mitosis and apoptotic bodies can be present
▶ Intraluminal features: crystalloids; blue mucin; pink amorphous secretion
▶ Cancer-specific features: mucinous fibroplasia (collagenous micronodules); glomeruloid formation; perineural invasion

Histologic Variants of Prostate Carcinoma

▶ Ductal adenocarcinoma
▶ Atrophic carcinoma
▶ Pseudohyperplastic carcinoma
▶ Foamy gland carcinoma
▶ Mucinous carcinoma
▶ Signet-ring carcinoma
▶ Small cell carcinoma
▶ Sarcomatoid carcinoma
▶ Urothelial carcinoma
▶ Squamous cell carcinoma
▶ Basaloid carcinoma

Gleason Grading System

▶ *Pattern 1:* Very well-circumscribed nodule of closely packed but separate glands that are of intermediate size and similar in size and shape
▶ *Pattern 2:* Less well-circumscribed nodule of medium-sized glands with some degree of variation in size and shape and looser arrangement. There may be minimal invasion of cancer glands into surrounding tissue
▶ *Pattern 3:* Cancer glands often infiltrate between the adjacent benign glands. They vary in size and shape and are often angular
▶ *Pattern 4:* Glands appear fused, cribriform, or poorly formed
▶ *Pattern 5:* Cancer cells forms solid sheets, strands, or single cells invading the stroma. Comedonecrosis may be present

Differential Diagnosis

▶ Normal prostatic/nonprostatic tissue (seminal vesicle/ejaculatory duct, verumontanum glands, Cowper's glands, paraganglia, mesonephric remnants)
▶ Benign conditions (atrophy, partial atrophy, postatrophic hyperplasia, urothelial/squamous metaplasia, basal cell hyperplasia, adenosis, sclerosing adenosis, inflammation, nonspecific granulomatous prostatitis, BPH)
▶ HGPIN
▶ Treatment effect (radiation atypia)

Architecture. Gland-forming prostate carcinomas are more crowded than benign glands and typically exhibit a haphazard growth pattern, with malignant glands oriented perpendicular to each other and irregularly separated by smooth muscle bundles. They also display "infiltrative growth pattern," with malignant glands situated between or flanking benign glands (Fig. 2-8A). When prostate carcinoma becomes less differentiated, it loses glandular differentiation and forms cribriform structures, fused glands, poorly delineated glands, solid sheets or cords, or even single tumor cells.

Cytoplasm. In contrast to benign glands with irregular and undulating luminal borders, prostate carcinoma glands are smaller and have straight luminal borders. They may have amphophilic, or darker, cytoplasm that is evident even at low magnification (Fig. 2-8B). However, low-grade prostate carcinoma often has pale-clear cytoplasm, indistinct from benign glands. Prostate carcinoma typically lacks lipofuscin pigment.

Nuclei. Typically, prostate carcinoma displays nuclear characteristics distinct from surrounding benign glands, including enlarged nuclei and prominent nucleoli (Fig. 2-8C,D). Some prostate carcinomas lack prominent nucleoli yet have enlarged and hyperchromatic nuclei. Mitoses and apoptotic bodies are more common in prostate carcinoma, although they are rarely found in benign glands and still not frequently seen in malignant glands. Cancer nuclei, even in poorly differentiated ones, show little variation in size and shape.

Intraluminal content. Crystalloids—dense eosinophilic, crystal-like structures found within the glandular lumina (Fig. 2-8D)—are found more commonly in cancer than in benign glands. However, they are also frequently found in adenosis, a benign condition that mimics low-grade prostate carcinoma. Intraluminal pink, acellular, dense secretions (Fig. 2-8C) and blue-tinged mucin (Fig. 2-8E) are additional findings seen preferentially in prostate carcinoma. In contrast, corpora amylacea are common in benign glands and are only rarely seen in prostate carcinoma.

Stroma. Ordinary prostate carcinoma does not elicit a stromal inflammatory or desmoplastic response. Ductal prostate adenocarcinoma, however, may induce such stromal reactions with fibrosis containing hemosiderin-laden macrophages.

Cancer-specific features. Three histologic features are diagnostic of prostate carcinoma, because they have not been described in benign glands. Mucinous fibroplasia, or collagenous micronodules, occur as a delicate fibrous tissue with ingrowth of fibroblasts within or adjacent to cancer glands (Fig. 2-8F). Glomeruloid formation is created by intraluminal proliferation of malignant cells and is often surrounded by a crescentic space, resembling a renal glomerulus (Fig. 2-8G). Perineural invasion with cancer glands completely or near-completely encircling the nerve is pathognomonic of prostate carcinoma (Fig. 2-8H). Benign glands can occasionally be found to abut a nerve; however, circumferential extension of benign glands entirely around a nerve has not been described.

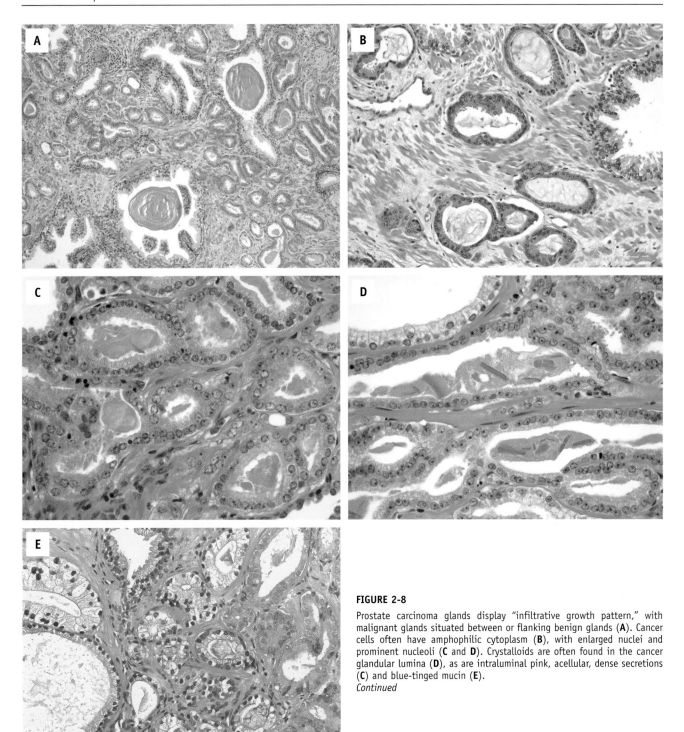

FIGURE 2-8

Prostate carcinoma glands display "infiltrative growth pattern," with malignant glands situated between or flanking benign glands (**A**). Cancer cells often have amphophilic cytoplasm (**B**), with enlarged nuclei and prominent nucleoli (**C** and **D**). Crystalloids are often found in the cancer glandular lumina (**D**), as are intraluminal pink, acellular, dense secretions (**C**) and blue-tinged mucin (**E**).
Continued

Gleason Grading System

The Gleason grading system, designed by Dr. Donald Gleason, is the predominant grading system for prostate carcinoma. It is based on the glandular architecture; nuclear atypia is not evaluated. The grading system defines five histologic patterns with decreasing glandular differentiation (Fig. 2-9A). The primary and sec- ondary patterns (in order of prevalence) are added to obtain a Gleason score or sum. If a prostate carcinoma only has one pattern, then that pattern is doubled to obtain the Gleason score. The primary and secondary patterns should be reported along with the Gleason score. Recently, several modifications have been made to the original Gleason grading scheme in an effort to

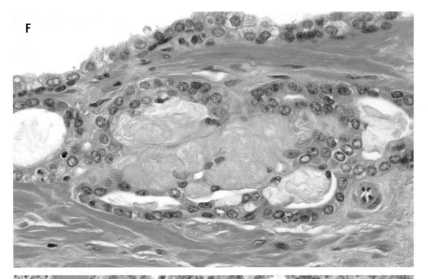

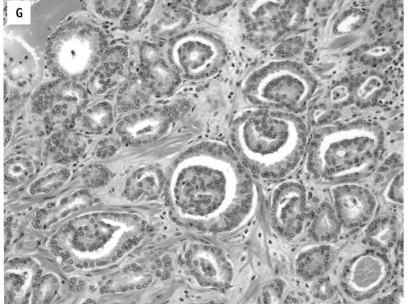

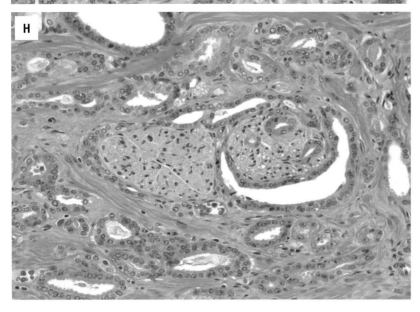

FIGURE 2-8, CONT'D

F, Mucinous fibroplasia consists of delicate fibrous tissue with ingrowth of fibroblasts within or adjacent to cancer glands. **G,** Glomeruloid formation is created by intraluminal proliferation of malignant cells and is often surrounded by a crescentic space. **H,** In perineural invasion, cancer glands entirely or partially encircle a nerve.

adapt this grading system to present-day practice in a uniform manner. The modified Gleason grading system is shown in Fig. 2-9B. The significant changes include a stricter definition of Gleason pattern 3 cribriform glands, and grading ill-defined glands with poorly formed glandular lumina as pattern 4 (see below).

Gleason Pattern 1. This pattern is composed of a very well-circumscribed nodule of closely packed but separate glands that do not infiltrate into adjacent tissue (Fig. 2-10). The glands are of intermediate size and are similar in size and shape. This pattern is exceed-

ingly rare and is usually only a minor component of prostate carcinoma when present. It is usually seen in transition zone prostate carcinoma. The new modified Gleason grading system states that "a Gleason score of $1 + 1 = 2$ is a grade that should not be diagnosed regardless of the type of specimen, with extremely rare exception".

Gleason Pattern 2. There is a less well-circumscribed nodule of medium-sized glands, with some degree of variation in size and shape and looser arrangement. There may be minimal invasion of cancer glands

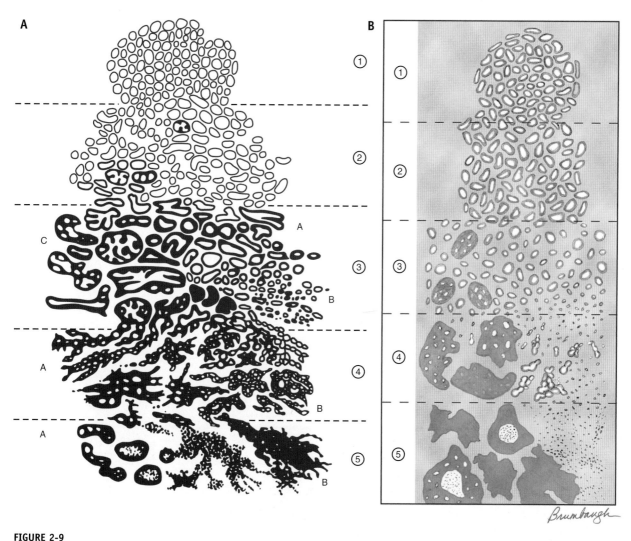

FIGURE 2-9

Gleason Grading System for Prostate Carcinoma. Original standardized drawing for grading prostate carcinoma (**A**) and modified Gleason grading system (**B**).

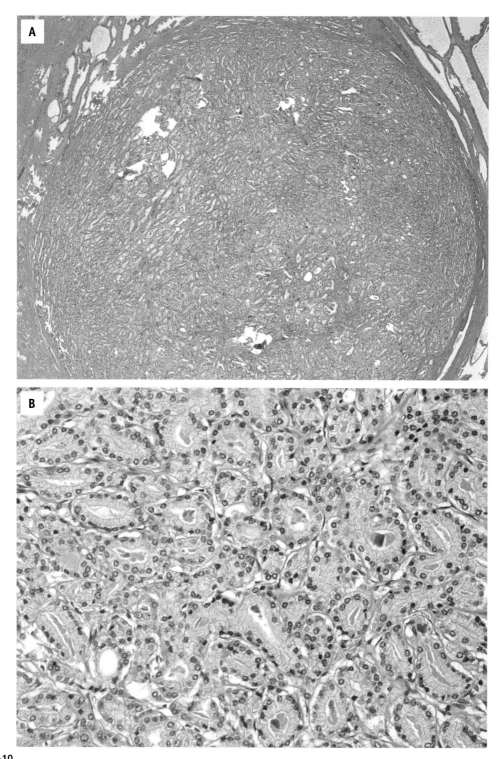

FIGURE 2-10

Gleason Pattern 1. Cancer glands, which are closely packed yet separated, of intermediate size, and similar in size and shape, form a circumscribed nodule.

into surrounding tissue (Fig. 2-11). Although the cytoplasm is not evaluated in the Gleason grading system, in Gleason patterns 1 and 2 cancer glands it tends to be abundant and pale-clear. Gleason pattern 2 cancer is often seen in the transition zone.

Gleason Pattern 3. This is the most common pattern. The cancer glands often infiltrate between the adjacent benign glands. They vary in size and shape and are often angular. Small glands are typical (Fig. 2-12A), but they may be large with papillary or cribriform (Fig. 2-12B) configuration. The Gleason pattern 3 cribriform glands have smooth, round contours, in contrast to the large, irregular Gleason pattern 4 cribriform glands (Fig. 2-13A).

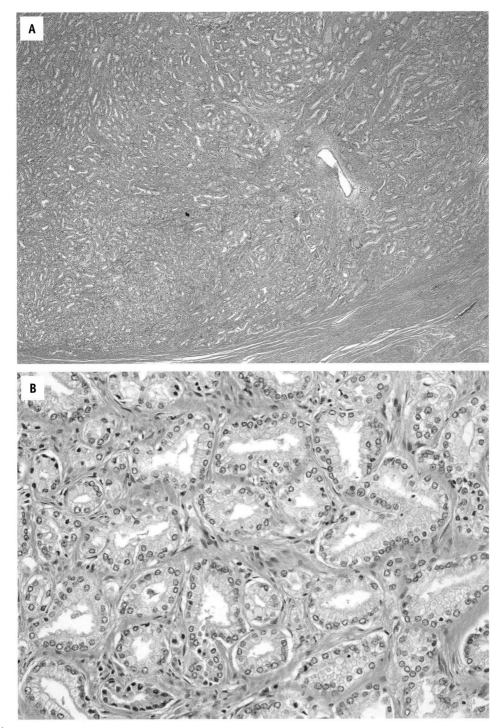

FIGURE 2-11

Gleason Pattern 2. Cancer glands are medium-sized, with some degree of variation in size and shape and looser arrangement (**B**). They form a less-well-circumscribed nodule (**A**).

Gleason Pattern 4. Glands appear fused, cribriform or poorly formed. Fused glands are composed of a group of glands that are no longer separated by stroma. Cribriform glands in pattern 4 are large and have irregular contour and jagged edges (Fig. 2-13A). The intraluminal cellular proliferation spans the entire diameter of the lumen. Poorly formed glands still have glandular configuration, but they have ill-formed glandular lumina (Fig. 2-13B). The hypernephromatoid pattern is a rare variant composed of fused glands with clear or very pale cytoplasm (Fig. 2-13C).

Gleason Pattern 5. Cancer cells form solid sheets (Fig. 2-14A), strands, or single cells (Fig. 2-14B) invading the stroma. Comedonecrosis may be present (Fig. 2-14C).

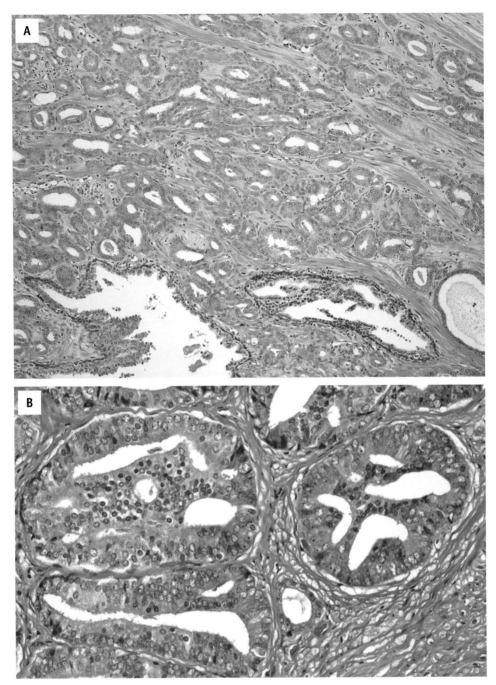

FIGURE 2-12

Gleason Pattern 3. The cancer glands infiltrate between the adjacent benign glands. Small glands are typical (**A**), but they may be large with papillary or cribriform (**B**) configuration. Cribriform glands are small and have smooth, round contours.

Tertiary Gleason pattern refers to a minor pattern occupying less than 5% of the tumor volume. In radical prostatectomy, the presence of a high-grade tertiary pattern adversely affects the prognosis. For example, the presence of a tertiary pattern 5 in a Gleason score 4 + 3 = 7 prostate carcinoma worsens the prognosis, compared with the same tumor without a tertiary high-grade component. However, the prognosis is not as poor as that of a 4 + 5 = 9 cancer. In prostate needle biopsies that harbor three patterns when the worst

pattern is the least common, the highest pattern should be incorporated as the secondary pattern.

Morphologic variants of prostate carcinoma are uncommon and often are mixed with ordinary prostate carcinoma. Grading such variants should be based on the underlying cancer glandular architecture. In general, ductal adenocarcinoma and mucinous adenocarcinoma behave more aggressively, comparable to Gleason score 8 acinar cancers, and signet-ring cell and sarcomatoid variants are even more aggressive, comparable to

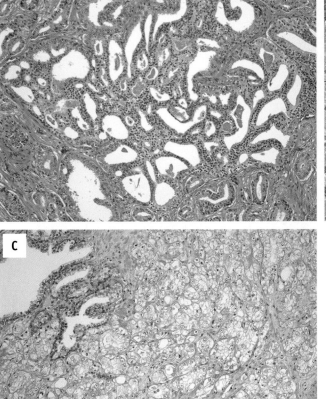

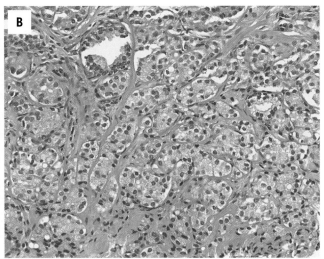

FIGURE 2-13

Gleason Pattern 4. Cribriform glands are large and have irregular contour and jagged edges (**A**). Poorly formed glands still have glandular configuration, but they have ill-formed glandular lumina (**B**). The hypernephromatoid pattern is composed of fused glands with clear or very pale cytoplasm (**C**).

Gleason score 9 or 10. On the other hand, squamous cell carcinoma, urothelial carcinoma, small cell carcinoma, and basaloid/adenoid cystic carcinoma are not assigned a Gleason grade.

Prostate carcinoma treated with hormonal ablation or radiation can appear artefactually to be of higher Gleason grade; therefore, Gleason grade should not be assigned to such cases. If no effect of the therapy is evident, a Gleason grade can be assigned.

Prostate carcinoma displays remarkable intratumoral grade heterogeneity; therefore, the biopsy Gleason grade may in some cases represent undergrading or overgrading compared with the radical prostatectomy. Nevertheless, the concordance between biopsy and prostatectomy Gleason scores is within one Gleason score in most cases.

Multiple studies have demonstrated that the Gleason grade is currently the most powerful prognostic indicator for prostate carcinoma. It correlates with all the important pathologic parameters in radical prostatec-

tomies, and with prognosis after radical prostatectomy and radiation therapy. The distinction between Gleason scores 6 and 7 is critical. Gleason 7 prostate carcinoma behaves significantly worse than Gleason 6 cancer but better than Gleason score 8 to 10 cancer. The following combination of Gleason scores results in groups with similar prognosis: Gleason score 2 to 4 (well-differentiated); Gleason score 5 to 6 (moderately differentiated); Gleason score 7 (moderately to poorly differentiated); and Gleason score 8 to 10 (poorly differentiated).

The importance of Gleason grade is evidenced by the use of various nomograms to predict pathologic stage and disease progression after surgery and radiotherapy. These nomograms, including Partin tables and Kattan nomograms, use preoperative biopsy Gleason score, tumor extent, clinical stage, and serum PSA to predict the risk of extraprostatic extension, seminal vesicle invasion, and lymph node metastasis and the probability of disease recurrence after treatment.

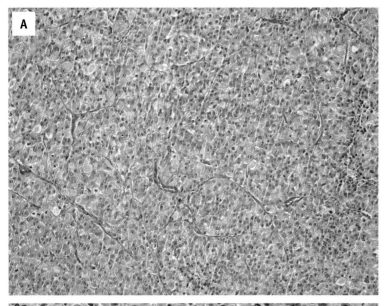

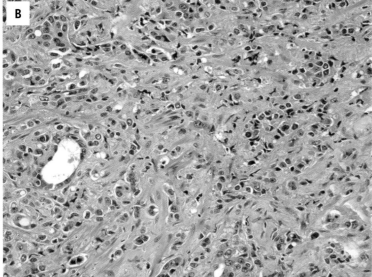

FIGURE 2-14
Gleason Pattern 5. Cancer cells forms solid sheets (**A**), strands, or single cells (**B**) invading the stroma. Comedonecrosis may be present (**C**).

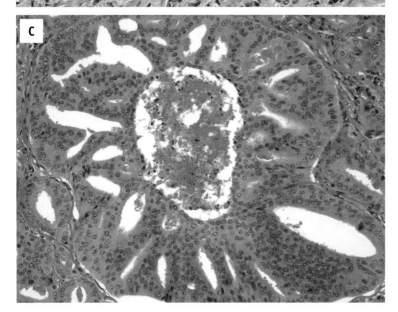

Histologic Variants of Prostate Carcinoma

Histologic variants of prostate carcinoma account for 5% to 10% of all the carcinomas in the prostate and are typically seen in association with ordinary acinar prostate carcinoma. These variants often differ from the latter in clinical, immunophenotypic, ultrastructural, and genetic features. Many also differ in prognosis and may prompt a different therapeutic approach. The following is a brief description of the histologic features of several variants. Other variants, including ductal adenocarcinoma, urothelial carcinoma, small cell carcinoma, squamous cell carcinoma, and basaloid carcinoma, are discussed separately.

Atrophic Carcinoma. The cancer glands have scant cytoplasm (Fig. 2-15A) and may be confused with

FIGURE 2-15

In atrophic prostate carcinoma, the cancer glands have scant cytoplasm (**A**); however, they display unequivocal malignant histologic features, including prominent nuclei and mucinous fibroplasia (**B**).

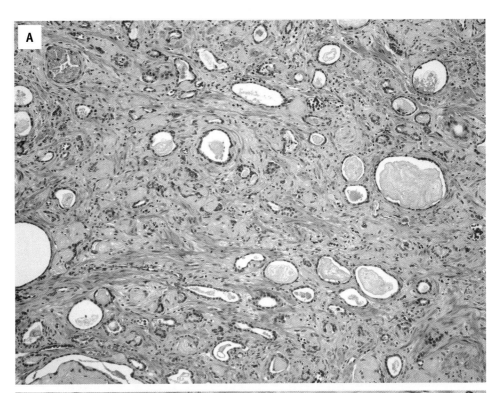

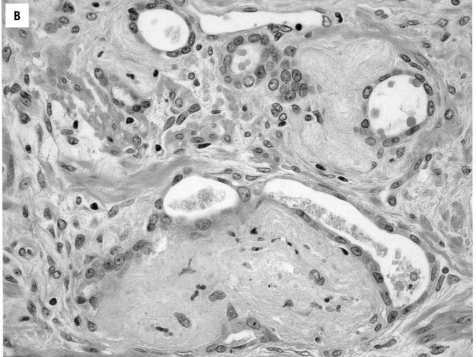

benign atrophy. The diagnosis is based on several features. First, atrophic prostate carcinoma displays an infiltrative growth pattern, with atrophic cancer glands intermingling with larger benign glands. In contrast, benign atrophy usually has a lobulated configuration. Atrophic prostate carcinoma has significant cytologic atypia, namely, nuclear enlargement and prominent nuclei (Fig. 2-15B). Finally, atrophic prostate carcinoma is often intermixed with nonatrophic ordinary prostate carcinoma.

Pseudohyperplastic Carcinoma. Resembling benign prostatic glands, pseudohyperplastic prostate carcinoma glands are large with branching and papillary infoldings (Fig. 2-16A). However, the malignant glands are much more closely packed than benign glands, and they display malignant nuclear features typical of prostate carcinoma (Fig. 2-16B). The diagnosis of pseudohyperplastic prostate carcinoma on needle biopsies is often difficult and requires immunohistochemistry to verify the absence of basal cells (Fig. 2-16C). Despite its benign appearance, pseudohyperplastic prostate carcinoma may be associated with typical intermediate-grade cancer and can exhibit aggressive behavior.

Foamy Gland Carcinoma. Cancer cells have abundant foamy or "xanthoma"-like cytoplasm with a very low nuclear/cytoplasmic ratio (Fig. 2-17A). Although the cytoplasm is xanthomatous in appearance, it contains empty vacuoles rather than lipid. The nuclei of foamy gland prostate carcinoma cells are typically small and hyperchromatic and lack the cytologic features of ordinary prostate carcinoma (Fig. 2-17B). The diagnosis of foamy gland prostate carcinoma is based on its architectural pattern of crowded and/or infiltrative glands, abundant foamy cytoplasm, and frequent intraluminal, dense, pink, acellular secretions. Basal cells are absent by immunohistochemistry. Despite its bland cytology, most of the cases that include an associated nonfoamy cancer are Gleason score 6 or greater. Foamy gland prostate carcinoma, therefore, appears best classified as an intermediate-grade carcinoma.

Mucinous (Colloid) Carcinoma. Mucinous prostate carcinoma is defined as a cancer in which 25% or more of the tumor consists of lakes of extracellular mucin. Prostate carcinoma with less than 25% mucinous component should be classified as having mucinous features, whereas prostate carcinoma with intraluminal mucin without lakes of extracellular mucin is not considered as mucinous prostate carcinoma. Clinically, the average age for mucinous prostate carcinoma is similar to that for the ordinary acinar prostate carcinoma, although the clinical stage at presentation is often advanced, with locally advanced or metastatic disease. Microscopically, tumor cells float in lakes of extracellular mucin that are sharply demarcated from the stroma (Fig. 2-18A). Tumor cells are arranged in cribriform configurations, cords, strands, acini, or tubules. Cytologically, they appear bland with occasional prominent nucleoli (Fig. 2-18B). They are positive for PSA and PSAP.

Signet-Ring-Like Carcinoma. Defined as 25% or more of tumor mass consisting of signet-ring-appearing cells, this histologic variant is a rare entity with an aggressive clinical course. Microscopically, the signet-ring-like tumor cells display nuclear displacement and indentation by clear cytoplasmic vacuoles (Fig. 2-19). In the majority of cases, these vacuoles contain lipid rather than mucin, as with true signet cells. The cancer cells grow in sheets, in small clusters, and as single cells. They are invariably mixed with ordinary acinar prostate carcinoma components. Immunostains for PSA and PSAP are positive in most cases, and stains for CK7, CK20, and HMWCK are negative in all cases. Before establishing a diagnosis of prostatic signet-ring carcinoma, a metastasis from other anatomic sites, including stomach, lung, colon, and pancreaticobiliary system, must be excluded. On the other hand, a prostatic signet-ring carcinoma should be considered when one encounters a signet-ring-cell carcinoma of unknown primary, especially if mucin stains are negative.

Sarcomatoid Carcinoma (Carcinosarcoma). Sarcomatoid prostate carcinoma is composed of both malignant epithelial and spindle cell elements. It may be a de novo diagnosis, or patients may have a previous history of prostate carcinoma treated with radiation or hormonal ablation therapy or both. Serum PSA is within normal limits in most cases, despite the frequent presence of nodal and distant metastases. The 5-year survival rate is less than 40%. Microscopically, sarcomatoid prostate carcinoma is biphasic, with a glandular component showing variable Gleason patterns and a sarcomatoid component often exhibiting nondescript malignant spindle cell proliferation (Fig. 2-20). Specific mesenchymal differentiation can also be present, including osteosarcoma, chondrosarcoma, and rhabdomyosarcoma. Immunohistochemically, the epithelial elements are positive for PSA and/or pancytokeratins, whereas the sarcomatoid elements react with markers of corresponding mesenchymal differentiation and variably express cytokeratins.

Treatment Effects

Treatment for prostate carcinoma, especially radiation and androgen ablation, can have profound effects on both benign and malignant prostate tissue.

Radiation Therapy Effects. Both cancer and benign glands respond variably to radiation, with some glands showing marked radiation effect and others showing no such effect. For benign prostatic tissue, the classic alterations are extensive glandular atrophy with stromal predominance. Glands retain their lobular architecture, although individual glands often assume irregular, angulated contours. Secretory cells are atrophic, and basal cells become hyperplastic and multilayered, with scattered, markedly atypical nuclei that appear degenerated (Fig. 2-21). These cells are positive for basal cell immunohistochemical markers. Radiation-treated prostate carcinoma, on the other hand, has a variable appearance, from no or minimal radiation effect to significant radiation-induced changes. The classic radiation-induced changes in prostate carcinoma are decrease in number of cancer glands, poorly formed glands and single cancer cells, abundant vacuolated cytoplasm, nuclear pyknosis, and stromal fibrosis

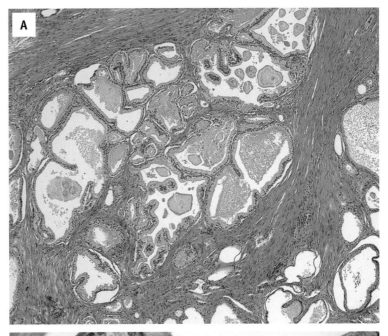

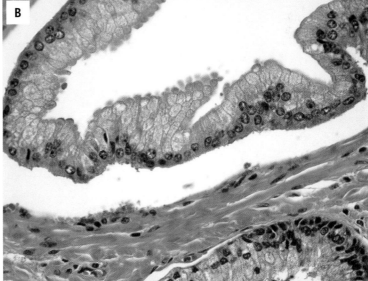

FIGURE 2-16

At low magnification, pseudohyperplastic prostate cancer glands are large with branching and papillary infoldings (**A**), resembling a hyperplastic nodule. However, the cancer glands display prominent nucleoli (**B**) and lack basal cells on p63 immunohistochemistry (**C**).

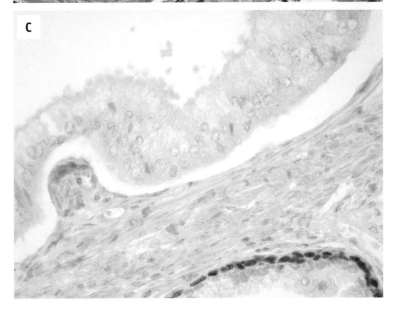

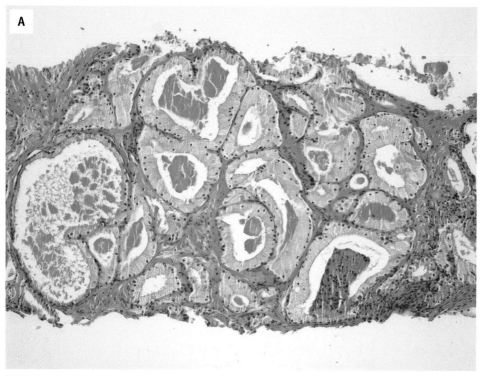

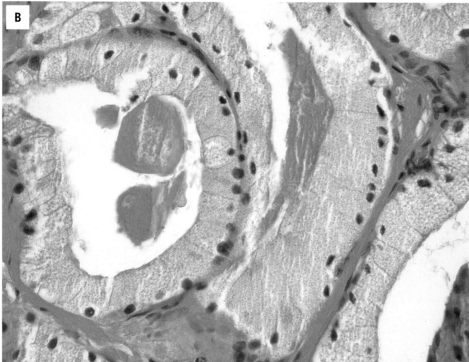

FIGURE 2-17

In foamy gland carcinoma, cancer glands frequently have intraluminal, dense, pink, acellular secretions, and cancer cells have abundant foamy cytoplasm (**A**). The nuclei are typically small and hyperchromatic (**B**).

(Fig. 2-22). Architecturally, the key feature for recognizing the radiated cancer is closely packed glands with a haphazard infiltrative growth pattern and the presence of infiltrating individual cancer cells, architectural findings that are inconsistent with a benign process. It may take up to 30 months for cancer to clear after radiation therapy. Therefore, rebiopsy should be performed no sooner than this time. Findings on rebiopsy predict the prognosis, with positive biopsies showing no treatment effect having a worse outcome than negative biopsies, and cancer with treatment effect having an intermediate prognosis.

Androgen Deprivation. Androgen deprivation by surgical castration or pharmacologic blockade has become a common treatment modality for patients with locally advanced or metastatic prostate carcinoma.

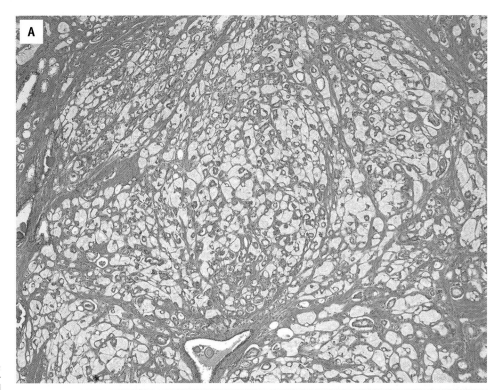

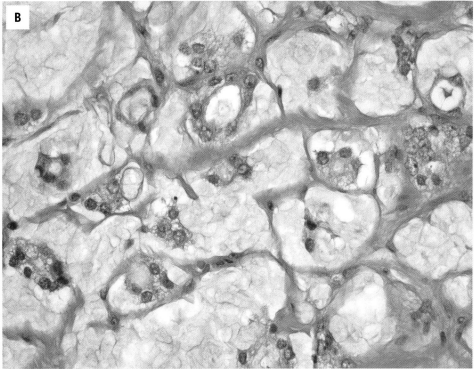

FIGURE 2-18

In mucinous prostate carcinoma, cancer cells float in lakes of extracellular mucin (**A**) and are arranged in cords and acini. Cytologically, they appear bland with occasional prominent nucleoli (**B**).

More recently, preoperative (neoadjuvant) hormonal ablation is sometimes used for clinically localized prostate carcinoma, to retard tumor growth before surgery if there is a delay between biopsy and definitive resection. In benign prostate tissue, androgen ablation results in pronounced glandular atrophy and stromal predominance. Luminal secretory cells become atrophic and exhibit nuclear pyknosis and cytoplasmic clearing. Basal cells undergo hyperplasia and squamous metaplasia. The histology of prostate carcinoma may be significantly altered after hormonal therapy. The neoplastic glands tend to be smaller and atrophic, with compressed or obliterated lumina (Fig. 2-23A). Tumor cells develop pyknotic nuclei and abundant foamy or

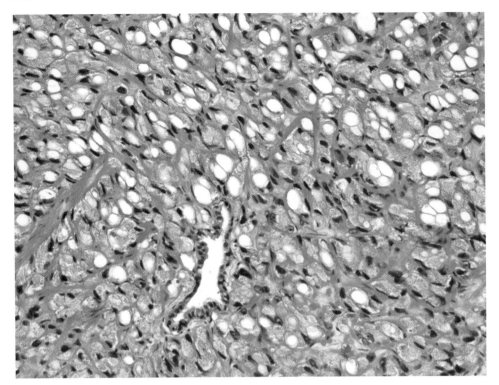

FIGURE 2-19
Signet-ring-like cancer cells display nuclear displacement and indentation by clear cytoplasmic vacuoles.

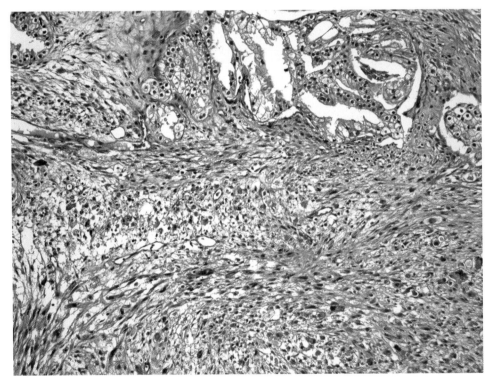

FIGURE 2-20
This sarcomatoid prostate carcinoma is biphasic, with a Gleason pattern 4 glandular component and a sarcomatoid component exhibiting malignant spindle cell proliferation.

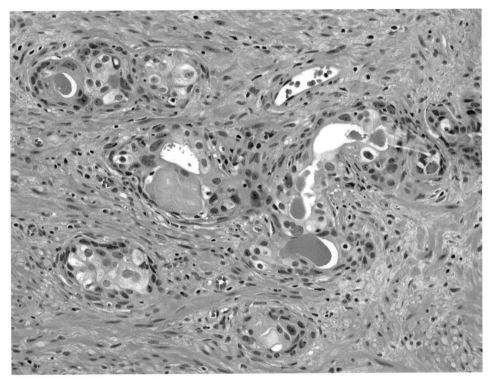

FIGURE 2-21
After radiation therapy, benign prostatic glands retain their lobular architecture, although individual glands assume irregular, angulated contours. Secretory cells are atrophic, and basal cells become multilayered, with scattered, markedly atypical nuclei that appear degenerated.

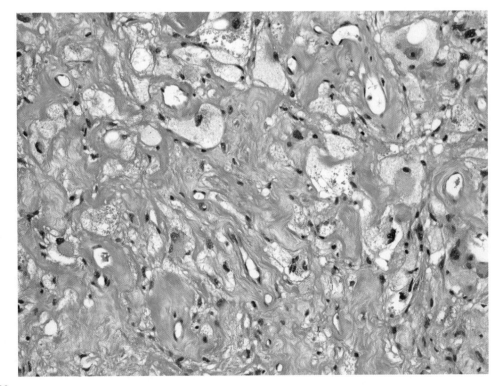

FIGURE 2-22
After radiation therapy, cancer glands become poorly formed, with single cells infiltrating in the fibrotic stroma. They have abundant vacuolated cytoplasm and pyknotic nuclei.

clear vacuolated cytoplasm (Fig. 2-23B). Sometimes, single tumor cells are widely scattered within the stroma, resembling histiocytes. There may also be complete dissolution of tumor cells, leaving empty clefts or mucin aggregates (Fig. 2-23C,D). Immunohistochemically, cancer cells after hormonal therapy are positive for pancytokeratins, PSA, and AMACR but negative for HMWCK, although the staining intensity for PSA and AMACR may be reduced.

ANCILLARY STUDIES

IMMUNOHISTOCHEMISTRY

Prostate-specific Antigen (PSA). PSA is detected in secretory cells of benign prostate glands in all anatomic zones, but not in basal cells, seminal vesicle/ejaculatory duct epithelium, or prostatic urothelial cells. The majority of prostate carcinomas also express PSA (Fig. 2-24A), although there is considerable intratumoral and intertumoral heterogeneity, and the expression is decreased in a minority of high-grade prostate carcinoma. After androgen deprivation and radiotherapy, some cancers can lose PSA expression. PSA immunoreactivity can be detected to variable degrees in some nonprostatic tissues and tumors, including urethral and periurethral glands, cystitis cystica and glandularis, urachal remnants, bladder adenocarcinoma, and extramammary Paget's disease of the penis.

Prostate-specific Acid Phosphatase (PSAP). PSAP has diagnostic utility similar to that of PSA, although it is in general more sensitive and less specific than the latter (Fig. 2-24B). Nonprostatic tumors that are reported to be positive for PSAP include some neuroendocrine tumors (pancreatic islet cell tumors and gastrointestinal carcinoids), urothelial carcinoma, and anal cloacogenic carcinoma.

Cytokeratins. Benign prostatic secretory and basal cells are immunoreactive for antibodies to broad-spectrum and low-molecular-weight cytokeratins (CKs). Negative

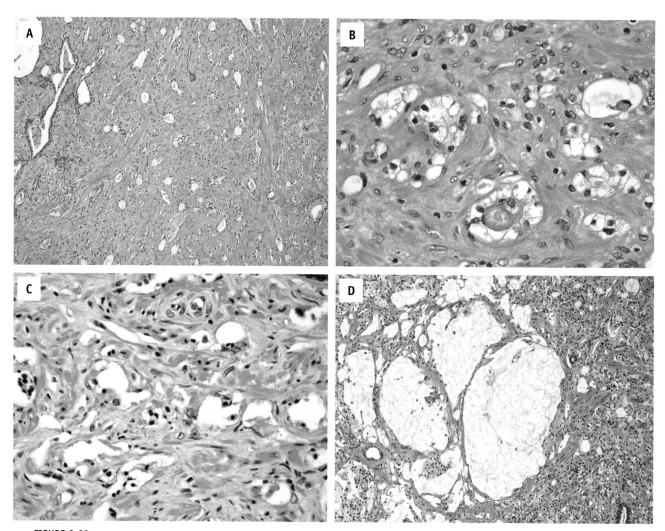

FIGURE 2-23

After hormonal ablation, both benign and malignant glands are markedly atrophic. The cancer glands are smaller, with compressed or obliterated lumina (**A**). Cancer cells have pyknotic nuclei and abundant foamy or clear vacuolated cytoplasm (**B**). They may be dissolved to leave empty clefts (**C**) or mucin aggregates (**D**).

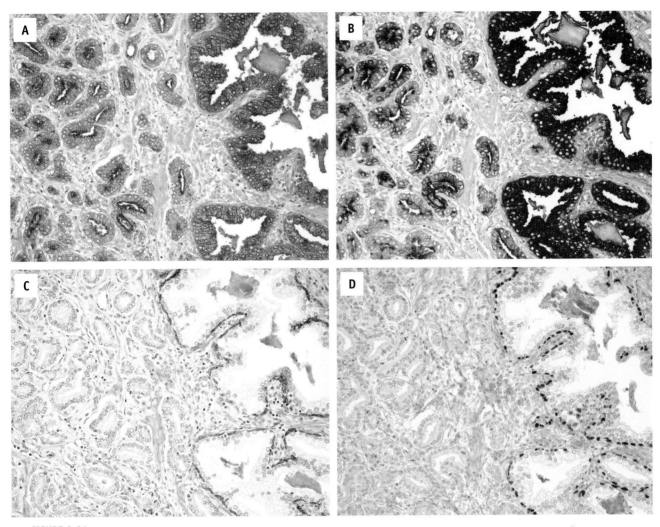

FIGURE 2-24

Benign prostatic glands *(right)* are positive for prostate-specific antigen (PSA) (**A**) and prostate-specific acid phosphatase (PSAP) (**B**). They have a basal cell layer as demonstrated by high-molecular-weight cytokeratin (HMWCK) (**C**) and p63 (**D**) immunostains. In contrast, cancer glands *(left)* are devoid of basal cells, although they are also positive for PSA and PSAP.

staining for both CK7 and CK20, which is typical of prostate cancer, is useful to differentiate prostate carcinoma from urothelial carcinoma, which is typically positive for both markers.

Basal Cell Markers. HMWCK, detected by antibody clone 34βE12 that recognizes CK1, CK5, CK10, and CK14, or by the antibody cocktail that recognizes CK5 and CK6, is expressed only by prostate basal cells, and not by secretory cells (Fig. 2-24C). Prostate carcinoma uniformly lacks a basal cell layer and therefore is negative for HMWCK (Fig. 2-24C). Absence of a basal lining is demonstrated by lack of immunostain for HMWCK and supports a diagnosis of prostate carcinoma in the context of suspicious architectural and/or cytologic features on routine H&E stains. However, prostate carcinoma can occasionally contain sparse tumor cells that are positive for 34βE12 yet not in a basal cell distribution, especially after radiation or hormonal therapy. Intraductal spread of prostate carcinoma or entrapped benign glands may also be mistaken as residual basal cells in prostate carcinoma. Conversely,

some benign conditions, including adenosis (atypical adenomatous hyperplasia) and partial atrophy, can sometimes have a discontinuous or even absent basal cell lining. P63 is a nuclear protein expressed in basal cells of pseudostratified epithelia, including prostate. It has similar diagnostic utility (Fig. 2-24D) and pitfalls as HMWCK but with the following advantages: (1) it stains a subset of basal cells that are negative for HMWCK, (2) it is less susceptible to staining variability, particularly in TURP specimens with cautery artifact, and (3) it is easier to interpret because of its strong and sharp nuclear staining.

α-Methylacyl-Coenzyme A Racemase. AMACR is an enzyme involved in the metabolism of branched-chain fatty acids and bile acid intermediates. It is overexpressed in the majority of prostate carcinomas (Fig. 2-25A,B). Because of its intratumoral heterogenous expression patterns, AMACR is positive in only 80% of prostate carcinomas in prostate needle biopsies. Several histologic variants of prostate carcinoma, such as foamy gland, atrophic, and pseudohyperplastic prostate

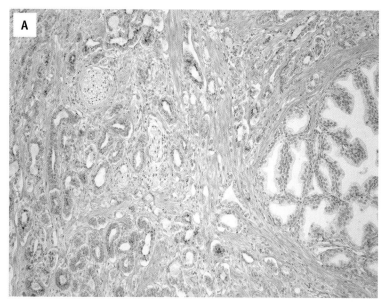

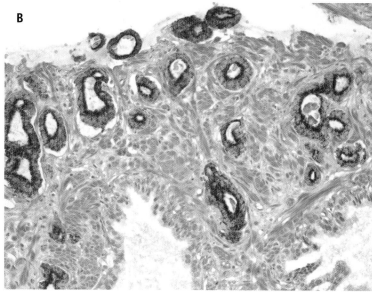

FIGURE 2-25

Cancer glands *(left)* are positive for α-methylacyl-coenzyme A racemase (AMACR) (**A**), with apical and cytoplasmic granular staining (**B**). Benign glands *(right)* are negative for AMACR (**A**).

carcinoma, show lower AMACR expression. AMACR is not entirely specific for prostate carcinoma, because it is present in HGPIN (> 90 %), adenosis (17.5 %), partially atrophic glands, and occasionally morphologically benign glands. AMACR can be used as a confirmatory staining for prostate carcinoma, in conjunction with H&E histology and basal cell markers.

Basal cell markers and AMACR can be combined in a single immunostaining reaction (Fig. 2-26). Such "cocktail" staining may be advantageous for working up a small focus of cancer that might be present only in one tissue section.

DIFFERENTIAL DIAGNOSIS

The differential diagnosis of prostate carcinoma is complex (Table 2-1). In many instances, the differential is with normal prostatic and nonprostatic structures, including seminal vesicles/ejaculatory duct epithelium, Cowper's gland, paraganglia, and mesonephric duct remnants. A wide variety of benign pathologic processes, such as inflammation, atrophy (simple atrophy, partial atrophy, and postatrophic hyperplasia), metaplasia (urothelial, squamous, and mucinous), basal cell hyperplasia, BPH, and radiation and hormonal treatment effects, can simulate prostate carcinoma to varying degrees. The prostate gland can rarely be involved by primary urothelial, small cell, mucinous, and signet-ring cell carcinoma. However, such a diagnosis should be made only after a metastasis from other sites is diligently excluded. On the other hand, prostate carcinoma can also mimic benign conditions. For example, a well-differentiated Gleason score 2 to 4 prostate carcinoma should always be differentiated from adenosis. Cribriform prostate carcinoma should be distinguished from benign cribriform hyperplasia or cribriform HGPIN. Atrophic and foamy gland prostate carcinoma

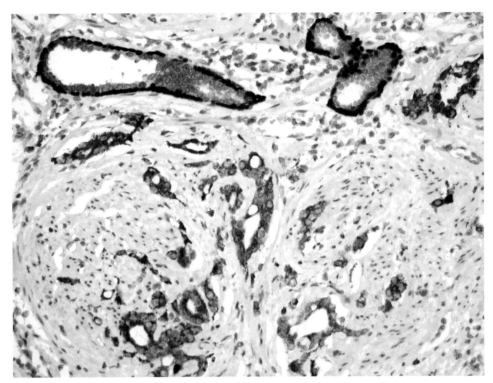

FIGURE 2-26
Stains for α-methylacyl-coenzyme A racemase (AMACR), high-molecular-weight cytokeratin (HMWCK), and p63 can be performed in a single reaction. Cancer glands *(lower half)* are negative for basal cell markers (HMWCK and p63, brown staining) but positive for AMACR *(red staining)*. Benign glands *(upper half)* are the opposite.

may be confused with benign atrophy and xanthoma, respectively. Pseudohyperplastic prostate carcinoma shares some architectural features with BPH, although the former invariably has significant nuclear atypia. Careful evaluation of the architectural and cytologic features and prudent use of basal cell markers and AMACR will lead to a correct diagnosis.

Sometimes a gland or a focus of glands is suspicious for prostate carcinoma, yet a definitive cancer diagnosis cannot be established due to the lack of sufficient architectural and cytologic atypia. The terms "atypical small acinar proliferation (ASAP)" and "focal atypical glands" have been used. Unlike HGPIN or prostate carcinoma, ASAP is a diagnostic term rather than a defined disease entity. It encompasses such lesions as HGPIN, benign mimickers of prostate cancer, reactive atypia, and many cases that in retrospect demonstrate focal cancer. ASAP found in needle biopsy denotes a high risk ($\sim 50\%$) of detecting prostate carcinoma in subsequent biopsies.

PROGNOSIS AND TREATMENT

The choice of therapeutic modalities for prostate carcinoma depends on the stage of the cancer, the patient's life expectancy, and comorbidity. Expectant management, or watchful waiting, in which patients are under close surveillance and definitive therapies are deferred until there is sign of disease progression, is most often selected for older men with a life expectancy of less than 10 years who have low or intermediate grade (Gleason score < 7), low-volume prostate carcinoma that is confirmed after extensive prostate sampling. For a man with clinically localized prostate carcinoma when curative intent is desired, radical prostatectomy and radiation therapy are options. Radical prostatectomy is the mainstay of primary treatment for clinically localized prostate carcinoma. It can also be performed after hormonal therapy and as salvage treatment after failure of radiation therapy. Radiation therapy, by external beam radiotherapy or implantation of radioactive seeds (brachytherapy), can also be used as a primary modality to treat prostate carcinoma. Hormonal ablation therapy, either by surgical castration (orchiectomy) or by pharmacologic blockade of androgen effect with luteinizing hormone-releasing hormone (LHRH) analogs or anti-androgen compounds, is the main modality of treatment for men with disseminated prostate carcinoma. However, such treatment is only palliative and not curative. Locally advanced prostate carcinoma is frequently managed by a combination of irradiation and hormonal ablation.

The prognosis for patients with prostate carcinoma is highly variable and depends on a variety of host, tumor, and treatment parameters. The College of American Pathologists classifies the prognostic factors into three categories. Category I includes factors that are proven to be of prognostic importance and useful in clinical management, including preoperative serum

TABLE 2-1

Differential Diagnosis of Prostate Carcinoma

Differential Diagnosis	Architectural Features	Cytologic Features	Immunohistochemistry
NORMAL PROSTATIC/NONPROSTATIC STRUCTURES			
Seminal vesicle or ejaculatory duct	Central irregular lumen with surrounding clusters of smaller glands	1. Scattered cells showing prominent degenerative nuclear atypia 2. Golden-brown lipofuscin pigment	1. Basal cells + by p63 and HMWCK 2. Secretory cells − PSA (monoclonal antibody) 3. + MUC6
Verumontanum mucosal gland hyperplasia	1. Closely packed small acini beneath urethral mucosa 2. Orange-brown dense luminal secretion	1. Prominent nucleoli − 2. Lipofuscin pigment + 3. Basal cells +	Basal cells + by HMWCK and p63
Cowper's glands	1. Noninfiltrative, lobular pattern 2. Dimorphic population of ducts and mucinous acini 3. Intermixed with skeletal muscle fibers	Acini with voluminous, pale cytoplasm	PSAP − PSA − or + in heterogeneous, clumpy fashion in minority of cases
Paraganglia	1. Small cluster or nest of clear cells with prominent vascular pattern 2. Intimately associated with nerve 3. Most common in periprostatic soft tissue	1. Clear or amphophilic, granular cytoplasm 2. Inconspicuous nucleoli	Neuroendocrine markers + PSA, PSAP −
BENIGN PROSTATIC LESIONS			
Mesonephric remnants	1. Lobular arrangement of small regular tubules 2. Dense, eosinophilic intraluminal secretion	Tubules lined with single layer of epithelium	PSA, PSAP − HMWCK +
Partial atrophy	1. Lobular configuration often maintained 2. Pale glands with irregular or angulated contour 3. Atrophy involving some glands, or part of a gland	May have mild nuclear atypia	Basal cell markers + but often patchy, or even absent in some glands
Postatrophic hyperplasia	Central dilated atrophic duct surrounded by fibrosis and clustered smaller atrophic glands	1. Atrophic cytoplasm 2. Inconspicuous nucleoli	Basal cell markers +
Urothelial metaplasia	1. Stratification of elongated cells underneath the secretory cells 2. Cells perpendicular to basement membrane	1. Elongated nuclei with nuclear grooves 2. Perinuclear clearing	Basal cell markers +
Squamous metaplasia	1. Associated with inflammation, infarction, or hormonal ablation therapy 2. Small, solid nests with admixed inflammation	1. Intercellular bridges 2. Squamoid cytoplasm 3. Keratin pearls may be present 4. Immature form may have prominent nucleoli	Basal cell markers +
Basal cell hyperplasia	1. More common in transition zone 2. Acinar, cribriform, and solid growth patterns 3. Lined with ≥2 layers of basal cells 4. May have squamous metaplasia or intraluminal calcifications, or intracytoplasmic eosinophilic globules	1. Bland oval or elongated cells 2. Occasionally have prominent nucleoli	PSA, PSAP − HMWCK, p63 +

BPH, benign prostatic hypertrophy; HGPIN, high-grade prostatic intraepithelial neoplasia; HMWCK, high-molecular-weight cytokeratins; PSA, prostate-specific antigen; PSAP, prostate-specific acid phosphatase.

TABLE 2-1

Differential Diagnosis of Prostate Carcinoma—cont'd

Differential Diagnosis	Architectural Features	Cytologic Features	Immunohistochemistry
BENIGN PROSTATIC LESIONS—CONT'D			
Adenosis	Small crowded glands admixed with larger glands in lobular configuration	1. Small glands share cytologic features with larger benign glands 2. Prominent nucleoli absent	Basal cells, detected by p63 or HMWCK antibody, may be patchy or absent in some small glands
Sclerosing adenosis	Mixture of well-formed glands, cords, or single cells and cellular spindle cells	Hyaline collarette around glands	Basal cells + for p63, HMWCK, S-100, and actin
Nonspecific granulomatous prostatitis	1. Acini or duct-centered process 2. Mixed inflammatory infiltrates containing lymphocytes, histiocytes, neutrophils, eosinophils, plasma cells, and giant cells	1. Epithelial cells may have conspicuous nucleoli 2. Histiocytes may have nucleoli	PSA, PSAP, and pancytokeratin – CD68 +
BPH	Nodular arrangement of small and large acini with papillary infoldings and projections	1. No cytologic atypia 2. Basal cells +	Basal cell markers +
RADIATION EFFECT IN BENIGN GLANDS	1. Lobular configuration 2. Individual glands with irregular, angulated contour 3. Multilayered cells	Scattered cells with marked degenerative nuclear atypia	Basal cell markers +
HGPIN	1. Glands similar to adjacent benign glands in size and shape and separated by stroma 2. Smooth glandular contour 3. Basal cell layer may be intact or discontinuous	1. Nuclear enlargement 2. Coarse chromatin 3. Nucleolar prominence	Basal cell markers highlight basal cell layers

PSA, Gleason grade, TNM stage, and surgical margin status. Category II includes factors that have been extensively studied biologically and clinically but whose importance remains to be validated in large multicenter trials. Factors included in this category are DNA ploidy, tumor volume, and histologic subtypes. Category III factors have not been sufficiently studied to demonstrate their prognostic value; they include perineural invasion, neuroendocrine differentiation, microvessel density, nuclear features other than ploidy, proliferation markers, and a variety of molecular markers.

DUCTAL ADENOCARCINOMA

CLINICAL FEATURES

Known previously as endometrial or endometrioid carcinoma of the prostate, this tumor is currently recognized as a variant of prostate adenocarcinoma.

The incidence of pure ductal adenocarcinoma is 1.3% of all prostate carcinomas. However, it is more commonly admixed with an ordinary acinar prostate carcinoma, with an incidence of 4.8% for mixed ductal-acinar prostate carcinoma. Affected men are of the same ages as those with acinar prostate carcinoma. Periurethral or centrally located tumor may manifest with urinary obstruction and hematuria, and peripherally located tumor may result in abnormal DRE findings. Serum PSA is usually elevated, although the level may be variable. Ductal adenocarcinoma often is diagnosed at a more advanced stage than acinar prostate carcinoma, and with a higher percentage of non-organ-confined disease.

PATHOLOGIC FEATURES

GROSS FINDINGS

Centrally occurring tumors may manifest as an exophytic polypoid or papillary mass projecting into the urethra, around the verumontanum. Peripherally loceted tumors have a gross appearance similar to that of acinar prostate carcinoma.

DUCTAL ADENOCARCINOMA—FACT SHEET

Definition
▶ Subtype of prostate carcinoma composed of large glands lined with pseudostratified columnar tumor cells

Incidence
▶ Pure ductal adenocarcinoma: 1.3% of all prostate cancer
▶ Mixed acinar and ductal adenocarcinoma: 4.8%

Gender, Race, and Age Distribution
▶ Same age as for acinar prostate carcinoma
▶ Mean age 63-72 years (range, 41-89 years)

Clinical Features
▶ Urinary obstruction and hematuria (central tumor)
▶ Abnormal DRE (peripheral tumor)
▶ PSA usually elevated

Prognosis and Treatment
▶ More aggressive than acinar prostate carcinoma
▶ Five-year survival rate: 15-43%
▶ Definitive therapy warranted even if only limited component is found on needle biopsies or TURP

DUCTAL ADENOCARCINOMA—PATHOLOGIC FEATURES

Gross Findings
▶ Central tumor—exophytic polypoid or papillary mass projecting into the urethra around the verumontanum
▶ Peripheral tumor—similar to acinar prostate carcinoma

Microscopic Findings
▶ Different growth patterns, often intermingled, including papillary, cribriform, single gland, and solid patterns
▶ True papillae with fibrovascular cores in papillary pattern
▶ Cribriform with slit-like spaces
▶ Glands lined with single or pseudostratified layers of tall columnar cells
▶ Cytologic atypia minimal or pronounced
▶ Stromal reactions, including fibrosis, inflammation, and hemosiderin deposition

Immunohistochemical Features
▶ + PSA, PSAP
▶ − HMWCK, p63 (usually); occasionally grows into ducts with retention of basal cell layer

Differential Diagnosis
▶ Acinar prostate carcinoma
▶ HGPIN
▶ Urothelial carcinoma
▶ Prostatic urethral polyp

MICROSCOPIC FINDINGS

Ductal adenocarcinoma can grow within and expand the prostatic urethra and periurethral ducts, or it can diffusely involve prostatic ducts and acini. It displays a variety of architectural patterns that are often intermingled, including papillary (Fig. 2-27A), cribriform (Fig. 2-27B), single gland (Fig. 2-27C), "endometrioid" (Fig. 2-27D), and solid patterns. In papillary ductal adenocarcinoma, the papillae have true fibrovascular cores (Fig. 2-27E). Stromal reactions, including fibrosis, inflammation, and hemosiderin deposition, are sometimes present. The malignant glands are lined by a pseudostratified layer of tall columnar cells with abundant amphophilic cytoplasm (Fig. 2-27E). Cytologic atypia is minimal in some cases, but in other cases mitoses and marked nuclear pleomorphism are common (Fig. 2-27F). Although ductal adenocarcinoma is typically not graded, it is most equivalent to Gleason pattern 4. Ductal adenocarcinoma may have a significant in situ component, with tumor cells extending into the pre-existing ducts and acini and preservation of a continuous or discontinuous basal cell layer.

ANCILLARY STUDIES

IMMUNOHISTOCHEMISTRY

Similar to ordinary acinar prostate carcinoma, ductal adenocarcinoma is positive for PSA and PSAP and negative for HMWCK and p63, although residual basal cells may be positive in the setting of intraductal growth.

DIFFERENTIAL DIAGNOSIS

Distinction of ductal adenocarcinoma from acinar prostate carcinoma with similar growth patterns may be difficult but is of little significance with regard to treatment decisions. HGPIN should also be distinguished from ductal adenocarcinoma, especially if residual basal cells are present in the latter. HGPIN typically does not have the same degree of glandular crowding, confluent growth pattern, true fibrovascular cores, and high-grade nuclear features as ductal adenocarcinoma. Prominent comedonecrosis, occasionally seen in ductal adenocarcinoma, is absent in HGPIN. Papillary urothelial carcinoma that arises in the prostatic urethra or involves prostatic ducts or acini may mimic ductal adenocarcinoma but often shows more pronounced cytologic atypia and lacks glandular formation. Tumor cells are positive for HMWCK and p63 but negative for PSA and PSAP. Finally, prostatic urethral polyp, a benign polypoid

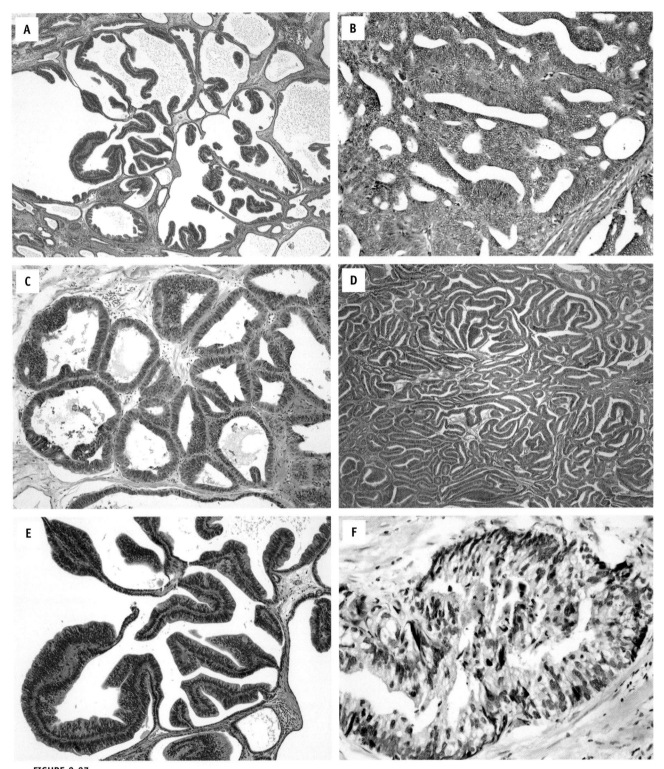

FIGURE 2-27

Ductal adenocarcinoma displays a variety of architectural patterns, including papillary (**A**), cribriform (**B**), single gland (**C**), and "endometrioid" (**D**). The papillae have true fibrovascular cores with pseudostratified columnar cells (**E**). Cytologic atypia is minimal in some cases (**E**), but in other cases mitoses and marked nuclear pleomorphism are common (**F**).

intraurethral growth, is composed of cytologically bland prostatic epithelium and does not have cribriform growth patterns or cytologic atypia.

PROGNOSIS AND TREATMENT

Ductal adenocarcinoma behaves more aggressively than acinar prostate carcinoma. Patients often present with large tumor and advanced disease, including bony metastases. Five-year survival rates range from 15% to 43%. Definitive therapy is warranted even when only limited ductal adenocarcinoma is found on needle biopsies.

UROTHELIAL CARCINOMA

CLINICAL FEATURES

Urothelial carcinomas of the prostate are infrequent, accounting for 2.8% of all prostate carcinomas. Primary urothelial carcinoma exclusively involving the prostate is even rarer, seen in only 1.1% of all prostate carcinomas. Most urothelial carcinomas (76% to 100%), including both carcinoma in situ (CIS) and invasive urothelial carcinoma, involve the prostate as a result of direct extension of the neoplastic process from the bladder. Most patients are of similar age to those with bladder carcinoma, with a mean age of 66 years (range, 45 to 91 years). They present with obstructive urinary symptoms and hematuria. DRE is variably abnormal, and serum PSA typically is not elevated.

PATHOLOGIC FEATURES

GROSS FINDINGS

In the setting of an invasive urothelial carcinoma directly invading the prostate, the prostatic urethral component can be polypoid-papillary on cystoscopy.

MICROSCOPIC FINDINGS

The majority of prostatic urothelial carcinomas are of high grade, with histologic features characteristic of urothelial carcinomas of the bladder. Urothelial carcinoma involving the prostate may be of three types. In CIS with intraductal spread from CIS in the bladder, prostatic ducts and acini are filled with malignant urothelial cells, often with central necrosis (Fig. 2-28A,B). Stromal invasion can be recognized as small irregular nests, cords, or single cells in a desmoplastic and inflamed stroma (Fig. 2-28C). In the second type, there is direct invasion from a large invasive urothelial carcinoma into the prostatic stroma (Fig. 2-28D). Finally, primary invasive urothelial carcinoma rarely arises in the prostate without concomitant bladder neoplasia. As in the bladder, squamous and glandular differentiation may be present. Both CIS and invasive urothelial carcinoma can spread along ejaculatory ducts into seminal vesicle. Metastases are to the regional lymph nodes and bone. Bony involvement is osteolytic, in contrast to the

---

UROTHELIAL CARCINOMA—FACT SHEET

Definition
▶ Urothelial carcinoma involving the prostate

Incidence
▶ Primary prostatic urothelial carcinoma rare (1.1% of prostate cancer)
▶ 76-100% associated with bladder or urethral urothelial carcinoma

Gender, Race, and Age Distribution
▶ Mean age, 66 years (range, 45-91)

Clinical Features
▶ Obstructive urinary symptoms
▶ Abnormal DRE

Prognosis and Treatment
▶ Prostatic stromal invasion significant worse prognosis (5-year survival 45% vs 100% urothelial carcinoma in situ after cystoprostatectomy)
▶ Radical prostatectomy or cystoprostatectomy
▶ Androgen deprivation therapy ineffective

UROTHELIAL CARCINOMA—PATHOLOGIC FEATURES

Gross Findings
▶ Shaggy and infiltrative, polypoid or papillary on cystoscopy

Microscopic Findings
▶ Identical to urothelial carcinoma of the bladder
▶ Prostatic stromal invasion recognized as small irregular nests, cords or single cells in desmoplastic stroma
▶ Osteolytic bony metastasis

Immunohistochemical Features
▶ – PSA, PAP
▶ + CK7, CK20, HMWCK and P63

Differential Diagnosis
▶ Poorly differentiated prostate carcinoma
▶ Secondary involvement by urothelial cells from the bladder or uretha
▶ Transitional cell metaplasia

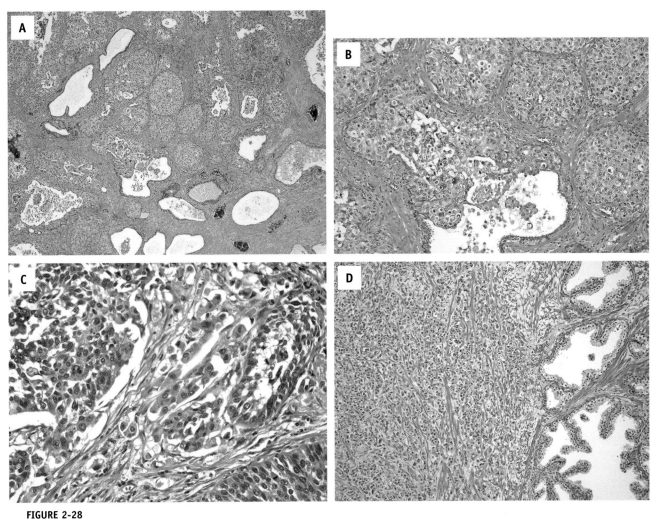

FIGURE 2-28

In urothelial carcinoma of the prostate, prostatic ducts and acini are filled with malignant urothelial cells (**A** and **B**). Stromal invasion can be recognized as small irregular nests, cords or single cells in a desmoplastic and inflamed stroma (**C**). Urothelial carcinoma can also directly invade into the prostatic tissue (**D**).

osteoblastic bony involvement seen in prostate carcinoma.

ANCILLARY STUDIES

IMMUNOHISTOCHEMISTRY

Prostate urothelial carcinoma cells are negative for PSA and PSAP but positive for CK7 and CK20. More than 50% of cases are also positive for p63, HMWCK, and thrombomodulin.

DIFFERENTIAL DIAGNOSIS

Prostatic urothelial carcinoma must be distinguished from a poorly differentiated prostate adenocarcinoma. Histologic clues for a urothelial carcinoma are the pre-

sence of rounded, solid nests of pleomorphic cells in an intensely inflamed background. Features that favor an invasive urothelial carcinoma include greater nuclear pleomorphism and mitotic activity, dense eosinophilic cytoplasm, and more prominent squamous differentiation. The diagnosis can be confirmed by immunohistochemistry. Most prostate urothelial carcinomas are diagnosed by TURP or, less frequently, by prostate needle biopsies. In cases without a known bladder primary, the possibility of secondary involvement from a primary bladder urothelial carcinoma should be excluded by random biopsies of the bladder. Urothelial metaplasia poses little diagnostic difficulty, because it is composed of bland metaplastic urothelial cells.

PROGNOSIS AND TREATMENT

The presence of prostatic stromal invasion significantly worsens the prognosis, with a 5-year survival rate of

45%, compared with 100% for patients with urothelial CIS after cystoprostatectomy. Radical prostatectomy or cystoprostatectomy is often recommended. Androgen deprivation therapy is ineffective.

NEUROENDOCRINE TUMORS

CLINICAL FEATURES

Neuroendocrine differentiation in prostate carcinoma has three forms: focal neuroendocrine differentiation, well-differentiated neuroendocrine carcinoma (carcinoid tumor), and small cell carcinoma. All prostate carcinomas show focal neuroendocrine differentiation, although most with only rare or sparse single neuroendocrine cells. Prostate carcinoid tumor that meets the diagnostic criteria for carcinoid tumors elsewhere is exceedingly rare. Small cell carcinoma of the prostate is also rare, accounting for 0.3% to 1% of all prostate carcinomas. About half of the cases exhibit pure small cell carcinoma, and in the other half small cell carcinoma is mixed with acinar prostate carcinoma. About one third of patients have a previous history of a hormonally treated acinar prostate carcinoma. Patients often present with advanced-stage disease with widespread metastasis. As the small cell carcinoma component predominates, serum PSA levels decline and may become undetectable. Although most small cell carcinomas of the prostate lack clinically evident hormone production, they account for the majority of prostatic tumors with clinical evidence of adrenocorticotropic hormone (ACTH) or antidiuretic hormone (ADH) production.

PATHOLOGIC FEATURES

GROSS FINDINGS

Small cell carcinoma usually extensively involves the prostate, with invasion into seminal vesicles, extraprostatic tissues, and bladder.

MICROSCOPIC FINDINGS

Prostate carcinoma with focal neuroendocrine differentiation may appear indistinguishable from ordinary prostate cancer, with the only evidence of neuroendocrine differentiation being evidenced immunohistochemically. Occasionally, sparse single cells or clusters of tumor cells have fine eosinophilic cytoplasmic granules (Fig. 2-29), which are immunoreactive for neuroendocrine markers. Prostate carcinoid shows classic architectural and cytologic features of carcinoid tumors. Small cell carcinoma histologically is identical to the lung counterpart (Fig. 2-30). In mixed small cell–acinar prostate carcinoma, the malignant glandular and small cell components may be intimately mixed.

SMALL CELL CARCINOMA—FACT SHEET

Definition
▶ Small cell neuroendocrine carcinoma that arises, either as an exclusive component or mixed with acinar prostate carcinoma, in the prostate gland

Incidence
▶ 0.3-1.0% of all prostate carcinoma

Gender, Race, and Age Distribution
▶ Mean age, 67 years (range, 28-89 years)

Clinical Features
▶ Patients present with advanced-stage disease with widespread metastases
▶ Low percentage have elevated serum PSA
▶ Previous history of prostate carcinoma treated with androgen ablation in one-third of cases
▶ Rarely endocrine paraneoplastic syndrome (Cushing's syndrome, ADH overproduction)

Prognosis and Treatment
▶ Median survival, 7-17 months
▶ Following biopsy treatment with chemotherapy

SMALL CELL CARCINOMA—PATHOLOGIC FEATURES

Gross Findings
▶ Extensively involves the prostate gland with invasion into seminal vesicles, extraprostatic tissue, and bladder

Microscopic Findings
▶ Identical to small cell carcinoma of other sites
▶ Malignant neuroendocrine cells can be intimately mixed with acinar prostate carcinoma

Immunohistochemical Features
▶ + neuroendocrine markers (synaptophysin, chromogranin A, CD57, NSA)
▶ − PSA, PSAP in small cell component

Differential Diagnosis
▶ Other small blue cell tumors (lymphoma, Ewing's sarcoma/PNET, neuroblastoma, rhabdomyosarcoma)
▶ Poorly differentiated prostate carcinoma
▶ Metastatic small cell carcinoma from other sites

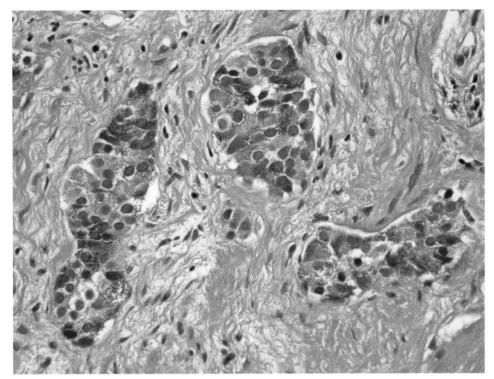

FIGURE 2-29
In prostate carcinoma with neuroendocrine differentiation, the cancer cells have bright red cytoplasmic granules.

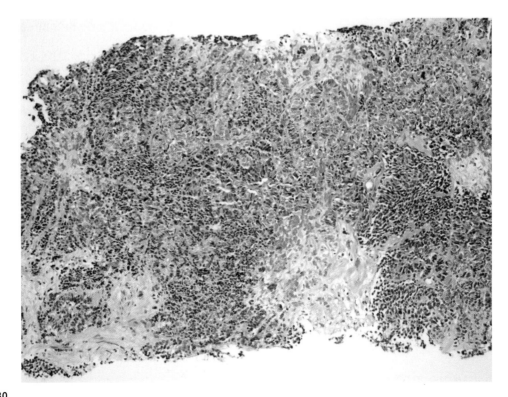

FIGURE 2-30
Small cell carcinoma of the prostate is composed of a relatively uniform population of cells with scant cytoplasm, hyperchromatic nuclei with fine chromatin, and inconspicuous nucleoli. Apoptotic bodies and mitotic figures are frequent.

ANCILLARY STUDIES

IMMUNOHISTOCHEMISTRY

Cancer cells with neuroendocrine differentiation are positive for neuroendocrine markers, including synaptophysin, chromogranin A, and CD57. Evidence of production of other hormones, including ACTH, calcitonin, serotonin, and ADH, can be demonstrated by immunostaining. PSA and PSAP are negative in the small cell component. TTF-1 expression does not discriminate between a small cell carcinoma arising in the prostate and a metastasis from the lung.

DIFFERENTIAL DIAGNOSIS

The differential diagnosis includes other small blue cell tumors (lymphoma, neuroblastoma, Ewing's sarcoma/primitive neuroectodermal tumor [PNET], and rhabdomyosarcoma), poorly differentiated prostate carcinoma, and small cell carcinoma from other sites. The patients' age, immunohistochemical markers, and clinical findings can resolve the diagnosis.

PROGNOSIS AND TREATMENT

The prognostic significance of neuroendocrine differentiation in an ordinary acinar prostate carcinoma is uncertain. Some studies have suggested a worse prognosis with neuroendocrine differentiation, but others have found no such correlation. The clinical outcome for small cell carcinoma, both pure and mixed forms, is extremely poor. The emergence of a small cell component during the course of acinar prostate carcinoma signals an aggressive terminal phase of the disease. The average median survival time after the diagnosis is 7 to 17 months. Treatment consists of chemotherapy, which may be followed by surgery.

BASALOID CARCINOMA

CLINICAL FEATURES

Basaloid carcinoma of the prostate is extremely rare and often manifests with urinary obstruction. Serum PSA is usually normal.

BASAL CELL CARCINOMA—FACT SHEET

Definition
▶ Malignant neoplasm exhibiting histologic and molecular features of prostate basal cells

Incidence
▶ Extremely rare

Gender, Race, and Age Distribution
▶ Mean age, 50 years (range, 28-72 years)

Clinical Features
▶ Symptoms of urinary obstruction
▶ Normal serum PSA

Prognosis and Treatment
▶ Uncertain
▶ May develop extraprostatic extension and distant metastasis

---

PATHOLOGIC FEATURES

GROSS FINDINGS

Basaloid carcinomas have no specific gross features.

MICROSCOPIC FINDINGS

Basaloid carcinoma grows in infiltrating nests, cords, trabeculae, and sheets (Fig. 2-31A) that may exhibit peripheral palisading (Fig. 2-31B). Some have extensive luminal formation with cribriform architecture

---

BASAL CELL CARCINOMA—PATHOLOGIC FEATURES

Gross Findings
▶ No specific gross findings

Microscopic Findings
▶ Infiltrating nests, cords, trabeculae, and sheets of tumor cells that may exhibit peripheral palisading
▶ May have extensive luminal formation with cribriform architecture—"adenoid cystic carcinoma" pattern
▶ Malignant features: infiltrative growth pattern, extraprostatic extension, perineural invasion, necrosis, and stromal desmoplasia

Immunohistochemical Features
▶ + HMWCK, p63
▶ − PSA, PSAP

Differential Diagnosis
▶ Basal cell hyperplasia
▶ Metastatic anal basaloid carcinoma

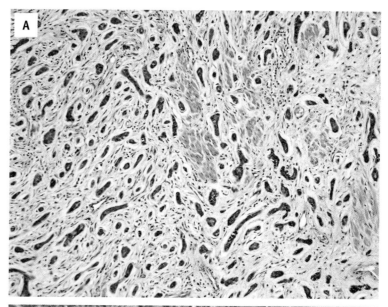

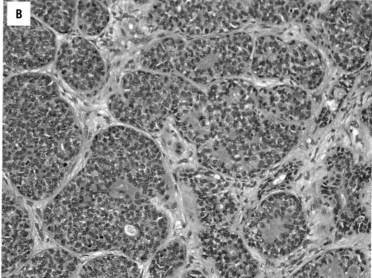

FIGURE 2-31

In basaloid carcinoma of the prostate, the cancer glands grow in small nests and cords, resembling basal cell hyperplasia except for prominent desmoplastic response and destruction of smooth muscle (**A**). Other patterns include solid sheets of cells with peripheral palisading and necrosis (**B**) and "adenoid cystic pattern" with cribriform architecture and perineural invasion (**C**).

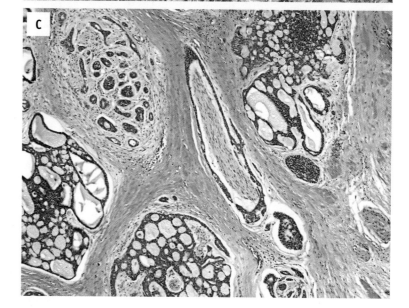

(Fig. 2-31C), a pattern that resembles adenoid cystic carcinoma of the salivary gland. The malignant features of basal cell carcinoma include infiltrative growth pattern, extraprostatic extension, perineural invasion, necrosis, and stromal desmoplasia.

ANCILLARY STUDIES

IMMUNOHISTOCHEMISTRY

Basal cells are positive for prostate basal cell markers, including HMWCK and p63, and are negative for PSA and PSAP.

DIFFERENTIAL DIAGNOSIS

Differentiation of basaloid carcinoma from basal cell hyperplasia depends on identifying unequivocal malignant features, which include tumor necrosis, perineural invasion, angiolymphatic invasion, and extraprostatic extension. Extension of anal basaloid carcinoma or adenoid cystic carcinoma of the Cowper's gland should also be excluded.

PROGNOSIS AND TREATMENT

The clinical outcome of basaloid carcinoma is uncertain due to insufficient data, although local extraprostatic extension and distant metastasis have been reported.

SQUAMOUS NEOPLASMS

CLINICAL FEATURES

Squamous cell carcinomas account for fewer than 0.6% of all the prostate cancers. An association between schistosomiasis and squamous cell carcinoma of the prostate and urinary tract has been documented. Adenosquamous carcinoma is even rarer and may arise in patients with prostate carcinoma after hormonal or radiation therapy. However, squamous and adenosquamous carcinoma may also involve the prostate without such predisposing factors. Clinically, patients present with symptoms and findings reminiscent of advanced-stage prostate carcinoma, including urinary obstruction, hematuria, bone pain, and markedly abnormal DRE findings. The PSA level is typically normal in squamous cell carcinoma but may be elevated in adenosquamous carcinoma.

SQUAMOUS NEOPLASMS—FACT SHEET

Definition
▶ Primary prostatic tumor with squamous cell differentiation

Incidence
▶ Squamous cell carcinoma <0.6% of all prostate cancers
▶ Adenosquamous carcinoma rarer

Gender, Race, and Age Distribution
▶ Mean age, 64 years (range, 52-79 years)

Clinical Features
▶ Urinary obstruction, hematuria, bone pain, and markedly abnormal DRE
▶ Normal PSA in squamous cell carcinoma
▶ PSA may be elevated in adenosquamous carcinoma
▶ Association between squamous cell carcinoma and schistosomiasis
▶ Adenosquamous cell carcinoma may arise after irradiation or hormonal ablation for prostate carcinoma

Prognosis and Treatment
▶ Extremely aggressive disease
▶ Resistant to androgen deprivation, irradiation, and chemotherapy
▶ Radical prostatectomy for organ-confined disease

PATHOLOGIC FEATURES

GROSS FINDINGS

The tumor is often bulky and replaces large portions of the prostate gland. Involvement of seminal vesicles, extraprostatic tissue, or bladder may be seen.

SQUAMOUS NEOPLASMS—PATHOLOGIC FEATURES

Gross Findings
▶ Bulky; replaces large portions of the prostate
▶ Involvement of seminal vesicles, extraprostatic tissue, and bladder may be seen

Microscopic Findings
▶ Squamous cell carcinoma is identical to squamous cell carcinoma of other anatomic sites
▶ Adenosquamous carcinoma harbors both malignant glandular and squamous components

Immunohistochemical Features
▶ Malignant squamous component is negative for PSA and PSAP but positive for HMWCK and p63
▶ Malignant glandular component expresses PSA and PSAP

Differential Diagnosis
▶ Squamous metaplasia
▶ Metastatic squamous cell carcinoma

MICROSCOPIC FINDINGS

Squamous cell carcinoma of the prostate is histologically identical to squamous cell carcinoma of other anatomic sites and does not contain any malignant glandular component. Adenosquamous carcinoma harbors both malignant glandular and squamous components that can be distinct or can exhibit direct transition from one pattern to another (Fig. 2-32).

ANCILLARY STUDIES

IMMUNOHISTOCHEMISTRY

The malignant squamous component is in most cases negative for PSA and PSAP but positive for HMWCK and p63. Malignant glandular components express PSA and PSAP.

DIFFERENTIAL DIAGNOSIS

Squamous cell carcinoma should be differentiated from squamous metaplasia that is secondary to hormonal or radiation therapy or adjacent to infarcts. Squamous metaplasia can have atypia adjacent to infarcts, and recognition of the associated infarct is critical to avoid a misdiagnosis of squamous cell carcinoma. Radiation change in the prostate also demonstrates squamous atypia, yet the atypia is degenerative in appearance and within preexisting benign glands, lacking the architectural disarray, destructive stromal reaction, and neoplastic nuclear atypia seen in squamous cell carcinoma. Secondary involvement of the prostate by a carcinoma with squamous differentiation from the bladder or other sites should be ruled out on clinical grounds.

PROGNOSIS AND TREATMENT

Prostatic squamous cell carcinoma and adenosquamous carcinoma are extremely aggressive diseases and are resistant to androgen deprivation, radiation therapy, and chemotherapy. In cases of organ-confined disease, radical prostatectomy or cystoprostatectomy with urethrectomy is recommended.

TUMORS OF SPECIALIZED PROSTATIC STROMA

CLINICAL FEATURES

The prostate gland contains a specialized stroma that is hormonally responsive and participates in the complex epithelial-stromal interaction during prostate organogenesis. Sarcoma and related proliferative lesions of the specialized stroma are rare and have been described by

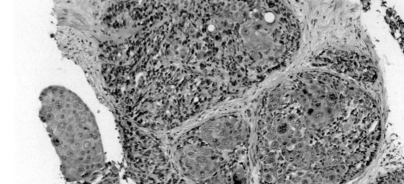

FIGURE 2-32

Adenosquamous carcinoma of the prostate, showing squamous differentiation within cancer glands.

various terms, including atypical stromal hyperplasia, phyllodes tumor, and prostatic cystic epithelial and stromal tumor. Currently, they are classified as either prostatic stromal proliferation of uncertain malignant potential (STUMP) or prostatic stromal sarcoma (PSS). Patients usually present with obstructive urinary symptoms, hematuria, and abnormal DRE findings. Rectal pain and a palpable rectal or abdominal mass are present in a minority of patients.

stroma without glandular elements (see Fig. 2-34E,F). The majority of STUMP specimens exhibit increased cellularity and cytologic atypia. Stromal overgrowth, necrosis, and increased mitosis are infrequently seen. Compared to STUMP, PSS has greater cellularity, cytologic atypia, mitotic figures, necrosis, and stromal overgrowth. The tumor cells show variable architectural patterns, ranging from diffuse sheets to short fascicles often with storiform arrangement.

PATHOLOGIC FEATURES

GROSS FINDINGS

Most tumors involves the posterior region of the prostate. Those that are larger protrude toward the vasa deferentia and seminal vesicles, compressing the adjacent bladder and rectum. Size can range from a few centimeters to 58 cm. The tumors are solid, cystic, or both solid and cystic (Fig. 2-33).

MICROSCOPIC FINDINGS

STUMP can have several patterns, including (1) hypercellular stroma with scattered atypical yet degenerative cells and normal glandular elements (Fig. 2-34A,B), (2) hypercellular stroma with normal glandular elements but without cytologically atypical cells (Fig. 2-34C), (3) stromal and glandular proliferation reminiscent of phyllodes tumors of the breast (Fig. 2-34D), and (4) extensive overgrowth of hypercellular

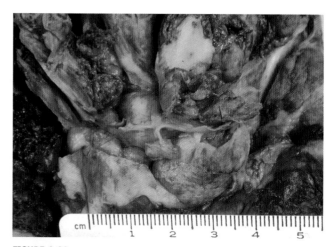

FIGURE 2-33

In prostatic stromal proliferation of uncertain malignant potential (STUMP), the prostate gland is diffusely involved by a solid, fibrous mass.

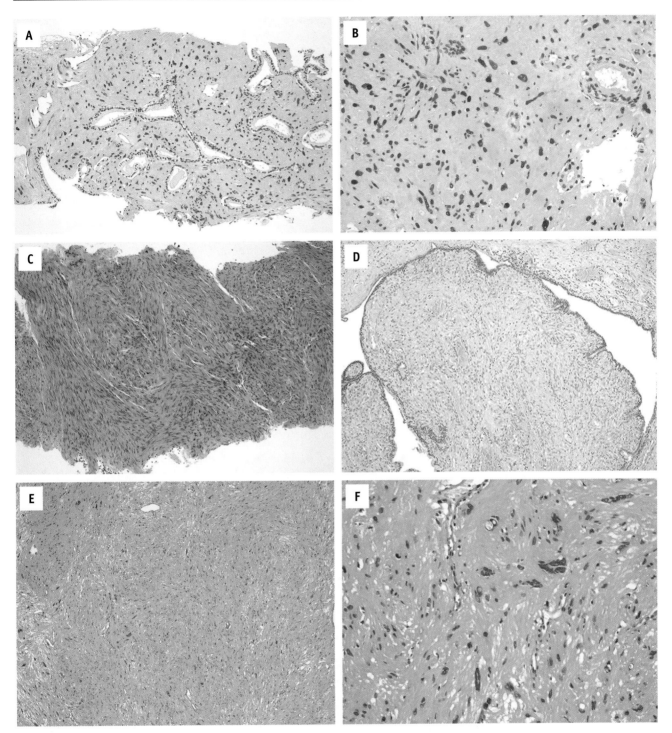

FIGURE 2-34

Histologic patterns of prostatic stromal proliferation of uncertain malignant potential (STUMP) include hypercellular stroma with scattered atypical cells and normal glandular elements (**A** and **B**), hypercellular stroma without cytologic atypia (**C**), stromal and glandular proliferation reminiscent of phyllodes tumors of the breast (**D**), and extensive overgrowth of hypercellular stroma without glandular elements (**E** and **F**).

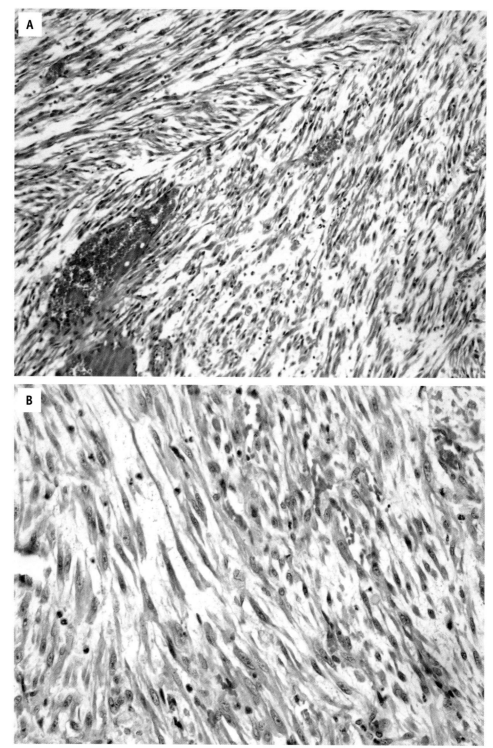

FIGURE 2-35
Inflammatory myofibroblastic tumor, showing spindle-cell proliferation in an edematous and inflamed myxoid stroma.

ANCILLARY STUDIES

IMMUNOHISTOCHEMISTRY

STUMP and PSS typically are positive for vimentin and CD34. They characteristically express progesterone receptors and uncommonly express estrogen receptors. Desmin, HHF-35, and SMA are often positive in STUMP but negative in PSS.

DIFFERENTIAL DIAGNOSIS

STUMP and PSS should be distinguished from other benign and malignant tumors with mesenchymal differentiation, including rhabdomyosarcoma, leiomyosarcoma, sarcomatoid carcinoma (carcinosarcoma), and inflammatory myofibroblastic tumor (IMT). Rhabdomyosarcomas contain cells with characteristic cytoplasmic cross-striations; they are positive for myogenic markers such as myogenin and MyoD and negative for CD34 and progesterone receptors. Desmin is not useful, because it can be positive in both prostatic stromal tumors and rhabdomyosarcoma. In leiomyosarcoma, the tumor cells are often arranged in short fascicles with cigar-shaped nuclei and paranuclear vacuoles. The cells are positive for actins HHF-35 and smooth muscle actin (SMA). IMT exhibits spindle-cell proliferation within an edematous and inflamed myxoid stroma (Fig. 2-35). Necrosis and mitoses may be present; however, frank nuclear atypia and atypical mitoses are not seen. Spindle cells are variably positive for SMA, and in a subset of cases are positive for anaplastic lymphoma kinase (ALK).

PROGNOSIS AND TREATMENT

STUMP is clinically heterogeneous. The majority does not behave in an aggressive fashion; however, occasionally it recurs rapidly after resection, and a minority progress to stromal sarcoma. If those lesions are extensive in biopsies or are associated with a palpable mass, definitive therapy may be considered. The biologic behavior of PSS is unclear, but some patients have developed distant metastasis. It is treated with therapies of curative intent.

OTHER PROSTATIC MESENCHYMAL TUMORS

Although rare, a wide variety of other mesenchymal tumors have been reported to arise in the prostate.

LEIOMYOMA—FACT SHEET

Definition
▶ Benign mesenchymal tumor with smooth muscle differentiation
▶ Lesion sharply circumscribed and ≥1 cm

Incidence
▶ Unknown
▶ Most common benign mesenchymal tumor of the prostate

Gender, Race, and Age Distribution
▶ Mean age at diagnosis: 60 years

Clinical Features
▶ Prostatism, urinary tract infection, or acute urinary retention

Prognosis and Treatment
▶ Benign
▶ Local recurrence rare

Benign mesenchymal tumors include leiomyoma, solitary fibrous tumor, hemangioma, chondroma, granular cell tumor, and neurofibroma, with leiomyoma being the most commonly encountered benign mesenchymal tumor. The most common malignant mesenchymal tumors are rhabdomyosarcoma (Figs. 2-36 and 2-37) in children and leiomyosarcoma (Fig. 2-38) in adults. Others include angiosarcoma, malignant peripheral nerve sheath tumor, malignant fibrous histiocytoma, and synovial sarcoma.

LEIOMYOMA—PATHOLOGIC FEATURES

Gross Findings
▶ Well-circumscribed with whorled cut surface

Microscopic Findings
▶ Similar to leiomyomas elsewhere
▶ Leiomyoma with degenerative nuclear atypia termed "atypical leiomyoma"
▶ Necrosis absent, rare to no mitoses

Immunohistochemical Features
▶ + desmin and actin

Differential Diagnosis
▶ Leiomyomatous stromal nodule (<1 cm)
▶ Leiomyosarcoma

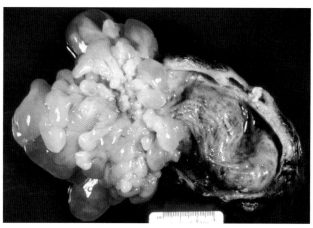

FIGURE 2-36

In rhabdomyosarcoma of the prostate, the prostate gland is replaced by clusters of edematous and myxoid polypoid masses (botryoides pattern). The urinary bladder *(right)* shows mucosal trabeculation due to outflow obstruction.

HEMATOLYMPHOID, SECONDARY, AND MISCELLANEOUS TUMORS

HEMATOLYMPHOID TUMORS

Rarely, the prostate gland may be involved by hematolymphoid malignancy, including leukemia, non-Hodgkin's lymphoma (Fig. 2-39), Hodgkin's disease, and multiple myeloma. The initial clinical presentation of leukemia or lymphoma is attributed to the prostatic involvement in only a few cases. The symptoms mimic prostatitis, BPH, or prostate carcinoma.

SECONDARY TUMORS INVOLVING THE PROSTATE

Malignant tumors of other anatomic sites can involve the prostate by direct extension or by metastasis via lymphovascular routes. In an autopsy study, approximately 44% of the secondary tumors in the prostate represented direct invasion by cancer from adjacent organs, most commonly bladder, urethra, or colon (Fig. 2-40). In 23% of patients with bladder urothelial carcinoma, the prostate is involved, by either direct extension, multifocal disease, or metastases. Secondary spread to the prostate is most often seen with hematolymphoid malignancies. Solid tumors rarely metastasize to the prostate, but metastases from the lung, skin (melanoma), gastrointestinal tract, kidney, and testis have been reported.

RHABDOMYOSARCOMA—FACT SHEET

Definition
- ► Sarcoma with skeletal muscle differentiation

Incidence
- ► Rare (<0.1% of primary prostate cancer)

Gender, Race, and Age Distribution
- ► Most common malignant prostate neoplasm in children and adolescents
- ► Most cases in young boys
- ► Median age at diagnosis: 3.5-6.5 years

Clinical Features
- ► Symptoms related to urinary obstruction
- ► Abnormal DRE
- ► Normal serum PSA

Radiologic Features
- ► Isoechoic by rectal ultrasound

Prognosis and Treatment
- ► Multimodal therapy improves survival of pediatric patients to 83% at 5 years
- ► Disease in adults is uniformly lethal
- ► Prognosis related to histologic subtypes and TNM stage
- ► Alveolar rhabdomyosarcoma—poor prognosis and necessitates aggressive chemotherapy

---

RHABDOMYOSARCOMA—PATHOLOGIC FEATURES

Gross Findings
- ► Bulky tumor often obliterating regional anatomy
- ► Solid with gelatinous cut surface

Microscopic Findings
- ► Embryonal subtype most common, with diffuse sheets or nests of small blue cells, "rhabdomyoblasts," or "strap" cells with cross-striation
- ► Alveolar subtype less common, with delicate anastomosing fibrous septa and tumor cells floating in the alveolar space

Immunohistochemical Features
- ► + desmin, MSA, myoglobin, MyoD, myogenin
- ► − cytokeratins, lymphoid markers

Genetic testing
- ► Two-thirds of alveolar rhabdomyosarcomas are positive for t(2;13) and t(1;13) translocation by cytogenetics or reverse transcriptase–polymerase chain reaction (RT-PCR)

Differential Diagnosis
- ► Other small round cell tumors, including leukemia, lymphoma, neuroblastoma, Ewing's sarcoma/PNET

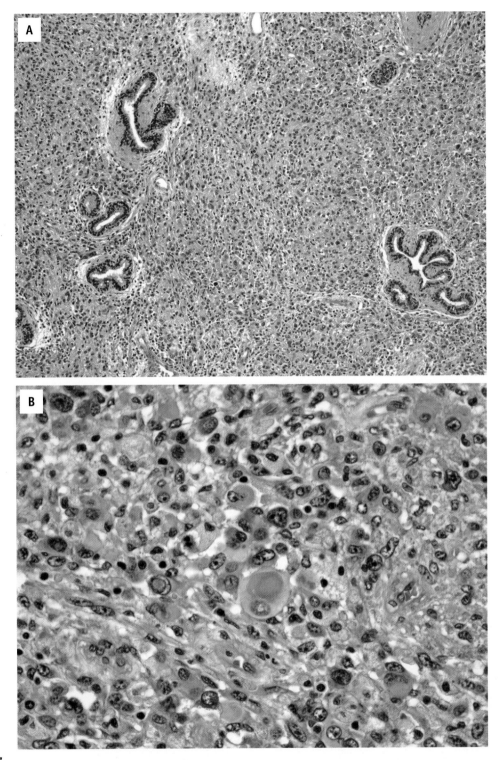

FIGURE 2-37

In rhabdomyosarcoma of the prostate, the prostate gland is diffusely infiltrated by small round tumor cells (**A**). Some tumor cells show characteristic rhabdomyoblastic differentiation (**B**).

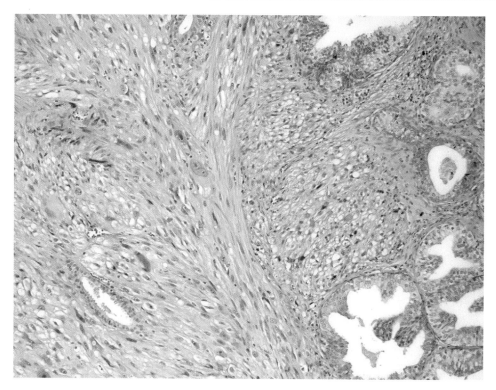

FIGURE 2-38

In leiomyosarcoma of the prostate, the prostate gland is infiltrated by fascicles of spindle cells with nuclear pleomorphism and mitoses.

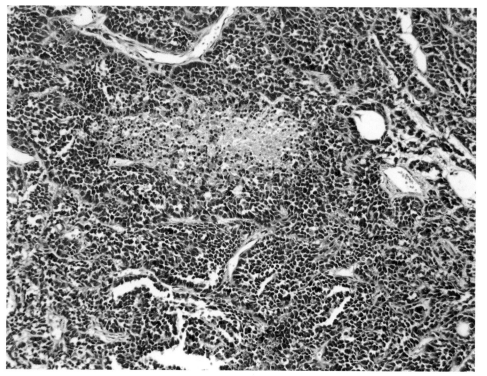

FIGURE 2-39

In lymphoma involving the prostate, the normal prostatic architecture is largely effaced by a monomorphic lymphocytic infiltrate.

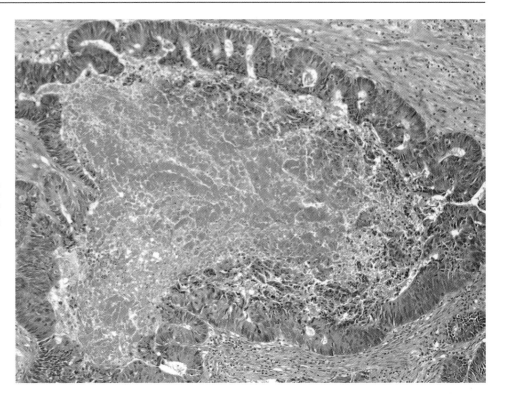

FIGURE 2-40
In colorectal adenocarcinoma metastasizing to the prostate, cancer glands are identical to those of primary colorectal adenocarcinoma with central necrosis.

MISCELLANEOUS TUMORS

Cystadenoma (multilocular cyst or giant multilocular prostatic cystadenoma) is a rare benign prostatic epithelial tumor. Other rare tumors that have reported to involve the prostate include Wilms' tumor, malignant

---

LEIOMYOSARCOMA—FACT SHEET

Definition
▶ Primary sarcoma demonstrating smooth muscle differentiation

Incidence
▶ Rare (~100 reported cases)
▶ Most common sarcoma arising in the adult prostate (30% of prostatic sarcoma)

Gender, Race, and Age Distribution
▶ Men age 57 years (range, 19-78 years)

Clinical Features
▶ Symptoms of urinary obstruction, hematuria, pelvic pain
▶ Normal serum PSA

Prognosis and Treatment
▶ Multimodality therapy with surgery, irradiation, and chemotherapy
▶ Multiple recurrences after treatment
▶ 50% develop distant metastases to lung and other organs
▶ Average survival 2-4 years

LEIOMYOSARCOMA—PATHOLOGIC FEATURES

Gross Findings
▶ Fleshy or firm
▶ May show hemorrhage, necrosis, or cystic degeneration

Microscopic Findings
▶ Smooth muscle tumor with hypercellularity, mitoses, and nuclear atypia

Immunohistochemical Features
▶ Majority + SMA and desmin
▶ Occasionally + cytokeratins

Differential Diagnosis
▶ Leiomyoma
▶ STUMP and PSS
▶ Inflammatory myofibroblastic tumor

---

rhabdoid tumor, germ cell tumor, clear cell adenocarcinoma, melanoma, and paraganglioma.

DISEASES OF THE SEMINAL VESICLE

Primary adenocarcinoma of the seminal vesicle is rare. The mean age is 62 years (range, 24 to 90 years). Patients usually present with obstructive uropathy

CYSTADENOMA—FACT SHEET

Definition
▶ Benign epithelial tumor of the prostate

Incidence and Location
▶ Rare, with <20 cases reported
▶ Intraprostatic, or attached to prostate by a pedicle, or pelvic without attachment to the prostate

Gender, Race, and Age Distribution
▶ Mean age, 56 years

Clinical Features
▶ Obstructive urinary symptoms and hematuria
▶ Palpable mass +/−

Prognosis and Treatment
▶ Complete surgical removal
▶ Benign
▶ May recur if incompletely excised

CYSTADENOMA—PATHOLOGIC FEATURES

Gross Findings
▶ Bosselated smooth external surface
▶ Multilocular cystic cut surface

Microscopic Findings
▶ Cysts lined with two-cell layered benign prostatic epithelium
▶ Hypocellular stroma with focal hyalinization and chronic inflammation
▶ May have prominent epithelial proliferation resembling florid BPH

Differential Diagnosis
▶ Benign prostatic cyst
▶ STUMP
▶ Multilocular peritoneal inclusion cyst, müllerian duct cyst, and seminal vesicle cyst
▶ BPH

caused by a nontender perirectal mass or, less commonly, with hematuria or hematospermia. Serum carcinoembryonic antigen (CEA) may be elevated. Grossly, tumors are usually large (3 to 5.0 cm) and often invade the bladder, ureter, or rectum. Microscopically, tumors have nonspecific histologic features with papillary, trabecular, and glandular patterns and varying degrees of differentiation. Rarely, tumors are undifferentiated or produce abundant extracellular mucin (colloid carcinoma). The diagnosis requires exclusion of secondary involvement by carcinomas of the prostate, bladder, or rectum, based on clinical information and judicial use of immunohistochemistry. Normal seminal vesicles and seminal vesicle adenocarcinomas are positive for CEA and CK7 and negative for PSA, PSAP, and CK20. The prognosis of primary seminal vesicle adenocarcinoma is poor. Most patients present with metastases, and in 95% of patients the survival time is less than 3 years

Cystadenoma is a rare benign tumor of the seminal vesicles. Patients range in age from 37 to 66 years and may be asymptomatic or symptomatic with bladder outlet obstruction. Ultrasound may reveal a complex, solid-cystic pelvic mass. Microscopically, the tumor is well circumscribed and contains glandular spaces of variable size with branching contours and cysts surrounded by a spindle-cell stroma. The glands contain pale intraluminal secretions and are lined by one or two layers of cuboidal to columnar cells. No significant cytologic atypia, mitotic activity, or necrosis is seen. The tumor has a benign outcome but may recur after incomplete resection.

Mixed epithelial-stromal tumors are composed of both neoplastic epithelial and stromal elements. They range in biologic behavior from benign lesions, such as adenofibroma and adenomyoma, to low-grade and high-grade mixed epithelial-stromal tumors, with the grade determined based on stromal cellularity, atypia, mitoses, and necrosis.

A variety of cysts may be seen in or adjacent to the seminal vesicles. They may be congenital and often are associated with ipsilateral abnormalities of the urinary tract, including renal, ureteral, and hemitrigone agenesis. They may also be acquired as a result of obstruction or inflammation. Both types of seminal vesicle cysts are usually unilateral and unilocular and histologically resemble dilated seminal vesicles lined with attenuated or papillary epithelium.

Localized amyloidosis of the seminal vesicles (senile amyloidosis) is usually asymptomatic and is observed in more than 20% of men older than 75 years of age. It is usually bilateral and consists of nodular subepithelial amyloid deposits (Fig. 2-41). In contrast, systemic amyloidosis, which rarely involves the seminal vesicles, is characterized by amyloid deposition in vascular walls and smooth muscle.

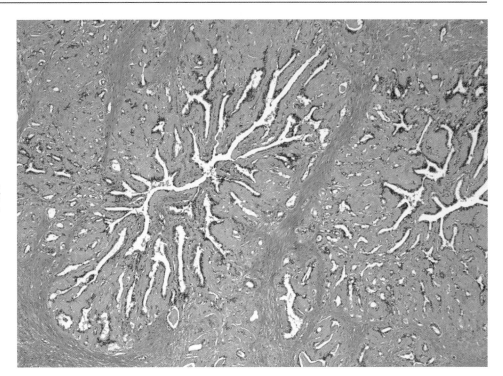

FIGURE 2-41

In amyloidosis of the seminal vesicle, pink, amorphous amyloid is diffusely deposited in the subepithelial areas. The lining epithelium is atrophic

SUGGESTED READINGS

Eble JN, Sauter G, Epstein JI, Sesterhenn IA: Pathology and Genetics: Tumours of the Urinary System and Male Genital Organs. IARC Press: Lyon, France, IARC Press, 2004.

Epstein JI, Yang XJ: Prostate Biopsy Interpretation, 3rd ed. Philadelphia, Williams & Wilkins, 2002.

Humphrey PA: Prostate Pathology. Chicago, AJCP Press, 2003.

Young RH, Srigley JR, Amin MB, et al: Tumors of the Prostate Gland, Seminal Vesicle, Male Urethra, and Penis, 3rd ed. Washington, DC, AFIP, 2000.

Prostatic Intraepithelial Neoplasia

Bishara T, Ramnani DM, Epstein JI (2004). High-grade prostatic intraepithelial neoplasia on needle biopsy: Risk of cancer on repeat biopsy related to number of involved cores and morphologic pattern. Am J Surg Pathol 2004;28:629–633.

Bostwick DG, Amin MB, Dundore P, et al: Architectural patterns of high-grade prostatic intraepithelial neoplasia. Hum Pathol 1993;24:298–310.

Bostwick DG, Foster CS: Predictive factors in prostate cancer: Current concepts from the 1999 College of American Pathologists Conference on Solid Tumor Prognostic Factors and the 1999 World Health Organization Second International Consultation on Prostate Cancer. Semin Urol Oncol 1999;17:222–272.

Bostwick DG, Qian J: High-grade prostatic intraepithelial neoplasia. Mod Pathol 2004;17:360–379.

Cohen RJ, McNeal JE, Baillie T: Patterns of differentiation and proliferation in intraductal carcinoma of the prostate: significance for cancer progression. Prostate 2000;43:11–19.

Davidson D, Bostwick DG, Qian J, et al: Prostatic intraepithelial neoplasia is a risk factor for adenocarcinoma: Predictive accuracy in needle biopsies. J Urol 1995;154:1295–1299.

Kronz JD, Allan CH, Shaikh AA, Epstein JI: Predicting cancer following a diagnosis of high-grade prostatic intraepithelial neoplasia on needle biopsy: Data on men with more than one follow-up biopsy. Am J Surg Pathol 2001;25:1079–1085.

Kronz JD, Shaikh AA, Epstein JI: High-grade prostatic intraepithelial neoplasia with adjacent small atypical glands on prostate biopsy. Hum Pathol 2001;32:389–395.

Schlesinger C, Bostwick DG, Iczkowski KA: High-grade prostatic intraepithelial neoplasia and atypical small acinar proliferation: predictive value for cancer in current practice. Am J Surg Pathol 2005;29:1201–1207.

Prostate Carcinoma

Deutsch E, Maggiorella L, Eschwege P, et al: Environmental, genetic, and molecular features of prostate cancer. Lancet Oncol 2004;5:303–313.

Epstein JI: PSA and PAP as immunohistochemical markers in prostate cancer. Urol Clin North Am 1993;20:757–770.

Epstein JI: Diagnosis and reporting of limited adenocarcinoma of the prostate on needle biopsy. Mod Pathol 2004;17:307–315.

Epstein JI, Allsbrook WC, Amin MB, et al: The 2005 International Society of Urological Pathology (ISUP) consensus conference on Gleason grading of prostate carcinoma. Am J Surg Pathol 2005;29:1228–1242.

Gaudin PB: Histopathologic effects of radiatin and hormonal therapies on benign and malignant prostate tissue. J Urol Pathol 1998;8:55–67.

Goldstein NS: Immunophenotypic characterization of 225 prostate adenocarcinomas with intermediate or high Gleason scores. Am J Clin Pathol 2002;117:471–477.

Gretzer MB, Partin AW: PSA markers in prostate cancer detection. Urol Clin North Am 2003;30:677–686.

Grignon DJ: Unusual subtypes of prostate cancer. Mod Pathol 2004;17:316–327.

Humphrey PA: Gleason grading and prognostic factors in carcinoma of the prostate. Mod Pathol 2004;17:292–306.

Jiang Z, Woda BA: Diagnostic utility of alpha-methylacyl CoA racemase (P504S) on prostate needle biopsy. Adv Anat Pathol 2004;11:316–321.

Shah RB, Zhou M, LeBlanc M, et al: Comparison of the basal cell-specific markers, 34betaE12 and p63, in the diagnosis of prostate cancer. Am J Surg Pathol 2002;26:1161–1168.

Srigley JR: Benign mimickers of prostatic adenocarcinoma. Mod Pathol 2004;17:328–348.

Thorson P, Humphrey PA: Minimal adenocarcinoma in prostate needle biopsy tissue. Am J Clin Pathol 2000;114:896–909.

Ductal Adenocarcinoma

Bostwick DG, Kindrachuk RW, Rouse RC: Prostatic adenocarcinoma with endometrioid features: Clinical, pathologic, and ultrastructural findings. Am J Surg Pathol 1985;9:595–609.

Brinker DA, Potter SR, Epstein JI: Ductal adenocarcinoma of the prostate diagnosed on needle biopsy: Correlation with clinical and radical prostatectomy findings and progression. Am J Surg Pathol 1999;23:1471–1479.

Christensen WN, Steinberg G, Walsh PC, Epstein JI: Prostatic duct adenocarcinoma: Findings at radical prostatectomy. Cancer 1991;67:2118–2124.

Epstein JI, Woodruff JM: Adenocarcinoma of the prostate with endometrioid features: A light microscopic and immunohistochemical study of ten cases. Cancer 1986;57:111–119.

Urothelial Carcinoma

Cheville JC: Urothelial carcinoma of the prostate: An immunohistochemical comparison with high grade prostatic adenocarcinoma and review of the literature. J Urol Pathol 1998;9:141–154.

Cheville JC, Dundore PA, Bostwick DG, et al: Transitional cell carcinoma of the prostate: Clinicopathologic study of 50 cases. Cancer 1998;82:703–707.

Mahadevia PS, Koss LG, Tar IJ: Prostatic involvement in bladder cancer: Prostate mapping in 20 cysto-prostatectomy specimens. Cancer 1986;58:2096–2102.

Oliai BR, Kahane H, Epstein JI: Clinicopathologic analysis of urothelial carcinomas diagnosed on prostate needle biopsy. Am J Surg Pathol 2001;25:794–801.

Neuroendocrine Tumors

Abrahamsson PA: Neuroendocrine differentiation in prostatic carcinoma. Prostate 1999;39:135–148.

Helpap B, Kollermann J, Oehler U: Neuroendocrine differentiation in prostatic carcinomas: Histogenesis, biology, clinical relevance, and future therapeutical perspectives. Urol Int 1999;62:133–1338.

Mackey JR, Au HJ, Hugh J, Venner P: Genitourinary small cell carcinoma: Determination of clinical and therapeutic factors associated with survival. J Urol 1998;159:1624–1629.

Ro JY, Tetu B, Ayala AG, Ordonez NG: Small cell carcinoma of the prostate. II. Immunohistochemical and electron microscopic studies of 18 cases. Cancer 1987;59:977–982.

Tetu B, Ro JY, Ayala AG, et al: Small cell carcinoma of the prostate. Part I. A clinicopathologic study of 20 cases. Cancer 1987;59:1803–1809.

Basaloid Carcinoma

Epstein JI, Armas OA: Atypical basal cell hyperplasia of the prostate. Am J Surg Pathol 1992;16:1205–1214.

Iczkowski KA, Ferguson KL, Grier DD, et al: Adenoid cystic/basal cell carcinoma of the prostate: Clinicopathologic findings in 19 cases. Am J Surg Pathol 2003;27:1523–1529.

McKenney JK, Amin MB, Srigley JR, et al: Basal cell proliferations of the prostate other than usual basal cell hyperplasia: A clinicopathologic study of 23 cases, including four carcinomas, with a proposed classification. Am J Surg Pathol 2004;28:1289–1298.

Rioux-Leclercq NC, Epstein JI: Unusual morphologic patterns of basal cell hyperplasia of the prostate. Am J Surg Pathol 2002;26:237–243.

Yang XJ, McEntee M, Epstein JI: Distinction of basaloid carcinoma of the prostate from benign basal cell lesions by using immunohistochemistry for bcl-2 and Ki-67. Hum Pathol 1998;29:1447–1450.

Squamous Neoplasms

Al Adani MS: Schistosomiasis-metaplasia and squamous cell carcinoma of the prostate: Histogenesis of squamous cancer cell determined by localization of specific markers. Neoplasm 1985;32:613–617.

Kanthan R, Torkian B: Squamous cell carcinoma of the prostate: A report of 6 cases. Urol Int 2004;72:28–31.

Orhan D, Sak SD, Yaman O, et al: Adenosquamous carcinoma of the prostate. Br J Urol 1996;78:646–647.

Parwani AV, Kronz JD, Genega EM, et al: Prostate carcinoma with squamous differentiation: An analysis of 33 cases. Am J Surg Pathol 2004;28:651–657.

Tumors of the Specialized Prostatic Stroma

Bostwick DG, Hossain D, Qian J, et al: Phyllodes tumor of the prostate: Long-term followup study of 23 cases. J Urol 2004;172:894–899.

Cohen MB: Atypical prostatic stromal lesions. Adv Anat Pathol 1998;5:359–366.

Gaudin PB, Rosai J, Epstein JI: Histopathologic effects of radiation and hormonal therapies on benign and malignant prostate tissue. J Urol Pathol 1998;8:55–67.

Shabaik A: Nonepithelial tumors and tumor-like lesions of the prostate gland. Crit Rev Clin Lab Sci 2003;40:429–472.

Other Prostatic Mesenchymal Tumors

Cheville JC, Dundore A, Nascimento AG, et al: Leiomyosarcoma of the prostate: Report of 23 cases. Cancer 1995;76:1422–1427.

Michaels MM, Brown HE, Favino CJ: Leiomyoma of prostate. Urology 1974;3:617–620.

Pins MR, Campbell SC, Laskin WB, et al: Solitary fibrous tumor of the prostate: A report of 2 cases and review of the literature. Arch Pathol Lab Med 2001;125:274–277.

Sexton WJ, Lance RE, Reyes AO, et al: Adult prostate sarcoma: The M.D. Anderson Cancer Center Experience. J Urol 2001;166:521–525.

Hematolymphoid, Secondary, and Miscellaneous Tumors

Bostwick DG, Iczkowski KA, Amin MB, et al: Malignant lymphoma involving the prostate: Report of 62 cases. Cancer 1998;83:732–738.

Kirsch AJ, Newhouse J, Hibshoosh H, et al: Giant multilocular cystadenoma of the prostate. Urology 1996;8:303–305.

Zein TA, Huben R, Lane W, et al: Secondary tumors of the prostate. J Urol 1985;133:615–616.

Diseases of the Seminal Vesicle

Baschinsky DY, Niemann TH, Maximo CB, Bahnson RR: Seminal vesicle cystadenoma: A case report and literature review. Urology 1998;51:840–845.

Maroun L, Jakobsen H, Kromann-Andersen B, Horn T: Amyloidosis of the seminal vesicle: A case report and review of the literature. Scand J Urol Nephrol 2003;37:519–521.

Mazur MT, Myers JL, Maddox WA: Cystic epithelial-stromal tumor of the seminal vesicle. Am J Surg Pathol 1987;11:210–217.

Ormsby AH, Haskell R, Ruthven SE, Mylne GE: Bilateral primary seminal vesicle carcinoma. Pathology 1996;28:196–200.

Patel B, Gujral S, Jefferson K, et al: Seminal vesicle cysts and associated anomalies. BJU Int 2002;90:265–271.

3

Non-Neoplastic Diseases of the Urinary Bladder

Ming Zhou • Cristina Magi-Galluzzi • Jonathan I. Epstein

ANATOMY AND HISTOLOGY

Located in the pelvis minor, the urinary bladder is shaped like an inverted pyramid. The superior surface, the dome, is covered by peritoneum. The most antero-superior point, the apex, is where the median umbilical ligament and the urachus insert. The posterior surface forms the base of the bladder. Between it and the rectum lie the lower vasa deferentia and seminal vesicles in males and the uterine cervix and upper vagina in females. The trigone is a triangular region located at the base of the bladder, between the ureteral orifices supero-laterally and the opening of the urethra inferiorly. Developmentally, the trigone is derived from the distal ureters and incorporated into the bladder wall. The bladder neck is the most distal portion of the bladder that opens into the urethra; it is formed by the convergence of the posterior and inferolateral walls. The musculature of the bladder neck is formed by the trigonal, detrusor, and urethral musculature. In males, the bladder neck merges with the prostate gland, and occasionally there may be prostatic tissue in this area.

The wall of the urinary bladder consists of four layers: urothelium, lamina propria, muscularis propria, and adventitia or serosa (Fig. 3-1). The urothelium, a specialized epithelium, varies in thickness from two to seven cells, depending on the extent of distention of the bladder. The most superficial or luminal layer consists of large, sometimes binucleated cells with abundant eosinophilic cytoplasm, termed umbrella cells. Significant nuclear atypia may be present in these cells. The urothelial cells of other layers are oriented perpendicular to the basement membrane. They have pale, sometimes clear, cytoplasm and small, uniform nuclei, frequently with grooves (Fig. 3-2). These cells are approximately twice the size of stromal lymphocytes.

Beneath the basement membrane is the lamina propria, a zone of loose connective tissue with delicate angiolymphatic vessels. In the midportion of the lamina propria are medium-sized arteries and veins (Fig. 3-1). Delicate bundles of smooth muscle fibers, referred to as muscularis mucosae, are often found associated with these vessels (Fig. 3-3). The muscularis mucosae of the bladder is variable, ranging from a sparse and incomplete array of smooth muscle fibers, to essentially a continuous layer. Beneath this layer is the muscularis

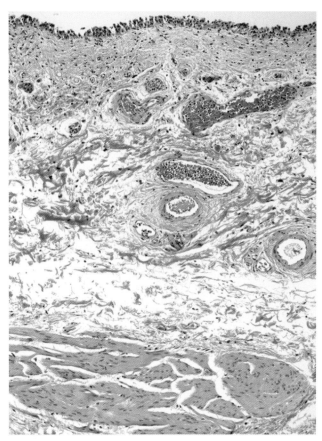

FIGURE 3-1
Normal bladder is composed of urothelium, lamina propria with medium-sized vessels, and thick muscle bundles of muscularis propria.

propria, or detrusor muscle, composed of large bundles of muscle fibers separated by connective tissue containing vessels, lymphatics, and nerves. Infrequently, small nests of paraganglia are present, usually associated with nerves and vessels. The outermost layer of the bladder wall is an adventitia of fibroadipose tissue. It is impossible to recognize the adventitia on biopsy, because adipose tissue may be seen at all levels of the bladder, including the lamina propria and muscularis propria.

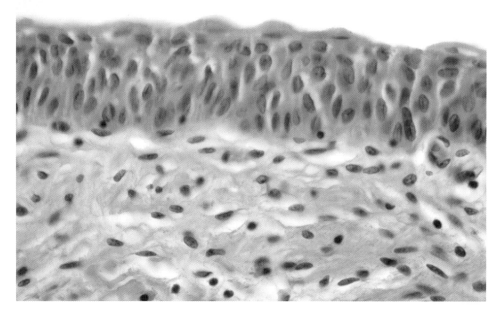

FIGURE 3-2
Urothelial cells are uniform with nuclear grooves. They are oriented perpendicular to the basement membrane.

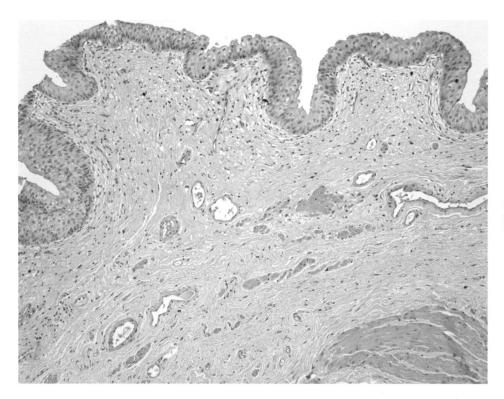

FIGURE 3-3
Delicate bundles of muscularis mucosae are associated with medium-sized vessels in the midportion of the lamina propria.

REACTIVE PROLIFERATIVE CHANGES OF THE UROTHELIUM

CLINICAL FEATURES

The urothelium may exhibit a host of morphologic variations, including von Brunn's nests, cystitis cystica, and cystitis glandularis. They are extremely common findings, present in 85% to 95%, 60%, and 71% of bladders, respectively, in several autopsy studies. They represent a continuum of reactive proliferative changes seen along the entire urinary tract, and it is common to see all three in the same specimen. They are considered as variants of normal urothelial histology. They may also occur as a result of local inflammation. There have been several reports of association between pelvic lipomatosis and the proliferative changes of the urothelium. There is no association between these proliferative changes and urothelial carcinoma.

PATHOLOGIC FEATURES

GROSS FINDINGS

Most von Brunn's nests are less than 5 mm in diameter and not visible grossly. At cystoscopy, large foci of cystitis cystica may appear as thin-walled, domed mucosal cysts or blebs and may contain clear yellow fluid. Florid cystitis glandularis can occasionally form irregular or nodular mucosal elevations. Rarely, it forms a large polypoid mass simulating a bladder cancer.

MICROSCOPIC FINDINGS

von Brunn's nests are solid nests of urothelial cells that lie beneath the urothelium and may be connected to the surface urothelium. These nests usually have a smooth, round contour and orderly spatial arrangement (Fig. 3-4). The cells in the von Brunn's nests lack cytologic atypia, although they may have slightly larger nuclei when compared with the overlying urothelial cells. Cystitis cystica consists of von Brunn's nests that

have become cystically dilated and acquired a luminal space due to degeneration of central cells (Fig. 3-5). The cysts are filled with eosinophilic fluid and may contain some inflammatory cells. Cystitis glandularis resembles cystitis cystica except that the cystic spaces are lined with cuboidal or columnar cells that secret mucin (Fig. 3-6). If the columnar epithelium acquires intestinal-type goblet cells, this variant is termed cystitis glandularis with intestinal or colonic metaplasia (Fig. 3-7), as opposed to the nonmucinous, typical type of cystitis glandularis. Rarely, von Brunn's nests, cystitis cystica, and cystitis glandularis are so prominent that they form grossly visible mass lesions (Fig. 3-8).

ANCILLARY STUDIES

IMMUNOHISTOCHEMISTRY

In the normal urothelium, cytokeratin 20 (CK20) immunoreactivity is detected in only the superficial umbrella cells and, occasionally, intermediate cells. CD44 stains only the basal cells. Nuclear p53 immunoreactivity varies from negative to weak and patchy in the basal layer. The immunostaining patterns of von Brunn's nests, cystitis cystica, and cystitis glandularis largely reflect the fact that the cells of these structures

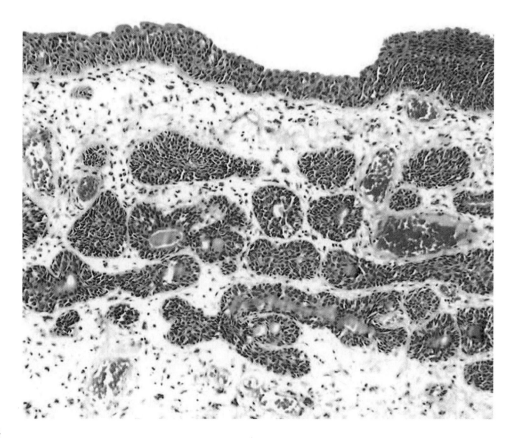

FIGURE 3-4
Solid von Brunn's nests of urothelial cells lie beneath the urothelium and have a smooth, round contour and orderly spatial arrangement. The nests with central cystic changes are cystitis cystica.

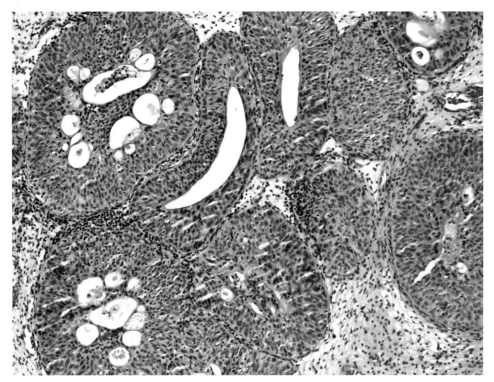

FIGURE 3-5
In cystitis cystica, nests of urothelial cells become cystically dilated and acquire a central luminal space.

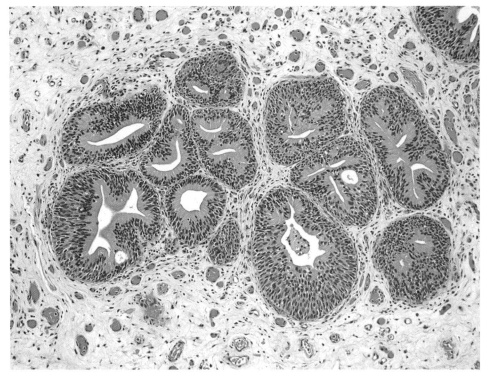

FIGURE 3-6
In cystitis glandularis, the cystic space is lined with columnar cells. Goblet cells are not present.

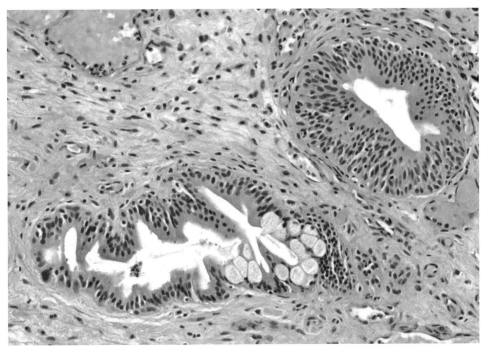

FIGURE 3-7
In cystitis glandularis with intestinal metaplasia, the lining cells are columnar with interspersed mucin-producing goblet cells.

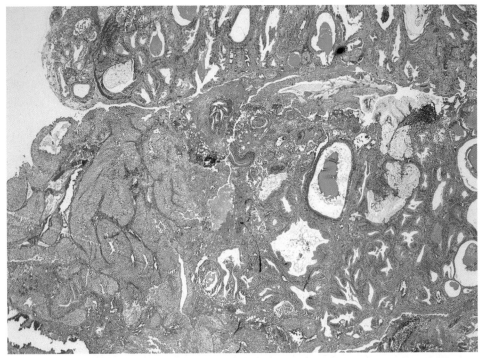

FIGURE 3-8
In florid proliferative cystitis, the lamina propria is expanded by von Brunn's nests, cystitis cystica, and cystitis glandularis.

are basal and intermediate urothelial cells, although the staining patterns are variable. For example, some von Brunn's nests are strongly positive for CK20, whereas others are completely negative.

DIFFERENTIAL DIAGNOSIS

Florid von Brunn's nests can be differentiated from the nested variant of urothelial carcinoma by its lobular or linear array of the nests, flat noninfiltrative base, and lack of cytologic atypia. Von Brunn's nests in the bladder are also in general larger, with a smooth, rounded contour and regular spacing. Cyst formation is often more pronounced, and apical glandular differentiation and eosinophilic secretions are also more common than in urothelial carcinoma. If von Brunn's nests are numerous and crowded, its distinction from inverted papilloma can be difficult and arbitrary. Urothelial carcinoma in situ (CIS) may involve von Brunn's nests and should not be mistaken as invasive urothelial carcinoma. Florid cystitis glandularis, especially of the intestinal type, may be confused with invasive adenocarcinoma. An irregular, haphazard arrangement of glands in the deeper lamina propria or muscularis propria and cytologic atypia should raise the suspicion for adenocarcinoma.

PROGNOSIS AND THERAPY

Considered as variants of normal histology or reactive changes in response to local inflammation, von Brunn's nests, cystitis cystica, and glandularis are entirely benign and do not require therapy.

METAPLASIA OF THE UROTHELIUM

Metaplastic changes of the urothelium occur as a response to chronic inflammatory stimuli such as infection, calculi, diverticula, and catheterization. Squamous, glandular, and nephrogenic metaplasia are most common, although osseous, chondroid, and myeloid metaplasia can occur rarely.

SQUAMOUS METAPLASIA

CLINICAL FEATURES

There are two types of squamous metaplasia of the urothelium, nonkeratinizing and keratinizing. The

---

SQUAMOUS METAPLASIA—FACT SHEET

Definition
- Replacement of normal urothelium with squamous epithelium

Incidence and Location
- Nonkeratinizing squamous metaplasia found in 85% women of reproductive age and 75% of postmenopausal women

Gender, Race, and Age Distribution
- Nonkeratinizing squamous metaplasia almost exclusively found in women
- Keratinizing squamous metaplasia more common in men

Clinical Features
- Nonkeratinizing squamous metaplasia: normal finding in women, occasionally seen in men receiving estrogen therapy
- Keratinizing squamous metaplasia: secondary to chronic irritation, including indwelling catheter, calculi, and schistosomiasis

Prognosis and Treatment
- Nonkeratinizing squamous metaplasia: benign, requires no treatment
- Keratinizing squamous metaplasia: increased risk for carcinoma in certain settings
- Increased risk for bladder contracture, ureteral obstruction. Requires close follow-up. Cystectomy may be indicated for extensive disease.

---

former is considered as a normal finding in females, present in the trigone and bladder neck in up to 85% of women of reproductive age and 75% of postmenopausal women. Very rare in men, this type of squamous metaplasia has been described in men receiving estrogen therapy for prostatic carcinoma. Keratinizing squamous metaplasia, also termed leukoplakia, is more common in men and is usually associated with chronic irritation, such as indwelling catheters, calculi, and schistosomiasis. It has been recognized as a significant risk factor for the development of carcinoma of the urinary mucosa, the majority of which are squamous cell carcinoma.

PATHOLOGIC FEATURES

GROSS FINDINGS

Cystoscopically, areas of squamous metaplasia appear gray-white (Fig. 3-9). An extensively keratinizing lesion may have a bulky, irregular appearance similar to carcinoma.

MICROSCOPIC FINDINGS

In nonkeratinizing squamous metaplasia, the normal urothelium is replaced with squamous epithelium with clear, glycogenated cytoplasm, resembling the vaginal

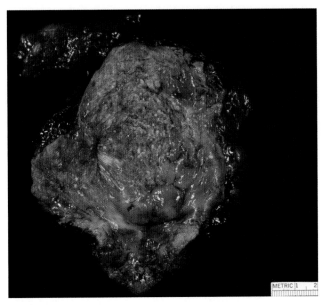

FIGURE 3-9
In keratinizing squamous metaplasia, the involved mucosa is gray with light brown flecks. (Courtesy of Dr. Greg MacLennan, Cleveland, Ohio.)

SQUAMOUS METAPLASIA—PATHOLOGIC FEATURES

Gross Findings
▶ White-gray area on cystoscopy
▶ Extensively keratinizing lesion may simulate cancer with an irregular bulky appearance

Microscopic Findings
▶ Nonkeratinizing squamous metaplasia: squamous epithelium with clear, glycogenated cells. No keratinization
▶ Keratinizing squamous metaplasia: squamous epithelium with hyperkeratosis and occasionally parakeratosis

---

squamous epithelium (Fig. 3-10A). The keratinizing squamous metaplasia features a squamous epithelium with hyperkeratosis and occasionally parakeratosis and even a granular layer (Fig. 3-10B). In most cases, there is no nuclear atypia. However, atypia as severe as in CIS can be seen.

PROGNOSIS AND THERAPY

Nonkeratinizing squamous metaplasia is essentially a normal finding in women and requires no treatment. Keratinizing squamous metaplasia, on the other hand, is a significant risk factor for bladder carcinoma and complications, such as bladder contracture and ureteral obstruction. The wide variation in lag time to the development of complications necessitates indefinite

follow-up. Cystectomy may be offered to selected patients with extensive bladder involvement and long life expectancy.

INTESTINAL METAPLASIA

CLINICAL FEATURES

The term intestinal metaplasia is used to describe the presence of isolated or aggregated goblet cells in cystitis glandularis, but it often refers to replacement of urothelium by epithelium resembling colonic mucosa. It usually occurs in chronically irritated bladders, such as those of paraplegics or in patients with stones or long-term catheterization.

PATHOLOGIC FEATURES

The surface of the bladder mucosa and glands in the lamina propria are lined by single layer of mucin-producing goblet cells (Fig. 3-11). Paneth cells may be identified at the base of crypt-like glands. The cells in

---

INTESTINAL METAPLASIA—FACT SHEET

Definition
▶ Focal or diffuse replacement of urothelium by colonic-like mucosa

Clinical Features
▶ Occurs in chronically irritated bladder (paraplegics, urinary lithiasis, indwelling catheter)

Prognosis and Treatment
▶ Association between diffuse intestinal metaplasia and bladder cancer uncertain

---

INTESTINAL METAPLASIA—PATHOLOGIC FEATURES

Microscopic Findings
▶ Surface and glands in the lamina propria lined with colonic-type epithelium
▶ May show at most moderate reactive glandular atypia
▶ Florid cases may minimally involve superficial muscularis propria and have mucin extravasation

Differential Diagnosis
▶ Invasive adenocarcinoma

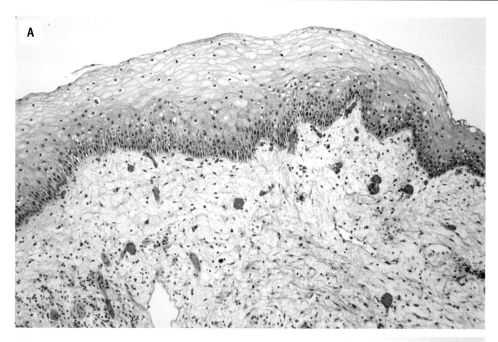

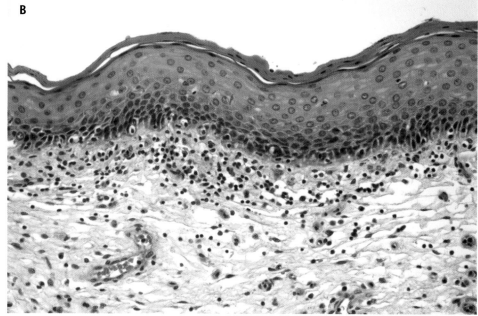

FIGURE 3-10

The nonkeratinizing type of squamous metaplasia has glycogenated clear cytoplasm (**A**), whereas the keratinizing type has a stratum corneum layer (**B**).

intestinal metaplasia may exhibit minimal reactive cytologic atypia, but moderate to severe atypia is absent. Florid cases may minimally involve superficial muscularis propria and have mucin extravasation; however, the change is usually focal and there are no free-floating cells in the mucin pools.

DIFFERENTIAL DIAGNOSIS

Diffuse intestinal metaplasia may be confused with invasive adenocarcinoma. Distinguishing the latter from intestinal metaplasia is the finding in adenocarcinoma of an infiltrative architectural pattern, extensive muscle invasion, and, most importantly, moderate to severe anaplasia.

PROGNOSIS AND THERAPY

The association between diffuse intestinal metaplasia and bladder cancer is uncertain. It had been associated with increased risk for development of bladder cancer, although a recent study found no such link.

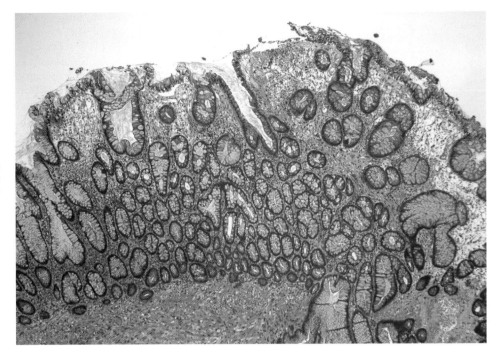

FIGURE 3-11
In intestinal metaplasia, the surface of the bladder mucosa is replaced by mucin-producing goblet cells, resembling colonic mucosa.

NEPHROGENIC ADENOMA OR METAPLASIA

CLINICAL FEATURES

Nephrogenic metaplasia (nephrogenic adenoma) is characterized by small tubular and papillary proliferation along the urothelial lining of the urinary tract. It often arises in the setting of an inflammatory insult and local injury, such as prior surgery, calculi, trauma, or infection. Eight percent of patients have a history of renal transplantation. Approximately two thirds of patients are male, and one third are younger than 30 years of age. Nephrogenic adenoma is often asymptomatic and detected incidentally, although it may manifest as a mass lesion simulating cancer. Named for its resemblance to the renal tubules, nephrogenic adenoma is considered to be a metaplastic process of the urothelium in response to injury. However, a recent study demonstrated that, at least in renal transplant recipients, these lesions are derived from shed renal tubular cells.

PATHOLOGIC FEATURES

GROSS FINDINGS

Nephrogenic adenoma is found throughout the urinary tract, with 55% localized in the bladder, 41% in the urethra, and the remaining 4% in the ureter. It may appear as a papillary or polypoid exophytic mass or

---

NEPHROGENIC METAPLASIA—FACT SHEET

Definition
▶ Metaplastic epithelial proliferation (that resembles the renal tubules) along the urothelial tract in response to chronic irritation and injury

Incidence and Location
▶ 55% in bladder, 41% in urethra, and 4% in ureter

Gender, Race, and Age Distribution
▶ Male/female ratio = 2:1
▶ One third of patients younger than 30 years of age

Clinical Features
▶ History of prior injury, calculi, trauma, or infection
▶ Increased risk in renal transplantation patients
▶ May present as a mass simulating cancer

Prognosis and Treatment
▶ Benign and reactive lesion
▶ May persist or recur
▶ No therapy necessary

---

velvety lesion (Fig. 3-12), most often smaller than 1 cm, although larger lesions may occasionally be seen.

MICROSCOPIC FINDINGS

Nephrogenic adenoma has a broad histologic spectrum. It may consist of papillae, small tubules, large

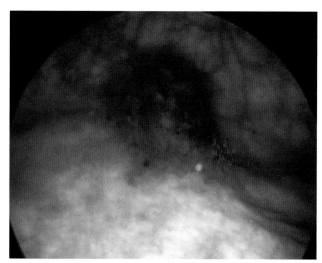

FIGURE 3-12

Cystoscopically, nephrogenic adenoma is a papillary lesion simulating cancer.

cystically dilated tubules with eosinophilic or basophilic intraluminal secretions, cords of cells, or single cells (Fig. 3-13A-D). Tubules are often surrounded by a layer of hyalinized basement membrane (Fig. 3-13D). A variable degree of acute and chronic inflammation and stromal edema are common in the background (Fig. 3-13B). The tubules and papillae are lined by cuboidal or low columnar epithelium. Prominent nucleoli can

---

NEPHROGENIC METAPLASIA—PATHOLOGIC FEATURES

Gross Findings
► Papillary or polypoid mass, or velvety lesion, or grossly invisible
► Most lesions <1 cm

Microscopic Findings
► Papillae, small tubules, large cystically dilated tubules lined with cuboidal and low columnar epithelium
► Tubules lined by flattened hobnail cells resembling vessels with reactive endothelium
► Small tubules with mucin resemble signet-ring cells
► Some tubules surrounded by thick hyalinized basement membrane
► Acute and chronic inflammation, stromal edema

Immunohistochemical Features
► Cytokeratin 7 +
► Focal and weak PSA and PSAP expression in a subset of cases
► Majority + for AMACR and PAX2, and − for high-molecular-weight cytokeratin (34βE12)

Differential Diagnosis
► Prostatic adenocarcinoma
► Papillary and nested variant urothelial carcinoma
► Signet-ring cell adenocarcinoma
► Clear cell adenocarcinoma
► Capillary hemangioma

---

be present, although nuclear atypia and mitoses are virtually absent. One characteristic finding is cystically dilated tubules lined with "hobnail" cells resembling endothelial-lined vascular spaces (Fig. 3-13B). Cells with oxyphilic or clear cytoplasm, or signet-ring-like cells, may also be seen. Different patterns are often admixed, although one pattern may predominate.

ANCILLARY STUDIES

IMMUNOHISTOCHEMISTRY

CK7 is positive in all nephrogenic adenomas. Focal and weak prostate-specific antigen (PSA) and prostate-specific acid phosphatase (PSAP) expression is detected in a subset of cases. The majority of cases are positive for α-methylacyl-coenzyme A racemase (AMACR) (Fig. 3-13E) and PAX2 (Fig. 3-13F) and negative for high-molecular-weight cytokeratin (34βE12).

DIFFERENTIAL DIAGNOSIS

Characteristic tubules lined with bland cuboidal or low columnar cells and surrounded by a prominent basement membrane in an inflammatory background readily suggest the correct diagnosis. However, nephrogenic adenomas in men may be confused with prostatic carcinoma, which consists of tubules with prominent nucleoli sometimes situated within muscle bundles. Atrophic cytoplasm, associated inflammation, a hyaline rim of connective tissue around some of the glands, other typical patterns of nephrogenic adenoma, and only weak positivity for PSA and PSAP should lead to the correct diagnosis. Nephrogenic adenomas should also be differentiated from the papillary and nested variants of urothelial carcinoma. Papillary urothelial neoplasms have delicate fibrovascular cores lined by stratified urothelium, in contrast to the edematous and inflamed cores covered with a single layer of bland cuboidal or low columnar cells in nephrogenic adenomas. The nested variant of urothelial carcinoma often has deceptively bland cytology; however, it usually exhibits greater atypia and increased mitoses at the deep invasive fronts. Nephrogenic adenoma may have a predominance of small tubules with mucin, resembling signet-ring-cell carcinoma. However, the thickened basement membrane, lack of nuclear atypia, and other patterns lead to the correct diagnosis. In female patients, nephrogenic adenoma can be differentiated from clear cell adenocarcinoma by its lack of widespread nuclear atypia, absent mitoses, infrequent presence of clear cells, and solid sheets of cells. Finally, nephrogenic adenoma may be confused with a capillary hemangioma because of the "vascular space"-like dilated tubules; however, the tubules are positive for CK7 and negative for endothelial markers such as CD31.

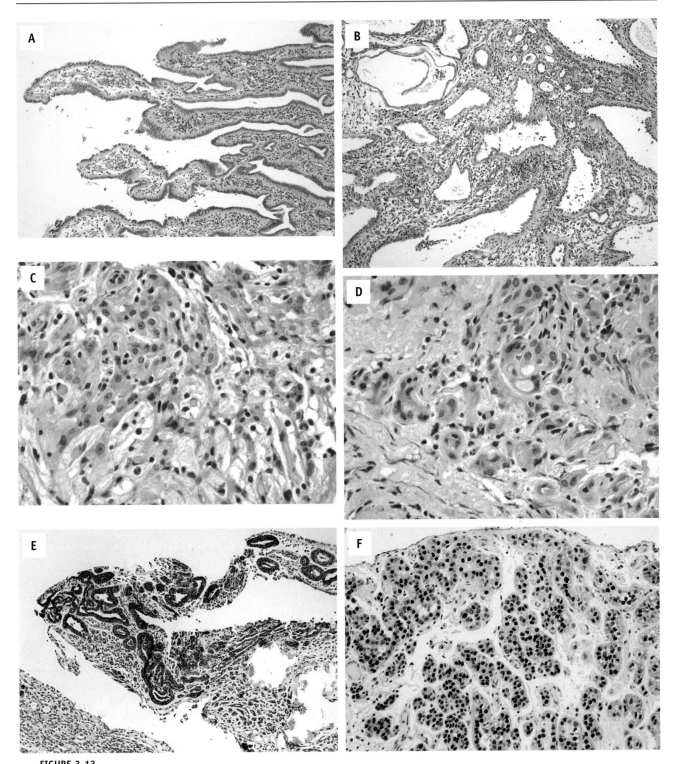

FIGURE 3-13

A variety of architectural patterns are seen in nephrogenic adenoma, including papillary (**A**), tubular (**B**), cords of cells (**C**), and single cells (**C**). Tubules are often surrounded by a layer of hyalinized basement membrane (**D**). Acute and chronic inflammation and stromal edema are common in the background (**B**). Nephrogenic adenoma is positive for AMACR (**E**, Courtesy of Dr. Rajal Shah, Ann Arbor, Michigan) and PAX2 (**F**, Courtesy of Dr. Guo-xia Tong, New York, New York).

PROGNOSIS AND THERAPY

Nephrogenic adenomas are benign, yet they may recur if the underlying cause persists. Therapy should be directed toward the underlying cause.

INFLAMMATION AND INFECTION

POLYPOID CYSTITIS

CLINICAL FEATURES

Polypoid cystitis is an inflammatory mucosal lesion that assumes polypoid configuration cystoscopically and microscopically. It arises as a reaction to any inflammatory insult to the bladder mucosa, most commonly in the clinical setting of indwelling catheters and vesical fistulas. It affects both genders equally, with an age range from 20 months to 79 years. Depending on the extent of edema of the lamina propria, there is a continuous morphologic spectrum from papillary cystitis (slender, finger-like papillae), to polypoid cystitis (broad-based, thick papillae), to bullous cystitis (papillae width greater than length).

PATHOLOGIC FEATURES

GROSS FINDINGS

Cystoscopically, polypoid cystitis appears as an area of friable mucosal irregularity or edematous broad

---

POLYPOID CYSTITIS—FACT SHEET

Definition
▶ Inflammatory lesion with lamina propria edema resulting in a polypoid configuration

Gender, Race, and Age Distribution
▶ Affects both genders equally
▶ Age 20 months to 79 years

Clinical Features
▶ Arises as a reaction to any inflammatory insult to the bladder mucosa

Prognosis and Treatment
▶ Benign
▶ No risk for bladder cancer

POLYPOID CYSTITIS—PATHOLOGIC FEATURES

Cystoscopic Findings
▶ Appears as friable mucosal irregularity or edematous broad papillae adjacent to inflamed area
▶ May be multifocal and can range up to 5 mm

Microscopic Findings
▶ Papillae have thick, edematous fibrovascular cores with vascular dilatation and acute and chronic inflammation in lamina propria
▶ Papillae lack branching
▶ At most reactive urothelial atypia
▶ Polypoid cystitis (broad-based, thick papillae with marked edema)
▶ Bullous cystitis (papillae with extensive edema such that width is greater than height)
▶ Papillary cystitis (end stage with slender finger-like papillae with more fibrosis)

Differential Diagnosis
▶ Papillary urothelial carcinoma—occasional papillary fronds in a lesion, out of context of the entire lesion, can resemble carcinoma

---

papillae adjacent to an inflamed area. Lesions may be multifocal and can range up to 5 mm. Urologists can in most cases readily distinguish polypoid cystitis from papillary urothelial neoplasms.

MICROSCOPIC FINDINGS

The papillae in polypoid cystitis have thick, edematous, fibrovascular cores with vascular dilatation and acute and chronic inflammation in the lamina propria (Fig. 3-14A,B). The papillae are simple without branching. The urothelium lining the edematous stalks may be normal, or it may show reactive atypia or squamous metaplasia. Bullous cystitis has extensive submucosal edema. Papillary cystitis often has less edematous and more fibrotic papillae.

DIFFERENTIAL DIAGNOSIS

Polypoid cystitis should be distinguished from papillary urothelial neoplasms. The fibrovascular cores in polypoid cystitis are edematous and broad based, in contrast to the thin, delicate fibrovascular cores of papillary urothelial neoplasms. In addition, the papillary fronds in polypoid cystitis do not branch into smaller papillae, as is seen in papillary urothelial neoplasms. Although there may be isolated papillary fronds in polypoid cystitis that can closely resemble those seen in a papillary urothelial neoplasm, one must interpret these fronds in the context of the rest of the lesion and diagnose the entire case as polypoid cystitis.

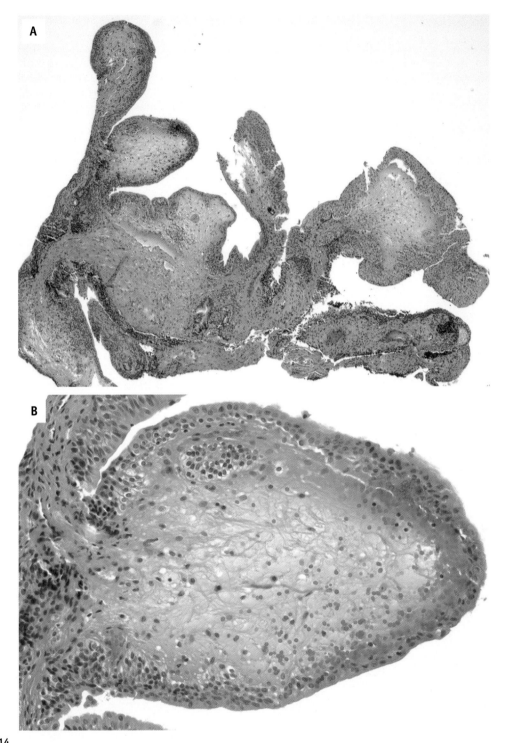

FIGURE 3-14
A, The low magnification shows a papillary configuration of the lesion of polypoid cystitis. **B,** The papillary frond is edematous with red blood cell extravasation and inflammation.

PROGNOSIS AND THERAPY

Polypoid cystitis is a benign lesion with no risk of evolving into carcinoma.

FOLLICULAR CYSTITIS

Follicular cystitis is a condition in which lymphoid follicles are present within the lamina propria, many with germinal centers (Fig. 3-15). It occurs frequently in patients with bladder cancer or urinary tract infection. The lesion may be seen grossly as white or gray nodules on erythematous mucosa. Malignant lymphoma is the most important differential diagnostic consideration.

GIANT CELL CYSTITIS

Giant cell cystitis is not a clinical entity; rather, it is a term used to describe the presence of atypical stromal cells in the lamina propria of the bladder. Such cells are common in bladder biopsies, including those without apparent pathology. Histologically, these cells often have bipolar or multipolar tapering eosinophilic processes and enlarged, hyperchromatic, or multiple nuclei (Fig. 3-16). Mitoses are absent or rare. Similar cells may be seen in the lamina propria after radiation therapy. If these cells are present in large numbers, suspicion for a sarcoma may be raised. However, these atypical stromal cells have nuclear atypia that appears degenerative, often multinucleated, and no mitotic activity.

INTERSTITIAL CYSTITIS

CLINICAL FEATURES

Interstitial cystitis is an enigmatic, essentially incurable condition characterized by a constellation of symptoms including urinary frequency, urgency, nocturia, suprapubic pressure, and pelvic and bladder pain. More than 90% of the patients are women, and the disease predominantly affects middle-aged and older women. Many patients have a history of autoimmune disease. The urine is sterile, and the cause remains unknown. It has been hypothesized that immunologic dysregulation, infection, trauma, and structural defects may play a role in pathogenesis.

The diagnosis of interstitial cystitis is primarily based on the clinical findings and exclusion of other possible causes, including other forms of cystitis and

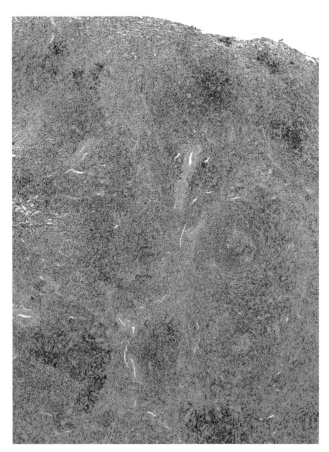

FIGURE 3-15
In follicular cystitis, the lamina propria contains many lymphoid follicles.

INTERSTITIAL CYSTITIS—FACT SHEET

Definition
▶ Chronic inflammatory process of the urinary bladder of uncertain etiology

Incidence and Location
▶ Female: 18.1 per 100,000
▶ Male: 1.2 per 100,000

Gender, Race, and Age Distribution
▶ >90% patients are women
▶ Affects middle-aged and older patients

Clinical Features
▶ Constellation of symptoms—urinary frequency, urgency, nocturia, suprapubic pressure, and pelvic and bladder pain
▶ No evidence of urothelial carcinoma or other forms of cystitis

Prognosis and Treatment
▶ Incurable with protracted course of exacerbations and remissions
▶ Palliative treatment for symptomatic relief

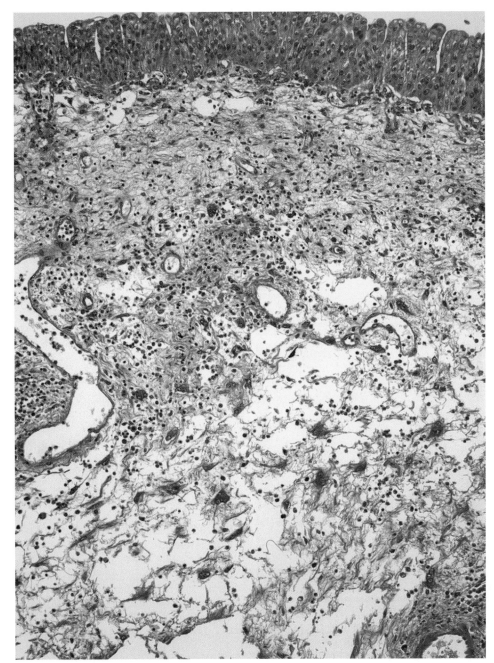

FIGURE 3-16

In giant cell cystitis, the lamina propria contains large stromal cells, some of which are multinucleated.

carcinoma. The role of pathologists in the management of interstitial cystitis is to rule out CIS and other forms of cystitis and to correlate pathologic results with clinical findings.

Interstitial cystitis is categorized as nonulcerative (early, nonclassic) or ulcerative (late, classic) disease based on cystoscopic findings. Transition from non-ulcerative to ulcerative disease is rare, and the two types may be completely separate entities pathologically.

PATHOLOGIC FEATURES

GROSS FINDINGS

The nonulcerative disease exhibits "glomerulations," which are petechial submucosal hemorrhages that occur after hydrodistention of the bladder (Fig. 3-17A). The ulcerative disease manifests as single or multiple patches of reddened mucosa, with small vessels radiat-

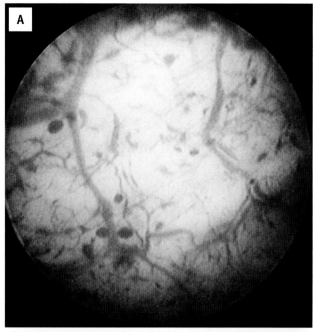

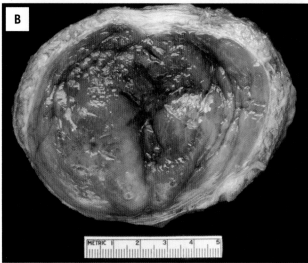

FIGURE 3-17

A, The nonulcerative form of interstitial cystitis exhibits petechial submucosal hemorrhage ("glomerulations") on cystoscopy. **B,** Hunner's ulcer. (B, Courtesy of Dr. Greg MacLennan, Cleveland, Ohio).

ing from a central scar called Hunner's ulcer (Fig. 3-17B). However, glomerulations are neither specific nor sensitive, and ulceration is extremely uncommon (< 5%) in interstitial cystitis.

MICROSCOPIC FINDINGS

There are no characteristic histologic features for interstitial cystitis. The nonulcerative disease has a relatively unaltered mucosa with a sparse inflammatory response. The main feature is multiple small mucosal ruptures and suburothelial hemorrhages (Fig. 3-18A). The bladder mucosa may be completely normal in some cases and in other cases denuded. In patients with

---

INTERSTITIAL CYSTITIS—PATHOLOGIC FEATURES

Gross Findings

► Glomerulations in nonulcerative type; neither sensitive nor specific

► Hunner's ulcer in ulcerative type; rare (<5%)

Microscopic Findings

► No characteristic histologic features
► Nonulcerative disease: multiple small mucosal ruptures and suburothelial hemorrhage
► Ulcerative disease: ulcer and marked inflammation in lamina propria
► Mast cell count not useful diagnostically

Differential Diagnosis

► Other forms of cystitis (hemorrhagic, radiation, eosinophilic, and infectious cystitis)
► Urothelial CIS (denuding cystitis)

Hunner's ulcer, the ulcer varies in thickness but usually involves the upper half of the lamina propria. It is often covered by debris, fibrin, inflammatory cells, and erythrocytes. The ulcer base is composed of granulation tissue. The rest of the lamina propria is moderately or markedly inflamed, with lymphoid aggregates. Perineural inflammation (Fig. 3-18B), or chronic perineuritis, is seen in 70% of patients. In long-standing disease, fibrosis and inflammation may be seen in the muscularis propria (Fig. 3-18C), a finding that correlates with the reduced bladder capacity seen in advanced disease. The perivesical fat usually lacks significant inflammation.

Mast cells have frequently been associated with interstitial cystitis. Activated mast cells may play an important role in the pathogenesis of interstitial cystitis. However, a high mast cell count in the detrusor muscle is not diagnostically useful, because the mast cell counts in interstitial cystitis overlap with those seen in patients with bladder inflammation of other causes, and they do not correlate with clinical symptoms, cystoscopic findings, or response to therapy.

DIFFERENTIAL DIAGNOSIS

A wide range of other diseases should be excluded before a diagnosis of interstitial cystitis is rendered. CIS is the most important diagnostic consideration. Cystoscopically, extensively denuded CIS ("denuding cystitis") can mimic interstitial cystitis. Histologically, denuding CIS exhibits ulceration, vascular congestion, and inflammation resembling interstitial cystitis. Multiple tissue sections should be examined to search for atypical cells. Other forms of cystitis, including hemorrhagic cystitis, radiation cystitis, eosinophilic

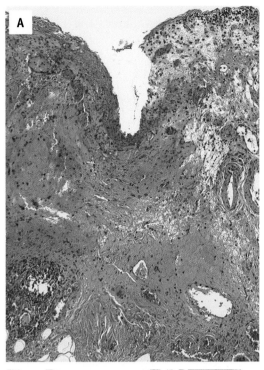

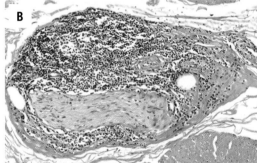

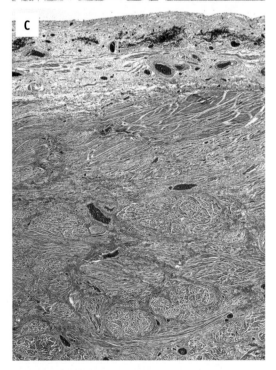

FIGURE 3-18

Microscopic features in interstitial cystitis. **A,** The bladder mucosa has a small mucosal rupture and subepithelial hemorrhage. **B,** Perineuritis is present. **C,** In long-standing cases, trichrome stain reveals extensive fibrosis of lamina propria and muscularis propria.

cystitis, and infectious cystitis, should be ruled out based on urinalysis, cytology, culture, and histologic examination.

PROGNOSIS AND THERAPY

Interstitial cystitis is incurable. Treatment offers symptomatic palliation. Most patients can be maintained in a satisfied, although not asymptomatic, state punctuated by exacerbations and remissions.

EOSINOPHILIC CYSTITIS

CLINICAL FEATURES

Eosinophilic cystitis is characterized by dense eosinophilic infiltrates in the bladder wall and lamina propria. It occurs in two clinical settings. It most commonly reflects a nonspecific, localized, self-limited, subacute inflammatory reaction to injury, such as that associated with transurethral resection or invasive cancer. Rarely, eosinophilic cystitis is associated with allergic disease; in most cases, patients also have asthma, eosinophilic gastroenteritis, or, rarely, parasitic infection. Patients range from newborn to elderly, and the female-to-male ratio is 2:1. Patients commonly present with frequency, dysuria, and hematuria. They may also have peripheral eosinophilia.

PATHOLOGIC FEATURES

GROSS FINDINGS

At cystoscopy, eosinophilic cystitis may appear as a polypoid lesion. Nodular, sessile lesions or ulcers may be seen.

MICROSCOPIC FINDINGS

The lamina propria is edematous, with a mixed inflammatory infiltrate in which eosinophils predominate (Fig. 3-19). Tissue eosinophilia is also commonly seen in the vicinity of an invasive urothelial carcinoma.

PROGNOSIS AND THERAPY

For eosinophilic cystitis associated with allergic disease, therapy is targeted toward the underlying disease.

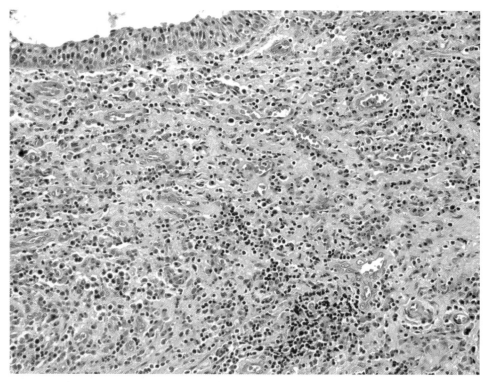

FIGURE 3-19
In eosinophilic cystitis, numerous eosinophils predominate in the inflammatory infiltrates in the lamina propria.

INFECTIOUS CYSTITIS

Infectious cystitis can be caused by various micro-organisms, including bacteria, fungi, viruses, and parasites. The diagnosis relies primarily on urinalysis, urine culture, and empirical antimicrobial therapy. In most cases, surgical pathologists play a limited role in diagnosis and management.

BACTERIAL CYSTITIS

Bacterial infection is the most common cause of cystitis, usually by *Escherichia coli, Staphylococcus saprophyticus, Klebsiella* species, *Proteus mirabilis,* or *enterococci.* Uncomplicated bacterial cystitis most commonly involves sexually active women between 20 and 40 years of age. Recurrent cystitis, on the other hand, affects patients with physiologic and structural abnormalities (including bladder exstrophy), urethral malformation, calculi, or systemic diseases such as diabetes, chronic renal disease, and immunosuppression. Patients present with dysuria, frequency, urgency, voiding of small urine volume, and suprapubic or lower abdominal pain.

VIRAL CYSTITIS

Both adenovirus and herpes simplex virus type 2 have been associated with hemorrhagic cystitis, especially in immunosuppressed patients after bone marrow transplantation. Herpes zoster and cytomegalovirus have also been rarely implicated in cystitis. Patients with human polyoma viruses and bladder involvement are usually immunocompromised after renal or bone marrow transplantation and have hemorrhagic cystitis. Although viruria and intranuclear inclusions are frequently present in urinary cytology samples, the identification of viral inclusions in tissue sections is rare (Fig. 3-20).

FUNGAL CYSTITIS

Fungal cystitis is uncommon and most often is caused by *Candida albicans.* Cystitis caused by *Aspergillus* and other fungi have rarely been reported. Most patients are debilitated or receiving antibiotic therapy, and many are diabetic. Women are predominantly affected. Dysuria, frequency, pyuria, and hematuria are common complaints. Microscopically, there is ulceration and inflammation in the lamina propria. The pseudohyphae and yeast forms may be seen in routine tissue sections or with periodic acid-Schiff (PAS) or silver stains.

TUBERCULOUS CYSTITIS

Despite the dramatically falling prevalence of pulmonary tuberculosis, the incidence of genitourinary tuberculosis remains constant in western countries, accounting for 7% of extrapulmonary cases. Most tuberculous cystitis is caused by *Mycobacterium tuberculosis* and follows renal tuberculosis. Urinary frequency, hematuria, and dysuria are common symptoms. Typi-

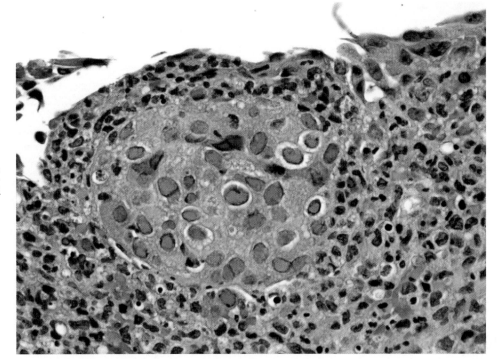

FIGURE 3-20

In herpes simplex viral cystitis, homogeneous intranuclear viral inclusions are present in the urothelial cells.

cally, the infection begins around the ureteral orifices with superficial ulceration, acute and chronic inflammation, and initially noncaseating granulomas. Larger caseating granulomas with central necrosis surrounded by multinucleated giant cells, plasma cells, and lymphocytes may ensue. Late complications include distortion and obstruction of the ureteral orifices and a small, scarred bladder with low capacity.

SCHISTOSOMIASIS

CLINICAL FEATURES

Schistosomiasis is most prevalent in the Middle East and in the African continent. Schistosomal involvement of the bladder is caused by larvae of *Schistosoma haematobium*. Adult male and female worm pairs dwell principally in the perivesical venous plexus in humans, where they mate and females lay eggs. Schistosomal disease results directly from the schistosome eggs and the granulomatous host response to them. Patients present with urinary frequency, terminal dysuria, hematuria, and chronic urinary tract infections. With greater chronicity, there is intense egg deposition involving all levels of the detrusor muscle with dense fibrosis. This results in "contracted bladder" syndrome, with intractable frequency, dysuria, urgency, and incompetence.

PATHOLOGIC FEATURES

GROSS FINDINGS

At the early active stage, the bladder mucosa has many erythematous, granular, sessile, and pedunculated polyps that are induced by a heavy burden of eggs. Ulceration may rarely be present. In the chronic stage, the characteristic changes are "sandy patches," with old, calcified schistosomal eggs buried immediately beneath the atrophic urothelial mucosa, resembling sand seen through shallow water. Stellate ulcers can also be present at this stage.

MICROSCOPIC FINDINGS

In the active phase, the schistosomal eggs are in the bladder wall with intense granulomatous inflammation and numerous eosinophils (Fig. 3-21A,B). As the disease evolves, the eggs are destroyed and calcified (Fig. 3-21C), inflammation subsides, and fibrosis ensues. The bladder mucosa frequently exhibits metaplastic changes, including keratinizing squamous metaplasia and intestinal metaplasia.

DIFFERENTIAL DIAGNOSIS

S. hematobium can be differentiated from other schistosomes, including *Schistosoma mansoni* and *Schistosoma japonicum*, by its terminal spines. However, these may be difficult to appreciate on tissue sections. Another feature that differentiates *S. hematobium* from other schistosomes is that *S. hematobium* egg shells are not acid-fast, whereas those of *S. mansoni* and *S. japonicum* eggs are.

URINARY SCHISTOSOMIASIS—FACT SHEET

Definition
▶ Schistosomal involvement of the bladder by larvae of *Schistosoma haematobium*

Incidence and Location
▶ Most prevalent in the Middle East and in most of the African continent

Clinical Features
▶ Urinary frequency, terminal dysuria, hematuria, and chronic urinary tract infection
▶ "Contracted bladder" syndrome with intractable frequency, dysuria, urgency, and incompetence as late complications

Prognosis and Treatment
▶ Morbidity and mortality determined by the overall parasitic burden and risk of reinfection
▶ Newer antischistosomal drugs dramatically improve the prognosis
▶ The major urinary tract complications are ureteral stricture, hydronephrosis, and nonfunctional kidneys
▶ Increased risk for squamous cell and urothelial carcinoma of the urinary tract, including bladder

---

URINARY SCHISTOSIMIASIS—PATHOLOGIC FEATURES

Gross Findings
▶ Early active stage: erythematous, granular, sessile and pedunculated polyps; rarely ulceration
▶ Chronic stage: characteristic "sandy patches"; stellate ulcers

Microscopic Findings
▶ Active stage: intense granulomatous inflammation with numerous eosinophils in response to schistosomal eggs
▶ Later in disease: schistosomal eggs are destroyed and calcified and inflammation subsides; fibrosis; urothelial mucosa frequently with metaplastic changes

Differential Diagnosis
▶ *S. hematobium* can be differentiated from other schistosomes, including *S. mansoni* and *S. japonicum*, by its terminal spines and lack of acid-fast staining in its egg shells

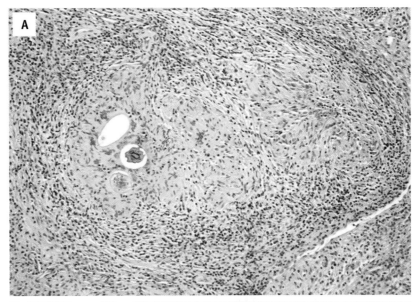

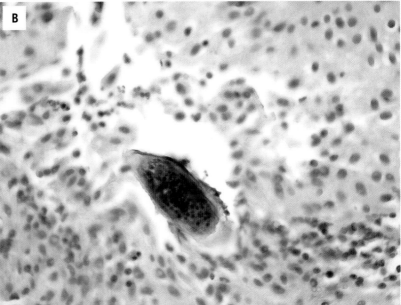

FIGURE 3-21

A, Granulomatous inflammation surrounds the schistosomal larvae. Eosinophils are abundant. **B**, The ovum of *Schistosoma haematobium* has a terminal spine. **C**, Calcified ova are seen in long-standing disease.   *Continued*

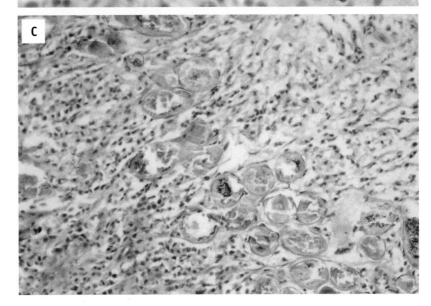

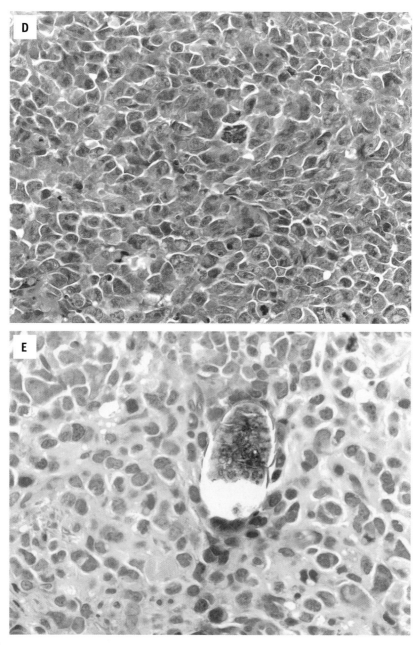

FIGURE 3-21, CONT'D

A case of high grade urothelial carcinoma with a predominant small cell carcinoma component (**D**) arises in a schistosomal-infected bladder. A schistosomal egg is embedded in the tumor (**E**).

PROGNOSIS AND THERAPY

The morbidity and mortality of schistosomiasis is determined by the overall parasitic burden and the risk of reinfection. Newer antischistosomal drugs have dramatically improved the prognosis. The major urinary tract complications include ureteral stricture, hydronephrosis, and nonfunctional kidneys. Patients are also at increased risk for squamous cell carcinoma of the urinary tract. We have also seen a case of urothelial carcinoma with a predominant small cell carcinoma component arising in a bladder infested with *S. hematobium* (Fig. 3-21D, E).

ENCRUSTED CYSTITIS

Encrusted cystitis refers to the deposition of inorganic salts in injured urothelial mucosa as the result of urine alkalization by urea-splitting bacteria. It is most common in women. Histologically, the lesions are covered with fibrin mixed with calcified necrotic debris and inflammatory cells, with deposits of calcium present in the lamina propria (Fig. 3-22).

EMPHYSEMATOUS CYSTITIS

Emphysematous cystitis consists of gas-filled blebs, which can be visualized at cystoscopy or at gross examination. It is typically more common in women, often diabetic, and is associated with bacterial infection with *E. coli* or *Aerobacter aerogenes*. Other predisposing conditions include trauma, fistula formation, instrumentation, and urinary stasis. Microscopically, the blebs consist of empty cavities in the lamina propria lined by attenuated cells (Fig. 3-23A). Frequently there are associated foreign body giant cells (Fig. 3-23B).

MALAKOPLAKIA

CLINICAL FEATURES

Derived from the Greek roots for soft (*malakos*) and plaque (*plakos*), malakoplakia is an uncommon histio-

---

MALAKOPLAKIA—FACT SHEET

Definition
▶ Uncommon histiocytic process that manifests as yellow-white soft plaques on the bladder mucosal surface

Incidence and Location
▶ Most commonly involves bladder
▶ Also involves other sites, including other genitourinary sites, gastrointestinal tract, skin, lungs, bone, and mesenteric lymph nodes

Gender, Race, and Age Distribution
▶ Patients usually older than 50 years
▶ Female/male ratio = 4:1

Clinical Features
▶ Patients present with the symptoms of bladder irritability and hematuria
▶ Bacteriuria with *Escherichia coli* and other gram-negative bacilli

Prognosis and Treatment
▶ Can cause significant mortality and morbidity depending on disease extent
▶ Treatment directed at control of the urinary tract infection

---

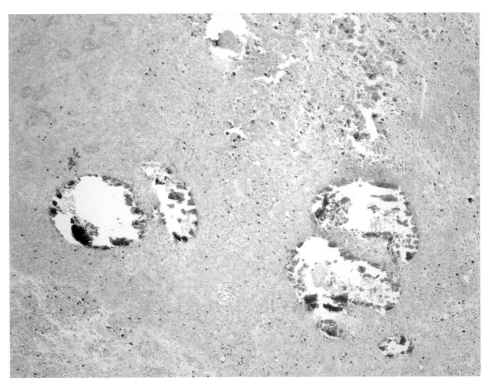

FIGURE 3-22
In encrusted cystitis, calcium salts are deposited within the necrotic debris in the lamina propria.

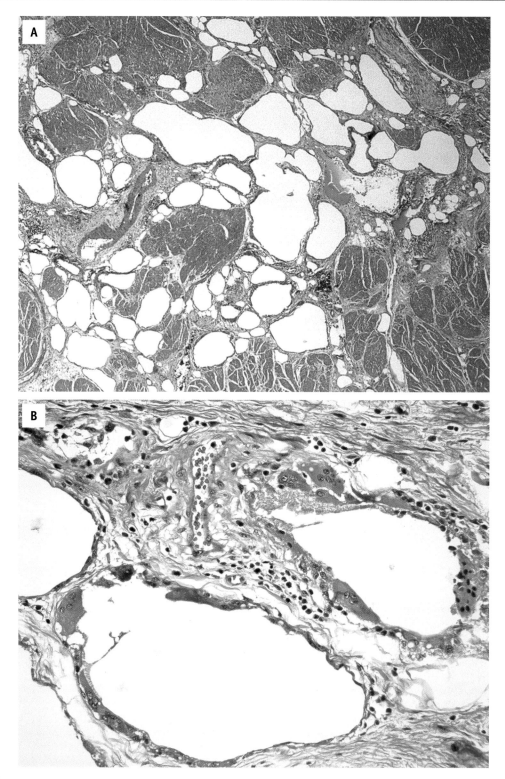

FIGURE 3-23

In emphysematous cystitis, the lamina propria and muscularis propria are dissected by numerous clear spaces (**A**), which are lined with attenuated cells and frequently with foreign body giant cells (**B**).

cytic process that manifests as yellow-white soft plaques on the mucosal surface. It results from impairment of mononuclear cells in their function of degrading phagocytosed bacteria. Most patients are older than 50 years of age, and there is a female predominance of 4:1. Patients often present with the symptoms of bladder irritability and hematuria. *E. coli* is most frequently isolated from the urine, but other gram-negative bacilli have also been implicated. Malakoplakia most commonly involves the bladder, although it can also involve other sites, including other genitourinary organs, gastrointestinal tract, skin, lungs, bone, and mesenteric lymph nodes.

PATHOLOGIC FEATURES

GROSS FINDINGS

Malakoplakia consists of usually multiple, soft yellow or yellow-brown plaques. The lesions are usually smaller than 2 cm in diameter. They may appear nodular and polypoid in rare cases (Fig. 3-24).

MICROSCOPIC FINDINGS

There is a collection of histiocytes with granular eosinophilic cytoplasm (von Hansemann histiocytes) in the superficial lamina propria (Fig. 3-25A). These cells contain characteristic intracytoplasmic inclusion bodies called Michaelis-Gutmann bodies. These inclusion bodies are typically spherical with concentric lamination, basophilic, and 5 to 8 μm in diameter (Fig. 3-25B). They are formed by precipitation of calcium or iron on bacteria or bacterial fragments. Michaelis-Gutmann bodies may be difficult to visualize on hematoxylin and

MALAKOPLAKIA—PATHOLOGIC FEATURES

Gross Findings
► Multiple, soft yellow or yellow-brown plaques on mucosal surface
► May appear nodular or polypoid

Microscopic Findings
► von Hansemann histiocytes with granular eosinophilic cytoplasm in the superficial lamina propria
► Characteristic intracytoplasmic inclusion bodies called Michaelis-Gutmann bodies that are typically spherical with concentric lamination, basophilic, and 5 to 8 μm in diameter
► Extensive fibrosis late in the disease process

Ultrastructural Features
► von Hansemann histiocytes contain many cytoplasmic phagolysosomes that contain fragments of bacterial cell wall
► Michaelis-Gutmann bodies range from 5 to 10 μm and have a dense crystalline core at the center that is surrounded by a homogeneous zone

Histochemical Stains
► von Kossa stain (calcium) and Perl's Prussian blue stain (iron) highlight Michaelis-Gutmann bodies

Differential Diagnosis
► Langerhans cell histiocytosis
► Xanthogranulomatous inflammation

eosin (H&E) staining, especially early in the disease process. Late in the disease, there may be extensive fibrosis.

ANCILLARY STUDIES

von Kossa calcium and Perl's Prussian blue iron stains highlight the Michaelis-Gutmann bodies (Fig. 3-26A,B). Ultrastructurally, von Hansemann histiocytes contain many cytoplasmic phagolysosomes with fragments of bacterial cell wall. Michaelis-Gutmann bodies have a dense crystalline core at the center that is surrounded by a homogeneous zone (Fig. 3-27).

DIFFERENTIAL DIAGNOSIS

Other diseases in which histiocytes or macrophages predominate, including Langerhans cell histiocytosis and xanthogranulomatous inflammation, should be differentiated from malakoplakia. Michaelis-Gutmann bodies are not present in the latter two entities. Langerhans cell histiocytes are positive for CD1a and

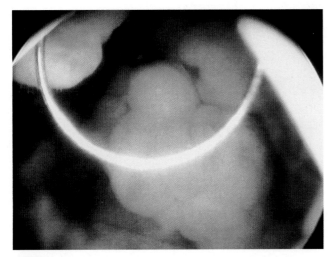

FIGURE 3-24
Malakoplakia appears as a polypoid, pink-tan mass covered with intact mucosa. (Courtesy of Dr. Greg MacLennan, Cleveland, Ohio.)

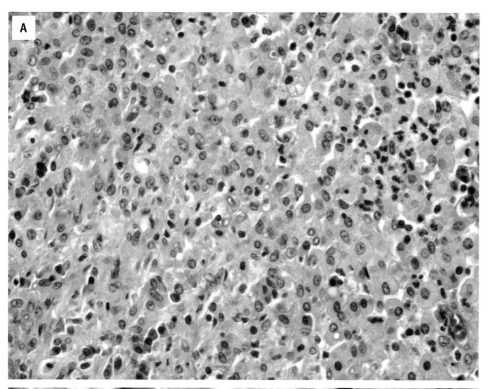

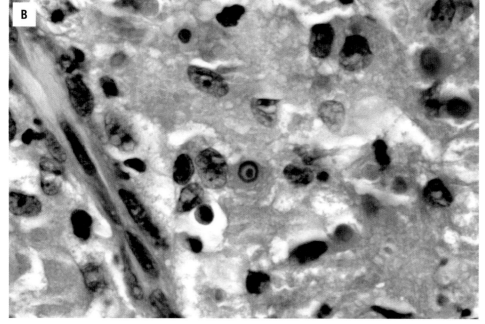

FIGURE 3-25

In malakoplakia, the lamina propria is filled with von Hansemann histiocytes (**A**). They contain Michaelis-Gutmann bodies (**A** and **B**).

S-100, whereas the histiocytes in malakoplakia are negative for these two markers.

PROGNOSIS AND THERAPY

Malakoplakia can cause significant mortality and morbidity depending on the disease extent. The treatment should be directed at control of the urinary tract infection, which should stabilize the disease process.

THERAPY-RELATED CHANGES

GRANULOMATOUS CYSTITIS AFTER BCG THERAPY

CLINICAL FEATURES

Bacille Calmette-Guérin (BCG) immunotherapy is the most effective form of intravesical therapy for prophy-

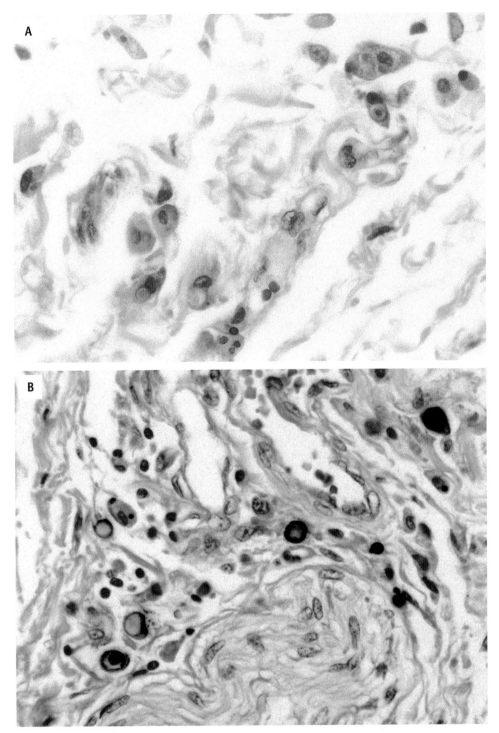

FIGURE 3-26
von Kossa calcium (**A**) and Perl's Prussian blue iron (**B**) stains highlight the Michaelis-Gutmann bodies.

laxis and treatment of urothelial CIS and superficially invasive urothelial carcinoma. After intravesical installation, most patients experience dysuria and urinary urgency and frequency. Hematuria is seen in one third of patients. Granulomatous inflammation may develop along the lower urinary tract, including bladder, prostate, and testis.

PATHOLOGIC FEATURES

MICROSCOPIC FINDINGS

Intense chronic inflammation with discrete, noncaseating granulomas containing epithelioid histiocytes and multinucleated giant cells is found in the superficial

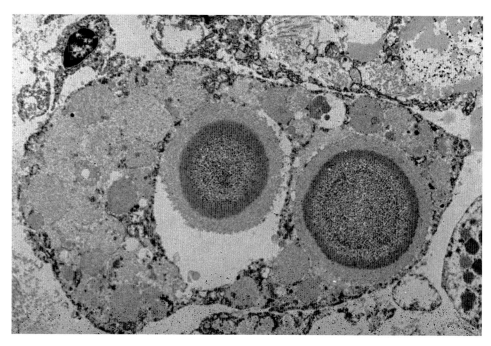

FIGURE 3-27
Ultrastructurally, Michaelis-Gutmann bodies have a dense crystalline central core surrounded by a homogeneous zone.

lamina propria (Fig. 3-28). The overlying urothelium may show reactive atypia or may be partially or entirely denuded.

commonly demonstrates inflammatory cells, including epithelioid histiocytes and occasional giant cells.

POSTSURGICAL GRANULOMAS

CLINICAL FEATURES

ANCILLARY STUDIES

Acid-fast staining rarely reveals organisms. In patients with a known history of BCG therapy, special stains for the organisms are not necessary. Urine cytology

A nonspecific granulomatous inflammation usually develops after transurethral resection of bladder

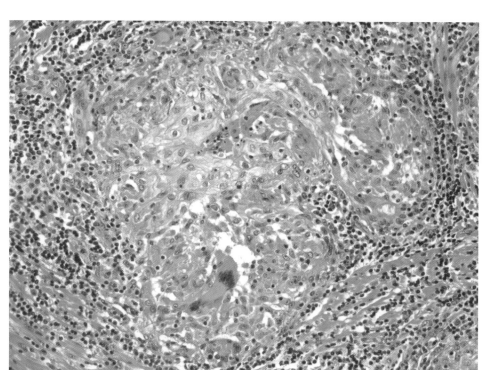

FIGURE 3-28
Granulomatous cystitis after bacille Calmette-Guérin (BCG) therapy shows intense chronic inflammation with discrete, noncaseating granulomas containing epithelioid histiocytes and multinucleated giant cells.

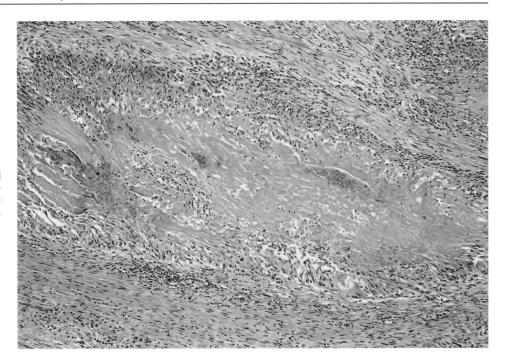

FIGURE 3-29
Postsurgical granulomas are rimmed with palisading histiocytes and surrounded by dense chronic inflammatory infiltrates with many eosinophils.

tumors. In approximately 10% of cases, the bladder develops necrobiotic granulomas. Similar lesions have also been reported after laser surgery. The frequency increases with the number of operations.

PATHOLOGIC FEATURES

Postsurgical necrobiotic granulomas typically have linear or serpiginous contours with central fibrinoid necrosis (Fig. 3-29), in which the necrotic outlines of tissue structures (i.e., vessels, stroma) can still be recognized. In contrast, caseating necrosis is granular and amorphous. Postsurgical necrobiotic granulomas are rimmed with palisading histiocytes, resembling rheumatoid nodules. Surrounding the granulomas is a dense chronic inflammatory infiltrate with many eosinophils. These granulomas will eventually evolve to fibrous scar with occasional dystrophic calcification.

RADIATION CYSTITIS

CLINICAL FEATURES

Radiation cystitis can occur any time the bladder is included in the radiation field. Acute symptoms of radiation damage typically occur 4 to 6 weeks after the initiation of the therapy and are marked by the onset of dysuria, urgency, and frequency. Symptoms usually subside 2 to 6 weeks after radiation therapy is completed. Six months to 2 years after irradiation, patients

RADIATION CYSTITIS—FACT SHEET

Definition
▶ Cystitis secondary to irradiation to the bladder

Clinical Features
▶ Acute symptoms occur 4 to 6 weeks after radiation therapy; marked by dysuria, urgency, frequency, and, rarely, hemorrhagic cystitis with profuse hematuria
▶ Subacute symptoms with sudden painless hematuria due to chronic cystitis with ulcer 6 months to 2 years after irradiation
▶ Late complications as the result of fibrosis and bladder contracture may develop up to 10 years after irradiation

may develop sudden painless hematuria due to chronic cystitis and ulcers. Late complications can develop up to 10 years after irradiation and are the result of fibrosis and bladder contracture. The clinical severity and histologic features of radiation cystitis are both time and dose dependent.

PATHOLOGIC FEATURES

GROSS FINDINGS

In acute radiation cystitis, there is diffuse mucosal erythema with petechial hemorrhage. Partial desquamation and ulceration are present in severe cases. In the subacute period, circumscribed atrophic areas, ulceration, and necrosis may be present. In the contracted bladder, mucosal atrophy is often prominent.

RADIATION CYSTITIS—PATHOLOGIC FEATURES

Gross Findings

▶ Acute phase: diffuse mucosal erythema with petechial hemorrhage; partial desquamation and ulceration in severe cases

▶ Subacute phase: circumscribed atrophic area, ulceration and necrosis

▶ Chronic phase: contracted bladder with prominent mucosal atrophy

Microscopic Findings

▶ Early changes: edema and vascular congestion in lamina propria; mucosal erosion and ulceration; pseudocarcinomatous hyperplasia in some cases; cytologic atypia in urothelial cells. Urothelial atypia should not persist >1 year after radiation

▶ Late effects: mucosal ulceration; collagenization of the lamina propria and detrusor muscles

Differential Diagnosis

▶ Urothelial carcinoma in situ

▶ Invasive urothelial carcinoma

MICROSCOPIC FINDINGS

The early changes of radiation cystitis are characterized by marked edema and vascular congestion in lamina propria. Mucosal erosion and ulceration are present. The urothelial cells may exhibit cytologic atypia that mimics and sometimes is indistinguishable from CIS (Fig. 3-30A). These atypical cells may have prominent, hyperchromatic, yet degenerative-appearing nuclei and abundant vacuolated cytoplasm. Giant cells and multinucleated cells are sometimes present. In some cases, there is pseudocarcinomatous hyperplasia with epithelial nests extending into the lamina propria (Fig. 3-30B). They are seen adjacent to ectatic vessels that frequently contain fibrin (Fig. 3-30C). The adjacent stroma is typically edematous with extravasated red blood cells, inflammation, and hemosiderin deposition. Late effects of radiation include collagenization of the lamina propria and detrusor muscles and myointimal proliferation or hyalinization of the media of arterioles (Fig. 3-30D). Mucosal ulceration with abundant fibrinous exudates is often present. Atypical fibroblasts are invariably present in the fibrotic lamina propria. The urothelium may be atrophic or hyperplastic, may undergo squamous metaplasia, and may still exhibit focal radiation-induced nuclear atypia.

DIFFERENTIAL DIAGNOSIS

Radiation-induced atypia in urothelial cells should be differentiated from residual urothelial CIS. Urothelial cells with radiation atypia often have abundant cytoplasm and a low nuclear/cytoplasmic ratio. Although they exhibit marked nuclear atypia, the altered urothelial cells are cytologically more bizarre than CIS cells, and their nuclei lack the crisp nuclear detail and appear degenerative. Mitoses are rare. Atypia present more than 1 year after cessation of radiation therapy strongly suggests neoplastic atypia, rather than radiation atypia.

Urothelial hyperplasia, or pseudocarcinomatous hyperplasia, may mimic invasive urothelial carcinoma, especially the nested variant. However, the finding of urothelial nests encircling vessels in the lamina propria associated with fibrin deposition is a characteristic feature of radiation-induced hyperplasia. Invasion of the detrusor muscle provides evidence that the lesion in question is malignant.

CHEMOTHERAPY-INDUCED CYSTITIS

CLINICAL FEATURES

Among the chemical agents that are important in bladder cancer, the most thoroughly studied are Cytoxan (cyclophosphamide), thiotepa, and mitomycin C. Cytoxan is administered systemically for a variety of cancers of nonurothelial origin, as well as autoimmune diseases. It causes hemorrhagic cystitis due to the topical effect of its active metabolite, which is concentrated in urine. The occurrence of hemorrhagic cystitis seems unrelated to dose and has been reported in roughly 8% of patients receiving the drug, although the incidence decreases dramatically when patients are well hydrated. Bladder cancer associated with Cytoxan has been reported, although it is relatively uncommon. Busulfan, another alkylating agent, has also been implicated as a rare cause of hemorrhagic cystitis.

Thiotepa and mitomycin C are given intravesically for urothelial CIS and superficially invasive urothelial

---

CHEMOTHERAPY-INDUCED CYSTITIS—FACT SHEET

Definition

▶ Cystitis and hyperplasia induced by systemically or topically administered chemotherapeutic or immunologic agents

Clinical Features

▶ Systemic use of Cytoxan causes hemorrhagic cystitis

▶ Intravesical thiotepa or mitomycin C causes mucosal denudation and cystitis

▶ Intravesical bacille Calmette Guérin (BCG) causes irritation and submucosal nodules

Prognosis and Treatment

▶ Forced fluids in patients receiving Cytoxan greatly reduces the risk of hemorrhagic cystitis

▶ Rarely, BCG immunotherapy can lead to systemic tuberculosis requiring triple-antibiotic therapy. Localized BCG cystitis does not require antibiotics

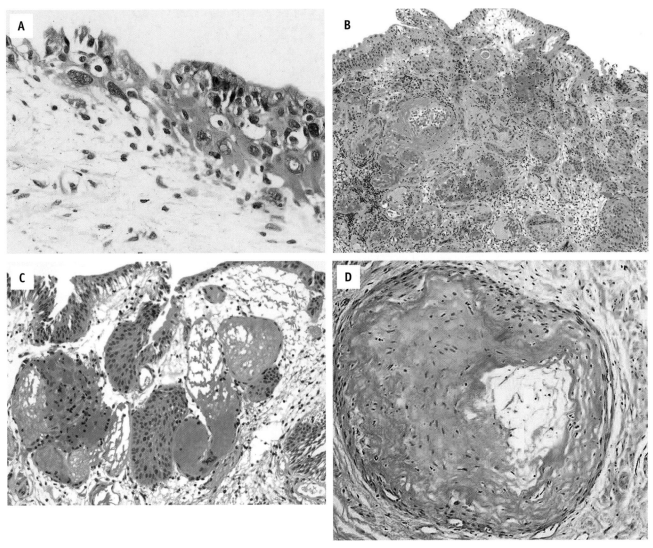

FIGURE 3-30

In radiation cystitis, the urothelial cells exhibit marked cytologic atypia that mimics carcinoma in situ (**A**). There may be epithelial hyperplasia with epithelial nests extending into the lamina propria (**B**). The stroma typically exhibits edema, hemorrhage, and ectatic vessels frequently containing fibrin (**C**). Late effects of irradiation include myointimal proliferation or hyalinization of the media of arterioles (**D**).

carcinoma. These agents act primarily as toxic substances to abrade the bladder mucosa, including tumors. Therefore, they result in mucosal denudation and symptoms of bladder irritation. They also cause cytologic atypia that is related to cellular degeneration and regeneration. The effect of the newer intravesical agent, gemcitabine, has not been well studied.

PATHOLOGIC FEATURES

GROSS FINDINGS

In Cytoxan-induced hemorrhagic cystitis, mucosal hyperemia, telangiectasia, hemorrhage, and focal necro-

sis may be observed. Bladder installed with thiotepa usually shows nonspecific findings, including dull erythematous patches, on cystoscopy.

MICROSCOPIC FINDINGS

In hemorrhagic cystitis, the bladder exhibits extensive ulceration and associated fibrinopurulent exudate. There is marked edema and hemorrhage throughout the lamina propria (Fig. 3-31A); the nonulcerated mucosa typically is thin with atypical cytology (Fig. 3-31B). During the regenerative phase, macrophages and fibroblasts populate the lamina propria, and the overlying epithelium exhibits increased mitoses, hyperplasia, and prominent cytologic atypia. Cytoxan produces cytologic atypia in the urothelium similar to that

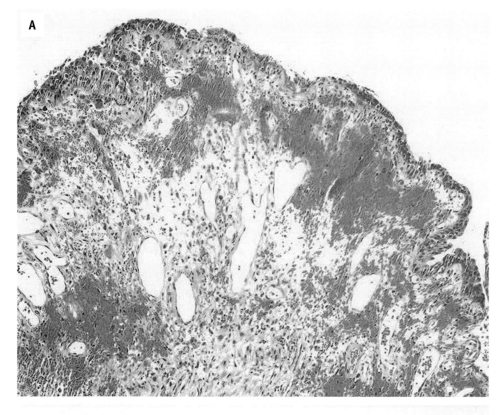

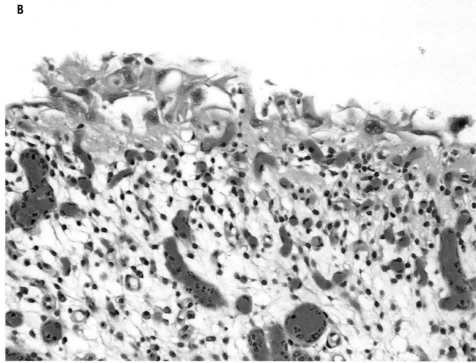

FIGURE 3-31

In chemotherapy-induced cystitis, there is focal mucosal denudation, diffuse hemorrhage, edema, and vascular ectasia in the lamina propria (**A**). Cytoxan produces cytologic atypia in the urothelium with cytoplasmic vacuolation, and nucleomegaly with degenerative changes (**B**).

CHEMOTHERAPY-INDUCED CYSTITIS—PATHOLOGIC FEATURES

Gross Findings

▶ Cytoxan-induced hemorrhagic cystitis: mucosal hyperemia, telangiectasia, hemorrhage, and focal necrosis
▶ Bladder installed with topical agents: nonspecific findings

Microscopic Findings

▶ Hemorrhagic cystitis: extensive ulceration and associated fibrinopurulent exudate; marked edema and hemorrhage throughout the lamina propria; nonulcerated mucosa with atypical cytology; occasionally pseudocarcinomatous hyperplasia with epithelial nests surrounding fibrin deposits
▶ Cystitis induced by topical agents: superficial urothelial cells with degenerative changes and nuclear atypia, mucosal denudation and regeneration
▶ BCG cystitis typically shows submucosal nonnecrotizing granulomas
▶ In all cystitis, reactive urothelial atypia may be present

Differential Diagnosis

▶ Urothelial dysplasia or carcinoma in situ

---

induced by irradiation, including cellular enlargement with cytoplasmic vacuolation, and nucleomegaly with degenerative changes and occasional multinucleation. Pseudocarcinomatous hyperplasia has been reported in several cases.

In patients treated with topical chemical agents, the urothelium shows degenerative changes in superficial cells, mucosal denudation, and regeneration. The lamina propria shows inflammation and edema. Cytologic atypia occurs only in the superficial cells. Umbrella cells have vacuolated cytoplasm, with enlarged and hyperchromatic nuclei containing degenerative, smudging chromatin. Mitotic figures are rare. Topical therapy for papillary urothelial carcinoma may result in truncated papillae lined with malignant cells, or papillae denuded of lining cells. In some cases, the urothelial neoplastic cells are destroyed on the surface but preserved in von Brunn's nests, cystitis cystica, or cystitis glandularis.

DIFFERENTIAL DIAGNOSIS

The criteria that distinguish Cytoxan-induced atypia from dysplasia or CIS is identical to that described earlier for differentiation of radiation atypia from neoplastic urothelial atypia. Topical intravesical chemotherapy atypia is limited to the umbrella cell layer, and the nuclear atypia appears degenerative without mitoses.

MÜLLERIAN LESIONS

ENDOMETRIOSIS

CLINICAL FEATURES

Involvement of the urinary tract occurs in approximately 1% of endometriosis case, and the bladder is the most common site of involvement. Classically, endometriosis affects women of reproductive age, with an average age of 35 years. However, it can rarely occur in postmenopausal women taking estrogen replacement therapy, or even in men treated with estrogen for prostate cancer. As many as 50% of patients have a history of prior pelvic surgery. Clinically, patients often present with urgency, frequency, and suprapubic pain, and occasionally with hematuria, although about 50% of patients have no vesical symptoms. Endometriosis involving the detrusor muscle may mimic interstitial cystitis.

PATHOLOGIC FEATURES

GROSS FINDINGS

At cystoscopy, the lesion usually appears as a domed, dark-colored cyst covered with hyperemic mucosa. The

---

ENDOMETRIOSIS—FACT SHEET

Definition

▶ Ectopic endometrial tissue in the bladder

Incidence and Location

▶ Bladder is the most common site of involvement along the urinary tract, accounting for 1% of endometriosis cases

Gender, Race, and Age Distribution

▶ Women of reproductive age
▶ Rarely in postmenopausal women or men receiving estrogen therapy

Clinical Features

▶ Urinary urgency, frequency, suprapubic pain, and occasionally hematuria
▶ 50% with history of pelvic surgery

Prognosis and Treatment

▶ Conservative surgery/hormonal therapy for women who desire fertility
▶ Definitive surgery for women beyond reproductive age

ENDOMETRIOSIS—PATHOLOGIC FEATURES

Gross Findings

▶ Dark-colored, domed cyst covered with hyperemic mucosa at cystoscopy

Microscopic Findings

▶ Endometrial glands, stromal cells, recent or old hemorrhage
▶ Can coexist with endosalpingiosis and endocervicosis, called "müllerianosis"

Differential Diagnosis

▶ Adenocarcinoma

adjacent bladder wall may be thickened due to inflammation and fibrosis. However, cystoscopy may be normal if the lesion is situated in muscularis propria or in serosa.

MICROSCOPIC FINDINGS

Lesions resemble those of endometriosis elsewhere (Fig. 3-32). The diagnosis relies on identification of at least two of the three components: endometrial glands, endometrial stromal cells, and recent or old hemorrhage.

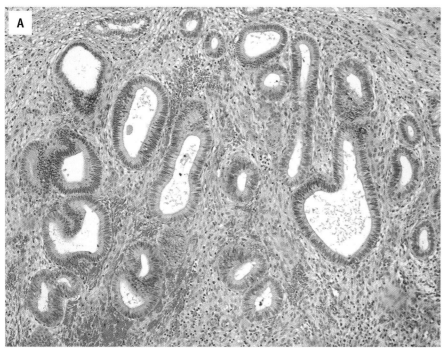

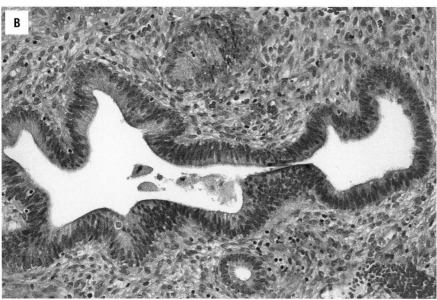

FIGURE 3-32

In endometriosis, large glands are embedded in cellular stroma (**A**). Glands are lined by pseudostratified columnar cells (**B**).

DIFFERENTIAL DIAGNOSIS

Endometriosis with minimal stroma, especially when it involves muscularis propria, should be differentiated from invasive adenocarcinoma of the bladder. Adenocarcinoma invariably has frank nuclear atypia.

PROGNOSIS AND THERAPY

In patients who desire future fertility, conservative surgery and/or hormonal therapy is often recommended. In women beyond reproductive age, definitive surgical treatment is preferred, with removal of the ectopic tissue, relief of obstruction, and removal of the ovaries with or without hysterectomy.

ENDOCERVICOSIS

CLINICAL FEATURES

Endocervicosis is a rare condition characterized by the presence of endocervical-like glands in the bladder wall. It affects women in their fourth and fifth decades. Patients often present with suprapubic pain, frequency, and dysuria. They often have a history of cesarean section.

PATHOLOGIC FEATURES

GROSS FINDINGS

Endocervicosis mainly involves the muscularis propria. Cystoscopy may show a submucosal nodule.

MICROSCOPIC FINDINGS

There is a haphazard proliferation of irregularly shaped glands (Fig. 3-33A) that are lined with columnar, mucin-secreting, endocervical-like epithelium (Fig. 3-33B). Ciliated cells are often present among the mucinous cells. Extravasation of mucin is present in all cases, secondary to gland rupture.

DIFFERENTIAL DIAGNOSIS

Because endocervicosis is often located deep within the bladder wall and an has a haphazard growth pattern, it may be mistaken for an invasive adenocarcinoma. However, it has no or at most minimal nuclear atypia, no mitoses, and no stromal tissue reaction.

PROGNOSIS AND THERAPY

This lesion is benign. Local treatment, including transurethral resection or partial cystectomy, typically suffices.

ENDOCERVICOSIS—FACT SHEET

Definition
► Presence of endocervical-like glands in the bladder wall

Incidence and Location
► Involves predominantly muscular wall of the bladder
► May also involve mucosa or serosa

Gender, Race, and Age Distribution
► Affects women of fourth and fifth decades

Clinical Features
► Suprapubic pain, frequency, and dysuria
► History of cesarean section

Prognosis and Treatment
► Benign
► Local treatment, including transurethral resection, or partial cystectomy

---

ENDOCERVICOSIS—PATHOLOGIC FEATURES

Gross Findings
► Cystoscopy: submucosal nodule

Microscopic Findings
► Haphazard proliferation of irregularly shaped glands lined with columnar, mucin-secreting, endocervical-like epithelium
► Ciliated cells are often present among the mucinous cells
► Extravasation of mucin present in all cases secondary to gland rupture
► Can coexist with endosalpingiosis and endometriosis, called "müllerianosis"

Differential Diagnosis
► Invasive adenocarcinoma

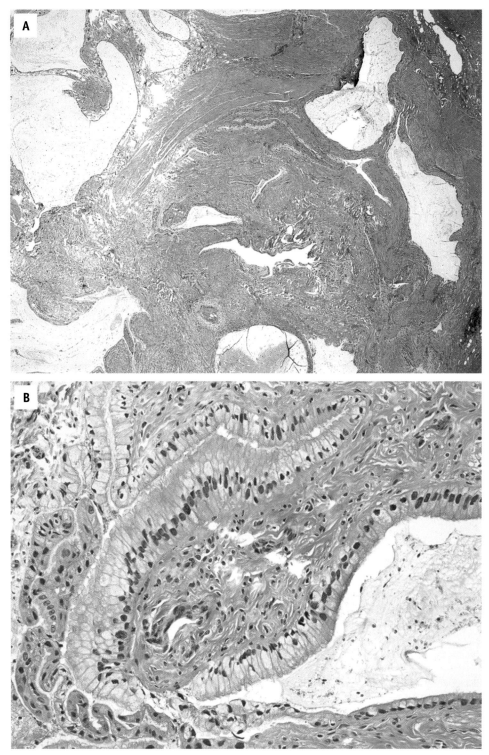

FIGURE 3-33

In endocervicosis, large, irregularly shaped glands are haphazardly arranged in the muscularis propria (**A**). Glands are lined with benign mucin-producing columnar cells (**B**).

DEVELOPMENTAL MALFORMATIONS

BLADDER EXSTROPHY

CLINICAL FEATURES

Bladder exstrophy is a congenital abnormality in which the bladder mucosa is everted to the surface of the lower abdominal wall. It results from defective lower abdominal development during embryogenesis. It is often accompanied by other malformations, such as epispadias, intestinal malformation, and defective spinal closure. The incidence of bladder exstrophy is estimated to be 3.3 cases per 100,000 live births. The male-to-female ratio is 2.3:1. The risk of a child being born with bladder exstrophy in a given family is 1 in 100 when there is an affected sibling, and 1 in 70 with an affected parent. The cause of bladder exstrophy is unknown.

PATHOLOGIC FEATURES

GROSS FINDINGS

In exstrophy, the urinary tract is open to the body wall from the urethral meatus to the umbilicus. The mucosa of the bladder and urethra is fused to the adjacent skin. At birth, the mucosa appears normal. Trauma and infection quickly ensue, and the mucosa shows ulceration, congestion, edema, and fibrosis.

BLADDER EXSTROPHY—FACT SHEET

Definition
▶ Congenital abnormality in which the bladder mucosa is everted to the surface of the lower abdominal wall

Incidence and Location
▶ 3.3 cases per 100,000 live births

Gender, Race, and Age Distribution
▶ Male/female ratio = 2.3:1

Clinical Features
▶ Risk of recurrence in a given family is 1 in 100 with an affected sibling, 1 in 70 with an affected parent

Prognosis and Treatment
▶ Surgical correction
▶ Untreated exstrophy predisposes patients to carcinoma, particularly adenocarcinoma

---

BLADDER EXSTROPHY—PATHOLOGIC FEATURES

Gross Findings
▶ Mucosa of the bladder and urethra fused to the adjacent skin
▶ Mucosa appears normal at birth
▶ Mucosal ulceration, congestion, edema, and fibrosis late in disease

Microscopic Findings
▶ Frequently acute and chronic inflammation with ulceration and squamous and glandular metaplastic changes resembling colon in the mucosa before surgical closure
▶ After closure, mucosa often remains inflamed, and metaplastic changes are common

---

MICROSCOPIC FINDINGS

The bladder mucosa frequently shows acute and chronic inflammation with ulceration and metaplastic changes at the time of surgical closure. Squamous and intestinal metaplasia are absent or minimal at birth but become extensive with time. After closure, the mucosa often remains inflamed and metaplastic changes are common.

PROGNOSIS AND THERAPY

The chronic inflammation and metaplasia in untreated exstrophy predisposes patients to carcinoma, particularly adenocarcinoma. With early surgical intervention, such exstrophy-associated carcinoma becomes rare.

URACHAL ANOMALY

CLINICAL FEATURES

During embryogenesis, the allantois and the superior end of the presumptive bladder undergo regression and are transformed into a ligamentous band (urachus or median umbilical ligament) that runs through the subperitoneal fat from the bladder dome to the umbilicus. Failure of part or all of the urachus to close results in one of the following conditions: patent urachus (Fig. 3-34A), umbilical urachal sinus (Fig. 3-34B), vesicourachal diverticulum (see Fig. 3-34C), or urachal cyst (Fig. 3-34D). Patent urachus is extremely rare, occurring in fewer than 3 per 1 million pediatric patients in one study, and accounting for 15% of urachal abnormalities. Urachal cyst is more common and accounts for 36% of urachal abnormalities. Symptoms include leakage of urine from the umbilicus, urinary tract infec-

URACHAL ANOMALY—FACT SHEET

Definition

▶ Developmental abnormality of urachus due to failure of part or all of the urachus to close

Incidence and Location

▶ Types of urachal abnormalities: patent urachus, umbilical urachal sinus, vesicourachal diverticulum, urachal cyst
▶ Extremely rare
▶ Urachal cyst most common

Clinical Features

▶ Urine leakage from the umbilicus
▶ Urinary tract infections
▶ Stone or carcinoma rare complications

Prognosis and Treatment

▶ Observation
▶ Surgery if symptomatic

URACHAL ANOMALY—PATHOLOGIC FEATURES

Gross Findings

▶ Urachal cysts may appear as thin-walled submucosal cysts in the bladder dome

Microscopic Findings

▶ Urachus or urachal cysts lined with urothelium or cuboidal epithelium
▶ Columnar epithelium may be present
▶ The lining of the urachal anomaly may be denuded and inflamed

Differential Diagnosis

▶ Omphalitis
▶ Patent omphalomesenteric duct
▶ Infected umbilical vessels

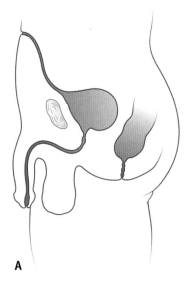

A

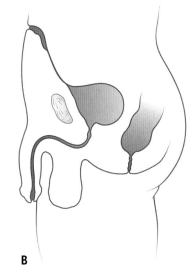

B

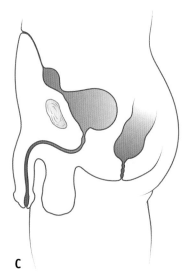

C

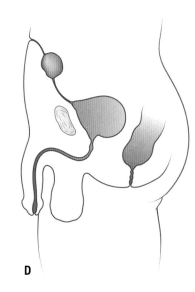

D

FIGURE 3-34

Urachal anomalies include patent urachus (**A**), umbilical urachal sinus (**B**), vesicourachal diverticulum (**C**), and urachal cyst (**D**).

tions, and peritonitis resulting from perforation of the patent urachus. Rarely, stones or carcinomas can arise within the urachal malformation.

PATHOLOGIC FEATURES

GROSS FINDINGS

Urachal cysts may appear as thin-walled, submucosal cysts in the bladder dome.

MICROSCOPIC FINDINGS

The urachus is usually lined with urothelium or cuboidal epithelium (Fig. 3-35), but columnar epithelium may be present. The lining may be denuded and inflamed (in the above-mentioned urachal abnormality).

DIFFERENTIAL DIAGNOSIS

Patent urachus should be differentiated from omphalitis, patent omphalomesenteric duct, and infected umbilical vessels. Analysis of the periumbilical fluid for creatinine and urea is useful in differentiating a patent urachus from these other conditions.

PROGNOSIS AND THERAPY

In the management of patent urachus, observation may be indicated for young infants with symptoms, because closure of the urachus is not complete at birth, and spontaneous closure can occur within the first few months of life. Treatment of the urachal cyst depends on the symptoms. In children with a small, asymptomatic mass, watchful waiting may be appropriate. However, definitive surgical excision is indicated for an infected urachal cyst.

BLADDER DIVERTICULUM

CLINICAL FEATURES

Most cases of bladder diverticulum result from increased intravesical pressure and occur in men older than 50 years of age who have urinary outflow obstruction due to benign prostatic hyperplasia. Infrequently, congenital diverticula occur in children associated with posterior urethral valves or neurogenic bladder without evidence of outflow obstruction. Occasionally, patients have genetic connective tissue

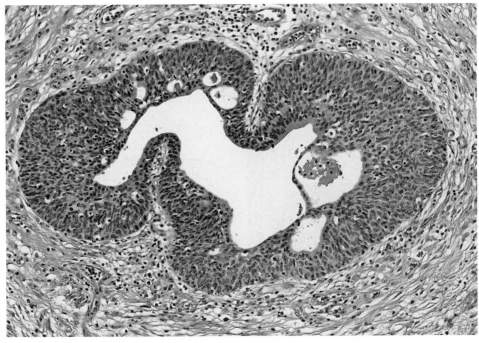

FIGURE 3-35
The urachus is frequently lined with urothelial cells with intraepithelial inflammatory cells.

a small bladder. Diverticula are most common in the vicinity of the ureteral orifices, the bladder dome, and the region of the urethral orifice. Diverticula may grossly distort the external surface of the bladder. The diverticulum and the bladder proper often are connected via a narrow orifice that traverses the inner muscularis propria layer (Fig. 3-36). The bladder mucosa adjoining the diverticulum is usually hyperemic or ulcerated, and the muscularis propria is hypertrophic.

MICROSCOPIC FINDINGS

In the wall of most acquired diverticula, few, if any, muscle layers are identified. Congenital diverticula may contain an attenuated outer layer of the muscularis propria. Infrequently, the urothelial lining of the diverticulum may undergo squamous or glandular metaplasia due to local irritation.

disorders with localized weakness and a defect in the detrusor muscles.

PATHOLOGIC FEATURES

GROSS FINDINGS

Acquired bladder diverticula are usually multiple and associated with urinary outlet obstruction. Congenital diverticula in children are often solitary and occur in

PROGNOSIS AND THERAPY

Small diverticula are usually asymptomatic. Larger diverticula may be associated with infection and stone formation. Carcinoma, mostly urothelial carcinoma, occurs in fewer than 10% of the cases. Surgical intervention may be required in the setting of recurring infections, persistent vesicoureteral reflux, bladder outlet obstruction, or significant ureteral obstruction.

AMYLOIDOSIS

CLINICAL FEATURES

The bladder can be secondarily involved in systemic amyloidosis or, rarely, affected by primary amyloidosis. In the latter situation, the disease manifests throughout adulthood but is more common after the fifth decade. In patients with systemic amyloidosis, hematuria is universal and usually severe. Although primary localized amyloidosis also manifests with hematuria, it is in general much less severe.

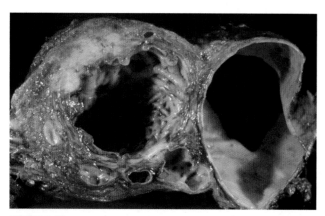

FIGURE 3-36
Multiple diverticula are present. The bladder proper has markedly trabeculated mucosa due to outflow obstruction. Note that there is an invasive urothelial carcinoma within the bladder wall.

AMYLOIDOSIS—FACT SHEET

Definition
▶ Deposition of amyloid protein in the bladder

Incidence and Location
▶ Rare

Gender, Race, and Age Distribution
▶ Throughout adulthood but more common after fifth decade

Clinical Features
▶ Hematuria
▶ Bladder involvement as part of systemic amyloidosis or primary localized disease

Prognosis and Treatment
▶ Primary localized amyloidosis may recur locally
▶ Laser ablation or surgical resection for localized amyloidosis

---

AMYLOIDOSIS—PATHOLOGIC FEATURES

Gross Findings
▶ Diffuse amyloidosis: mucosal erythema, sometimes with petechial hemorrhage or necrosis
▶ Localized amyloidosis: mucosa-lined domed mass

Microscopic Findings
▶ Deposition of eosinophilic amorphous amyloid proteins in lamina propria and the connective tissue surrounding muscle fascicles
▶ Deposition in vascular wall less common and usually in systemic amyloidosis
▶ Congestion and hemorrhage, scant inflammation

Ultrastructural Features
▶ Randomly arranged, rigid, nonbranching, 8- to 10-nm fibrils are diagnostic of amyloidosis

Immunohistochemical and Histochemical Features
▶ Congo red birefringence by polarizing microscopy is the most specific stain
▶ Fluorescence of thioflavine T is the most sensitive stain
▶ Serum amyloid P component is present in the majority of cases by immunohistochemistry
▶ Immunoglobulin light chain λ or κ also frequently present
▶ Transthyretin occasionally detected

PATHOLOGIC FEATURES

GROSS FINDINGS

If the bladder is widely involved, diffuse mucosal erythema, sometimes with petechial hemorrhage or necrosis, can be seen at cystoscopy. A localized amyloidoma appears as a submucosal domed mass covered by urothelium.

MICROSCOPIC FINDINGS

Amyloid protein appears as eosinophilic amorphous material deposited preferentially in the lamina propria and extending into the connective tissue surrounding muscle fascicles (Fig. 3-37A). Deposition in the vascular wall is less common and usually is seen in systemic amyloidosis (Fig. 3-37B). Congestion and hemorrhage are common because of damage to the blood vessels, but inflammation is scant.

ANCILLARY STUDIES

Congo red birefringence by polarizing microscopy is the most specific stain for amyloidosis (Fig. 3-37C), and fluorescence of thioflavine T is the most sensitive stain. Immunohistochemistry detects serum amyloid P component (SAP) in the majority of cases. Immunoglobulin light chain λ or κ is also frequently present, and transthyretin is occasionally detected. Randomly arranged, rigid, nonbranching 8- to 10-nm fibrils are virtually diagnostic of amyloidosis by ultrastructural study.

PROGNOSIS AND THERAPY

For small, localized lesions, fulguration or laser therapy seems to be a reasonable approach. For larger lesions, transurethral resection or partial cystectomy may be necessary. Dimethyl sulfoxide has been used to solubilize amyloid deposits with dubious effect. Regular cystoscopic follow-up is necessary, because local recurrence is not uncommon in primary localized amyloidosis.

ECTOPIC PROSTATE TISSUE

CLINICAL FEATURES

Polyps composed of prostate tissue are rarely found in the bladder. They predominantly occur in young men, and the presenting symptom is usually hematuria.

PATHOLOGIC FEATURES

GROSS FINDINGS

Most lesions arise in the trigone. There is usually a single, papillary or polypoid mass covered with urothelial mucosa.

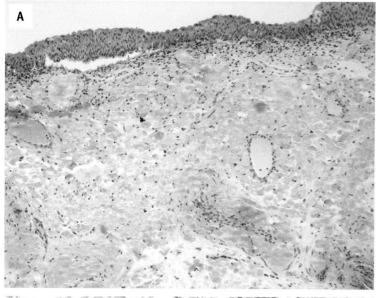

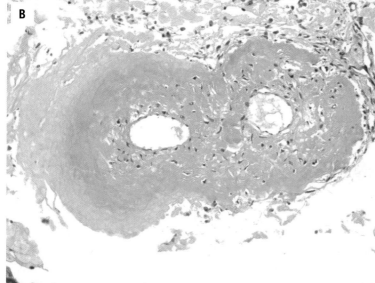

FIGURE 3-37

Lamina propria and detrusor muscle are effaced with eosinophilic amorphous amyloid protein (**A**). Amyloidosis also involves a blood vessel (**B**), confirmed by the presence of "apple green" birefringence demonstrated by Congo red staining (**C**).

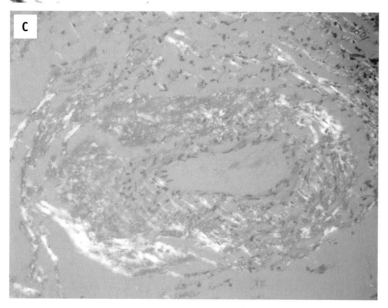

ECTOPIC PROSTATE—FACT SHEET

Definition
► Normal prostatic tissue outside the prostate gland

Incidence and Location
► Most arise in the trigone

Gender, Race, and Age Distribution
► Occurs in young men

Clinical Features
► Hematuria

Prognosis and Treatment
► Benign
► Complete removal by transurethral resection

MICROSCOPIC FINDINGS

The surface is lined by urothelial cells, prostatic glandular epithelium, or a combination of both. The submucosal component is composed of stroma and prostatic glands that may show focal crowding or cystic dilatation.

ANCILLARY STUDIES

IMMUNOHISTOCHEMISTRY

The prostatic epithelial cells on the surface and in the submucosa are characteristically positive for PSA and PSAP.

ECTOPIC PROSTATE—PATHOLOGIC FEATURES

Gross Findings
► Usually single, papillary or polypoid lesion covered with urothelial mucosa

Microscopic Findings
► Surface lined with urothelial cells, prostatic glandular epithelium, or both
► Submucosal component composed of stroma and prostatic glands that may show focal crowding or cystic dilatation

Immunohistochemical Features
► PSA and PSAP +

Differential Diagnosis
► Prostatic urethral polyp
► "Middle lobe" benign prostatic hyperplasia

DIFFERENTIAL DIAGNOSIS

Prostatic urethral polyps are identical to ectopic prostatic tissue within the bladder, yet the former are restricted to the prostatic urethra. Benign prostatic hyperplasia, especially "middle lobe" hyperplasia that predominantly involves the periurethral zone at the bladder neck, may expand into the bladder lumen and mimic ectopic prostate tissue.

PROGNOSIS AND THERAPY

Ectopic prostate tissue is benign. Complete removal of the lesion by transurethral resection suffices.

SUGGESTED READINGS

Bostwick DG, Eble JN: Prostate Urological Surgical Pathology. St. Louis, Mosby, 1997.
Eble JN, Sauter G, Epstein JI, Sesterhenn IA: Pathology and Genetics: Tumours of the Urinary System and Male Genital Organs. Lyon, France, IARC Press, 2004.
Epstein JI, Amin MB, Reuter VE: Bladder Biopsy Interpretation. Philadelphia, Lippincott Williams & Wilkins, 2004.
Murphy WM, Grignon DJ, Perlman EJ: Tumors of the Kidney, Bladder, and Related Urinary Structures, 4th ed. Washington, DC, AFIP, 2004.

Anatomy and Histology

Philip AT, Amin MB, Tamboli P, et al: Intravesical adipose tissue: Quantitative study of its presence and location with implications for therapy and prognosis. Am J Surg Pathol 2000;24:1286–1290.
Reuter VE: Urinary bladder and ureter. In Sternberg SS (ed): Histology for Pathologists, 2nd ed. New York, Raven Press, 1997, pp 835–847.
Ro JY, Ayala AG, El-Naggar A: Muscularis mucosa of urinary bladder: Importance for staging and treatment. Am J Surg Pathol 1987;11:668–673.

Reactive Proliferative Changes of the Urothelium

Ito N, Hirose M, Shirai T, et al: Lesions of the urinary bladder epithelium in 125 autopsy cases. Acta Pathol Jpn 1981;31:545–557.
Masumori N, Tsukamoto T: Pelvic lipomatosis associated with proliferative cystitis: Case report and review of the Japanese literature. Int J Urol 1999;6:44–49.
Volmar KE, Chan TY, De Marzo AM, Epstein JI: Florid von Brunn nests mimicking urothelial carcinoma: A morphologic and immunohistochemical comparison to the nested variant of urothelial carcinoma. Am J Surg Pathol 2003;27:1243–1252.
Wiener DP, Koss LG, Sablay B, Freed SZ: The prevalence and significance of Brunn's nests, cystitis cystica and squamous metaplasia in normal bladders. J Urol 1979;122:317–321.

Metaplasia of the Urothelium

Allan CH, Epstein JI: Nephrogenic adenoma of the prostatic urethra: A mimicker of prostate adenocarcinoma. Am J Surg Pathol 2001;25:802–808.
Bullock PS, Thoni DE, Murphy WM: The significance of colonic mucosa (intestinal metaplasia) involving the urinary tract. Cancer 1987;59:2086–2090.
Corica FA, Husmann DA, Churchill BM, et al: Intestinal metaplasia is not a strong risk factor for bladder cancer: Study of 53 cases with long-term follow-up. Urology 1997;50:427–431.

Gupta A, Wang HL, Policarpio-Nicolas ML, et al: Expression of alpha-methylacyl-coenzyme A racemase in nephrogenic adenoma. Am J Surg Pathol 2004;28:1224–1229.

Jacobs LB, Brooks JD, Epstein JI: Differentiation of colonic metaplasia from adenocarcinoma of urinary bladder. Hum Pathol 1997;28:1152–1157.

Khan MS, Thornhill JA, Gaffney E, et al: Keratinising squamous metaplasia of the bladder: Natural history and rationalization of management based on review of 54 years experience. Eur Urol 2002;42:469–474.

Lopez-Beltran A, Cheng L, Andersson L, et al: Preneoplastic non-papillary lesions and conditions of the urinary bladder: An update based on the Ancona International Consultation. Virchows Arch 2002;440:3–11.

Mazal PR, Schaufler R, Altenhuber-Muller R, et al: Derivation of nephrogenic adenomas from renal tubular cells in kidney-transplant recipients. N Engl J Med 2002;29:653–659.

Skinnider BF, Oliva E, Young RH, Amin MB: Expression of alpha-methylacyl-CoA racemase (P504S) in nephrogenic adenoma: A significant immunohistochemical pitfall compounding the differential diagnosis with prostatic adenocarcinoma. Am J Surg Pathol 2004;28:701–705.

Young RH, Bostwick DG: Florid cystitis glandularis of intestinal type with mucin extravasation: A mimic of adenocarcinoma. Am J Surg Pathol 1996;20:1462–1468.

Inflammation and Infection

Benson MC, Kaplan MS, O'Toole K, Romagnoli M: A report of cytomegalovirus cystitis and a review of other genitourinary manifestations of the acquired immune deficiency syndrome. J Urol 1988;140:153–154.

Boldorini R, Veggiani C, Barco D, Monga G: Kidney and urinary tract polyomavirus infection and distribution: Molecular biology investigation of 10 consecutive autopsies. Arch Pathol Lab Med 2005;129:69–73.

Curran FT: Malakoplakia of the bladder. Br J Urol 1987;59:559–563.

Giannakopoulos S, Alivizatos G, Deliveliotis C, et al: Encrusted cystitis and pyelitis. Eur Urol 2001;39:446–448.

Hansson S, Hanson E, Hjalmas K, et al: Follicular cystitis in girls with untreated asymptomatic or covert bacteriuria. J Urol 1990;143:330–332.

Itano NM, Malek RS: Eosinophilic cystitis in adults. J Urol 2001;165:805–807.

Koga S, Shindo K, Matsuya F, et al: Acute hemorrhagic cystitis caused by adenovirus following renal transplantation: Review of the literature. J Urol 1993;149:838–839.

Lenk S, Schroeder J: Genitourinary tuberculosis. Curr Opin Urol 2001;11:93–98.

Long JP Jr, Althausen AF: Malakoplakia: A 25-year experience with a review of the literature. J Urol 1989;141:1328–1331.

Meria P, Desgrippes A, Arfi C, Le Duc A: Encrusted cystitis and pyelitis. J Urol 1998;160:3–9.

Ohtsuki Y, Furihata M, Iwata J, et al: Multinucleated giant cells in submucosal layer of human urinary bladder: An immunohistochemical and electron microscopic study. Pathol Res Pract. 2000;196:293–298.

Patel NP, Lavengood RW, Fernandes M, et al: Gas-forming infections in genitourinary tract. Urology 1992;39:341–345.

Paul JF, Verma S, Berry K: Urinary schistosomiasis. Emerg Med J 2002;19:483–484.

Quint HJ, Drach GW, Rappaport WD, Hoffmann C: Emphysematous cystitis: A review of the spectrum of disease. J Urol 1992;147:134–137.

Rice SJ, Bishop JA, Apperley J, Gardner SD: BK virus as cause of haemorrhagic cystitis after bone marrow transplantation. Lancet 1985;12:844–845.

Rosamilia A, Igawa Y, Higashi S: Pathology of interstitial cystitis. Int J Urol 2003;10(Suppl):S11–S15.

Tomaszewski JE, Landis JR, Russack V, et al; Interstitial Cystitis Database Study Group: Biopsy features are associated with primary symptoms in interstitial cystitis: Results from the Interstitial Cystitis Database study. Urology 2001;57(Suppl 1):67–81.

Verhagen PC, Nikkels PG, de Jong TP: Eosinophilic cystitis. Arch Dis Child 2001;84:344–346.

Warren JW, Keay SK: Interstitial cystitis. Curr Opin Urol 2002;12:69–74.

Wise GJ, Silver DA: Fungal infections of the genitourinary system. J Urol 1993;149:1377–1388.

Wise GJ, Marella VK: Genitourinary manifestations of tuberculosis. Urol Clin North Am 2003;30:111–121.

Wise GJ, Talluri GS, Marella VK: Fungal infections of the genitourinary system: Manifestations, diagnosis, and treatment. Urol Clin North Am 1999;26:701–718,vii.

Young RH: Papillary and polypoid cystitis: A report of eight cases. Am J Surg Pathol 1988;12:542–546.

Therapy-related Changes

Baker PM, Young RH: Radiation-induced pseudocarcinomatous proliferations of the urinary bladder: A report of 4 cases. Hum Pathol 2001;31:678–683.

Bhan R, Pisharodi LR, Gudlaugsson E, Bedrossian C: Cytological, histological, and clinical correlations in intravesical bacillus Calmette-Guérin immunotherapy. Ann Diagn Pathol 1998;2:55–60.

Chan TY, Epstein JI: Radiation or chemotherapy cystitis with "pseudocarcinomatous" features. Am J Surg Pathol 2004;28:909–913.

Crew JP, Jephcott CR, Reynard JM: Radiation-induced haemorrhagic cystitis. Eur Urol 2001;40:111–123.

Eble JN, Banks ER: Post-surgical necrobiotic granulomas of urinary bladder. Urology 1990;35:454–457.

Lage JM, Bauer WC, Kelley DR, et al: Histological parameters and pitfalls in the interpretation of bladder biopsies in bacillus Calmette-Guérin treatment of superficial bladder cancer. J Urol 1986;135:916–919.

Lopez-Beltran A, Luque RJ, Mazzucchelli R, et al: Changes produced in the urothelium by traditional and newer therapeutic procedures for bladder cancer. J Clin Pathol 2002;55:641–647.

Murphy WM, Soloway MS, Finebaum PJ: Pathological changes associated with topical chemotherapy for superficial bladder cancer. J Urol 1980;126:461–464.

Spagnolo DV, Waring PM: Bladder granulomata after bladder surgery. Am J Clin Pathol 1986;86:430–437.

Suresh UR, Smith VJ, Lupton EW, Haboubi NY: Radiation disease of the urinary tract: Histological features of 18 cases. J Clin Pathol 1993;46:228–231.

Müllerian Lesions

Clement PB, Young RH: Endocervicosis of the urinary bladder: A report of six cases of a benign mullerian lesion that may mimic adenocarcinoma. Am J Surg Pathol 1992;16:533–542.

Comiter CV: Endometriosis of the urinary tract. Urol Clin North Am 2002;29:625–635.

Parker RL, Dadmanesh F, Young RH, Clement PB: Polypoid endometriosis: A clinicopathologic analysis of 24 cases and a review of the literature. Am J Surg Pathol 2004;28:285–297.

Young RH: Pseudoneoplastic lesions of the urinary bladder and urethra: A selective review with emphasis on recent information. Semin Diagn Pathol 1997;14:133–146.

Young RH, Clement PB: Mullerianosis of the urinary bladder. Mod Pathol 1996;9:731–737.

Developmental Malformation

Bauer SB, Retik AB: Urachal anomalies and related umbilical disorders. Urol Clin North Am 1978;5:195–211.

Eble JN: Abnormalities of the rrachus. In Young RH (ed): Pathology of the Urinary Bladder. New York, Churchill Livingstone, 1989.

Mildenberger H, Kluth D, Dziuba M: Embryology of bladder exstrophy. J Pediatr Surg 1988;23:166–170.

Rudin L, Tannenbaum M, Lattimer JK: Histologic analysis of the exstrophied bladder after anatomical closure. J Urol 1972;108:802–807.

Smeulders N, Woodhouse CR: Neoplasia in adult exstrophy patients. BJU Int 2001;87:623–628.

Bladder Diverticulum

Melekos MD, Asbach HW, Barbalias GA: Vesical diverticula: Etiology, diagnosis, tumorigenesis, and treatment. Analysis of 74 cases. Urology 1987;30:453–457.

Micic S, Ilic V: Incidence of neoplasm in vesical diverticula. J Urol
    1983;129:734–735.
Schiff M Jr, Lytton B: Congenital diverticulum of the bladder. J Urol
    1970;104:111–115.

Amyloidosis

Khan SM, Birch PJ, Bass PS, et al: Localized amyloidosis of the lower
    genitourinary tract: A clinicopathological and immunohistochemical
    study of nine cases. Histopathology 1992;21:143–147.
Tirzaman O, Wahner-Roedler DL, Malek RS, et al: Primary localized
    amyloidosis of the urinary bladder: A case series of 31 patients. Mayo
    Clin Proc 2000;75:1264–1268.

Ectopic Prostate Tissue

Dogra PN, Ansari MS, Khaitan A, et al: Ectopic prostate: an unusual
    bladder tumor. Int Urol Nephrol 2002;34:525–526.
Remick DG Jr, Kumar NB: Benign polyps with prostatic-type epithelium
    of the urethra and the urinary bladder: A suggestion of histogenesis
    based on histologic and immunohistochemical studies. Am J Surg
    Pathol 1984;8:833–839.

4

Neoplasms of the Urinary Bladder

Cristina Magi–Galluzzi • Ming Zhou • Jonathan I. Epstein

Tumors of the urinary bladder include neoplasms of virtually all types of tissue derivation, and the 2004 World Health Organization (WHO) Classification of tumors of the urinary system and male genital organs reflects the diversity (Table 4-1). The histologic classification of tumors of the urinary tract comprises urothelial tumors, squamous neoplasms, glandular neoplasms, neuroendocrine tumors, melanocytic tumors, mesenchymal tumors, hematopoietic and lymphoid tumors, and miscellaneous tumors. For practical pur-

---

TABLE 4-1

WHO histological classification of tumors of the urinary tract

UROTHELIAL TUMORS

Infiltrating urothelial carcinoma
With squamous differentiation
With glandular differentiation
With trophoblastic differentiation
Nested
Microcystic
Micropapillary
Lymphoepithelioma-like
Lymphoma-like
Plasmacytoid
Sarcomatoid
Giant Cell
Undifferentiated

Non-invasive urothelial neoplasms
Urothelial carcinoma in-situ (CIS)
Non-invasive papillary urothelial carcinoma, high grade
Non-invasive papillary urothelial carcinoma, low grade
Non-invasive papillary urothelial neoplasm of low
  malignant potential
Urothelial papilloma
Inverted urothelial papilloma

SQUAMOUS NEOPLASMS

Squamous cell carcinoma
Verrucous carcinoma
Squamous cell papilloma

GLANDULAR NEOPLASMS

Adenocarcinoma
Enteric

Mucinous
Signet-ring cell
Villous adenoma

NEUROENDOCRINE TUMORS

Small cell carcinoma
Carcinoid
Paraganglioma

MELANOCYTIC TUMORS

Malignant melanoma
Nevus

MESENCHYMAL TUMORS

Rhabdomyosarcoma
Leiomyosarcoma
Angiosarcoma
Osteosarcoma
Malignant fibrous histiocytoma
Leiomyoma
Hemangioma
Other

HEMATOPOIETIC AND LYMPHOID TUMORS

Lymphoma
Plasmacytoma

MISCELLANEOUS TUMORS

Carcinoma of Skene, Cowper, and Littre glands
Metastatic tumors and tumors extending from other organs

poses, we will divide lesions into epithelial neoplasms of the urinary bladder and nonepithelial neoplasms of the urinary bladder.

EPITHELIAL NEOPLASMS OF THE URINARY BLADDER

Bladder cancer is the seventh to ninth most common cancer worldwide, and the fourth most common cancer among American men. Approximately 330,000 new cases and more than 130,000 deaths per year have been reported. Cancer of the urinary bladder accounts for about 3.2% of all cancers worldwide. It is more common in men than in women, with a ratio of 3.5:1.

Bladder cancer is primarily attributable to smoking, which accounts for 65% of male and 30% of female cases in some developed countries. Other less important causes include analgesic abuse (phenacetin), some types of cancer chemotherapy, and occupational exposure to chemicals such as 2-naphthylamine. In Egypt and some Asian regions, chronic cystitis caused by *Schistosoma haematobium* infection is a major risk factor. The treatment of bladder cancer often permits long-term survival in developed countries, where 65% of patients live for at least 5 years after diagnosis.

UROTHELIAL NEOPLASMS (TRANSITIONAL CELL TUMORS)

The category of urothelial neoplasms of the urinary bladder encompasses a group of rather diverse entities all of which share the common origins from a transformed urothelial cell. Approximately 90% of bladder tumors are classified as urothelial carcinoma, also referred to as transitional cell carcinoma (TCC), and are believed to originate from transformation of the normal urothelium. Localized proliferation of transformed cells can give rise to a carcinoma in-situ, which may take several clinical forms, not necessarily associated with high grade or high risk of progression. Invasion can occur by growth into the lamina propria and muscularis propria of the bladder, as occurs in 25% of the cases. The non-invasive form of urothelial lesions can be further subdivided in two subgroups: flat and papillary.

Flat Urothelial Lesions

In 1998, the World Health Organization/ International Society of Urological Pathology (WHO/ISUP) published a consensus classification that included the following categories for flat urinary bladder lesions: reactive atypia, atypia of unknown significance, dysplasia (low-grade intraepithelial neoplasia), and carcinoma in situ (high-grade intraepithelial neoplasia). Because the 2004 WHO has accepted the nomenclature used in 1998, the system is currently referred to as WHO/ISUP.

REACTIVE ATYPIA

Reactive atypia, also known as inflammatory atypia, consists of nuclear abnormalities occurring in acutely or chronically inflamed urothelium.

CLINICAL FEATURES

A history of instrumentation, stones, or therapy is often present.

PATHOLOGIC FEATURES

GROSS FINDINGS

Reactive urothelium may be denuded.

MICROSCOPIC FINDINGS

Nucleomegaly is the most prominent finding (Fig. 4-1). The cells often have a single prominent nucleolus and evenly distributed vesicular chromatin. Nuclei are round, and pleomorphism is lacking. Architecturally, the cells maintain their polarity perpendicular to the basement membrane. Mitotic figures may be increased, predominantly in the basal and middle urothelium; however, atypical mitoses are not seen. Acute or chronic inflammation is commonly identified.

ANCILLARY STUDIES

IMMUNOHISTOCHEMISTRY

Distinction of urothelial carcinoma in situ (CIS) from reactive atypia on the basis of morphology alone may be difficult in some cases. Similarly to normal urothelium, reactive urothelium shows cytokeratin 20

REACTIVE ATYPIA—FACT SHEET

Definition
► Nuclear abnormalities occurring in acutely or chronically inflamed urothelium

Clinical Features
► History of instrumentation, stones, or therapy is often present

Prognosis and Treatment
► Benign lesion
► Conservative management

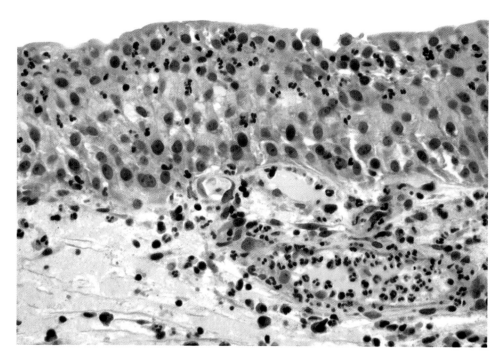

FIGURE 4-1

Nucleomegaly is the most prominent finding in reactive atypia. Nuclei are round, and pleomorphism is lacking. Architecturally, the cells maintain their polarity perpendicular to the basement membrane. Acute or chronic inflammation is commonly identified.

(CK20) immunoreactivity in only the umbrella cell layer, and p53 nuclear staining is predominantly negative, with occasional weak positivity in the basal and parabasal intermediate cells. CD44 is expressed either in the entire reactive urothelium or focally in intermediate cells.

REACTIVE ATYPIA—PATHOLOGIC FEATURES

Gross Findings

▶ Reactive urothelium may be denuded or associated with ulcers

Microscopic Findings

▶ Nucleomegaly is the most prominent finding
▶ Cells have a single prominent nucleolus and evenly distributed vesicular chromatin
▶ Nuclei are frequently round
▶ Pleomorphism is lacking (each cell looks identical to others)
▶ Architecturally, the cells maintain their polarity
▶ Atypical mitoses are not seen
▶ Acute or chronic inflammation is commonly identified

Immunohistochemical Features

▶ CK20 immunoreactivity in umbrella cell layer
▶ p53 is predominantly negative, with occasional weak positivity in the basal and parabasal intermediate cells
▶ CD44 is expressed either in the entire reactive urothelium or focally in intermediate cells

Differential Diagnosis

▶ Urothelial carcinoma in situ

DIFFERENTIAL DIAGNOSIS

In contrast to CIS, the nuclei in reactive atypia are vesicular with prominent nucleoli and are uniform in size and shape.

PROGNOSIS AND TREATMENT

This is a benign lesion. The underlying source of inflammation and reactive atypia should be addressed.

FLAT UROTHELIAL HYPERPLASIA

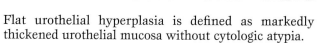

Flat urothelial hyperplasia is defined as markedly thickened urothelial mucosa without cytologic atypia.

CLINICAL FEATURES

Flat urothelial hyperplasia may be seen in the flat mucosa adjacent to a low-grade papillary urothelial lesion. When seen by itself, there is no evidence suggesting that it has premalignant potential.

FLAT UROTHELIAL HYPERPLASIA—FACT SHEET

Definition
▶ Markedly thickened urothelial mucosa without cytologic atypia

Morbidity and Mortality
▶ Urothelial lesion without malignant potential
▶ Controversial role as early neoplastic lesion in the multistep development of urothelial carcinoma

Clinical Features
▶ It may be seen in the flat mucosa adjacent to low-grade papillary urothelial lesion

Prognosis and Treatment
▶ Patients may have concomitant papillary tumors
▶ Follow-up and conservative management

FLAT UROTHELIAL HYPERPLASIA—PATHOLOGIC FEATURES

Gross Findings
▶ Nonspecific

Microscopic Findings
▶ Markedly thickened urothelium
▶ Lacks cytologic atypia

Cytogenetics
▶ Frequent deletions of chromosome 9 detected by FISH

Differential Diagnosis
▶ Urothelial carcinoma in situ
▶ Urothelial dysplasia

PATHOLOGIC FEATURES

GROSS FINDINGS

There are no specific gross findings.

MICROSCOPIC FINDINGS

Morphologically, flat urothelial hyperplasia consists of markedly thickened urothelium that lacks cytologic atypia (Fig. 4-2). Rather than requiring a specific number of cell layers, marked thickening is needed to diagnose flat hyperplasia.

ANCILLARY STUDIES

CYTOGENETICS

Frequent deletions of chromosome 9, detected by fluorescence in situ hybridization (FISH), have been reported in flat urothelial hyperplasia found in patients with papillary bladder cancer. In addition to deletions at chromosome 9, further genetic alterations have been detected by comparative genomic hybridization (CGH), including changes frequently found in invasive papillary bladder cancer: loss of chromosomes 2q, 4, 8p,

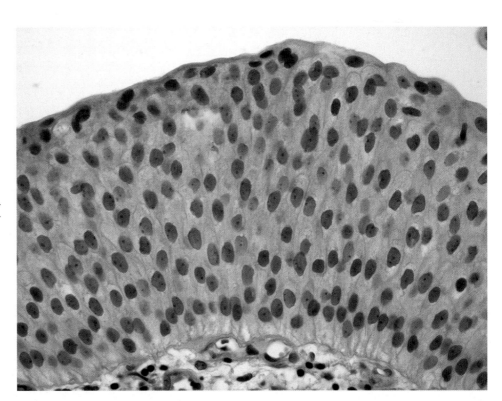

FIGURE 4-2
Flat urothelial hyperplasia is characterized by markedly thickened urothelium that lacks cytologic atypia.

and 11p; gain of chromosome 17; and amplification at 11q12q13. Although there is considerable genetic heterogeneity between hyperplasia and papillary tumors, loss of heterogeneity (LOH) and/or CGH analyses suggest a clonal relationship in half of the cases.

DIFFERENTIAL DIAGNOSIS

Differential diagnosis includes urothelial dysplasia and CIS.

PROGNOSIS AND TREATMENT

Flat urothelial hyperplasia is regarded in the new WHO classification as a urothelial lesion without malignant potential. Molecular analysis has shown that urothelial hyperplasia in bladder cancer patients may be chronologically related to papillary tumors. In the absence of an associated papillary urothelial neoplasm, no treatment or follow-up is required.

UROTHELIAL DYSPLASIA

Neoplastic atypical urothelial changes that fall short of CIS are diagnosed as urothelial dysplasia. Urothelial dysplasia is usually a histologic diagnosis and is seen most commonly in patients with bladder neoplasia, in whom the incidence is 22% to 86%. The incidence approaches 100% in patients with invasive carcinoma.

CLINICAL FEATURES

In most cases, the diagnosis of bladder cancer precedes that of dysplasia. In this setting, dysplasia is usually clinically and cystoscopically silent. Little is known about primary (de novo) dysplasia. De novo dysplasia affects predominantly middle-aged men, who occasionally present with irritative bladder symptoms with or without hematuria.

PATHOLOGIC FEATURES

GROSS FINDINGS

Macroscopically, the lesion may be inapparent, or it may be associated with erythema, erosion, or, rarely, ulceration.

UROTHELIAL DYSPLASIA—FACT SHEET

Definition
▶ Spectrum of neoplastic atypical urothelial changes that fall short of CIS

Incidence and Location
▶ Usually seen in patients with bladder neoplasia
▶ Incidence is 22-86% in patients with bladder neoplasia, 100% in patients with invasive carcinoma

Morbidity and Mortality
▶ Dysplasia in patients with noninvasive papillary neoplasms indicates urothelial instability and a marker for progression or recurrence
▶ De novo dysplasia progresses to urothelial neoplasia in 5-19% of patients

Gender, Race, and Age Distribution
▶ Primary (de novo) dysplasia affects predominantly middle-aged men

Clinical Features
▶ Clinically and cystoscopically silent when preceded by cancer
▶ Primary (de novo) dysplasia may manifest with irritative bladder symptoms with or without hematuria

Prognosis and Treatment
▶ Frequently present with invasive cancer, which determines the outcome

---

UROTHELIAL DYSPLASIA—PATHOLOGIC FEATURES

Gross Findings
▶ May be inapparent or associated with erythema, erosion, or, rarely, ulceration

Microscopic Findings
▶ Thickness of urothelium is usually normal, but it may be increased or decreased
▶ Loss of cell polarity
▶ Cytologic atypia is not severe enough to merit a diagnosis of CIS
▶ Nuclei with irregular nuclear borders and mildly altered chromatin distribution
▶ Inconspicuous nucleoli and rare mitoses

Immunohistochemistry
▶ Aberrant CK20 expression
▶ Overexpression of p53 and Ki-67

Cytogenetics
▶ Frequent alteration of chromosome 9 and p53
▶ Allelic losses

Differential Diagnosis
▶ Urothelial carcinoma in situ
▶ Reactive atypia

MICROSCOPIC FINDINGS

Dysplastic lesions show variable, often appreciable, loss of cell polarity with nuclear crowding and cytologic atypia that is not severe enough to merit a diagnosis of CIS. The cells may have mildly altered chromatin distribution, slightly enlarged nuclei, inconspicuous nucleoli, and rare mitoses (Fig. 4-3). The degree of atypia is comparable to that seen within noninvasive, low-grade papillary urothelial carcinoma. Pleomorphism, prominent nucleoli throughout the urothelium, and upper-level mitoses argue for a CIS diagnosis. The thickness of the urothelium in dysplastic lesions is usually normal; however, it may be increased or decreased. The lamina propria is usually unaltered, but it may contain increased inflammation or neovascularity. Denudation with atypical cells clinging to the submucosa is not a common feature of dysplasia.

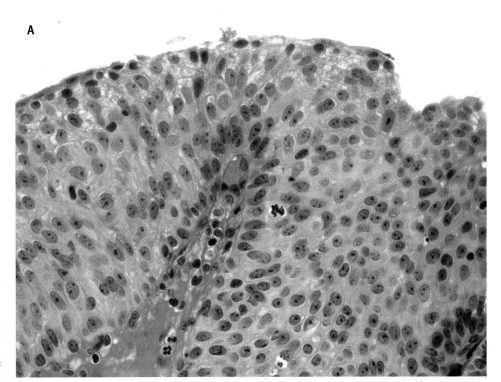

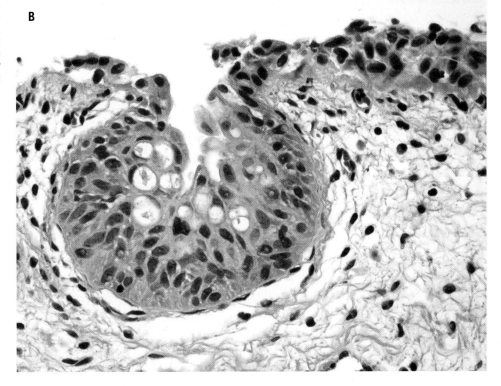

FIGURE 4-3

A, Dysplastic lesions show variable, often appreciable, loss of cell polarity with nuclear crowding and cytologic atypia that is not severe enough to merit a diagnosis of carcinoma in situ. The cells may have mildly altered chromatin distribution, slightly enlarged nuclei, inconspicuous nucleoli, and rare mitoses. The thickness of the urothelium in dysplastic lesions is usually normal; however, it may be increased or decreased. **B,** Urothelial dysplasia may involve von Brunn's nests.

Urothelial dysplasia may involve von Brunn's nests (Fig. 4-3).

ANCILLARY STUDIES

IMMUNOHISTOCHEMISTRY

Distinguishing CIS and dysplasia from reactive atypia on the basis of histologic features alone is often difficult. Aberrant CK20 expression in urothelial cells and overexpression of p53 and Ki-67 are indicators of dysplastic change in urothelial mucosa.

CYTOGENETICS

Alteration of chromosome 9 and p53 allelic losses have been demonstrated in urothelial dysplasia.

DIFFERENTIAL DIAGNOSIS

Because reactive inflammatory atypia and even normal urothelium may mimic dysplasia, a diagnosis of primary dysplasia (no prior history or concomitant urothelial neoplasia) should be made with great caution. Comparison with normal-appearing urothelium, if present in the same biopsy specimen or in another specimen obtained simultaneously, may help in assessing features such as nucleomegaly and loss of polarity. The presence of pleomorphism, prominent nucleoli throughout the urothelium, and upper-level mitosis argue for a diagnosis of urothelial CIS.

PROGNOSIS AND TREATMENT

The finding of dysplasia in patients with noninvasive papillary neoplasms indicates urothelial instability and a marker for progression or recurrence. Urothelial dysplasia is frequently present with invasive cancer, whose characteristics determine the outcome. De novo dysplasia progresses to urothelial neoplasia in 5% to 19% of patients. The diagnosis of dysplasia should not be used as a default diagnosis when there is no CIS and the cytologic or architectural atypia that is present is so mild that it may just represent normal urothelium with dark staining, mild reactive atypia, or thick sectioning.

UROTHELIAL CARCINOMA IN SITU

Urothelial CIS is a nonpapillary (i.e., flat) lesion in which the surface epithelium contains cells that are cytologically malignant. The term "carcinoma in situ"

is synonymous with "high-grade intraurothelial neoplasia." De novo (primary) CIS accounts for fewer than 1% to 3% of urothelial neoplasms but is seen with 45% to 65% of invasive urothelial carcinomas. It is present with 7% to 15% of papillary neoplasms.

CLINICAL FEATURES

CIS patients are usually in their fifth to sixth decade of life. They may be asymptomatic or symptomatic with dysuria, frequency, urgency, or even hematuria. In patients with associated invasive urothelial carcinoma, the symptoms are usually those of the associated invasive carcinoma. CIS is commonly multifocal and may be diffuse. It can involve several sites in the urinary tract synchronously or metachronously.

UROTHELIAL CARCINOMA IN SITU—FACT SHEET

Definition
► Flat lesion in which the surface epithelium contains cytologically malignant cells

Incidence and Location
► De novo (primary) CIS accounts for less than 1-3% of urothelial neoplasms
► CIS is present in 45-65% of invasive urothelial carcinomas (secondary CIS)
► Present in 7-15% of papillary neoplasms
► Commonly multifocal, it may be diffuse

Morbidity and Mortality
► De novo CIS is less likely to progress to invasive disease than is secondary CIS
► 45-65% of patients with concomitant invasive tumors die
► 7-15% of patients with concomitant noninvasive tumors die

Gender, Race, and Age Distribution
► Patients are usually in their fifth or sixth decade of life

Clinical Features
► Asymptomatic or symptomatic with dysuria, frequency, urgency, or even hematuria

Prognosis and Treatment
► Extensive lesions associated with marked symptoms have a guarded prognosis
► Intravesical chemotherapy reduces both short-term (20%) and long-term (7%) tumor recurrence
► BCG immunotherapy remains the most effective treatment and prophylaxis; it reduces tumor recurrence, disease progression, and mortality

PATHOLOGIC FEATURES

GROSS FINDINGS

Macroscopically, the mucosa may be unremarkable, or it may be erythematous and edematous (Fig. 4-4). Mucosal erosions may also be present.

UROTHELIAL CARCINOMA IN SITU—PATHOLOGIC FEATURES

Gross Findings

► Urothelial mucosa may be unremarkable or erythematous and edematous
► Mucosal erosion may also be present

Microscopic Findings

► Nuclear anaplasia identical to high-grade urothelial carcinoma
► Enlarged nuclei, pleomorphic, hyperchromatic with coarse or condensed chromatin
► Large nucleoli may be present
► Complete loss of polarity, marked crowding
► Mitoses, including atypical ones, are common and can extend into the upper cell layers
► Presence of any malignant cells suffices for CIS, ranging from isolated cells (pagetoid) to full-thickness atypia
► Umbrella cells usually absent but rarely present
► Urothelium may be denuded with discohesion, diminished in thickness, of normal thickness, or hyperplastic

Immunohistochemical Features

► Intense CK20 and p53 positivity in the majority of malignant cells
► CD44 detects residual basal cells; however, the neoplastic cells are negative

Differential Diagnosis

► Urothelial dysplasia
► Squamous cell carcinoma in situ
► Reactive atypia

MICROSCOPIC FINDINGS

Unequivocal severe cytologic atypia is necessary for the diagnosis of CIS. CIS shows nuclear anaplasia identical to high-grade papillary urothelial carcinoma. The anaplasia is usually obvious, although a spectrum of severity may exist. The urothelium may be denuded, diminished in thickness, of normal thickness, or even hyperplastic. There may be complete loss of polarity, marked crowding, and pleomorphism (Fig. 4-5A,B). The enlarged nuclei are frequently hyperchromatic and have a coarse or condensed chromatin distribution. The most atypical CIS nuclei are approximately four to five times the size of adjacent stromal lymphocytes, compared with normal urothelium in which they are only two times the size of stromal lymphocytes. Large nucleoli may be present. Mitoses, including atypical ones, are common and can extend into the upper cell layers. The cytoplasm is often eosinophilic or amphophilic. The neoplastic change may or may not involve the entire thickness of the epithelial layer, and umbrella cells may be present. Additionally, there are varied cytologic and architectural patterns in the histologic presentation of CIS, with pleomorphic large cell, nonpleomorphic large cell, small cell, clinging, and pagetoid features. Loss of intercellular cohesion may result in a denuded surface (denuding cystitis) (Fig. 4-5C). Von Brunn's nests and cystitis cystica may be completely or partially replaced by the cytologically malignant cells (Fig. 4-5D). The lamina propria usually shows an inflammatory infiltrate, some degree of edema, and vascular congestion.

ANCILLARY STUDIES

IMMUNOHISTOCHEMISTRY

CIS frequently shows diffuse strong cytoplasmic reactivity for CK20 (Fig. 4-6A). Nuclear reactivity for

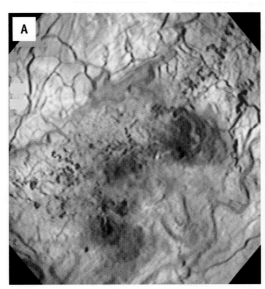
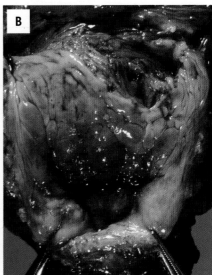

FIGURE 4-4

A, Endoscopic image of urinary bladder with urothelial carcinoma in situ (CIS). The lesion is characterized by irregularly hyperemic mucosa (Courtesy of Dr. Stephen Jones, Cleveland, Ohio.) **B,** Gross photograph of surgically resected urinary bladder with extensive urothelial CIS.

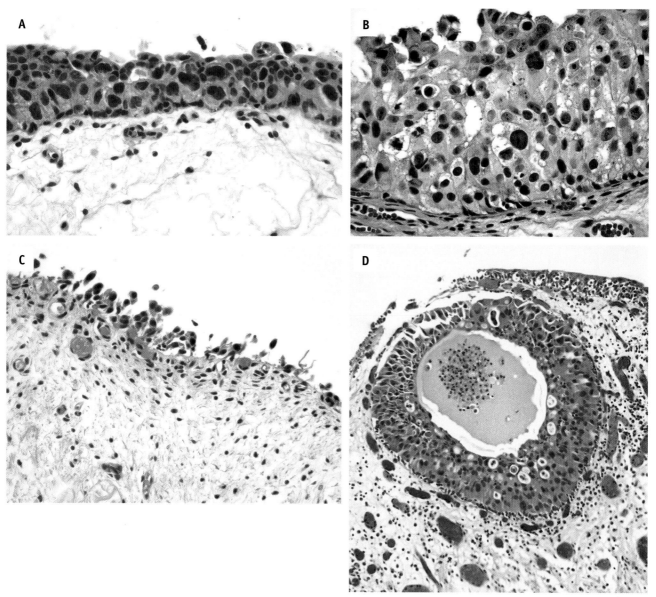

FIGURE 4-5

A, Unequivocal severe cytologic atypia is necessary for the diagnosis of carcinoma in situ (CIS). The most atypical CIS nuclei are four to five times the size of adjacent stromal lymphocytes. **B,** The urothelium may show complete loss of polarity, marked crowding, and pleomorphism. The enlarged nuclei are frequently hyperchromatic and have a coarse or condensed chromatin distribution. Mitoses, including atypical ones, are common and can extend into the upper cell layers. **C,** Loss of intercellular cohesion may result in a denuded surface (denuding cystitis). **D,** Von Brunn's nests are replaced by cytologically malignant cells of CIS.

p53 may be diffuse throughout the full thickness of the urothelium (Fig. 4-6B). CD44 reactivity is limited to a residual basal cell layer of normal urothelium if present, but it is often absent in urothelial CIS.

ones) in the upper urothelium favors the diagnosis of CIS over dysplasia. Distinction of CIS from reactive conditions can be difficult, although in most instances it is straight forward based on nuclear characteristics.

DIFFERENTIAL DIAGNOSIS

The distinction of dysplasia from CIS is based on the degree of atypia. The presence of pleomorphism comparable to that seen with high-grade papillary carcinoma, discohesion, or mitoses (particularly atypical

PROGNOSIS AND TREATMENT

Data suggest that de novo urothelial CIS is less likely than secondary CIS to progress to invasive disease. Between 45% and 65% of patients with CIS and concomitant invasive tumors die of the disease, compared

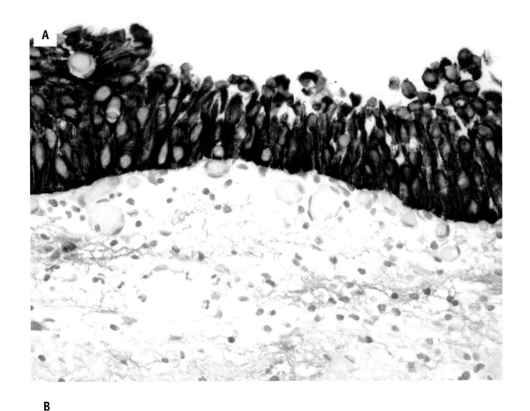

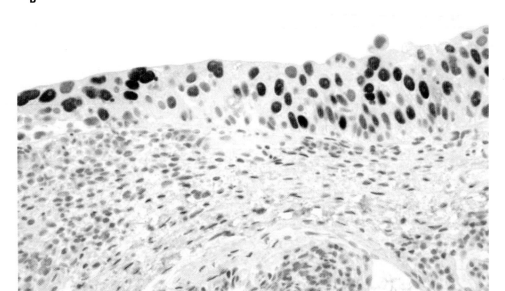

FIGURE 4-6

Immunohistochemical features of urothelial carcinoma in situ. **A,** Diffuse strong cytoplasmic reactivity for cytokeratin 20. **B,** Nuclear reactivity for p53 in individual cells throughout the full thickness of the urothelium.

with 7% to 15% of patients who have CIS and concomitant noninvasive tumor. Extensive lesions associated with marked symptoms have a guarded prognosis. Intravesical chemotherapy reduces short-term tumor recurrence by about 20% and long-term recurrence by about 7%. Presently, bacille Calmette-Guérin (BCG) immunotherapy remains the most effective treatment and prophylaxis for CIS, reducing tumor recurrence, disease progression, and mortality.

Papillary Urothelial Lesions

The WHO/ISUP classification of noninvasive papillary urothelial lesions comprises papillary hyperplasia, urothelial papilloma and inverted papilloma, papillary neoplasm of low malignant potential, and low-grade and high-grade papillary urothelial carcinoma. To simplify the WHO (1973) system and avoid an intermediate cancer grade group (grade II), the WHO/ISUP system

TABLE 4-2

Comparison of WHO/ISUP diagnosis of papillary urothelial neoplasms with other grading systems

WHO/ISUP	Previous WHO	Murphy
Papilloma	Papilloma	Papilloma
Papillary urothelial neoplasm of low malignant potential	Most grade I/III	Some papilloma Some carcinoma, low grade
Papillary urothelial carcinoma, low grade	Some grade I/III Most grade II/III	Most carcinoma, low grade
Papillary urothelial carcinoma, high grade	Carcinoma, grade III/III Some carcinoma, grade II/III	Carcinoma, high grade

classifies papillary urothelial carcinoma into only two grades: low-grade papillary urothelial carcinoma and high-grade papillary urothelial carcinoma (Table 4-2).

PAPILLARY UROTHELIAL HYPERPLASIA

A proportion of papillary urothelial hyperplasia likely represents the precursor lesion to low-grade papillary urothelial neoplasms.

CLINICAL FEATURES

Typically, papillary urothelial hyperplasia is discovered on routine follow-up cystoscopy for papillary urothelial neoplasms; less frequently, it is found during the workup for microhematuria or urinary obstructive symptoms.

PATHOLOGIC FEATURES

GROSS FINDINGS

In most cases, at cystoscopy, a focally elevated lesion is identified and is described as papillary, raised, sessile, or bleb-like.

MICROSCOPIC FINDINGS

Histologically, papillary urothelial hyperplasia consists of undulating urothelium arranged into narrow papillary mucosal folds of varying height (Fig. 4-7A). Both the urothelium within papillary hyperplasia and the adjacent flat mucosa are often thicker than normal. The cytologic findings in typical papillary hyperplasia

---

PAPILLARY UROTHELIAL HYPERPLASIA—FACT SHEET

Definition
► Undulating folds of thicker than normal, cytologically benign urothelium

Morbidity and Mortality
► De novo hyperplasia: increased risk yet not invariable progression to low-grade papillary urothelial neoplasia
► Secondary hyperplasia: indicates early recurrence of papillary urothelial neoplasia

Clinical Features
► Discovered on routine follow-up cystoscopy for papillary urothelial neoplasms or, less frequently, in the workup for microhematuria or urinary obstructive symptoms

Prognosis and Treatment
► Patients should be closely monitored

PAPILLARY UROTHELIAL HYPERPLASIA—PATHOLOGIC FEATURES

Gross Findings
► Focally elevated lesion: papillary, raised, sessile, or bleb-like

Microscopic Findings
► Thicker than normal urothelium
► Tenting, undulating folds without detached-appearing papillary fronds
► Cytologic findings similar to normal urothelium
► Increased vascularity in the stroma at the base of the papillary folds

Immunohistochemistry
► p53 is consistently negative
► Ki-67 labeling index: 1.1%

Differential Diagnosis
► Urothelial papilloma

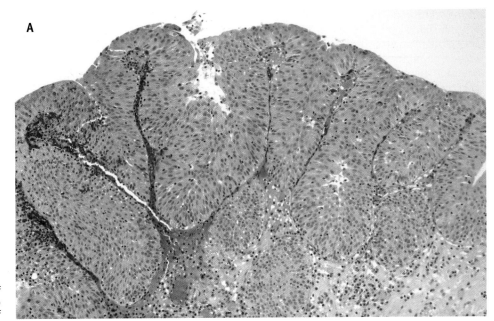

FIGURE 4-7

A, Papillary hyperplasia consists of undulating urothelium arranged into narrow papillary mucosal folds of varying height. Both the urothelium within papillary hyperplasia and the adjacent flat mucosa are often thicker than normal. **B,** Some cases show increased vascularity in the stroma at the base of the papillary folds. The well-developed, branching fibrovascular cores of a papillary neoplasm are not evident.

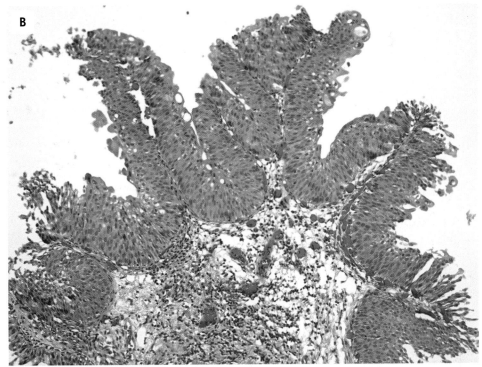

are similar to those characteristic of normal urothelium. Some cases show increased vascularity in the stroma at the base of the papillary folds. Well-developed, branching fibrovascular cores of a papillary neoplasm are not evident (Fig. 4-7B).

ANCILLARY STUDIES

IMMUNOHISTOCHEMISTRY

Papillary hyperplasia lacks p53 positivity, and the reported Ki-67 labeling index is 1.1%.

DIFFERENTIAL DIAGNOSIS

Papillary hyperplasia is distinguished from papillary urothelial neoplasms by a lack of arborization and the absence of detached-appearing papillary fronds.

PROGNOSIS AND TREATMENT

Large studies with sufficient follow-up to evaluate the clinical significance of de novo papillary hyperplasia are lacking. Although de novo papillary hyperplasia does not invariably progress to urothelial neoplasia, it is reasonable to suggest that patients should be monitored, because papillary hyperplasia may be the harbinger of low-grade papillary urothelial neoplasms. If papillary hyperplasia is diagnosed in someone with a history of urothelial neoplasia (secondary), most likely it indicates early recurrence of papillary neoplasia and warrants either continued close follow-up or additional intravesical therapy, depending on the preference of the urologist.

UROTHELIAL PAPILLOMA

The WHO/ISUP system has very restrictive histologic features for the diagnosis of papilloma, requiring papillary fronds to be lined by normal-appearing urothelium. Most papillomas manifest as single lesions that are relatively small; however, multifocal tumors and larger lesions may be seen. The incidence of urothelial papilloma is low, usually ranging from 1% to 4% of bladder tumors. The male-to-female ratio is 1.9:1. Papillomas tend to occur in younger patients and are seen in children.

CLINICAL FEATURES

The most common locations for urothelial papillomas are (1) the posterior or lateral walls of the bladder close to the ureteral orifices and (2) the urethra. Gross or microscopic hematuria is the main symptom.

PATHOLOGIC FEATURES

GROSS FINDINGS

The cystoscopic appearance is essentially identical to that of other low-grade papillary urothelial neoplasms.

MICROSCOPIC FINDINGS

Microscopically, papillary fronds are lined by normal-appearing urothelium, lacking atypia. Most papillomas have a simple, nonbranching or minimally branching arrangement and slender fibrovascular stalks with a predominantly exophytic pattern (Fig. 4-8A,B). The stroma may show edema or scattered inflammatory cells, or both. Superficial umbrella cells are often prominent, varying from inconspicuous to cuboidal cells with slightly enlarged nuclei and paler cytoplasm, to hobnail cells with abundant eosinophilic cytoplasm, to cells with prominent vacuolization (Fig. 4-8C,D). Mitoses are absent to rare; if present, they are basal in location and not abnormal.

UROTHELIAL PAPILLOMA—FACT SHEET

Definition
▶ Delicate fibrovascular core lined by normal-appearing urothelium

Incidence and Location
▶ The incidence is low (1-4% of bladder tumors)
▶ Most common locations: posterior or lateral walls of bladder, close to ureteral orifices, and urethra

Morbidity and Mortality
▶ Rarely recur (8% of the cases)
▶ Rarely progress to higher-grade disease (8% of the cases)

Gender, Race, and Age Distribution
▶ Male predominance (M/F ratio, 1.9:1)
▶ Tend to occur in younger patients
▶ Seen in children

Clinical Features
▶ Gross or microscopic hematuria

Prognosis and Treatment
▶ Clinical course is typically favorable
▶ Complete TUR is the treatment of choice

UROTHELIAL PAPILLOMA—PATHOLOGIC FEATURES

Gross Findings
▶ Cystoscopic appearance is essentially identical to other low-grade papillary urothelial neoplasms

Microscopic Findings
▶ Normal-appearing urothelium lacking atypia
▶ Superficial umbrella cells are often prominent
▶ Nonbranching or minimally branching arrangement, slender fibrovascular stalks, predominantly exophytic pattern
▶ Stroma may show edema and/or scattered inflammatory cells
▶ Mitoses are absent to rare; if present, they are basal in location and not abnormal

Immunohistochemical Features
▶ Ki-67 demonstrates low proliferation rate
▶ p53 is always negative
▶ CK20 expression is confined to umbrella cells

Differential Diagnosis
▶ Papillary neoplasm of low malignant potential (PUNLMP)
▶ Low-grade papillary urothelial carcinoma

ANCILLARY STUDIES

IMMUNOHISTOCHEMISTRY

Urothelial papillomas are diploid lesions with rare mitoses and a low proliferation rate as determined by

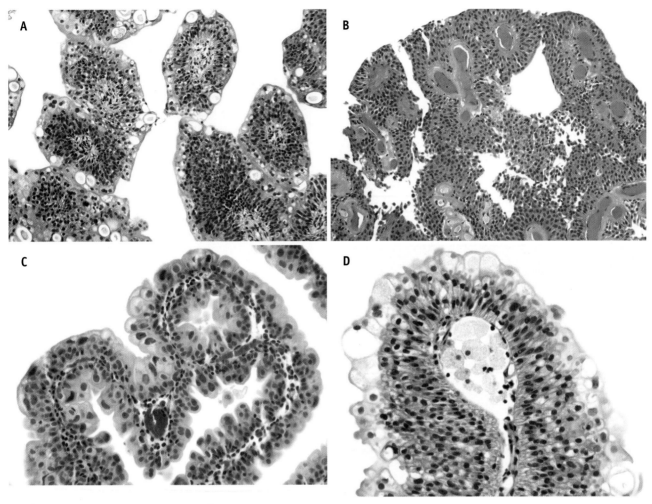

FIGURE 4-8

A, In urothelial papilloma, papillary fronds are lined by normal-appearing urothelium, lacking atypia. **B,** Most papillomas have a simple, non-branching or minimally branching arrangement and slender fibrovascular stalks with a predominantly exophytic pattern. **C,** Superficial umbrella cells are often prominent, varying from inconspicuous to cuboidal cells with slightly enlarged nuclei and paler cytoplasm to hobnail cells with abundant eosinophilic cytoplasm. **D,** Prominent vacuolization of the umbrella cells may also be seen.

immunohistochemical assessment of Ki-67 expression. CK20 expression is confined to the umbrella cells, as in normal urothelium. Alteration of p53 is not seen in urothelial papillomas.

DIFFERENTIAL DIAGNOSIS

Urothelial atypia, other than what can be seen in umbrella cells, excludes the diagnosis of papilloma. Urothelial papillomas must be distinguished from papillary urothelial neoplasm of low malignant potential (PUNLMP). PUNLMP lesions do not have cytologic features of malignancy, but they have thickened urothelium as compared with papilloma. Mitoses may rarely be present but are confined to the basal layers.

PROGNOSIS AND TREATMENT

Although the clinical course is typically favorable, urothelial papillomas rarely recur and can also progress to higher-grade disease (approximately 8% of the cases). Complete TUR is the treatment of choice.

INVERTED PAPILLOMA

Inverted papilloma is a benign tumor of the urinary bladder comprising less than 1% of urothelial neoplasms. The cause of inverted papilloma of the urinary tract remains unknown. Lesions occur in a wide age range (10 to 94 years), with a peak frequency in the sixth and seventh decades. There is a striking male predilection: the male-to-female ratio is 4:1 to 5:1. Tumor size varies from small to 8.0 cm. Most lesions are solitary and manifest with hematuria.

CLINICAL FEATURES

Patients with inverted papillomas usually present with hematuria or irritative symptoms but infrequently may have obstructive symptoms. More than 70% of the reported cases are located in the bladder, but inverted papillomas may also be found in ureter, renal pelvis, and urethra. Most bladder cases are located in the trigone.

PATHOLOGIC FEATURES

GROSS FINDINGS

Cystoscopically, inverted papillomas appear as solitary, sessile, pedunculated, or, rarely, polypoid lesions with a smooth surface.

INVERTED PAPILLOMA—PATHOLOGIC FEATURES

Gross Findings

► Solitary, sessile, or pedunculated; rarely, polypoid lesions with a smooth surface
► Tumor size varies from <1.0 cm to 8.0 cm

Microscopic Findings

► Islands and cords of normal urothelial cells
► May invaginate extensively into lamina propria but not into muscular wall
► Base of the lesion is well circumscribed
► Central portion of cords contains urothelial cells, and periphery contains palisades of basal cells
► Foci of nonkeratinizing squamous metaplasia may be seen
► Cytologic atypia is minimal to absent
► Mitotic figures are rare and are seen at the periphery of the trabeculae
► Inflammation absent

Differential Diagnosis

► Florid proliferation of von Brunn's nests
► Florid cystitis cystica and cystitis glandularis
► Urothelial carcinoma with inverted pattern of growth

INVERTED PAPILLOMA—FACT SHEET

Definition

► Benign urothelial tumor characterized by inverted growth pattern with normal to minimal cytologic atypia

Incidence and Location

► Fewer than 1% of urothelial neoplasms
► Most cases (70%) are located in the bladder
► Trigone is the most common location
► Can be found in ureter, renal pelvis, and urethra

Morbidity and Mortality

► Most lesions are solitary and self-limited
► Infrequent recurrence and extremely rare progression

Gender, Race, and Age Distribution

► Occurs in a wide age range (10-94 years)
► Peak frequency in sixth and seventh decades
► Striking male predilection (M/F ratio, 4-5:1)

Clinical Features

► Patients present with hematuria or irritative symptoms; infrequently may produce obstructive symptoms
► Urine cytology may show atypical cells

Prognosis and Treatment

► Benign tumor
► Complete TUR is the treatment of choice

MICROSCOPIC FINDINGS

Inverted papilloma is characterized by anastomosing islands and cords of normal urothelial cells that originate from the overlying mucosa and grow downward into the stroma (Fig. 4-9A). The urothelial cells may invaginate extensively from the surface into the lamina propria but not into the muscular bladder wall. The base of the lesion is well circumscribed. In contrast to conventional papillary urothelial neoplasms, the central portion of the cords contains urothelial cells and the periphery demonstrates palisading basal cells (Fig. 4-9B). The stromal component is mostly minimal and lacks inflammation. Foci of nonkeratinizing squamous metaplasia are often seen in inverted papillomas. Cytologic atypia is minimal to absent, although in rare cases multinucleated cells with degenerative atypia, pagetoid cells, and small foci resembling CIS may be present. Mitotic figures are rare and are only seen at the periphery of the trabeculae.

DIFFERENTIAL DIAGNOSIS

Inverted papilloma must be distinguished principally from other polypoid lesions with predominantly subsurface growth pattern, such as florid proliferation of von Brunn's nests and urothelial carcinoma with inverted pattern of growth. A prominent exophytic

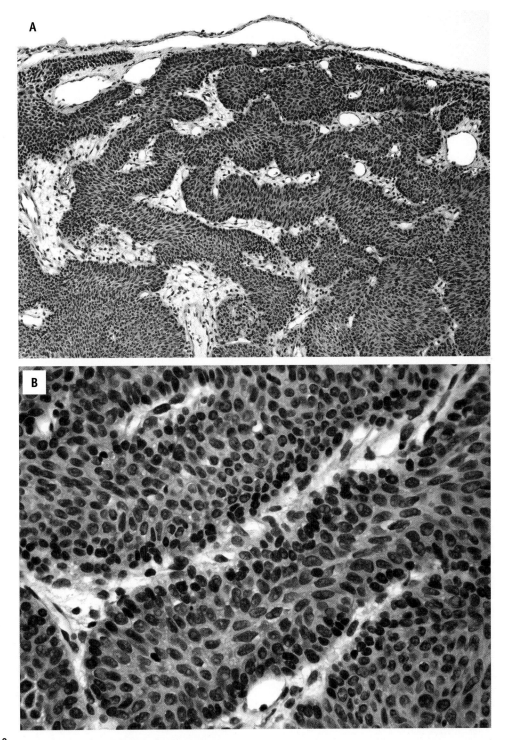

FIGURE 4-9

A, In inverted papilloma, at low power, anastomosing islands and cords of normal urothelial cells originating from the overlying mucosa are growing downward into the stroma. **B,** At high power, the central portion of the cords contains urothelial cells and the periphery demonstrates palisading basal cells. The stromal component is mostly minimal and lacks inflammation. Cytologic atypia is minimal to absent.

component, considerable cytologic atypia, irregularity of proliferating nests with large rounded nests, and invasion rule out an inverted papilloma. Von Brunn's nests tend to be round, without the anastomosing pattern of inverted papilloma, although isolated cases have overlapping features.

PROGNOSIS AND TREATMENT

If the diagnosis of inverted papilloma is strictly confined to the criteria described, these tumors are benign with infrequent recurrence. An association with papillary urothelial carcinoma has been described, although it is unresolved whether there is an increased risk of this relationship. Complete TUR is the treatment of choice.

PAPILLARY UROTHELIAL NEOPLASM OF LOW MALIGNANT POTENTIAL

PUNLMP is a papillary urothelial tumor that resembles exophytic urothelial papilloma but shows increased thickness of the urothelium. Most studies demonstrate prognostic differences between PUNLMP and papillary low-grade urothelial carcinoma, with recurrence in 25% to 47% of the former and 48% to 77% of the latter. Although it may occasionally be difficult to reliably distinguish between those two entities, the distinction is still useful in that it provides a noncancerous diagnosis for a group of patients with indolent disease.

CLINICAL FEATURES

The incidence is 3 per 100,000 individuals per year. The male-to-female ratio is 5:1, and the mean age at diagnosis is 64.6 years (range, 29 to 94 years). Most patients present with gross or microscopic hematuria. Urine cytology is negative in most cases. The lateral and posterior walls of the bladder, close to the ureteral orifices, are the preferred sites.

PATHOLOGIC FEATURES

GROSS FINDINGS

Cystoscopy reveals a papillary tumor that may be small to 2.0 cm in diameter.

MICROSCOPIC FINDINGS

The papillae of PUNLMP are discrete and slender and are lined by a thickened, multilayered urothelium with minimal to absent cytologic atypia (Fig. 4-10A,B). The cell density appears to be increased compared with that of normal urothelium. The polarity is preserved. The basal layers show palisading, and the umbrella cell layer is often preserved (Fig. 4-10C,D). Mitoses are rare and have a basal location.

DIFFERENTIAL DIAGNOSIS

PUNLMP is distinguished by urothelium that is thicker than that of urothelial papilloma. In contrast to noninvasive low-grade papillary urothelial carcinoma, PUNLMP has a proliferation of monotonous, bland-appearing cells and lacks the scattered cells with enlarged hyperchromatic nuclei seen in carcinoma. More than a rare mitotic figure favors the diagnosis of carcinoma.

PAPILLARY UROTHELIAL NEOPLASM OF LOW MALIGNANT POTENTIAL—FACT SHEET

Definition
▶ PUNLMP is a papillary tumor that resembles exophytic papilloma but shows increased cellular proliferation exceeding the thickness of normal urothelium

Incidence and Location
▶ Incidence is 3/100,000 individuals per year
▶ Lateral and posterior walls of the bladder, close to the ureteral orifices

Morbidity and Mortality
▶ Indolent disease
▶ Recurrences occur (25-47%), but at a significantly lower frequency than in noninvasive papillary carcinomas
▶ Not associated with concurrent invasive carcinoma

Gender, Race, and Age Distribution
▶ Male predominance (M/F ratio, 5:1)
▶ Mean age at diagnosis is 64.6 years (range, 29-94 years)

Clinical Features
▶ Gross or microscopic hematuria
▶ Urine cytology is negative in most cases

Prognosis and Treatment
▶ Prognosis is excellent
▶ TUR is the treatment of choice

PAPILLARY UROTHELIAL NEOPLASM OF LOW MALIGNANT POTENTIAL—PATHOLOGIC FEATURES

Gross Findings
▶ Cystoscopy reveals a 1.0-2.0 cm delicate papillary tumor

Microscopic Findings
▶ The papillae are discrete and slender and are lined by multilayered urothelium thicker than papilloma
▶ Minimal to absent cytologic atypia with very monotonous size, shape, and chromatin
▶ Cell density appears to be increased compared to normal
▶ Polarity is preserved
▶ Mitoses are rare and have a basal location

Differential Diagnosis
▶ Urothelial papilloma
▶ Noninvasive low-grade papillary urothelial carcinoma

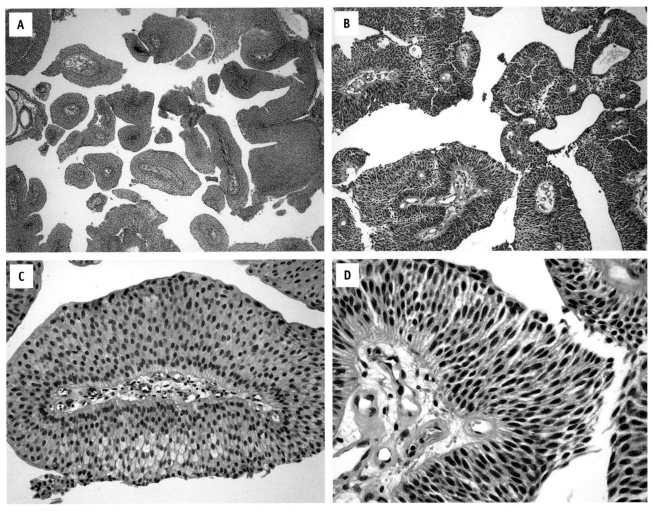

FIGURE 4-10

A and **B,** At low power, the papillae of papillary urothelial neoplasm of low malignant potential (PUNLMP) are discrete and slender and are lined by a thickened multilayered urothelium with minimal to absent cytologic atypia. **C** and **D,** At high power, the cell density appears to be increased compared to normal. The polarity is preserved. The basal layers show palisading, and the umbrella cell layer is often preserved.

PROGNOSIS AND TREATMENT

The prognosis for patients with PUNLMP is excellent. Recurrences occur but at a significantly lower frequency than with noninvasive papillary carcinoma. Invasion is not seen. Transurethral resection is the treatment of choice.

NONINVASIVE LOW-GRADE PAPILLARY UROTHELIAL CARCINOMA

Low-grade papillary carcinoma is a neoplasm of the urothelium lining the papillary fronds that is characterized by an overall orderly appearance but with easily recognizable variation in architectural and cytologic features.

CLINICAL FEATURES

The incidence is 5 per 100,000 individuals per year. The male-to-female ratio is 2.9:1, and the mean age is 69.2 years (range, 28 to 90 years). The lesion predominantly involves the posterior or lateral wall of the bladder, close to the ureteral orifices. Gross or microscopic hematuria is the main symptom.

PATHOLOGIC FEATURES

GROSS FINDINGS

The endoscopic appearance is similar to that of PUNLMP. In most cases the tumor is single, but in 22% of the cases there are two or more lesions.

NONINVASIVE LOW-GRADE PAPILLARY UROTHELIAL CARCINOMA—FACT SHEET

Definition
▶ Neoplasm of the urothelium lining papillary fronds, characterized by an overall orderly appearance but with easily recognizable variation in architectural and cytologic features

Incidence and Location
▶ Incidence is 5/100,000 individuals per year
▶ Predominantly involves posterior or lateral wall of the bladder, close to the ureteral orifices

Morbidity and Mortality
▶ Single lesion in most cases
▶ Two or more tumors in 22% of cases

Gender, Race, and Age Distribution
▶ Male predominance (M/F ratio, 2.9:1)
▶ Mean age is 69.2 years (range, 28-90 years)

Clinical Features
▶ Gross or microscopic hematuria is the main symptom

Prognosis and Treatment
▶ Progression to invasion and cancer death occurs in <5% of cases
▶ Recurrence is common and occurs in approximately 48-71%
▶ TUR is the treatment of choice
▶ Treatment with intravesical therapy in cases with multifocal, large, or recurrent tumors

NONINVASIVE LOW-GRADE PAPILLARY UROTHELIAL CARCINOMA—PATHOLOGIC FEATURES

Gross Findings
▶ The endoscopic appearance is similar to that of PUNLMP

Microscopic Findings
▶ Slender papillary fronds that show frequent branching and minimal fusion
▶ Orderly appearance, with easily recognizable architectural and cytologic variation
▶ Nuclei are uniformly enlarged, with mild differences in shape, contour, and chromatin distribution
▶ Nucleoli may be present but inconspicuous
▶ Mitoses are infrequent and may occur at any level but are usually limited to the lower half

Immunohistochemical Features
▶ Superficial CK20 expression
▶ p53 detected in some cases

Differential Diagnosis
▶ Papillary urothelial neoplasm of low malignant potential (PUNLMP)
▶ Non-invasive high-grade papillary urothelial carcinoma

MICROSCOPIC FINDINGS

Low-grade papillary urothelial carcinoma is characterized by slender papillary fronds that show frequent branching and minimal fusion (Fig. 4-11A,B). The lesion shows an orderly appearance with easily recognizable variations in architectural and cytologic features (Fig. 4-11C). The nuclei are uniformly enlarged, with mild differences in shape, contour, and chromatin distribution (Fig. 4-11D). Nucleoli may be present but inconspicuous. Mitoses are infrequent and may occur at any level but are usually limited to the lower half.

ANCILLARY STUDIES

IMMUNOHISTOCHEMISTRY

The expression of p53 and Ki-67 immunostaining is intermediate between that of PUNLMP and non-invasive high-grade papillary urothelial carcinoma. The lesion is usually diploid.

DIFFERENTIAL DIAGNOSIS

The finding of scattered hyperchromatic nuclei and more than a rare mitotic figure best distinguishes low-grade papillary urothelial carcinoma from PUNLMP. If the tumor is predominantly low grade and there is a high-grade component occupying more than 5% of the tumor, it should be classified as high-grade papillary carcinoma. For the uncommon case with a very minor (<5%) high-grade component, the lesion is diagnosed as low grade with a comment as to the presence of focal higher-grade tumor, the significance of which is unknown.

PROGNOSIS AND TREATMENT

Progression to invasion and cancer death occurs in fewer than 5% of cases of low-grade papillary urothelial carcinomas. In contrast, recurrence is common and occurs in approximately 48% to 71% of patients. Transurethral resection is the treatment of choice. Multifocal or recurrent disease is sometimes also treated with intravesical immunotherapy.

NONINVASIVE HIGH-GRADE PAPILLARY UROTHELIAL CARCINOMA

High-grade papillary urothelial carcinoma is a neoplasm of urothelium lining the papillary fronds that is

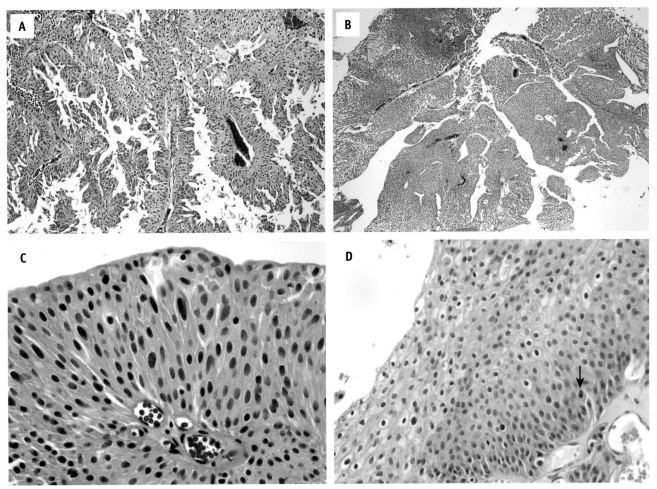

FIGURE 4-11
A and **B,** At low power, the lesion of noninvasive low-grade papillary urothelial carcinoma is characterized by slender papillary fronds that show frequent branching and minimal fusion. **C,** At high power, urothelial cells show an orderly appearance with easily recognizable variations in architectural and cytologic features. **D,** The nuclei are uniformly enlarged, with mild differences in shape, contour, and chromatin distribution. Scattered hyperchromatic nuclei and occasional mitoses are present *(arrow)*. Nucleoli may be present but inconspicuous.

characterized by a disorderly appearance resulting from marked architectural and cytologic abnormalities, recognizable at low magnification.

CLINICAL FEATURES

Gross or microscopic hematuria is the main symptom.

PATHOLOGIC FEATURES

GROSS FINDINGS

The endoscopic appearance varies from papillary to nodular/solid sessile lesion. Patients may have single or multiple tumors (Fig. 4-12).

NONINVASIVE HIGH-GRADE PAPILLARY UROTHELIAL CARCINOMA— FACT SHEET

Definition
► Neoplasm of the urothelium lining papillary fronds, characterized by a disorderly appearance resulting from marked architectural and cytologic abnormalities

Morbidity and Mortality
► High risk of association with invasive disease at the time of presentation

Clinical Features
► Gross or microscopic hematuria is the main symptom

Prognosis and Treatment
► Progression to invasion occurs in 15-40% of cases
► TUR and fulguration are mainstay of treatment
► Intravesical chemotherapy (thiotepa and mitomycin-C)
► Intravesical immunotherapy (BCG)

NONINVASIVE HIGH-GRADE PAPILLARY UROTHELIAL CARCINOMA—PATHOLOGIC FEATURES

Gross Findings

▶ The endoscopic appearance varies from papillary to nodular/solid sessile lesion
▶ Patients may have single or multiple lesions

Microscopic Findings

▶ Easily recognizable architectural and cytologic variation (scanning magnification)
▶ The papillae are frequently fused and branching, although some may be delicate
▶ Cytologic pleomorphism ranging from moderate to marked
▶ Chromatin tends to be clumped, and nucleoli may be prominent
▶ Mitotic figures are frequently seen at all levels of the urothelium
▶ Urothelium thickness may vary considerably, often with cell discohesion

Immunohistochemical Features

▶ Diffuse CK20 expression
▶ p53 detected in half of cases

Differential Diagnosis

▶ Noninvasive low-grade papillary urothelial carcinoma
▶ Invasive high-grade urothelial carcinoma

MICROSCOPIC FINDINGS

High-grade papillary urothelial carcinoma shows a predominant pattern of disorder with variations in architectural and cytologic features that are easily recognizable even at scanning magnification. The papillae are frequently fused and branching, although some may be delicate (Fig. 4-13A). Cytologically, there is a spectrum of pleomorphism ranging from moderate to marked (Fig. 4-13B). The chromatin tends to be clumped, and nucleoli may be prominent. Mitotic figures, including atypical forms, are frequently seen at all levels of the urothelium, including the surface. The thickness of the urothelium may vary considerably, often with cell discohesion. In tumors with variable histology, the tumor should be graded according to the highest grade (see earlier discussion in the section on Noninvasive Low-Grade Papillary Urothelial Carcinoma).

ANCILLARY STUDIES

IMMUNOHISTOCHEMISTRY

Detection of p53 and Ki-67 is more frequent in high-grade papillary urothelial carcinomas than in low-grade tumors. High-grade papillary carcinomas are usually aneuploid.

DIFFERENTIAL DIAGNOSIS

In contrast to noninvasive low-grade papillary urothelial carcinoma, it is easy to recognize in high-grade carcinomas more marked variation in nuclear polarity, size, shape, and chromatin pattern. Invasion both within the papillary cores and at the base of the lesions is commonly present and should be ruled out.

PROGNOSIS AND TREATMENT

High-grade papillary urothelial carcinomas carry a much higher risk of progression than low-grade lesions do, with figures varying from 15% to 40%. These tumors also have a high risk of association with invasive disease at the time of presentation. The surrounding flat urothelial mucosa may also demonstrate CIS. The mainstay of treatment for noninvasive high-grade papillary urothelial carcinoma is TUR and fulguration of the visible tumor. In patients at high risk for recurrence and progression, a variety of adjuvant therapies have been applied, such as intravesical chemotherapy with Thiotepa and mitomycin-C and intravesical immunotherapy with BCG.

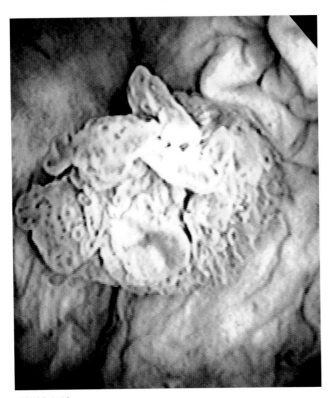

FIGURE 4-12

The endoscopic appearance of noninvasive high-grade papillary urothelial carcinoma of the urinary bladder is characterized by fused, thick papillary fronds. (Courtesy of Dr. Stephen Jones, Cleveland, Ohio.)

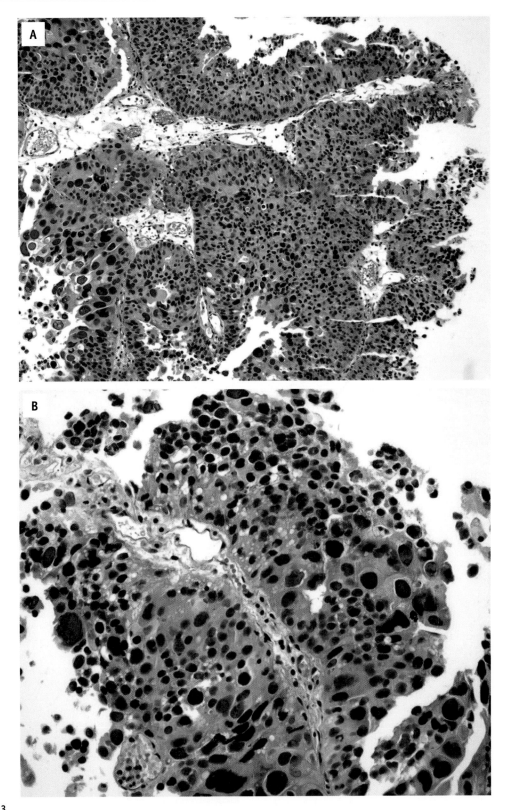

FIGURE 4-13
A, At low power, the lesion of noninvasive high-grade papillary urothelial carcinoma shows a predominant pattern of disorder with easily recognizable variations in architectural and cytologic atypia. The papillae are frequently fused and branching, although some may be delicate. **B,** At high power, there is a spectrum of pleomorphism ranging from moderate to marked. The chromatin tends to be clumped, and nucleoli may be prominent. The thickness of the urothelium may vary considerably, and cell discohesion is often present.

INVASIVE UROTHELIAL CARCINOMA

Invasive urothelial carcinoma, also known as transitional cell carcinoma, is defined as a urothelial tumor that invades beyond the basement membrane. Urothelial carcinoma is the most common type of bladder cancer in developed countries, and it constitutes more than 90% of bladder cancer cases in United States, France, and Italy. This neoplasm usually arises in male patients older than 50 years of age.

ETIOLOGY OF UROTHELIAL BLADDER CANCER

Cigarette smoking and occupational exposure to aromatic amines are the most important risk factors for bladder cancer. The risk of bladder cancer attributed to tobacco smoking is an estimated 66% for men and 30% for women, and it is two to six times greater than the risk for nonsmokers. The risk increases with increasing duration and intensity of smoking. The risk of bladder cancer 15 years after stopping smoking is similar to the risk in nonsmokers. Bladder cancer is also associated with occupational exposures. It has been estimated that contact with carcinogens such as aniline dye and aromatic amines (benzidine and 2-naphthylamine) causes up to 25% of all bladder tumors. Chronic abuse of analgesics containing phenacetin enhances the risk of developing urothelial carcinoma.

MOLECULAR BIOLOGY

Invasive urothelial carcinoma of the bladder is characterized by the presence of a high number of genetic alterations involving many different chromosomal regions. Most frequently observed are losses in 2q, 5q, 8p, 9p, 9q, 10q, 11p, 18q, and Y and gains in 1q, 5p, 8q, and 17q. *ERBB2* (HER-2/NEU) is amplified in 10% to 20% of the cases and overexpressed in 10% to 50%. *HRAS* mutations have been reported in up to 45% of bladder cancers, without association to tumor stage or grade. p53 alterations are not uncommon. Currently, there is no validated molecular parameter with sufficient predictive power to have clinical value.

GENETIC SUSCEPTIBILITY

Although urothelial carcinoma is not considered to be a familial disease, there are studies describing families with multiple cases. A 1.5- to 2-fold increased risk among first-degree relatives of patients has been reported. Glutathione *S*-transferase M1 (GSTM1) null status is associated with a small increase in bladder cancer risk.

CLINICAL FEATURES

Urothelial carcinoma accounts for 84% of bladder cancers in men and 79% of those in women. The type and severity of clinical signs and symptoms depend on the extent and location of the tumor. The most common presenting symptom is painless gross hematuria, which occurs in 85% of patients. Dysuria, urgency, and frequency may occur in large tumors, in tumors located at the bladder neck, or in cases of extensive CIS. Hydronephrosis may occur in tumors that infiltrate the ureteral orifice, and it is considered a poor prognostic finding. Upper tract tumors occur in fewer than 10% of patients with bladder tumors, and two thirds of them are located in the distal ureter.

IMAGING FEATURES

Various imaging modalities are used not only for detection but also for staging of urothelial carcinoma.

INVASIVE UROTHELIAL CARCINOMA—FACT SHEET

Definition
- ▶ Urothelial tumor that invades beyond the basement membrane

Incidence and Location
- ▶ Seventh to ninth most common cancer worldwide, fourth most common among American men
- ▶ 330,000 new cases and more than 130,000 deaths per year
- ▶ Accounts for 84% of bladder cancers in men and 79% in women

Morbidity and Mortality
- ▶ 20-30% of patients with newly diagnosed bladder cancer present with muscle-invasive disease

Gender, Race, and Age Distribution
- ▶ Male predominance (M/F ratio, 3.5:1)
- ▶ More common in patients >50 years of age
- ▶ Incidence is higher in United States, France, and Italy
- ▶ Among African countries, Algeria and Tunisia have a higher incidence

Clinical Features
- ▶ Painless gross hematuria occurs in 85% of patients
- ▶ Dysuria, urgency, and frequency may occur
- ▶ Hydronephrosis may occur in tumors infiltrating the ureteral orifice (poor prognostic sign)

Prognosis and Treatment
- ▶ T1 disease: TUR with or without adjuvant intravesical therapy; 5-year survival rate is about 70%
- ▶ T2-T4 disease: total cystectomy or cystoprostatectomy; variable survival rates

The staging accuracy with transabdominal ultrasonography is less than 70% for infiltrating bladder tumors. Although intravenous urography (IVU) is reliable in diagnosing intraluminal processes, it fails to detect the extent of extramural tumor; therefore, it has increasingly been replaced by computed tomography (CT) and magnetic resonance imaging (MRI). The staging accuracy of CT has been described as approximately 55%, and that of MRI as approximately 83%.

TUMOR SPREAD AND STAGING

Urothelial carcinoma is classified as invading the subepithelial connective tissue or lamina propria (pT1); the muscularis propria (pT2), superficial (pT2a) and deep (pT2b); the perivesical adipose tissue (pT3); and adjacent organs such as prostate, uterus, vagina, pelvic wall, and abdominal wall (pT4) (Table 4-3). Most pT1 tumors are low- or high-grade papillary urothelial carcinomas, whereas most pT2 to pT4 carcinomas are nonpapillary and of high grade. Tumor infiltrating muscle is not equivalent to muscularis propria invasion, because small, wispy fascicles of muscle are frequently present in lamina propria (muscularis mucosae). Tumor infiltrating adipose tissue is not always indicative of extravesical extension, because fat may be normally present in all layers of the bladder wall.

PATHOLOGIC FEATURES

GROSS FINDINGS

Urothelial carcinoma grossly may be papillary, polypoid, nodular (Fig. 4-14A), solid, ulcerative, or showing a transmural diffuse growth (Fig. 4-14B). The lesion may be solitary or multifocal. The remaining mucosa may be normal or erythematous, which sometimes corresponds to microscopic areas of CIS.

MICROSCOPIC FINDINGS

Urothelial carcinoma is graded as low grade or high grade depending on the degree of nuclear anaplasia and architectural abnormalities. With rare exceptions (i.e., nested or tubular variants), invasive urothelial carcinoma is high grade. The most important element in the pathologic evaluation of urothelial carcinoma is the recognition of the presence and extent of invasion. In early invasive urothelial carcinomas (pT1), foci of invasion are characterized by nests, clusters of single cells within the papillary cores and/or lamina propria (Fig. 4-15A). These invasive foci often are associated with retraction artifacts, mimicking vascular invasion. In more advanced stages, the tumor may infiltrate

---

TABLE 4-3

TNM Classification of carcinomas of the urinary bladder

TNM classification		N2	Metastasis in a single lymph node more than 2 cm but not more than 5 cm in greatest dimension, or multiple lymph nodes, none more than 5 cm in greatest dimension	
T-	Primary Tumor			
TX	Primary tumor cannot be assessed			
T0	No evidence of primary tumor	N3	Metastasis in a lymph node more than 5 cm in greatest dimension	
Ta	Non-invasive papillary carcinoma	M -	Distant Metastasis	
Tis	Carcinoma in-situ: "flat tumor"	MX	Distant metastasis cannot be assessed	
T1	Tumor invades subepithelial connective tissue	M0	No distant metastasis	
T2	Tumor invades muscle	M1	Distant metastasis	
T2a	Tumor invades superficial muscle (inner half)	**STAGE GROUPING**		
T2b	Tumor invades deep muscle (outer half)			
T3	Tumor invades perivesical tissue	Stage 0a	Ta	N0	M0
T3a	Microscopically	Stage 0is	Tis	N0	M0
T3b	Macroscopically (extravesical mass)	Stage I	T1	N0	M0
T4	Tumor invades any of the following: prostate, uterus, vagina, pelvic wall, abdominal wall	Stage II	T2a, b	N0	M0
T4a	Tumor invades prostate, uterus, or vagina	Stage III	T3, a, b	N0	M0
			T4	N0	M0
T4b	Tumor invades pelvic wall or abdominal wall	Stage IV	T4b	N0	M0
N	Regional Lymph Nodes	Any T	N1, N2, N3	M0
NX	Regional lymph nodes cannot be assessed	Any T	Any N	M1
N0	No regional lymph node metastasis			
N1	Metastasis in a single lymph node 2 cm or less in greatest dimension			

INVASIVE UROTHELIAL CARCINOMA—PATHOLOGIC FEATURES

Gross Findings

▶ Papillary, polypoid, nodular, solid, ulcerative, or transmural diffuse growth
▶ The remaining mucosa may be normal or erythematous

Microscopic Findings

▶ Most have significant nuclear anaplasia and architectural abnormalities and are classified as high grade
▶ Nests, clusters of single neoplastic cells within papillary cores and/or lamina propria (pT1), and muscularis propria (pT2)
▶ Invasive nests variably induce a desmoplastic stromal reaction
▶ Histologic variants: with squamous differentiation—21%; with glandular differentiation—6%; nested, which lacks prominent atypia—rare; microcystic, often coexisting with nested—rare; micropapillary variant—rare; lymphoepithelioma-like—rare; plasmacytoid—rare; and sarcomatoid (with/without heterologous elements)

Immunohistochemical Features

▶ Frequently positive for CK7, CK20, and p63
▶ Negative for PSA

Differential Diagnosis

▶ Noninvasive urothelial carcinoma
▶ von Brunn's nests versus nested variant
▶ Nephrogenic adenoma versus urothelial carcinoma with glandular differentiation
▶ Prostate carcinoma
▶ Lymphoma

---

muscularis propria (detrusor muscle) (Fig. 4-15B) or adipose tissue (Fig. 4-15C). Vascular invasion is often present (Fig. 4-15D).

Another feature of invasive cancers is that they often have more abundant eosinophilic cytoplasm than the adjacent noninvasive component (paradoxical differentiation). The invasive nests may induce a desmoplastic stromal reaction, which is occasionally pronounced and may mimic a malignant spindle-cell component, a feature known as pseudosarcomatous stromal reaction.

HISTOLOGIC VARIANTS

Urothelial carcinoma has a propensity for divergent differentiation, with the most common forms being squamous followed by glandular. Divergent differentiation frequently parallels high-grade and high-stage lesions. If small cell differentiation is present, even focally, it should be diagnosed as small cell carcinoma. Clear cell changes may also occur (Fig. 4-16).

Infiltrating Urothelial Carcinoma with Squamous Differentiation

Urothelial carcinoma with squamous differentiation occurs in 21% of urothelial carcinomas of the bladder and in 44% of tumors of the renal pelvis (Fig. 4-17A,B). The clinical significance of squamous differentiation remains uncertain, although it seems that, stage for stage, squamous differentiation does not seem to affect prognosis.

Infiltrating Urothelial Carcinoma with Glandular Differentiation

Glandular differentiation, defined as the presence of true glandular spaces within the urothelial component, may be present in about 6% of urothelial carcinomas of the bladder. It may consist of tubular or enteric glands with mucin secretions (Fig. 4-18A,B). Intracytoplasmic mucin, present in 14% to 64% of urothelial carcinomas, is not considered to represent glandular differentiation. One must also distinguish urothelial carcinoma with gland-like lumina, which represents microcystic change within urothelial carcinoma that often contains mucin yet lacks the apical cytoplasm and basally situated nuclei of true glandular differentiation. The clinical significance of glandular differentiation and mucin positivity in urothelial carcinomas is still uncertain, but, as with squamous differentiation, it does not seem to affect prognosis once stage is accounted for.

Infiltrating Urothelial Carcinoma, Nested Variant

The nested variant of urothelial carcinoma is an uncommon aggressive neoplasm, with a mortality rate

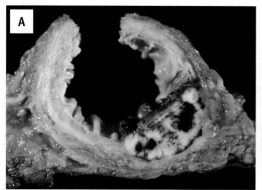
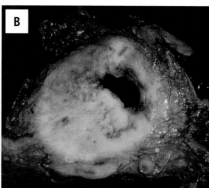

FIGURE 4-14

Gross photograph of surgically resected urinary bladder with invasive urothelial carcinoma. **A,** Nodular solid growth. **B,** Transmural diffuse growth.

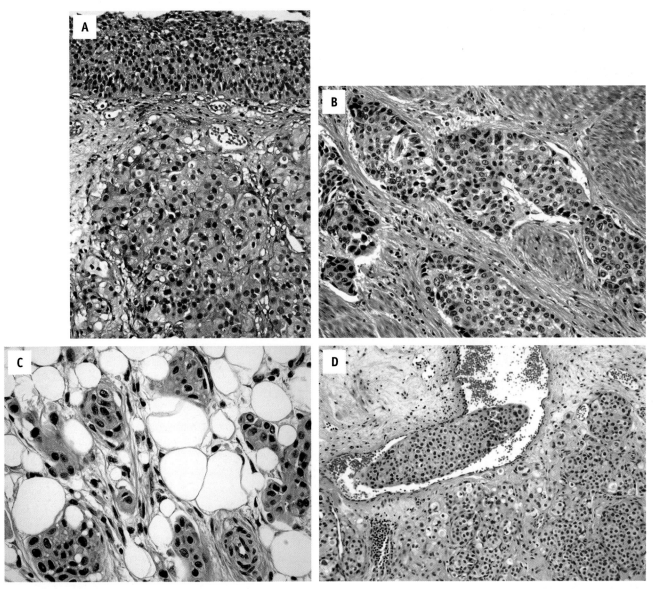

FIGURE 4-15

A, In early invasive urothelial carcinomas, foci of invasion are characterized by nests or clusters of single cells within the lamina propria. **B,** In more advanced stages, the tumor may infiltrate muscularis propria (detrusor muscle). **C,** It may also infiltrate adipose tissue, which can represent extravesical extension. **D,** Vascular invasion may be present and must be distinguished from retraction artifact, by the presence of either an endothelial cell lining, associated red blood cells, or a muscle wall.

of 70% at 4 to 40 months after diagnosis, despite therapy. There is a marked male predominance. This variant of urothelial carcinoma has a deceptively benign appearance that closely resembles von Brunn's nests infiltrating the lamina propria (Fig. 4-19A). The presence of muscle invasion (Fig. 4-19B), smaller nests than von Brunn's nests, irregularly invading crowded nests, and the tendency for increasing atypia (Fig. 4-19C) in the deeper portion of the lesion are useful features in recognizing this lesion as malignant.

Infiltrating Urothelial Carcinoma, Microcystic Variant

Urothelial carcinoma may occasionally show a striking cystic pattern, with cysts ranging from microscopic up to 1 to 2 mm in diameter (Fig. 4-20A). The cysts may contain necrotic material or pink, pale secretions (Fig. 4-20B). The cyst lining may be absent, flattened, or urothelial and may show differentiation toward mucinous cells (Fig. 4-20C). The differential diagnosis includes urothelial carcinoma with glandular differentiation and benign processes such as cystitis cystica, cystitis glandularis, and nephrogenic adenoma. Urothelial carcinoma with microcystic pattern often coexists with the nested variant of urothelial carcinoma and is unrelated to primary adenocarcinoma of the urinary bladder.

Infiltrating Urothelial Carcinoma, Micropapillary Variant

This rare variant of urothelial carcinoma resembles papillary serous carcinoma of the ovary. There is a

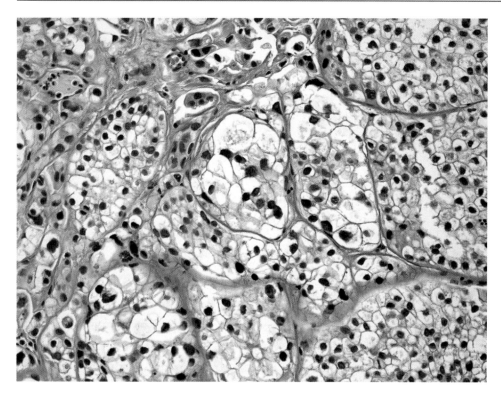

FIGURE 4-16
Clear cell changes may be seen in invasive urothelial carcinoma.

male predominance, and patient age ranges from the fifth through the ninth decades (mean age, 66 years). The micropapillary pattern exhibits two distinct morphologic features. The surface of the tumors exhibits slender, delicate papillary and villiform processes, often with a central vascular core. In contrast, the invasive portion is characterized by minute nests of cells or fine papillae contained within tissue retraction spaces, simulating lymphatic spaces (Fig. 4-21A). The tumors are invariably muscle-invasive, high-grade (Fig. 4-21B), high-stage cancers with high incidence of metastasis and morbidity.

Infiltrating Urothelial Carcinoma, Lymphoepithelioma-like

A few cases of urothelial carcinoma resembling lymphoepithelioma of the nasopharynx have recently been described in the urinary bladder (Fig. 4-22). These tumors show a male predominance and tend to occur in late adulthood. The proportion of lymphoepithelioma-like carcinoma should be reported. The behavior of these carcinomas is uncertain, because only few cases have been reported, but if only focal lymphoepithelioma-like disease is present, the behavior is similar to conventional urothelial carcinoma of the same grade and stage. The pure form of lymphoepithelioma-like carcinoma is responsive to chemotherapy.

Lymphoma-Like and Plasmacytoid Variants

In the lymphoma-like and plasmacytoid variants of urothelial carcinoma the malignant cells resemble those of malignant lymphoma or plasmacytoma (Fig. 4-23). Only a few cases have been reported, most of which had a component of high-grade urothelial carcinoma in addition to the single malignant cells. The tumor cells express cytokeratin, CK7 and, in some cases, CK20, but lymphoid markers are consistently negative.

Sarcomatoid Variants with and without Heterologous Elements

The term *sarcomatoid variant* of urothelial carcinoma should be used for all biphasic malignant neoplasms exhibiting morphologic and/or immunohistochemical evidence of epithelial and mesenchymal differentiation. The mean age is 66 years, and most patients present with hematuria. The mesenchymal component most frequently observed is an undifferentiated high-grade spindle-cell neoplasm. The most common heterologous element is osteosarcoma, followed by chondrosarcoma (Fig. 4-24), rhabdomyosarcoma, and leiomyosarcoma. Nodal and distant organ metastasis at the time of diagnosis are common. The mortality rate is 70% 1 to 48 months (mean survival time, 17 months).

ANCILLARY STUDIES

IMMUNOHISTOCHEMISTRY

Most urothelial carcinomas show diffuse cytoplasmic positivity for CK7, and a subset of cases are also positive for CK20 (Fig. 4-25A,B). Positive staining for both CK7 and CK20 favors the diagnosis of urothelial carcinoma. In addition, most of urothelial carcinomas show nuclear immunoreactivity for p63 (Fig. 4-25C).

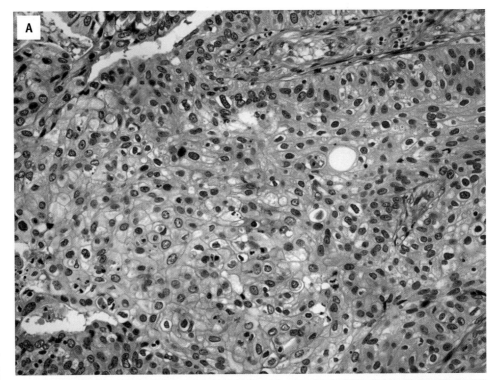

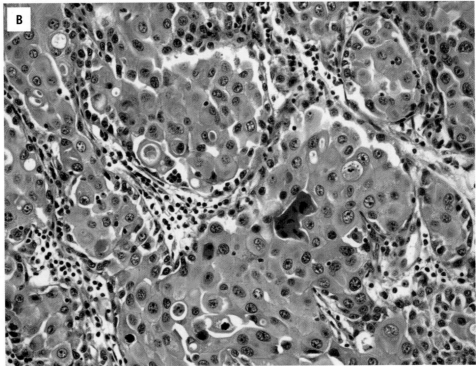

FIGURE 4-17

A, In infiltrating urothelial carcinoma with squamous differentiation, the presence of intercellular bridges can be appreciated at low power. **B,** High-power view shows intercellular bridges and keratinization.

DIFFERENTIAL DIAGNOSIS

The nested variant of urothelial carcinoma can occasionally cause some difficulty in its distinction from von Brunn's nests. The glandular component of urothelial carcinoma with glandular differentiation in rare cases consists of small, relatively regular tubules, suggesting the possibility of a nephrogenic adenoma. A poorly differentiated bladder cancer in a male patient should raise the possibility of prostate carcinoma, particularly if the specimen is obtained from the trigone or bladder neck. Immunoperoxidase staining can be very helpful, because prostate carcinoma stains positive for prostate-specific antigen (PSA) and is negative for p63 and thrombomodulin. Occasionally, urothelial carcinoma

Text continued on page 189

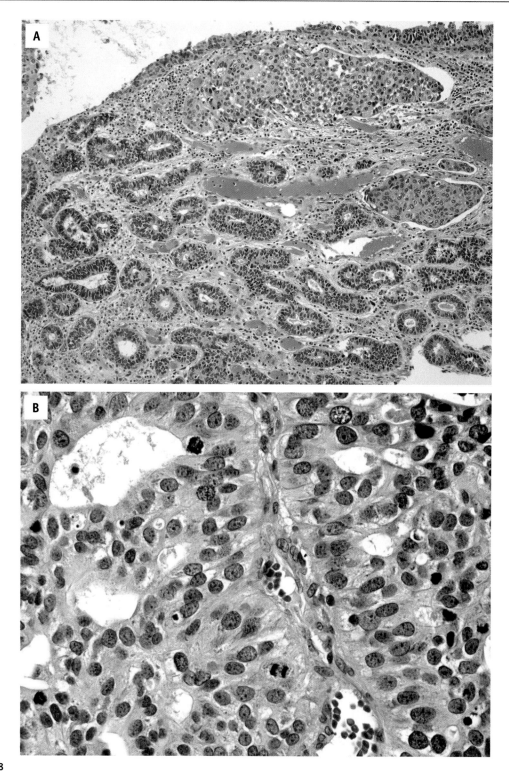

FIGURE 4-18

A, Glandular differentiation, defined as the presence of true glandular spaces within the urothelial component, may be present in urothelial carcinoma. It may consist of tubular or enteric glands with mucin secretion. **B,** At high power, apical cytoplasm and basally situated nuclei characteristic of true glandular differentiation are observed.

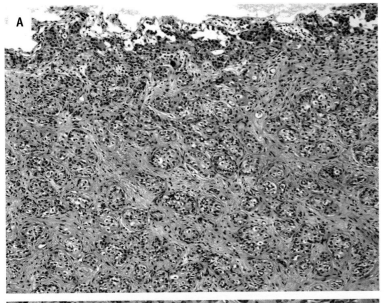

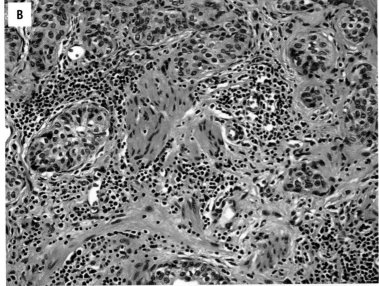

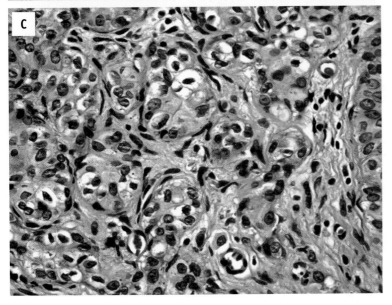

FIGURE 4-19
A, At low power, the nested variant of infiltrating urothelial carcinoma has a deceptively benign appearance that closely resembles von Brunn's nests infiltrating the lamina propria. **B,** Crowded nests are seen irregularly invading muscle fibers. **C,** At high power, the cytologic atypia increases in the deeper portion of the lesion.

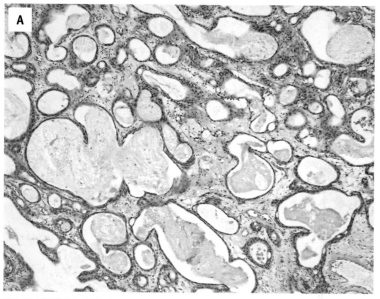

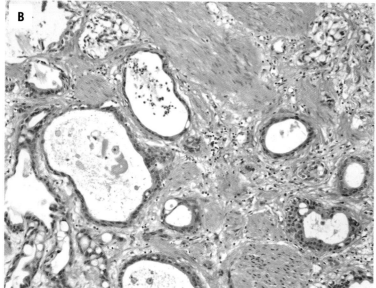

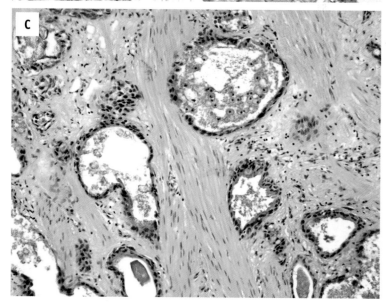

FIGURE 4-20

A, At low power, the tumor of infiltrating urothelial carcinoma may occasionally show a striking cystic pattern. **B,** At high power, the cysts may contain necrotic material or pink, pale secretions. The cyst lining may be absent, flattened, or urothelial. **C,** The cyst lining may show differentiation towards mucinous cells (mucicarmine stain).

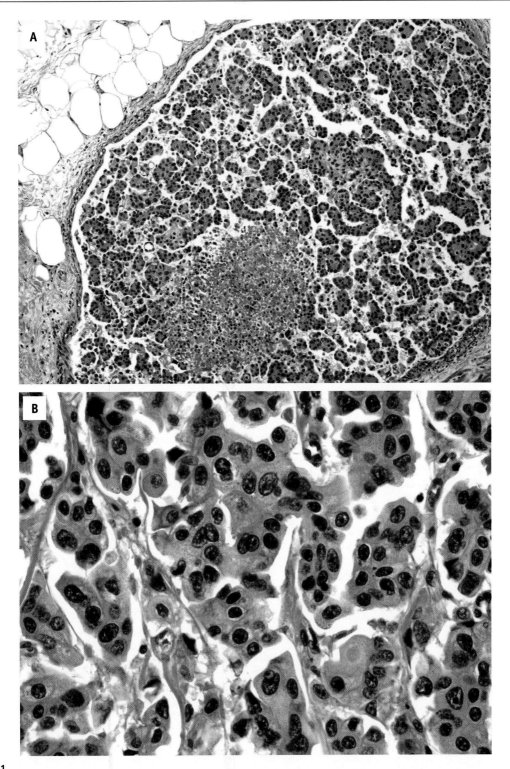

FIGURE 4-21
A, The invasive portion of the micropapillary variant of infiltrating urothelial carcinoma is characterized by fine papillae contained within tissue retraction spaces, simulating lymphatic spaces. **B,** At high power, the cytologic features are invariably high grade.

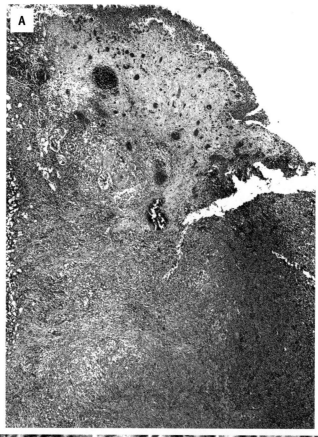

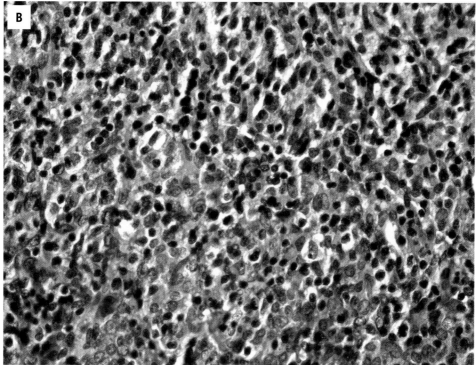

FIGURE 4-22

A, At low power, the lesion of the lymphoepithelioma-like variant of infiltrating urothelial carcinoma is characterized by a prominent inflammatory background. **B,** At high power, the tumor is composed of sheets of undifferentiated cells with large nuclei. The cytoplasmic borders are poorly defined, imparting a syncytial appearance.

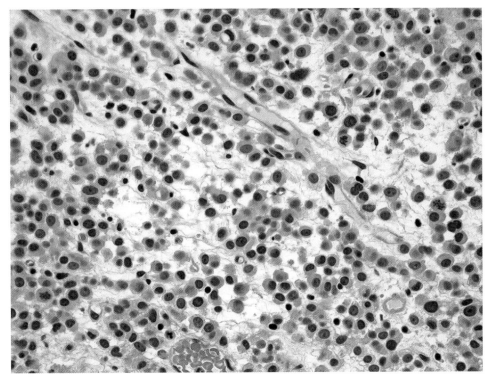

FIGURE 4-23

The plasmacytoid variant of infiltrating urothelial carcinoma is characterized by the presence of single malignant cells in a loose or myxoid stroma. The tumor cells have eosinophilic cytoplasm and eccentrically placed, enlarged hyperchromatic nuclei.

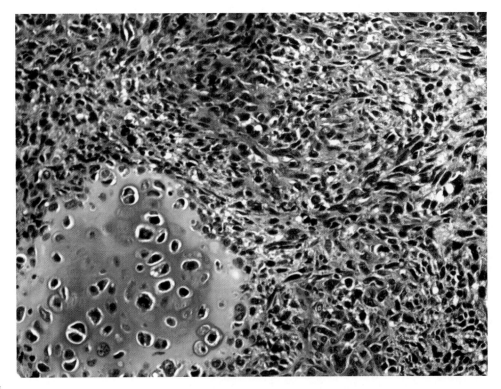

FIGURE 4-24

The mesenchymal component of this sarcomatoid urothelial carcinoma demonstrates an undifferentiated, high-grade spindle cell neoplasm with heterologous elements of chondrosarcoma, showing binucleation and atypical chondrocytes within lacunae.

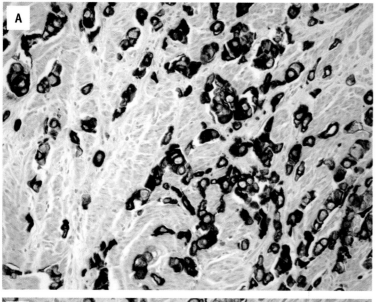

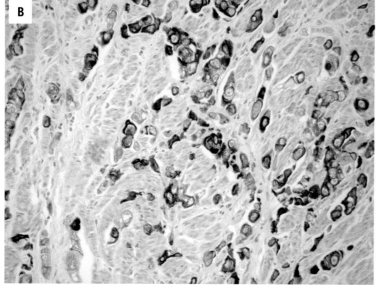

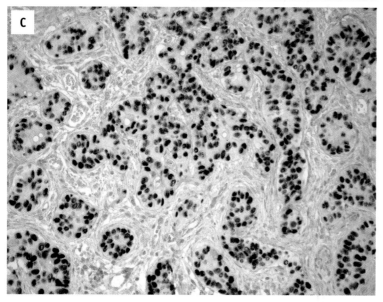

FIGURE 4-25

A, Clusters and individual tumor cells infiltrating muscularis propria showing diffuse, strong cytoplasmic reactivity for cytokeratin 7 (CK7). **B,** Diffuse cytoplasmic staining for CK20 is shown. **C,** The nested variant of urothelial carcinoma shows strong nuclear immunoreactivity for p63.

may resemble malignant lymphoma. Special stains for epithelial and lymphoid markers may aid in the diagnosis.

PROGNOSIS AND TREATMENT

Transurethral resection of all visible lesions down to the base is required for accurate assessment of the depth of tumor invasion. Invasion of lamina propria (pT1) without extension into the muscularis propria does not require radical surgery. Those patients are treated by TUR with or without adjuvant intravesical therapy. The 5-year survival rate is about 70%. The standard treatment for muscle-invasive (pT2 to pT4) bladder cancer is total cystectomy or cystoprostatectomy. Survival rates after total cystectomy vary depending on stage.

SQUAMOUS CELL CARCINOMA

Squamous cell carcinoma (SCC) of the urinary bladder is a malignant neoplasm derived from the urothelium that shows a histologically pure squamous cell phenotype. SCC of the bladder is much less frequent than urothelial carcinoma, constituting about 1.3% of bladder tumors in men and 3.4% in women, worldwide. SCC accounts for fewer than 5% of bladder carcinomas in areas where schistosomiasis is not endemic and 75% in areas where the infection with *S. haematobium* is endemic. SCC of the bladder predominates in west, east, and southeast Africa and in Egypt. In South Africa, the marked difference in histology between blacks (36% SCC, 41% urothelial carcinoma) and whites (2% SCC, 94% urothelial carcinoma) is related to the prevalence of infection with *S. haematobium*.

CLINICAL FEATURES

Tobacco is an important risk factor for SCC of the bladder. It has been estimated that the relative risk for current smokers is about five times that of nonsmokers. Infection with *S. haematobium* is the classic condition wherein chronic inflammation is associated with SCC, but there are other examples of this association, such as calculi and urethral stricture. SCC accounts for approximately 20% of tumors arising within bladder diverticula, 50% of tumors occurring in patients with nonfunctioning bladder, and 15% of tumors in patients who have undergone renal transplantation.

SCC of the bladder manifests with irritative symptoms and the occasional passage of keratinous material in the urine.

SQUAMOUS CELL CARCINOMA—FACT SHEET

Definition
► Malignant neoplasm derived from the urothelium showing histologically pure squamous cell phenotype

Incidence and Location
► 75% of bladder tumors in areas where schistosomiasis is endemic
► <5% of bladder tumors in areas where schistosomiasis is not endemic (1.3% in men, 3.4% in women)
► 20% of tumors arising within bladder diverticula
► 50% of tumors occurring in nonfunctioning bladder
► 15% of tumors in renal transplant patients

Gender, Race, and Age Distribution
► Predominates in west, east, and southeast Africa and in Egypt
► In South Africa, more common among blacks

Clinical Features
► Associated with *Schistosoma haematobium* infection
► Presents with irritative symptoms and occasional passage of keratinous material in the urine

Prognosis and Treatment
► Overall 5-year survival rate is 56% (67% for organ-confined and 19% for non-organ-confined disease)
► Radical surgery appears to improve survival compared with radiation therapy and/or chemotherapy
► Neoadjuvant radiation improves outcome in locally advanced tumors

---

PATHOLOGIC FEATURES

GROSS FINDINGS

Most SCCs are bulky, polypoid, solid, necrotic masses often filling the bladder lumen. The presence of necrotic material and keratin debris on the surface is relatively constant.

MICROSCOPIC FINDINGS

The diagnosis of SCC is restricted to pure tumors. The presence of keratinizing squamous metaplasia in the adjacent flat epithelium supports the diagnosis of SCC. The invasive tumor may be well differentiated, with islands of squamous cells demonstrating keratinization, prominent intercellular bridges, and minimal nuclear pleomorphism, or poorly differentiated, with marked nuclear pleomorphism and only focal evidence of squamous differentiation (Fig. 4-26).

DIFFERENTIAL DIAGNOSIS

Many vesical SCCs are well to moderately differentiated and have only mild to moderate cytologic atypia.

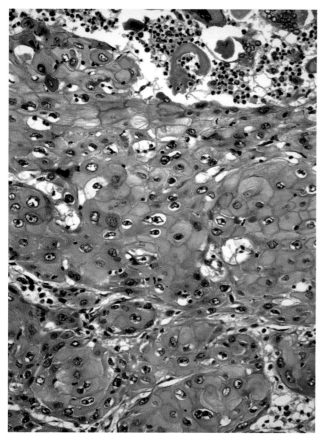

FIGURE 4-26
Well-differentiated invasive squamous cell carcinoma with islands of squamous cells demonstrating keratinization, prominent intercellular bridges, and minimal nuclear pleomorphism.

Squamous papilloma and condyloma can be distinguished from SCC by the lack of cytologic atypia and invasion, and, in the case of condyloma, by the presence of koilocytic cells.

SQUAMOUS CELL CARCINOMA—PATHOLOGIC FEATURES

Gross Findings
▶ Bulky, polypoid, solid, necrotic masses often filling the bladder lumen
▶ Necrotic material and keratin debris on the surface are relatively constant

Microscopic Findings
▶ Diagnosis of SCC is restricted to pure tumors
▶ Keratinizing squamous metaplasia in the adjacent flat epithelium supports the diagnosis
▶ SCC, well-differentiated: defined islands of squamous cells with keratinization, prominent intercellular bridges, and minimal nuclear pleomorphism
▶ SCC, poorly differentiated: marked nuclear pleomorphism and only focal evidence of squamous differentiation

Differential Diagnosis
▶ Urothelial carcinoma with focal squamous differentiation

PROGNOSIS AND TREATMENT

Tumor stage, lymph node involvement, and tumor grade have been shown to be of independent prognostic value. The overall 5-year survival rate is 56% (67% for patients with organ-confined tumors, and 19% for those with nonorgan-confined tumors). Radical surgery appears to result in improved survival, compared with radiation therapy, chemotherapy, or both, whereas neoadjuvant radiation improves the outcome in locally advanced tumors.

ADENOCARCINOMA (NONURACHAL)

Bladder adenocarcinoma is a malignant neoplasm derived from the urothelium that shows a histologically pure glandular phenotype. This tumor is uncommon, accounting for fewer than 2% of all malignant urinary bladder tumors. Adenocarcinoma can be of urachal origin, associated with exstrophy, associated with endometriosis, or unassociated (nonurachal). Nonurachal adenocarcinoma is the most common type, accounting for approximately two thirds of adenocarcinomas of the bladder. Approximately 15% of tumors arise in patients with a nonfunctioning bladder, and 85% are associated with exstrophy.

CLINICAL FEATURES

Adenocarcinoma of the urinary bladder occurs more commonly in men than in women, with a ratio of 2.6:1, and it affects adults, with a peak incidence in the sixth decade of life. Hematuria is the most common symptom, followed by dysuria, but mucosuria is rarely seen.

PATHOLOGIC FEATURES

GROSS FINDINGS

These tumors may be exophytic, papillary, sessile, ulcerating, or infiltrating and may exhibit a gelatinous appearance. They typically occur in the bladder base or dome but can appear anywhere in the bladder.

MICROSCOPIC FEATURES

Histologically, adenocarcinomas of the urinary bladder are subclassified by their histology: adenocarcinoma not otherwise specified (27%), mucinous (24%), enteric (19%), signet-ring cell (17%), and mixed (13%). The enteric type resembles adenocarcinoma of the colon (Fig. 4-27A,B). Tumors that show abundant mucin with tumor cells floating within the mucin are

---

ADENOCARCINOMA (NONURACHAL)—FACT SHEET

Definition
▶ Malignant neoplasm derived from the urothelium showing histologically pure glandular phenotype

Incidence and Location
▶ Uncommon (< 2% of all malignant urinary bladder tumors)
▶ Two thirds of bladder adenocarcinomas
▶ 15% arise in patients with nonfunctioning bladder
▶ 85% are associated with exstrophy
▶ Typically occurs in the bladder base or dome

Gender, Race, and Age Distribution
▶ Male predominance (M/F ratio, 2.6:1)
▶ Affects adults (peak incidence: sixth decade of life)

Clinical Features
▶ Hematuria is the most common symptom, followed by dysuria
▶ Mucosuria is rarely seen

Prognosis and Treatment
▶ Poor prognosis (5-year survival rate varies from 18% to 47%)
▶ Management includes partial or radical cystectomy
▶ Chemotherapy or radiation therapy should be considered according to the extent of the lesion

DIFFERENTIAL DIAGNOSIS

The most important differential diagnosis includes metastatic disease or direct extension, most commonly from colorectum or prostate. Secondary involvement of the urinary bladder is more common than primary adenocarcinoma of the bladder.

The vast majority of adenocarcinomas of the bladder have readily identifiable cytologic atypia, in contrast to endometriosis, endocervicosis, and cystitis glandularis.

PROGNOSIS AND TREATMENT

Adenocarcinoma of the bladder generally has a poor prognosis, with the 5-year survival rate varying from 18% and 47%. Management includes partial or radical cystectomy followed by consideration of chemotherapy or radiation therapy according to the extent of the lesion. Advanced stage at diagnosis is associated with a poor prognosis.

---

classified as mucinous or colloid type. The signet-ring cell variant (Fig. 4-27C) may be diffuse or mixed. Adenocarcinoma in situ may be found alone or in combination with invasive adenocarcinoma. The urothelial mucosa is replaced by glandular structures with definite nuclear atypia. Three different adenocarcinoma in situ patterns have been described: papillary, cribriform, and flat. Adenocarcinoma in situ, when unaccompanied by invasive adenocarcinoma, may also be seen with CIS, micropapillary urothelial carcinoma, or small cell carcinoma of the bladder.

ANCILLARY STUDIES

IMMUNOHISTOCHEMISTRY

The immunohistochemical profile of bladder adenocarcinoma is variable and closely matches that of colonic adenocarcinomas. CK7 positivity is variable, whereas CK20 is reported to be positive in most bladder adenocarcinomas. Villin has recently been reported to be positive in the enteric type. According to one study, positive nuclear staining for β-catenin is detected in the majority of colorectal adenocarcinomas secondarily involving the bladder but in none of the primary bladder tumors. Adenocarcinomas primary in the bladder may be positive for prostate-specific acid phosphatase (PSAP) but are negative for PSA.

ADENOCARCINOMA (NONURACHAL)—PATHOLOGIC FEATURES

Gross Findings
▶ Tumor may be exophytic, papillary, sessile, ulcerating, or infiltrating
▶ It may exhibit a gelatinous appearance

Microscopic Findings
▶ Urothelial mucosa replaced by glandular structures with definite nuclear atypia
▶ Adenocarcinoma in situ may be found alone or in combination with invasive adenocarcinoma
▶ Three different patterns: papillary, cribriform, and flat
▶ Microscopic subgroups: adenocarcinoma not otherwise specified—28%; mucinous—24%; enteric—19%; signet-ring cell—17%; and mixed—13%

Immunohistochemical Features
▶ Variable CK7 positivity
▶ Frequently positive for CK20
▶ Villin is positive in the enteric type
▶ Nuclear staining for β-catenin is negative
▶ Negative for PSA and PSAP

Differential Diagnosis
▶ Metastatic adenocarcinoma
▶ Direct extension, most commonly from colorectum or prostate
▶ Endometriosis
▶ Endocervicosis
▶ Cystitis glandularis

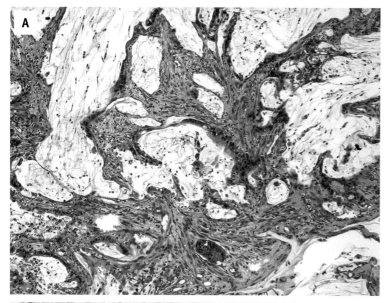

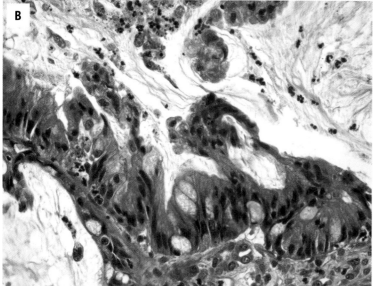

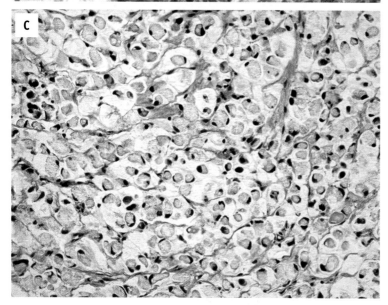

FIGURE 4-27

A, The enteric type of nonurachal adenocarcinoma resembles adenocarcinoma of the colon, with abundant mucin and tumor cells floating within the mucin. **B,** At high power, cells show different degrees of cytologic atypia. **C,** The signet-ring cell variant shows diffuse infiltration by single cells.

URACHAL CARCINOMA

Urachal carcinoma is a primary carcinoma derived from the urachal remnants. The vast majority of urachal carcinomas are adenocarcinomas, although urothelial and squamous carcinomas may also occur. Urachal adenocarcinoma is far less common than nonurachal adenocarcinoma of the bladder. Most cases occur in the fifth or sixth decade of life; the mean patient age is 50 years, which is about 10 years less than for nonurachal bladder adenocarcinoma. Urachal adenocarcinoma occurs slightly more frequently in men than in women, with a ratio of approximately 1.8:1. Patients may present with a suprapubic mass. Mucosuria occurs in approximately 25% of the cases, and its presence should raise the suspicion of urachal adenocarcinoma, although this finding may also be seen with villous adenoma.

PATHOLOGIC FEATURES

GROSS FINDINGS

Urachal carcinoma usually involves the bladder dome. The tumor mass may be discrete, but it can also involve urachal remnants, forming a large mass in the anterior abdominal wall (Fig. 4-28). Mucinous lesions tend to calcify, and these calcifications may be detected on a plain radiographic films of the abdomen.

MICROSCOPIC FINDINGS

Urachal adenocarcinomas are subdivided into different subtypes, similar to nonurachal adenocarcinomas (Fig. 4-29). The criteria to classify a tumor as urachal are (1) location in the dome or anterior wall of the bladder; (2) sharp demarcation between tumor and normal surface epithelium; (3) lack of in situ adenocarcinoma; (4) typically, lack of prominent cystitis glandularis in adjacent mucosa; (5) bulk of tumor in the bladder wall rather than luminal; and (6) exclusion of primary adenocarcinoma located elsewhere that has spread secondarily to the bladder. The majority of urachal adenocarcinomas are muscle invasive at the time of diagnosis.

DIFFERENTIAL DIAGNOSIS

Bladder nonurachal adenocarcinoma may be histologically very difficult to differentiate from urachal adenocarcinoma and requires clinical correlation.

URACHAL CARCINOMA—FACT SHEET

Definition
▶ Primary carcinoma derived from urachal remnants

Incidence and Location
▶ Uncommon (one third of bladder adenocarcinomas)
▶ Involves the bladder dome or anterior wall; may also involve urachal remnants (mass involving anterior abdominal wall)

Morbidity and Mortality
▶ Recurrences are common, especially after a partial cystectomy
▶ Majority of tumors are muscle-invasive disease

Gender, Race, and Age Distribution
▶ Slight male predominance (M/F ratio, 1.8:1)
▶ Most cases occur in the fifth and sixth decade of life (mean age, 50 years)

Clinical Features
▶ Suprapubic mass
▶ Mucosuria occurs in approximately 25% of the cases

Prognosis and Treatment
▶ Poor prognosis (5-year survival rate varies from 25% to 61%)
▶ Partial or radical cystectomy, including resection of the umbilicus, is a treatment of choice

---

URACHAL CARCINOMA—PATHOLOGIC FEATURES

Gross Findings
▶ Tumor mass may be discrete, but it may also involve the urachal remnants, forming a large mass in the anterior abdominal wall

Microscopic Findings
▶ Criterion 1—Dome or anterior wall of the bladder
▶ Criterion 2—Sharp demarcation between tumor and normal surface epithelium without in situ component
▶ Criterion 3—Typically not associated with prominent cystitis glandularis
▶ Criterion 4—Primarily located in the muscularis propria with little mucosal involvement
▶ Criterion 5—Bulk of tumor in bladder wall rather than luminal (i.e., muscle-invasive disease)
▶ Criterion 6—Exclusion of primary adenocarcinoma located elsewhere that has spread secondarily to the bladder

Immunohistochemical Features
▶ See nonurachal adenocarcinoma

Differential Diagnosis
▶ Nonurachal adenocarcinoma
▶ Metastatic adenocarcinoma
▶ Direct extension, most commonly from colorectum and prostate

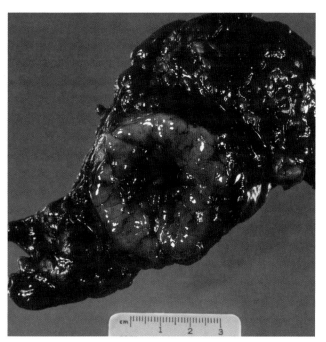

FIGURE 4-28
Gross photograph of surgically resected partial cystectomy specimen including urachal carcinoma tumor and connective tissue between bladder and anterior abdominal wall.

PROGNOSIS AND TREATMENT

Complete eradication of the lesion is the proper management. Partial or radical cystectomy, including resection of the umbilicus, is a treatment of choice.

Recurrences are common, especially in cases in which a partial cystectomy is done. The 5-year survival rate has been reported to range from 25% to 61%.

SMALL CELL CARCINOMA

Small cell carcinoma of the urinary bladder is a malignant neuroendocrine neoplasm derived from the urothelium that mimics its pulmonary counterpart. It accounts for almost 0.5% of malignant tumors of the bladder. Approximately 85% of patients are male, with a mean age of 69 years.

CLINICAL FEATURES

Almost all small cell carcinomas of the urinary tract arise in the urinary bladder. Gross hematuria is the most common presenting symptom. All tumors are invasive at presentation, and approximately half of patients have metastatic disease at the time of diagnosis. Peripheral neuropathy, attributed to a paraneoplastic syndrome associated with tumor production of anti-neuronal autoantibodies, may also be a clinical sign of metastatic disease. Hypercalcemia, hypophosphatemia, and ectopic secretion of adrenocorticotropic hormone (ACTH) have also been reported as part of the paraneoplastic syndrome associated with small cell carcinoma of the bladder.

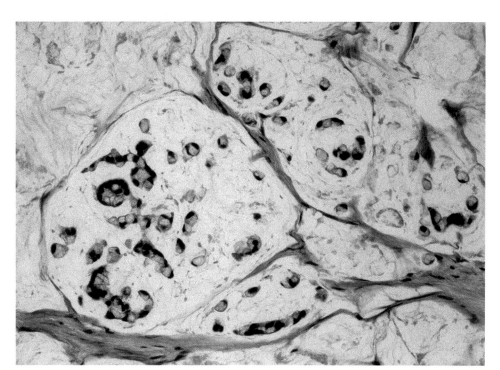

FIGURE 4-29
Urachal adenocarcinoma manifests as a mucinous adenocarcinoma with clusters of signet-ring cells floating within the mucin.

SMALL CELL CARCINOMA—FACT SHEET

Definition
▶ Malignant neuroendocrine neoplasm derived from urothelium, with histology similar to that of the pulmonary counterpart

Incidence and Location
▶ Uncommon (0.5% of malignant tumors of the bladder)
▶ Urinary bladder is the most common location in the urinary tract
▶ Lateral wall and dome of bladder are the most frequent locations
▶ 5% of cases arise in diverticula

Morbidity and Mortality
▶ All tumors are invasive at presentation
▶ Half of patients present with metastatic disease at the time of diagnosis

Gender, Race, and Age Distribution
▶ Male predominance (85% of patients)
▶ Mean age, 69 years

Clinical Features
▶ Gross hematuria
▶ Paraneoplastic syndrome (peripheral neuropathy, hypercalcemia, hypophosphatemia, ectopic secretion of ACTH)

Prognosis and Treatment
▶ Aggressive clinical behavior and poor prognosis
▶ 5-year survival rate for patients with local disease is as low as 8%
▶ Typically treated with aggressive combination chemotherapy
▶ Localized residual disease after chemotherapy is treated by radical cystectomy

PATHOLOGIC FEATURES

GROSS FEATURES

The tumor may appear as a large solid, isolated, polypoid, nodular mass and may extensively infiltrate the bladder wall. The lateral walls of the urinary bladder and the dome are the most frequent locations; approximately 5% of small cell carcinoma arise in diverticula.

MICROSCOPIC FINDINGS

The cells are small, rather uniform, with nuclear molding, scant cytoplasm, and nuclei with finely stippled chromatin and inconspicuous nucleoli. Mitoses are present and may be frequent (Fig. 4-30). Necrosis is common. Approximately 50% of small cell carcinomas of the bladder show areas of urothelial carcinoma; less frequently, they may have areas of squamous cell carcinoma (SCC) and/or adenocarcinoma. The diagnosis of small cell carcinoma can be made on morphologic grounds alone, even if neuroendocrine differentiation cannot be demonstrated immunohistochemically.

ANCILLARY STUDIES

IMMUNOHISTOCHEMISTRY

Neuron-specific enolase (NSE) and CD56 (Fig. 4-31) is expressed in most instances, with chromogranin seen only in a third of cases.

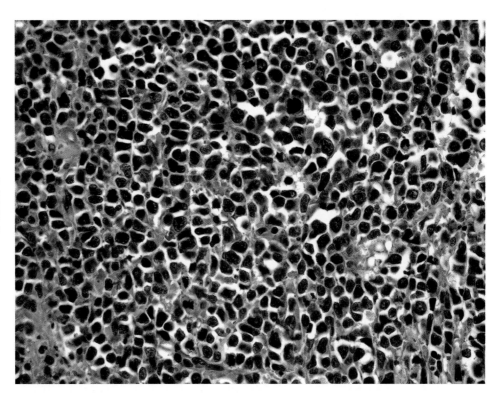

FIGURE 4-30

In small cell carcinoma, the cells are small, rather uniform, with nuclear molding, scant cytoplasm, and nuclei with finely stippled chromatin and inconspicuous nucleoli. Mitoses are present and may be frequent.

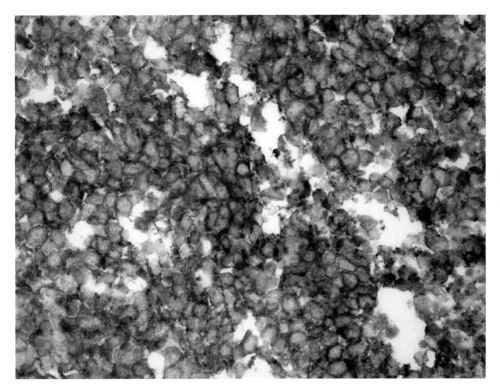

FIGURE 4-31
Diffuse cytoplasmic expression of CD56 in small cell carcinoma of the bladder.

SMALL CELL CARCINOMA—PATHOLOGIC FEATURES

Gross Findings

▶ Large solid, isolated, polypoid, nodular mass
▶ It may extensively infiltrate the bladder wall

Microscopic Findings

▶ Cells are small and rather uniform, with scant cytoplasm
▶ Nuclear molding, nuclei with finely stippled chromatin and inconspicuous nucleoli
▶ Mitoses may be frequent
▶ Necrosis is common
▶ Approximately 50% of tumors show areas of in situ or invasive urothelial carcinoma or, less commonly, SCC and/or adenocarcinoma

Immunohistochemical Features

▶ NSE, CD56 expressed in most cases
▶ Chromogranin is positive in one third of cases

Differential Diagnosis

▶ Metastatic small cell carcinoma from another site
▶ Malignant lymphoma
▶ Lymphoepithelioma-like carcinoma
▶ Plasmacytoid urothelial carcinoma
▶ Poorly differentiated urothelial carcinoma

DIFFERENTIAL DIAGNOSIS

The differential diagnosis includes metastatic small cell carcinoma from another site, malignant lymphoma, lymphoepithelioma-like carcinoma, plasmacytoid carcinoma, and poorly differentiated urothelial carcinoma.

PROGNOSIS AND TREATMENT

Small cell carcinoma of the urinary bladder is characterized by an aggressive clinical behavior and poor prognosis. The overall 5-year survival rate for patients with local disease is reported to be as low as 8%. Initial treatment is with aggressive chemotherapy; if the tumor responds but local disease persists, this may be followed by radical cystectomy.

Papillary Nonurothelial Lesions

CONDYLOMA ACUMINATA

Condyloma acuminata are common, sexually transmitted benign tumors caused by human papillomavirus

(HPV). On rare occasions, they may involve the urinary bladder. Typically only the distal urethra is involved, but occasionally there is extension to the proximal urethra and the urinary bladder.

CLINICAL FEATURES

Most cases of condyloma acuminata of the urinary bladder reported in the literature were associated with coexistent condylomata of the external genitalia, and some required pelvic exenteration for uncontrolled expansile growth. Although the lesion may be discrete, there is a tendency for diffuse involvement. Condyloma acuminata of the urinary tract can cause irritative symptoms and hematuria.

PATHOLOGIC FEATURES

GROSS FEATURES

The lesions are smooth, pink-tan, and papillary (Fig. 4-32).

MICROSCOPIC FEATURES

The lesions are characterized by papillary fronds lined by hyperplastic, metaplastic squamous epithelium, which may be hyperkeratotic (Fig. 4-33A). Many of the epithelial cells have a perinuclear halo (koilocytes) (Fig. 4-33B).

CONDYLOMA ACUMINATA—PATHOLOGIC FEATURES

Gross Findings
► Smooth, pink-tan, papillary lesions

Microscopic Findings
► Papillary fronds lined by hyperplastic, metaplastic squamous epithelium, which may be hyperkeratotic
► Many of the epithelial cells with irregular, crinkly, occasionally multinucleated nuclei with perinuclear halo (koilocytes)

Differential Diagnosis
► Verrucous carcinoma

DIFFERENTIAL DIAGNOSIS

In contrast to condyloma acuminata, verrucous carcinoma lacks koilocytes, and the nests and columns of squamous epithelium invade irregularly into the underlying tissue.

PROGNOSIS AND TREATMENT

Discrete lesions are managed by TUR, but diffuse disease usually requires more radical surgery. Rare cases have been associated with malignant transformation.

CONDYLOMA ACUMINATA—FACT SHEET

Definition
► Benign HPV-induced papilloma

Incidence and Location
► Rarely involves urinary bladder (typically only distal urethra is involved)

Morbidity and Mortality
► Rare risk of malignant transformation

Clinical Features
► Can cause irritative symptoms and hematuria

Prognosis and Treatment
► TUR

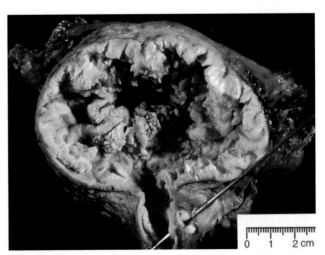

FIGURE 4-32

Gross photograph of surgically resected cystectomy specimen of condyloma acuminata, showing diffuse involvement by papillary fronds.

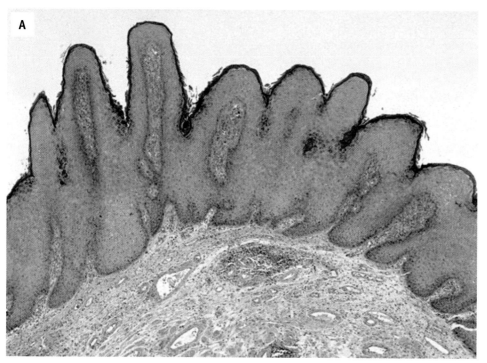

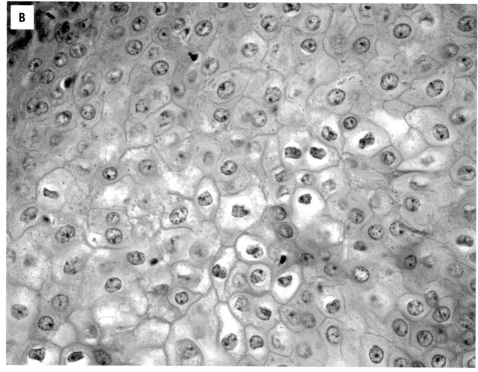

FIGURE 4-33

A, The lesion of condyloma acuminata is characterized by papillary fronds lined by thickened squamous epithelium, which may be hyperkeratotic. **B,** Many of the epithelial cells have a perinuclear halo (koilocytes).

SQUAMOUS PAPILLOMA

Squamous papilloma of the urinary tract is a very rare lesion. It is characterized by a proliferation of mature and benign-appearing squamous epithelium surrounding a central fibrovascular core. Koilocytes are not present. The lesions occur in elderly women and follow a benign clinical course with infrequent recurrence. Clinically, the symptoms are nonspecific. Cystoscopy shows a solitary papillary lesion. The lesion is not associated with HPV infection.

VILLOUS ADENOMA

Villous adenoma is a rare glandular neoplasm of the urinary bladder that histologically mimics its enteric counterpart.

CLINICAL FEATURES

There is a male predilection. The lesion occurs in elderly patients (mean age, 65 years), and the most common locations are the urachus, dome, and trigone of the urinary bladder. Patients often present with hematuria and/or irritative symptoms, occasionally with mucosuria.

PATHOLOGIC FEATURES

GROSS FINDINGS

The lesion is a papillary tumor indistinguishable from papillary urothelial carcinoma.

VILLOUS ADENOMA—FACT SHEET

Definition
▶ Benign glandular neoplasm of the urinary bladder that histologically mimics its enteric counterpart

Incidence and Location
▶ Rare
▶ Most common locations: urachus, dome, and trigone of the urinary bladder

Morbidity and Mortality
▶ Often coexists with in situ and invasive adenocarcinoma

Gender, Race, and Age Distribution
▶ Male predilection
▶ Elderly patients (mean age, 65 years)

Clinical Features
▶ Hematuria and/or irritative symptoms
▶ Occasionally mucosuria

Prognosis and Treatment
▶ Isolated lesions have an excellent prognosis
▶ Complete resection is the treatment of choice

VILLOUS ADENOMA—PATHOLOGIC FEATURES

Gross Findings
▶ Papillary lesion indistinguishable from papillary urothelial carcinoma

Microscopic Findings
▶ Blunt, finger-like papillary architecture with central fibrovascular cores, lined by pseudostratified columnar epithelium
▶ Cells display nuclear stratification, crowding, hyperchromasia, and occasional prominent nucleoli
▶ May coexist with in situ and/or invasive adenocarcinoma

Immunohistochemical Features
▶ Always positive for CK20
▶ Often positive for CK7, CEA, and acid mucin
▶ Occasionally positive for EMA

Differential Diagnosis
▶ Invasive/metastatic adenocarcinoma from colon can mimic bladder villous adenoma; colon lesion needs to be ruled out clinically

---

MICROSCOPIC FINDINGS

The tumor is characterized by blunt, finger-like papillary architecture with central fibrovascular cores (Fig. 4-34A), lined by pseudostratified columnar epithelium. The epithelial cells display nuclear stratification, crowding, hyperchromasia, and occasional prominent nucleoli (Fig. 4-34B). Invasion of the underlying stroma precludes the diagnosis of villous adenoma. Villous adenoma of the bladder often coexists with in situ and/or invasive adenocarcinoma.

ANCILLARY STUDIES

IMMUNOHISTOCHEMISTRY

Villous adenomas are always positive for CK20, often positive for CK7 and CEA, and occasionally positive for epithelial membrane antigen (EMA). Stains for acid mucin are also frequently positive.

DIFFERENTIAL DIAGNOSIS

Villous adenoma of the urinary bladder must be distinguished from invasive adenocarcinoma; the criteria employed are identical to those used in analogous colonic lesions. Spread to the bladder from an invasive colonic adenocarcinoma can also mimic villous adenoma of the bladder.

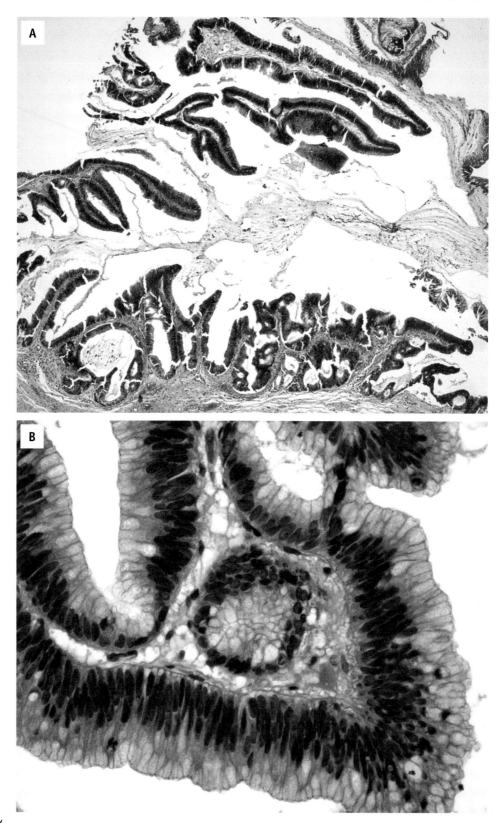

FIGURE 4-34

Villous adenoma. **A,** The tumor is characterized by blunt, finger-like papillary architecture with central fibrovascular cores. **B,** The papillae are lined by pseudostratified columnar epithelium. The epithelial cells display nuclear stratification, crowding, hyperchromasia, and occasional prominent nucleoli.

PROGNOSIS AND TREATMENT

Patients with an isolated lesion have an excellent prognosis. The entire specimen should be processed to exclude invasive disease.

NONEPITHELIAL NEOPLASMS OF THE URINARY BLADDER

Benign Mesenchymal Lesions

Rare cases of benign mesenchymal neoplasms of the urinary tract have been described, although they are less common than their malignant counterparts. Leiomyoma is the most common benign mesenchymal tumor of the bladder.

INFLAMMATORY MYOFIBROBLASTIC TUMOR

The term "postoperative spindle-cell nodule" was used in the past to describe a spindle-cell proliferation that occurs in the bladder, typically after TUR. Other lesions with overlapping morphology were observed in patients without a prior history of surgery; although there were numerous terms for this entity, it was most commonly referred to as pseudosarcomatous fibromyxoid tumor. Currently, these two types of lesions are thought to be related and are designated inflammatory myofibroblastic tumors (IMT).

CLINICAL FEATURES

IMTs of the genitourinary tract are neoplastic proliferations that can infiltrate the bladder wall and even extend into perivesical adipose tissue. Surgery-related lesions arise within months after a TUR and are typically small (< 1.0 cm.). IMTs not associated with prior surgery tend to be larger, up to 9.0 cm.

PATHOLOGIC FEATURES

GROSS FINDINGS

The lesions are either pedunculated or polypoid.

MICROSCOPIC FINDINGS

IMTs are characterized by myofibroblastic cells resembling tissue-culture fibroblasts. The cells may be

---

INFLAMMATORY MYOFIBROBLASTIC TUMOR—FACT SHEET

Definition
▶ Spindle-cell proliferation that occurs in the bladder typically after TUR

Incidence and Location
▶ Rare neoplasm
▶ Can infiltrate bladder wall and even extend into perivesical adipose tissue

Morbidity and Mortality
▶ Once resected, even incompletely, typically tends to regress or stay stable

Clinical Features
▶ Cases that arise after surgery appear within months of a TUR

Prognosis and Treatment
▶ Typically tends to regress or stay stable
▶ Occasionally may recur, causing local morbidity and potentially even necessitating radical surgery
▶ Close follow-up is recommended

INFLAMMATORY MYOFIBROBLASTIC TUMOR— PATHOLOGIC FEATURES

Gross Findings
▶ Either pedunculated or polypoid

Microscopic Findings
▶ Characterized by myofibroblastic cells resembling tissue-culture fibroblasts
▶ Cells may be arranged in fascicles or more haphazardly
▶ Nuclei tend to be enlarged and ovoid, with vesicular chromatin and prominent nucleoli
▶ Prominent delicate network of small vessels in edematous or myxoid stroma with little-to-moderate collagen deposition
▶ Mitotic figures may be present and even frequent, but they are not atypical
▶ Surface epithelium is usually ulcerated, with a superficial acute inflammatory infiltrate
▶ Chronic inflammatory cells and extravasated red blood cells are scattered throughout the remainder of the lesion

Immunohistochemical Features
▶ Often positive for cytokeratin, vimentin, and actin
▶ Negative for caldesmon and EMA
▶ Two thirds express anaplastic lymphoma kinase (ALK)

Differential Diagnosis
▶ Leiomyosarcoma
▶ Sarcomatoid carcinoma
▶ Invasive urothelial or metastatic carcinoma

arranged in fascicles resembling a smooth muscle tumor (more common in postoperative lesions) or more haphazardly (more commonly without prior surgery). Nuclei tend to be enlarged and ovoid, with vesicular chromatin and prominent nucleoli. Nuclei tend to be more uniform in postoperative lesions, with greater variation in size and shape in lesions not associated with surgery. A prominent delicate network of small vessels in an edematous or myxoid stroma with little to moderate collagen deposition is a prominent feature (Fig. 4-35). Mitotic figures may be present and even frequent, but they are not atypical. The surface epithelium is usually ulcerated with a superficial acute inflammatory infiltrate. Chronic inflammatory cells and extravasated red blood cells are scattered throughout the remainder of the lesion.

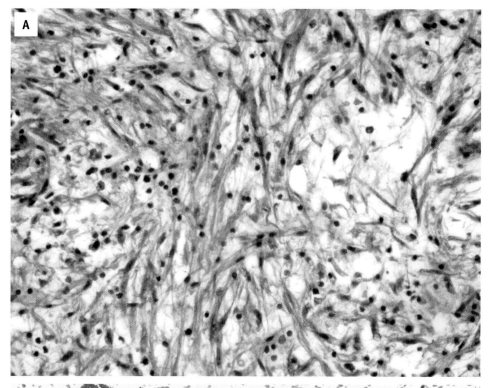

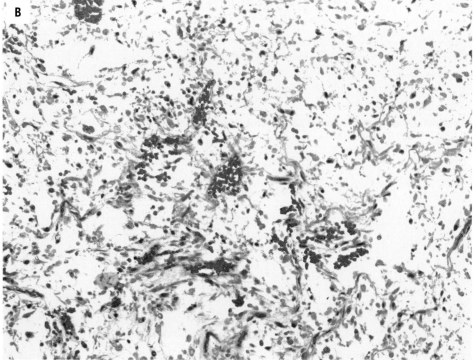

FIGURE 4-35

A, Inflammatory myofibroblastic tumor is characterized by myofibroblastic cells resembling tissue culture fibroblasts. The cells are arranged in fascicles with moderate collagen deposition. **B,** Prominent delicate network of small vessels in an edematous stroma.

ANCILLARY STUDIES

IMMUNOHISTOCHEMISTRY

Proliferative myofibroblasts may be positive for cytokeratin, vimentin, and actin, although they are negative for caldesmon and EMA. IMTs express anaplastic lymphoma kinase (ALK) by immunohistochemistry in about two thirds of cases (Fig. 4-36). The overexpression of ALK in those tumors is associated with the finding of a translocation involving chromosome 2p23, site of the ALK gene.

DIFFERENTIAL DIAGNOSIS

The differential diagnosis is with leiomyosarcoma and sarcomatoid carcinoma. Invasive urothelial or metastatic carcinoma may also incite a pseudosarcomatous stromal reaction that could be confused with a myofibroblastic proliferation or with sarcoma. The best clues to the benign nature are tissue culture-like cells, lack of nuclear hyperchromasia, delicate but abundant vascular network, absence of atypical mitotic figures, edematous and myxoid stroma, and sprinkling of chronic inflammatory cells and erythrocytes.

PROGNOSIS AND TREATMENT

Typically these tumors once resected, even incompletely, tend to regress or stay stable. However, they may recur, causing local morbidity and potentially even necessitating radical surgery. We have also seen rare cases of IMT which, upon recurrence, have dedifferentiated into sarcoma. Close follow-up is recommended.

LEIOMYOMA

Leiomyoma is the most common benign mesenchymal neoplasm of the urinary bladder. There is a female predilection (male/female ratio, 1:2). The majority occur in adults, although rare examples in children are reported. Grossly and microscopically, leiomyomas of the urinary bladder resemble their more common uterine counterparts.

CLINICAL FEATURES

Obstructive symptoms are common because of a ball-valve effect of the pedunculated tumors. Less often, the tumor produces pelvic pain or ureteral obstruction with hydronephrosis.

PATHOLOGIC FEATURES

GROSS FINDINGS

The gross appearance of leiomyomas varies according to their location: two thirds of cases are submucosal, producing a polypoid or pedunculated mass. Less com-

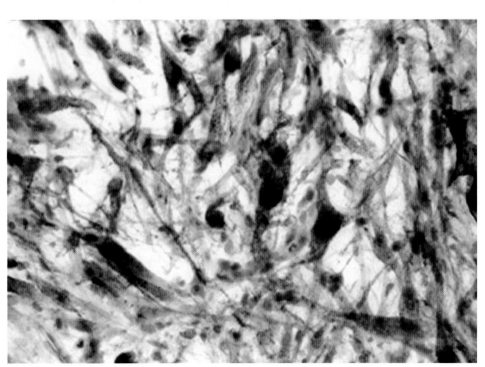

FIGURE 4-36

Cytoplasmic expression of anaplastic lymphoma kinase (ALK) in inflammatory myofibroblastic tumor.

LEIOMYOMA—FACT SHEET

Definition
▶ Benign smooth muscle neoplasm

Incidence and Location
▶ Most common benign mesenchymal neoplasm

Morbidity and Mortality
▶ Can recur if incompletely resected

Gender, Race, and Age Distribution
▶ Female predilection (M/F ratio, 1:2)
▶ Typically occurs in adults, although reported in children

Clinical Features
▶ Obstructive symptoms (pedunculated tumors)
▶ Pelvic pain or ureteral obstruction with hydronephrosis

Prognosis and Treatment
▶ Treated conservatively
▶ TUR or segmental resection

monly, they arise within the wall or subserosally. The overlying epithelium is usually intact. Most of the tumors are 1.0 to 4.0 cm in diameter, although tumors as large as 25.0 cm have been described. The cut surface is typically circumscribed and bulging, with a whorled grey-white appearance.

MICROSCOPIC FINDING

The lesion is characterized by fascicles of spindle-shaped cells with fusiform, blunt-ended nuclei and eosinophilic cytoplasm. There is minimal atypia, and few mitotic figures are present. In tumors with any atypical features (nuclear pleomorphism, more than rare mitotic figures, or necrosis), no criteria allow precise discrimination between benign and malignant

LEIOMYOMA—PATHOLOGIC FEATURES

Gross Findings
▶ Polypoid or pedunculated mass

Microscopic Findings
▶ Fascicles of spindle-shaped cells
▶ Fusiform, blunt-ended nuclei
▶ Eosinophilic cytoplasm
▶ Minimal atypia and few mitotic figures

Differential Diagnosis
▶ Low-grade leiomyosarcoma

lesions. It has been recommended that smooth muscle tumors with rare or absent mitotic figures and an infiltrative pattern should be considered as low-grade leiomyosarcomas or as smooth muscle tumors of uncertain malignant potential.

DIFFERENTIAL DIAGNOSIS

The presence of an infiltrative pattern argues against a diagnosis of leiomyoma. Focal myxoid change can occur in leiomyoma. However, a prominent myxoid background is more likely in leiomyosarcomas.

PROGNOSIS AND TREATMENT

Leiomyomas are treated conservatively. Depending on the size of the lesion, TUR or segmental resection is indicated. In cases with atypical features, complete resection with proper evaluation of margins may be appropriate. In most cases, the treatment is curative, although leiomyomas can recur if incompletely excised.

NEUROFIBROMA

Neurofibroma is a benign mesenchymal tumor consisting of a mixture of cell types including Schwann cells, perineurial-like cells, and fibroblasts. Neurofibromas of the urinary bladder are uncommon. The tumor typically occurs in young patients with neurofibromatosis type 1. The mean age at diagnosis is 17 years, and the male-to-female ratio is 2.3:1.

CLINICAL FEATURES

Patients typically exhibit physical stigmata of neurofibromatosis type 1. The urinary bladder is the most common site of genitourinary involvement in neurofibromatosis, and the involvement of the bladder is often extensive. Clinical signs include hematuria, irritative voiding symptoms, and pelvic mass.

PATHOLOGIC FEATURES

GROSS FINDINGS

The tumors frequently are transmural, showing a diffuse or plexiform pattern of growth.

NEUROFIBROMA—FACT SHEET

Definition
▶ Benign mesenchymal tumor consisting of a mixture of cell types including Schwann cells, perineurial-like cells, and fibroblasts

Incidence and Location
▶ Uncommon
▶ Bladder is the most common site of genitourinary involvement

Gender, Race, and Age Distribution
▶ Typically occurs in young patients with neurofibromatosis type 1
▶ Male predominance (M/F ratio, 2.3:1)
▶ Mean age at diagnosis is 17 years

Clinical Features
▶ Stigmata of neurofibromatosis type 1
▶ Hematuria, irritative voiding symptoms, and pelvic mass

Prognosis and Treatment
▶ Cystectomy is necessary in approximately one third of cases

MICROSCOPIC FINDINGS

The tumor is characterized by a proliferation of spindle cells with ovoid or elongated nuclei in a collagenized matrix (Fig. 4-37A) that stains positive for Alcian blue. Diffuse neurofibroma is more common than the plexiform type. Cellular neurofibromas lack significant cytologic atypia or mitotic figures. The finding of rare mitotic figures is not sufficient for a diagnosis of malignancy (Fig. 4-37B).

NEUROFIBROMA—PATHOLOGIC FEATURES

Gross Findings
▶ Transmural lesion, showing a diffuse or plexiform pattern of growth

Microscopic Findings
▶ Proliferation of spindle cells with ovoid or elongated nuclei
▶ Collagenized matrix (Alcian blue positive)
▶ Lack of significant cytologic atypia or mitotic figures

Immunohistochemical Features
▶ Cytoplasmic processes of tumor cells are S-100 positive

Differential Diagnosis
▶ Low-grade malignant peripheral nerve sheath tumor
▶ Leiomyoma
▶ Postoperative spindle nodule
▶ Inflammatory myofibroblastic tumor
▶ Leiomyosarcoma
▶ Rhabdomyosarcoma

ANCILLARY STUDIES

IMMUNOHISTOCHEMISTRY

The cytoplasmic processes of tumor cells stain positive for S-100 protein.

DIFFERENTIAL DIAGNOSIS

Neurofibroma must be differentiated from low-grade malignant peripheral nerve sheath tumor, and the diffuse pattern of neurofibroma from fibrosis in the lamina propria.

PROGNOSIS AND TREATMENT

Because of the often extensive involvement of the urinary bladder, cystectomy is necessary in approximately one third of cases. Approximately 7% of tumors, none of which occurred in children, have undergone malignant transformation.

HEMANGIOMA

Hemangioma of the urinary bladder is a rare benign tumor that arises from the endothelium of blood vessels. There is a male predominance (male/female ratio, 3.7:1), and the mean age at presentation is 58 years (range, 17 to 76 years). These tumors may be associated with the Klippel-Trenaunay-Weber or Sturg-Weber syndromes.

CLINICAL FEATURES

Patients often present with microscopic hematuria. The tumor has a predilection for the posterolateral wall of the bladder; it may be single or multiple, and it may be superficial or extend through the full thickness of the bladder wall. The majority of the tumors are small (1 to 2.0 cm).

PATHOLOGIC FEATURES

GROSS FINDINGS

The presence of a sessile, blue, multiloculated mass at cystoscopy is highly suggestive of hemangioma.

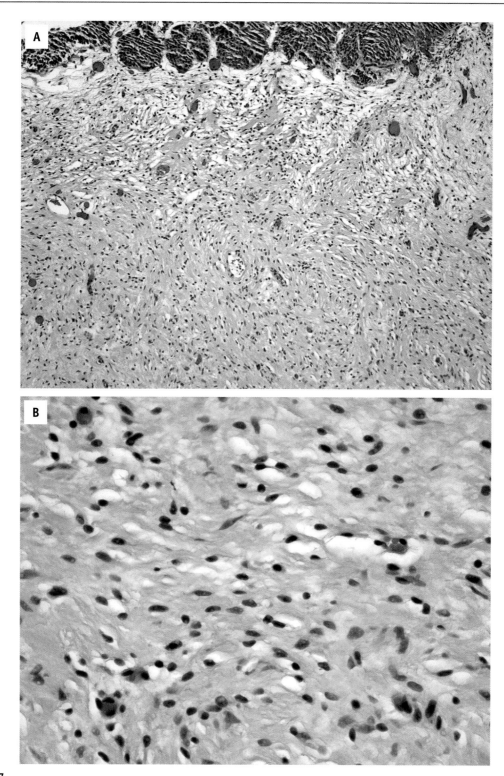

FIGURE 4-37

A, At low power, neurofibroma is characterized by a proliferation of spindle cells in a collagenized matrix. **B,** At high power, the cells have ovoid or elongated nuclei and lack significant cytologic atypia or mitotic figures.

HEMANGIOMA—FACT SHEET

Definition
▶ Benign tumor that arises from the endothelium of blood vessels

Incidence and Location
▶ Predilection for posterolateral walls of bladder

Gender, Race, and Age Distribution
▶ Male predominance (M/F ratio, 3.7:1)
▶ Mean age at presentation is 58 years (range, 17-76 years)

Clinical Features
▶ Patients often present with microscopic hematuria

Prognosis and Treatment
▶ Partial cystectomy or local excision is recommended
▶ Obliteration with the Nd:YAG laser has been successful

HEMANGIOMA—PATHOLOGIC FEATURES

Gross Findings
▶ Sessile, blue, multiloculated mass at cystoscopy is highly suggestive of hemangioma

Microscopic Findings
▶ Histologic subtypes: cavernous (most common type), capillary, and arteriovenous

Differential Diagnosis
▶ Angiosarcoma
▶ Kaposi's sarcoma
▶ Papillary cystitis
▶ Granulation tissue

MICROSCOPIC FINDINGS

Hemangioma is classified in three histologic subtypes: cavernous, capillary, and arteriovenous, with cavernous being the most common type (Fig. 4-38). Morphologically, these tumors are identical to their counterparts in other organs.

DIFFERENTIAL DIAGNOSIS

The major differential diagnostic considerations are angiosarcoma and Kaposi's sarcoma. Exuberant vascular proliferation may also be observed in papillary cystitis and granulation tissue. However, these reactive lesions contain prominent inflammatory cells, which are either not present or less pronounced in hemangioma.

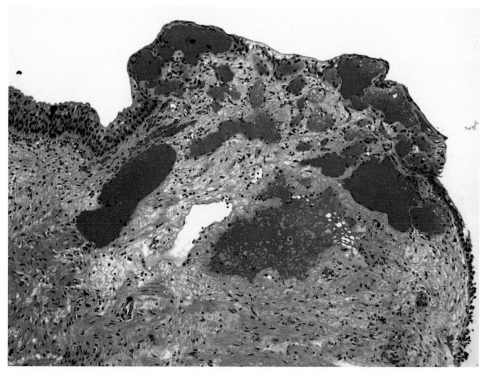

FIGURE 4-38
Hemangioma is characterized by lack of cytologic atypia and by well-circumscribed growth.

PROGNOSIS AND TREATMENT

Treatment depends on the size and location of the tumor. Most investigators recommend partial cystectomy or local excision. Recently, obliteration with the neodymium:yttrium-aluminum-garnet (Nd:YAG) laser has been successful.

SOLITARY FIBROUS TUMOR

Solitary fibrous tumor (SFT) is a distinct spindle-cell tumor arising mainly in the pleura; however, it may originate within the pelvis, including bladder and prostate. SFT is a mesenchymal tumor that shows fibroblastic differentiation. The lesion occurs most often in adults in the fifth and sixth decades of life.

CLINICAL FEATURES

The tumor may be asymptomatic, or it may be associated with hematuria, obstruction, or pelvic pain.

PATHOLOGIC FEATURES

GROSS FINDINGS

SFT of the bladder manifests as a submucosal mass and may be ulcerated.

SOLITARY FIBROUS TUMOR—FACT SHEET

Definition
▶ Benign mesenchymal tumor showing fibroblastic differentiation

Incidence and Location
▶ Rare lesion
▶ It may originate within the pelvis, including the bladder

Morbidity and Mortality
▶ Incompletely resected and unresectable cases recur locally

Gender, Race, and Age Distribution
▶ Adults in the fifth or sixth decade of life

Clinical Features
▶ Asymptomatic or associated with hematuria, obstruction, or pelvic pain

Prognosis and Treatment
▶ Most behave in a benign fashion, but malignant variants occur
▶ Complete excision is the treatment of choice

SOLITARY FIBROUS TUMOR—PATHOLOGIC FEATURES

Gross Findings
▶ Submucosal mass; it may be ulcerated

Microscopic Findings
▶ Spindle cells arranged in a haphazard or storiform pattern
▶ Zones of hypocellularity and hypercellularity
▶ Deposition of intercellular collagen
▶ Malignant examples with pleomorphism and high mitotic rate have been described

Immunohistochemical Features
▶ Positive for CD34 and bcl-2
▶ Cytokeratins, EMA, smooth muscle markers are negative

Differential Diagnosis
▶ Other sarcomas
▶ Sarcomatoid carcinoma
▶ Neurofibroma

MICROSCOPIC FINDINGS

The microscopic features are identical to those seen in other sites, including spindle cells arranged in a haphazard or styliform pattern, zones of hypocellularity and hypercellularity, and deposition of intercellular collagen. Malignant examples with cellular pleomorphism and a high mitotic rate have been described.

ANCILLARY STUDIES

IMMUNOHISTOCHEMISTRY

SFTs are positive for CD34 and bcl-2. Cytokeratins, EMA, and smooth muscle markers are negative.

DIFFERENTIAL DIAGNOSIS

Despite the classic cytologic and growth pattern characteristics observed in most cases, SFT is often misdiagnosed as malignant sarcoma or sarcomatoid carcinoma. Immunohistochemistry is a useful aid in the classification.

PROGNOSIS AND TREATMENT

Although the exact biologic behavior of these tumors has not been clarified, most of the reported cases in the bladder have had a benign clinical course after complete excision. Incompletely resected and unresectable lesions may recur locally.

Malignant Mesenchymal Tumors

Primary sarcomas of the urinary bladder are rare. They are more common in men than in women. Most are of muscle origin and comprise less than 0.04% of all malignant tumors of the urinary bladder. Rhabdomyosarcoma is the most frequent tumor of the bladder in children, whereas leiomyosarcoma is the most frequent sarcoma in adults. Other sarcomas, including malignant fibrous histiocytoma, angiosarcoma, osteosarcoma, fibrosarcoma, and liposarcoma, have been described in the bladder. Although those tumors may arise in the urinary bladder, they are more likely to originate in other sites and to involve the bladder secondarily. The possibility that those malignant sarcomas represent elements of heterologous differentiation in a sarcomatoid carcinoma should also be ruled out by sampling. The development of a tumor a few years after radiation therapy should raise the possibility of a postradiation sarcoma.

RHABDOMYOSARCOMA

Rhabdomyosarcomas are malignant tumors that recapitulate the morphologic and molecular features of skeletal muscle. They are the most common urinary bladder tumors in childhood and adolescence. In children, 20% to 25% of rhabdomyosarcomas arise in the genitourinary tract, with bladder, prostate, and paratesticular regions as primary sites in boys, bladder and vagina in girls. The mean age at diagnosis for vesical rhabdomyosarcomas is 4 years. There is a male predominance (male/female ratio, 3:2). Most bladder rhabdomyosarcomas are of embryonal subtype and exophytic (polypoid), with or without a botryoid component. The genetically distinct alveolar subtype is extremely rare in these sites. In adults, rhabdomyosarcoma is rare and usually of the pleomorphic type.

PATHOLOGIC FEATURES

GROSS FINDINGS

Grossly, embryonal rhabdomyosarcoma can be divided into two basic forms with prognostic impact: polypoid, mostly intraluminal tumors associated with favorable prognosis (botryoid subtype), and deeply invasive tumors involving the entire bladder wall and usually adjacent organs, which show a worse prognosis.

MICROSCOPIC FINDINGS

The tumor cells of embryonal rhabdomyosarcoma are usually small and round and often are set in a myxoid stroma. The botryoid subtype has a condensation of tumor cell beneath the covering surface epithelium, called the "cambium layer." The underlying stroma is hypocellular and myxoid. Typical rhabdomyoblasts and cross-striations are seen frequently in embryonal rhabdomyosarcomas but rarely in the spindle-cell and alveolar types.

RHABDOMYOSARCOMA—FACT SHEET

Definition
▸ Malignant tumors recapitulating morphologic and molecular features of skeletal muscle

Incidence and Location
▸ Most common urinary bladder tumor in childhood and adolescence
▸ Primary sites in male: bladder, prostate, and paratesticular region
▸ Primary sites in female: bladder and vagina

Morbidity and Mortality
▸ Exophytic tumors have a better prognosis than those diffusely infiltrating bladder wall

Gender, Race, and Age Distribution
▸ Mean age at diagnosis is 4 years
▸ Male predominance (M/F ratio, 3:2)

Prognosis and Treatment
▸ Poor prognosis in adults
▸ Combined surgery and chemotherapy have greatly improved survival in pediatric group

---

RHABDOMYOSARCOMA—PATHOLOGIC FEATURES

Gross Findings
▸ Polypoid or deeply invasive tumors

Microscopic Findings
▸ Embryonal type is most common in the bladder: cells are small, round, often set in a myxoid stroma; rhabdomyoblasts and cross-striations are frequently seen; condensation of tumor cell beneath surface epithelium ("cambium layer"); underlying stroma is hypocellular and myxoid
▸ Alveolar type is extremely rare in bladder
▸ Pleomorphic type is common in adults

Immunohistochemical Features
▸ Myogenin (myf4) and MyoD1 are positive
▸ Desmin and pan-actin (HHF-35) can also be positive
▸ Myosin and myoglobin can be negative

Differential Diagnosis
▸ Reactive myofibroblastic proliferations
▸ Inflammatory myofibroblastic tumor

ANCILLARY STUDIES

IMMUNOHISTOCHEMISTRY

Rhabdomyosarcoma cells express myogenin (myf4) and MyoD1 in the nucleus. Highly differentiated tumors can lack myogenin expression. Desmin and muscle-specific actin (HHF-35) can also be detected in almost all lesions but are not specific. Staining for myosin and myoglobin is usually found in well-differentiated tumors, but can be negative in less differentiated ones.

DIFFERENTIAL DIAGNOSIS

Rhabdomyosarcoma should enter in the differential diagnosis of all spindle and myxoid lesions of the genitourinary tract in the pediatric age group. In particular, in children IMT must be differentiated from rhabdomyosarcoma.

PROGNOSIS AND TREATMENT

In general, rhabdomyosarcomas have a poor prognosis in adults. Combination therapy with surgery and chemotherapy has greatly improved survival in the pediatric age group. Exophytic rhabdomyosarcomas have a better prognosis than those diffusely infiltrating the bladder wall. Morphologic evidence of "maturation" is a common finding in treated tumors.

LEIOMYOSARCOMA

Leiomyosarcoma is a rare malignant mesenchymal tumor arising from urinary bladder smooth muscle.

CLINICAL FEATURES

Although leiomyosarcoma is the most common sarcoma of the urinary bladder, it accounts for much less than 1% of all bladder malignancies. Leiomyosarcomas are most commonly seen in adults in their sixth to eighth decade. They occur more frequently in men than in women, with a ratio of 2:1. Leiomyosarcoma can occur anywhere within the bladder and very rarely can involve the ureter or renal pelvis. Hematuria is the most common presenting symptom; occasionally, patients have a palpable pelvic mass, abdominal pain, or urinary tract obstruction.

LEIOMYOSARCOMA—FACT SHEET

Definition
► Malignant mesenchymal tumor arising from smooth muscle

Incidence and Location
► Most common sarcoma of the urinary bladder (adults)
► Rare (<1% of all bladder tumors)
► Can occur anywhere within the bladder; very rarely can involve ureter or renal pelvis

Gender, Race, and Age Distribution
► Commonly seen in adults in their sixth to eighth decade
► Male predominance (M/F ratio, 2:1)

Clinical Features
► Hematuria is the most common presenting symptom
► A palpable pelvic mass, abdominal pain, or urinary tract obstruction can occur

Prognosis and Treatment
► Poor prognosis
► Recurrent or metastatic disease resulting in death in almost half of the patients

---

PATHOLOGIC FEATURES

GROSS FINDINGS

The lesion is typically a large (mean size, 7.0 cm), infiltrating mass. Gross and microscopic necrosis is frequently found in high-grade tumors (Fig. 4-39).

MICROSCOPIC FINDINGS

The tumor is composed of infiltrative, interlacing fascicles of spindle cells, with variable amounts of eosinophilic cytoplasm with mild-to-marked nuclear atypia (Fig. 4-40). Low-grade leiomyosarcoma exhibits mild to moderate cytologic atypia; the mitotic activity is less than 5 mitoses per 10 high-power fields (HPF). In contrast, high-grade tumors show marked cytologic atypia and in most cases have more than 5 mitoses per 10 HPF.

ANCILLARY STUDIES

IMMUNOHISTOCHEMISTRY

More than two thirds of tumors demonstrate immunoreactivity for both smooth muscle actin (SMA) and muscle-specific actin (HHF-35). Desmin is positive in less than 50% of cases, Cytokeratin (CK) and EMA may be positive.

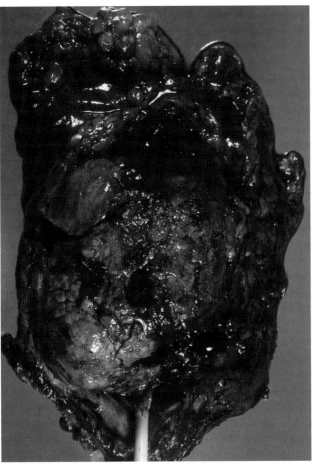

FIGURE 4-39
Gross photograph of surgically resected cystectomy specimen of leiomyosarcoma, showing a large infiltrating mass with extensive necrosis.

LEIOMYOSARCOMA—PATHOLOGIC FEATURES

Gross Findings
► Large infiltrating mass
► Necrosis is frequently found in high-grade tumors

Microscopic Findings
► Interlacing fascicles of spindle cells
► Variable amounts of eosinophilic cytoplasm
► Low-grade leiomyosarcoma: mild-to-moderate cytologic atypia; <5 mitoses per 10 HPF
► High-grade leiomyosarcoma: marked cytologic atypia; >5 mitoses per 10 HPF

Immunohistochemical Features
► SMA and HHF-35 are frequently positive
► Desmin is often positive
► CK and EMA can be positive
► Caldesmon is positive

Differential Diagnosis
► Sarcomatoid carcinoma
► Reactive spindle cell lesions
► Inflammatory myofibroblastic tumor

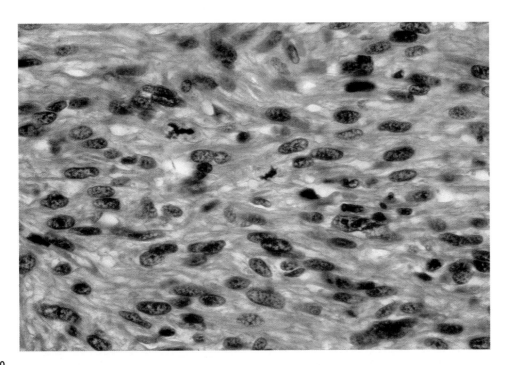

FIGURE 4-40
Leiomyosarcoma is composed of interlacing fascicles of spindle cells with variable amounts of eosinophilic cytoplasm with mild-to-marked nuclear atypia and mitotic activity.

DIFFERENTIAL DIAGNOSIS

Sarcomatoid carcinoma may mimic leiomyosarcoma and must be excluded by adequate sampling. Sarcomatoid carcinoma is usually associated with a malignant epithelial component. Leiomyosarcoma exhibits greater cytologic atypia, with nuclear hyperchromasia, abnormal mitoses, less inflammation and vascularity, absence of tissue culture-like cells, and an arrangement in compact cellular fascicles, in contrast to IMT.

PROGNOSIS AND TREATMENT

Most patients with leiomyosarcoma of the urinary bladder develop recurrent or metastatic disease resulting in death in almost half of the patients.

GERM CELL TUMORS

TROPHOBLASTIC

Urothelial carcinoma may exhibit trophoblastic differentiation in several patterns. Typical urothelial carcinoma may contain scattered syncytiotrophoblastic giant cells. More rarely, choriocarcinoma may arise in the bladder and must be differentiated from anaplastic urothelial carcinoma, which expresses human chorionic gonadotropin (HCG) immunohistochemically and in the serum.

DERMOID CYST

A few dermoid cysts of the urinary bladder have been described in women 30 to 49 years of age who typically had symptoms of long duration. The lesions were cystic and contained hair and calcified material. Ovarian dermoid cysts may perforate into the bladder, so secondary involvement of the bladder from the ovary must be excluded before a primary dermoid cyst of the bladder is diagnosed.

YOLK SAC TUMOR

A yolk sac tumor of the bladder was described in a 1-year-old boy with hematuria, a markedly elevated serum α-fetoprotein level, and a polypoid, red, gelatinous, focally hemorrhagic and necrotic tumor. The

patient underwent a partial cystectomy followed by chemotherapy. He was well 14 months postoperatively.

Hematologic Malignancies

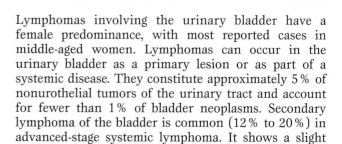

LYMPHOMA

Lymphomas involving the urinary bladder have a female predominance, with most reported cases in middle-aged women. Lymphomas can occur in the urinary bladder as a primary lesion or as part of a systemic disease. They constitute approximately 5% of nonurothelial tumors of the urinary tract and account for fewer than 1% of bladder neoplasms. Secondary lymphoma of the bladder is common (12% to 20%) in advanced-stage systemic lymphoma. It shows a slight male predominance and may occur in children.

CLINICAL FEATURES

The most frequent symptom of urinary tract lymphomas is gross hematuria, followed by dysuria, urinary frequency, nocturia, and abdominal or back pain. Bladder lymphoma as the first sign of disseminated

---

LYMPHOMA—FACT SHEET

Definition
▶ Malignant neoplasm of lymphoid cells

Incidence and Location
▶ 5% of nonurothelial tumors of the urinary tract, <1% of bladder neoplasms
▶ 90% affect the urinary bladder

Morbidity and Mortality
▶ Worse prognosis with disseminated and recurrent lymphoma

Gender, Race, and Age Distribution
▶ Female predominance
▶ Most reported cases have been in middle-aged women

Clinical Features
▶ Gross hematuria is most common symptom
▶ Dysuria, urinary frequency, nocturia, and abdominal or back pain may occur

Prognosis and Treatment
▶ Primary MALT lymphoma has an excellent prognosis after local therapy
▶ Other primary, disseminated, and recurrent lymphomas have a worse prognosis

disease is termed "nonlocalized lymphoma" and has a much better prognosis than "secondary (recurrent) lymphoma" in patients with a history of lymphoma elsewhere.

PATHOLOGIC FEATURES

GROSS FINDINGS

Frequently, the lesions appear as solitary submucosal masses. The urothelium is typically intact, although ulceration has been reported. The tumor may form a solitary mass (70%), multiple masses (20%), or diffuse thickening (10%) of the bladder wall. Ulceration is rare (<20%) in primary tumors but common in secondary urinary tract lymphomas.

MICROSCOPIC FINDINGS

Low grade mucosa-associated lymphoid tissue (MALT) lymphoma is the most frequent primary lymphoma in the urinary bladder. Burkitt's lymphoma, T-cell lymphoma, Hodgkin's lymphoma, and plasmocytoma are very rare. Among secondary urinary tract lymphomas, diffuse large B-cell lymphoma is the single most frequent histologic subtype, followed by follicular, small cell, low-grade MALT, mantle cell, Burkitt's, and Hodgkin's lymphomas.

DIFFERENTIAL DIAGNOSIS

The differential diagnosis is with undifferentiated carcinoma. Immunohistochemistry may be necessary to resolve rare challenging cases.

PROGNOSIS AND TREATMENT

Primary MALT lymphoma of the urinary tract has an excellent prognosis after local therapy, with virtually no tumor-related deaths. Nonlocalized lymphomas and secondary lymphomas have a worse prognosis (median survival time, 9 years and 0.6 years, respectively) comparable to that of patients with advanced lymphomas of respective histologic type elsewhere.

Miscellaneous Lesions

MELANOMA

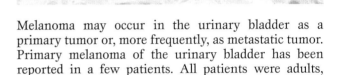

Melanoma may occur in the urinary bladder as a primary tumor or, more frequently, as metastatic tumor. Primary melanoma of the urinary bladder has been reported in a few patients. All patients were adults, ranging in age from 48 to 65 years, and men and women were equally affected.

CLINICAL FEATURES

Gross hematuria is the most frequent presenting symptom, but some patients present with symptoms related to metastatic disease. Before assuming that a melanoma

---

LYMPHOMA—PATHOLOGIC FEATURES

Gross Findings
▶ Solitary submucosal masses (70%)
▶ Multiple masses (20%)
▶ Diffuse thickening (10%)

Microscopic Findings
▶ Low-grade MALT lymphoma is the most frequent primary lymphoma in the bladder
▶ Diffuse large B-cell lymphoma is the most frequent subtype among secondary lesions

Differential Diagnosis
▶ Poorly differentiated carcinoma

MELANOMA—FACT SHEET

Definition
▶ Malignant melanocytic neoplasm that may occur as a primary or, more frequently, as a metastatic tumor

Incidence and Location
▶ Extremely rare

Morbidity and Mortality
▶ Most patients have a poor prognosis reflecting late diagnosis

Gender, Race, and Age Distribution
▶ Adults, ranging from 48 to 65 years of age
▶ Men and women are equally affected

Clinical Features
▶ Gross hematuria is the most frequent presenting symptom

Prognosis and Treatment
▶ Poor (two thirds of patients are dead of metastatic disease within 3 years)

is primary in the bladder, a metastasis from a skin lesion must be ruled out. Cystoscopically, the differential diagnostic considerations for pigmented raised lesions include endometriosis, melanoma, and sarcoma.

PATHOLOGIC FEATURES

GROSS FINDINGS

Almost all tumors have a dark pigmented appearance at cystoscopy and on gross pathologic evaluation. The size of the lesion ranges from less than 1.0 cm to a few centimeters.

MICROSCOPIC FINDINGS

The majority of tumors show pleomorphic nuclei, spindle and polygonal cytoplasmic contours, and melanin pigment (Fig. 4-41). Pigment production can be variable and may even be absent. A few of the tumors may be associated with melanosis of the vesical epithelium.

ANCILLARY STUDIES

IMMUNOHISTOCHEMISTRY

Similarly to melanomas in other location, these tumors stain positive for Melan A (Fig. 4-42A), S-100 (Fig. 4-42B), and HMB-45.

MELANOMA—PATHOLOGIC FEATURES

Gross Findings
▶ Dark, pigmented, raised lesion

Microscopic Findings
▶ Pleomorphic nuclei
▶ Spindle and polygonal cytoplasmic contour
▶ Melanin pigment production is variable and may be absent
▶ Melanosis of vesical epithelium may be present

Immunohistochemical Features
▶ Positive for S-100, HMB-45, and MELAN A

Differential Diagnosis
▶ Endometriosis
▶ Sarcoma

DIFFERENTIAL DIAGNOSIS

One can not reliably differentiate a primary from a metastatic melanoma based on histologic grounds, as metastatic disease can extend onto the mucosa, mimicking a primary lesion. Immunoreactivity for S-100 protein and HMB-45 may be helpful in distinguishing melanoma from poorly differentiated sarcoma or carcinoma.

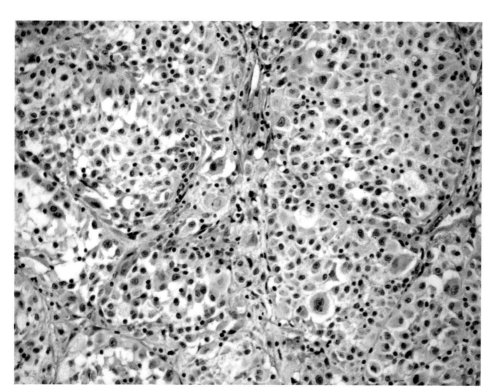

FIGURE 4-41

Melanoma of the bladder shows an alveolar and nesting pattern. The cells have pleomorphic nuclei, polygonal cytoplasmic contours, and eosinophilic cytoplasm.

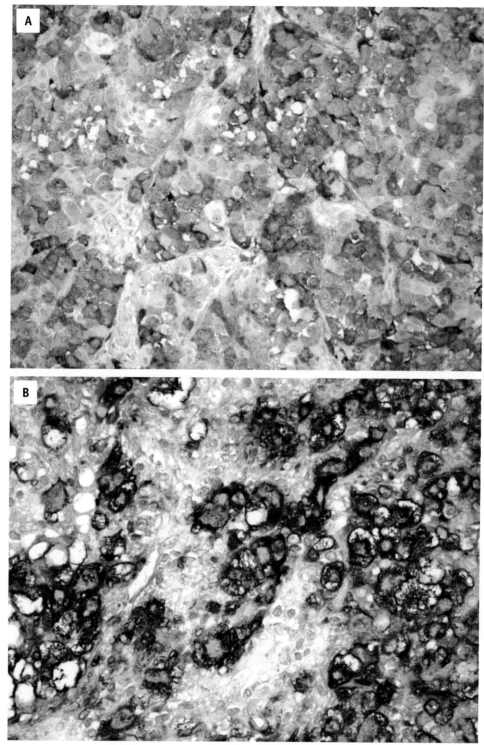

FIGURE 4-42
A, Melanoma, showing nests of Melan A–positive cells. **B,** S-100 positive cells.

PROGNOSIS AND TREATMENT

Two thirds of patients with melanoma of the urinary bladder were dead of metastases within 3 years after diagnosis. Those patients still alive at the time of the report had been observed for less than 2 years, so the long-term prognosis is most likely even worse.

PARAGANGLIOMA

Paraganglioma of the urinary bladder (also designated as bladder pheochromocytoma) is a neoplasm derived from paraganglia cells in the bladder wall. Histologically, these tumors are identical to paragangliomas at other sites. The incidence is approximately 0.06% to 0.1% of all bladder tumors.

CLINICAL FEATURES

These tumors occur over a wide age range (10 to 88 years), with a mean age of 41 years. There is a female predominance, with a male-to-female ratio of 2:3. The tumors are usually hormonally active, causing hypertension in two thirds of the patients. Almost half of the patients have associated symptoms of headache, palpitations, hypertension, blurred vision, and/or sweating (micturition attack). Hematuria is a clinical presentation in approximately half of the patients. The lesion may occur in any part of the bladder, at any level of the bladder wall. The muscularis propria is the most common location for those lesions.

PATHOLOGIC FEATURES

GROSS FINDINGS

Most paragangliomas are circumscribed or multinodular tumors, usually less than 4.0 cm in size (Fig. 4-43).

MICROSCOPIC FINDINGS

Paragangliomas usually show nests of cells in a *Zellballen* pattern, but this feature is not always conspicuous, and some tumors show a diffuse pattern of growth (Fig. 4-44A). The cells are round, with clear, amphophilic or most characteristically acidophilic cytoplasm. Nuclei are ovoid, with variable nuclear pleomorphism and mitotic activity (Fig. 4-44B). Paraganglioma of the bladder can invade deeply into the muscle or show vascular invasion.

PARAGANGLIOMA—FACT SHEET

Definition
► Neoplasm derived from paraganglia cells in the bladder wall

Incidence and Location
► Rare (0.06-0.1% of all bladder tumors)
► May occur in any part of the bladder and at any level of the bladder wall
► Muscularis propria is the most common location

Morbidity and Mortality
► Distant metastases are rare and can occur many years later

Gender, Race, and Age Distribution
► Age ranges from 10 to 88 years (mean age, 41 years)
► Slight female predominance (M/F ratio, 2:3)

Clinical Features
► Hypertension (two thirds of the patients)
► Half of the patients have associated symptoms of headache, palpitations, hypertension, blurred vision, and/or sweating (micturition attack)
► Hematuria is a clinical presentation in half of the cases

Prognosis and Treatment
► 10-15% of bladder paragangliomas are malignant
► Localized tumors are treated with TUR, wedge resection, or partial cystectomy
► Malignant tumors are treated with radical cystectomy and removal of metastases if possible

---

PARAGANGLIOMA—PATHOLOGIC FEATURES

Gross Findings
► Circumscribed or multinodular tumors typically with intact urothelium, usually <4.0 cm in size

Microscopic Findings
► Nests of cells in the *Zellballen* pattern or diffuse pattern of growth
► Prominent, thin-walled vascular network
► Cells are round with clear, acidophilic, amphophilic (most characteristic) cytoplasm and ovoid nuclei
► Variable degree of nuclear pleomorphism and mitotic activity
► Can invade deeply into the muscle or show vascular invasion

Immunohistochemical Features
► Always negative for CK
► Frequently positive for chromogranin, NSE, and synaptophysin
► Sustentacular cells stain with S-100 protein

Differential Diagnosis
► Invasive urothelial carcinoma

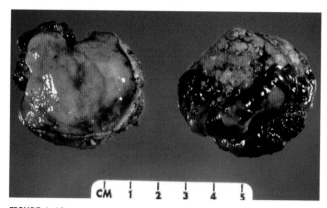

FIGURE 4-43

Gross photograph of surgically resected circumscribed paraganglioma of the urinary bladder.

ANCILLARY STUDIES

IMMUNOHISTOCHEMISTRY

The tumor is negative for epithelial markers (CK) and positive for neuroendocrine markers such as chromogranin, NSE, and synaptophysin. Flattened sustentacular cells can sometimes be highlighted in the periphery of the cell nests with S-100 protein.

DIFFERENTIAL DIAGNOSIS

When the *Zellballen* pattern of this tumor is conspicuous, the diagnosis should come to mind. Invasive

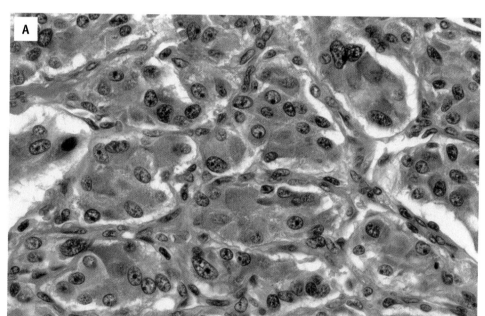

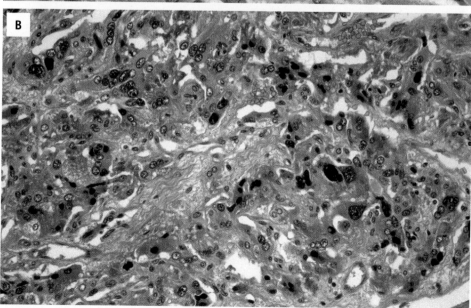

FIGURE 4-44

A, Paraganglioma consists of nests of cells in a *Zellballen* pattern. The cells are round, with clear, amphophilic or acidophilic cytoplasm. **B,** Nuclear pleomorphism may be present.

urothelial carcinoma occasionally grows in a nested pattern reminiscent of paraganglioma; however, urothelial tumors are likely to be associated with CIS or noninvasive papillary carcinoma.

PROGNOSIS AND TREATMENT

Approximately 10% to 15% of bladder paragangliomas are malignant; in absence of metastases, malignancy cannot be reliably predicted based on histologic features. Sometimes local recurrences develop over a period of many years before extravesical spread occurs. Distant metastases are rare and can occur many years later. Localized tumors are treated with TUR, wedge resection, or partial cystectomy. The treatment for malignant paraganglioma of the bladder is radical cystectomy with removal of metastases if possible.

CARCINOID TUMORS

A few cases of carcinoid tumors have been reported in the urinary bladder of adults ranging from 30 to 75 years of age. Carcinoid syndrome was not present in any of the cases. The tumors were small, submucosal, and within the bladder neck, and the patients presented with hematuria.

At cystoscopy, carcinoids are smooth-surfaced, sessile, polypoid nodules covered by urothelium. Microscopically, they are similar to carcinoid tumors in other organs.

Neuroendocrine differentiation can be confirmed by stains for chromogranin, synaptophysin, and neural cell adhesion molecule (CD56/NCAM). Some urothelial carcinomas grow in nests, which may superficially resemble those of a carcinoid.

GRANULAR CELL TUMORS

Granular cell tumor is rare in the urinary bladder, with only few cases reported in the literature. It occurs in adult patients between 23 and 70 years of age, with no gender predilection.

The tumors are usually solitary, well-circumscribed or encapsulated, yellow-white nodules up to 12.0 cm in diameter. Microscopically, the lesion consists of spindle- to polygonal-shaped cells with abundant granular eosinophilic cytoplasm and vesicular nuclei (Fig. 4-45). The granules are periodic acid-Schiff (PAS) positive and diastase resistant. The tumor cells are positive for S-100 protein, similarly to granular cell tumor elsewhere. To date, only one malignant granular cell tumor of the bladder has been described. Conservative treatment is suggested, given the benign course of the majority of the cases.

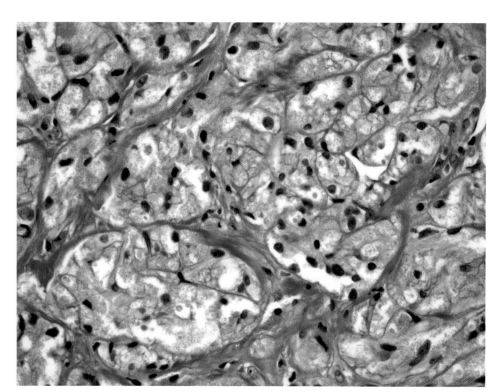

FIGURE 4-45
Granular cell tumor, showing nests of polygonal cells with abundant granular eosinophilic cytoplasm and vesicular nuclei.

METASTATIC TUMORS AND SECONDARY EXTENSION

The urinary bladder may be involved secondarily by direct extension of tumors from adjacent sites such as prostate, seminal vesicles, lower intestinal tract, and female genital tract or by metastases from a distant site. The most frequent locations of metastases to the bladder are bladder neck and trigone. Excluding hematopoietic malignancies, other secondary tumors account for approximately 15% of malignant bladder tumors. Direct extensions or metastases from colonic carcinomas (Fig. 4-46) are most frequent and represent 21% of the cases, followed by those from carcinoma of the prostate (19%), rectum (12%), and uterine cervix (11%). Much less frequent is metastatic spread from stomach, skin, breast, and lung cancers.

CLINICAL FEATURES

GROSS FINDINGS

The lesions may mimic a primary urothelial carcinoma, or they may manifest as multiple submucosal nodules.

MICROSCOPIC FINDINGS

Tumors with less characteristic histologic features, such as poorly differentiated or undifferentiated high-grade tumors, require immunohistochemical workup. Multifocality, prominent vascular involvement, absence

of mucosal abnormality, and unusual morphology should raise the suspicion of metastatic tumors.

ANCILLARY STUDIES

IMMUNOHISTOCHEMISTRY

Immunostains may be helpful in differentiating between prostate cancer involving the bladder and a primary bladder urothelial cancer. PSA and PSAP are

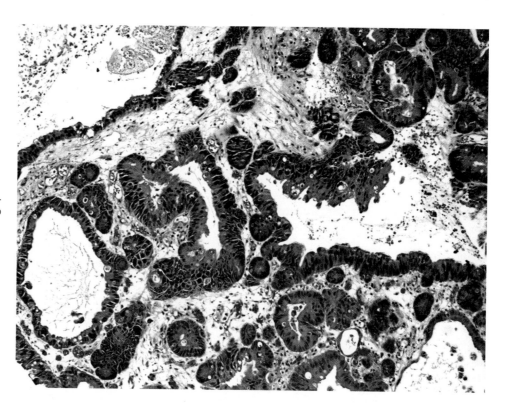

FIGURE 4- 46
Moderately differentiated adenocarcinoma of the colon metastatic to urinary bladder.

METASTATIC TUMORS AND SECONDARY EXTENSION—PATHOLOGIC FEATURES

Gross Findings
► May mimic a primary urothelial carcinoma or may manifest as multiple nodules

Microscopic Findings
► Multifocality
► Prominent vascular involvement
► May show absence of mucosal abnormality
► May show involvement of muscularis propria only
► Metastatic colon adenocarcinoma may be identical to primary adenocarcinoma or primary villous adenoma with growth onto mucosa mimicking in situ adenocarcinoma
► Unusual morphology

Immunohistochemical Features
► Prostate adenocarcinoma: PSA and PSAP positive; HMWCK, p63 and thrombomodulin negative
► Colonic primary adenocarcinoma: β-catenin positive

Differential Diagnosis
► Primary adenocarcinoma of the bladder
► Urothelial carcinoma with enteric differentiation

---

positive in prostate cancer. Thrombomodulin, high-molecular-weight cytokeratin (HMWCK), and p63 are positive in urothelial carcinoma and negative in prostatic adenocarcinoma. Although there is overlap in CK7 and CK20 expression in prostate adenocarcinoma and bladder urothelial carcinoma, negative immunoreactivity for CK7 favors a prostatic primary.

DIFFERENTIAL DIAGNOSIS

It is difficult to impossible to distinguish between a metastasis from the colon and a bladder primary (primary adenocarcinoma and urothelial carcinoma with enteric differentiation), because metastatic colonic tumors can even involve the mucosa and secondarily colonize it, to create a villous architecture that would suggest a primary bladder tumor. A recent study suggested that β-catenin is expressed in cases of colonic primary tumor and is absent in primary bladder adenocarcinoma.

SUGGESTED READINGS

Eble JN, Young RH: Tumors of the urinary tract. In Fletcher CDM (ed): Diagnostic Histopathology of Tumors, 2nd ed. New York, Churchill Livingston, 2000.
Epstein JI, Amin MB, Reuter VE: Bladder biopsy interpretation. Biopsy Interpretation Series. Philadelphia, Lippincott Williams & Wilkins, 2004.

Epstein JI, Amin MB, Reuter VR, Mostofi FK: (1998). The World Health Organization/International Society of Urological Pathology consensus classification of urothelial (transitional cell) neoplasms of the urinary bladder. Bladder Consensus Conference Committee. Am J Surg Pathol 1998;22:1435–1448.
Grignon DJ: Neoplasms of the urinary bladder. In Bostwich DG, Eple NJ (eds): Urologic Surgical Pathology. St. Louis, Mosby, 1997.
Murphy WM: Atlas of Tumor Pathology: Tumors of the Kidney, Bladder, and Related Urinary Structures, 3rd ed. Washington, DC, AFIP, 1994.
World Health Organization: WHO World Cancer Report. Geneva, WHO, 2003.
World Health Organization: Classfications of Tumors: Pathology and Genetics. Tumors of the Urinary System and Male Genital Organs. Lyon, France, IARC Press, 2004.

Reactive Urothelial Atypia

McKenney JK, Desai S, Cohen C, Amin MB: Discriminatory immunohistochemical staining of urothelial carcinoma in situ and non-neoplastic urothelium: An analysis of cytokeratin 20, p53, and CD44 antigens. Am J Surg Pathol 2001;25:1074–1078.

Flat Urothelial Hyperplasia

Obermann EC, Junker K, Stoehr R, et al: Frequent genetic alterations in flat urothelial hyperplasias and concomitant papillary bladder cancer as detected by CGH, LOH, and FISH analyses. J Pathol 2003;199:50–57.
Taylor DC, Bhagavan BS, Larsen MP, et al: Papillary urothelial hyperplasia: A precursor to papillary neoplasms. Am J Surg Pathol 1996;20:1481–1488.

Urothelial Dysplasia

Amin MB, McKenney JK: An approach to the diagnosis of flat intraepithelial lesions of the urinary bladder using the World Health Organization/International Society of Urological Pathology consensus classification system. Adv Anat Pathol 2002;9:222–232.
Amin MB, Young RH: Intraepithelial lesions of the urinary bladder with a discussion of the histogenesis of urothelial neoplasia. Semin Diagn Pathol 1997;14:84–97.
Cheng L, Cheville JC, Neumann RM, Bostwick DG: Natural history of urothelial dysplasia of the bladder. Am J Surg Pathol 1999;23:443–447.
Cheng L, Cheville JC, Neumann RM, Bostwick DG: Flat intraepithelial lesions of the urinary bladder. Cancer 2000;88:625–631.
Czerniak B, Li L, Chaturvedi V, et al: Genetic modeling of human urinary bladder carcinogenesis. Genes Chromosomes Cancer 2000;27:392–402.
Harnden P, Eardley I, Joyce AD, Southgate J: Cytokeratin 20 as an objective marker of urothelial dysplasia. Br J Urol 1996;78:870–875.
Hartmann A, Schlake G, Zaak D, et al: Occurrence of chromosome 9 and p53 alterations in multifocal dysplasia and carcinoma in situ of human urinary bladder. Cancer Res 2002;62:809–818.
Mallofre C, Castillo M, Morente V, Sole M: Immunohistochemical expression of CK20, p53, and Ki-67 as objective markers of urothelial dysplasia. Mod Pathol 2003;16:187–191.
Murphy WM, Soloway MS: Urothelial dysplasia. J Urol 1982;127:849–854.
Zuk RJ, Rogers HS, Martin JE, Baithun SI: Clinicopathological importance of primary dysplasia of bladder. J Clin Pathol 1988;41:1277–1280.

Urothelial Carcinoma In Situ

Cordon-Cardo C, Cote RJ, Sauter G: Genetic and molecular markers of urothelial premalignancy and malignancy. Scand J Urol Nephrol Suppl 2000;205:82–93.
Cordon-Cardo C, Wartinger D, Petrylak D, et al: Altered expression of the retinoblastoma gene product: Prognostic indicator in bladder cancer. J Natl Cancer Inst 1992;84:1251–1256.
Elliott GB, Moloney PJ, Anderson GH: "Denuding cystitis" and in situ urothelial carcinoma. Arch Pathol 1973;96:91–94.
Esrig D, Elmajian D, Groshen S, et al: Accumulation of nuclear p53 and tumor progression in bladder cancer. N Engl J Med

1994;331:1259–1264.

Grossman HB, Schmitz-Drager B, Fradet Y, Tribukait B: Use of markers in defining urothelial premalignant and malignant conditions. Scand J Urol Nephrol Suppl 2000;205:94–104.

Murphy WM, Busch C, Algaba F: Intraepithelial lesions of urinary bladder: Morphologic considerations. Scand J Urol Nephrol Suppl 2000;205:67–81.

Norming U, Tribukait B, Gustafson H, et al: Deoxyribonucleic acid profile and tumor progression in primary carcinoma in situ of the bladder: A study of 63 patients with grade 3 lesions. J Urol 1992;147:11–15.

Orozco RE, Martin AA, Murphy WM: Carcinoma in situ of the urinary bladder: Clues to host involvement in human carcinogenesis. Cancer 1994;74:115–122.

Prout GR Jr, Griffin PP, Daly JJ, Heney NM: Carcinoma in situ of the urinary bladder with and without associated vesical neoplasms. Cancer 1983;52:524–532.

Sarkis AS, Dalbagni G, Cordon-Cardo C, et al: Association of P53 nuclear overexpression and tumor progression in carcinoma in situ of the bladder. J Urol 1994;152:388–392.

Schenkman E, Lamm DL: Superficial bladder cancer therapy. Scientific World Journal 2004;4(Suppl 1):387–399.

Weinstein RS, Miller AW 3rd, Pauli BU: Carcinoma in situ: Comments on the pathobiology of a paradox. Urol Clin North Am 1980;7:523–531.

Papillary Urothelial Hyperplasia

Cina SJ, Lancaster-Weiss KJ, Lecksell K, Epstein JI: Correlation of Ki-67 and p53 with the new World Health Organization/International Society of Urological Pathology Classification System for Urothelial Neoplasia. Arch Pathol Lab Med 2001;125:646–651.

Swierczynski SL, Epstein JI: Prognostic significance of atypical papillary urothelial hyperplasia. Hum Pathol 2002;33:512–517.

Urothelial Papilloma

Cheng L, Neumann RM, Bostwick DG: Papillary urothelial neoplasms of low malignant potential: Clinical and biologic implications. Cancer 1999;86:2102–2108.

Magi-Galluzzi C, Epstein JI: Urothelial papilloma of the bladder: A review of 34 de novo cases. Am J Surg Pathol 2004;28:1615–1620.

McKenney JK, Amin MB, Young RH: Urothelial (transitional cell) papilloma of the urinary bladder: A clinicopathologic study of 26 cases. Mod Pathol 2003;16:623–629.

van Rhijn BW, Montironi R, Zwarthoff EC, et al: Frequent FGFR3 mutations in urothelial papilloma. J Pathol 2002;198:245–251.

Inverted Papilloma

Cameron KM, Lupton CH: Inverted papilloma of the lower urinary tract. Br J Urol 1976;48:567–577.

Kunze E, Schauer A, Schmitt M: Histology and histogenesis of two different types of inverted urothelial papillomas. Cancer 1983;51:348–358.

Summers DE, Rushin JM, Frazier HA, Cotelingam JD: Inverted papilloma of the urinary bladder with granular eosinophilic cells: An unusual neuroendocrine variant. Arch Pathol Lab Med 1991;115:802–806.

Papillary Urothelial Neoplasm of Low Malignant Potential

Alsheikh A, Mohamedali Z, Jones E, et al: Comparison of the WHO/ISUP classification and cytokeratin 20 expression in predicting the behavior of low-grade papillary urothelial tumors. World/Health Organization/International Society of Urologic Pathology. Mod Pathol 2001;14:267–272.

Malmstrom PU, Busch C, Norlen BJ: Recurrence, progression and survival in bladder cancer: A retrospective analysis of 232 patients with greater than or equal to 5-year follow-up. Scand J Urol Nephrol 1987;21:185–195.

Pich A, Chiusa L, Formiconi A, et al: Biologic differences between noninvasive papillary urothelial neoplasms of low malignant potential

and low-grade (grade 1) papillary carcinomas of the bladder. Am J Surg Pathol 2001;25:1528–1533.

Noninvasive Low-Grade and High-Grade Papillary Urothelial Carcinoma

Desai S, Lim SD, Jimenez RE, et al: Relationship of cytokeratin 20 and CD44 protein expression with WHO/ISUP grade in pTa and pT1 papillary urothelial neoplasia. Mod Pathol 2000;13:1315–1323.

Holmang S, Johansson SL: The nested variant of transitional cell carcinoma: A rare neoplasm with poor prognosis. Scand J Urol Nephrol 2001;35:102–105.

Holmang S, Johansson SL: Stage Ta-T1 bladder cancer: The relationship between findings at first followup cystoscopy and subsequent recurrence and progression. J Urol 2002;167:1634–1637.

Urist MJ, Di Como CJ, Lu ML, et al: Loss of p63 expression is associated with tumor progression in bladder cancer. Am J Pathol 2002;161:1199–1206.

Invasive Urothelial Carcinoma

Amin MB, Ro JY, Lee KM, et al: Lymphoepithelioma-like carcinoma of the urinary bladder. Am J Surg Pathol 1994;18:466–473.

Andresen R, Wegner HE: Intravenous urography revisited in the age of ultrasound and computerized tomography: Diagnostic yield in cases of renal colic, suspected pelvic and abdominal malignancies, suspected renal mass, and acute pyelonephritis. Urol Int 1997;58:221–226.

Datta SN, Allen GM, Evans R, et al: Urinary tract ultrasonography in the evaluation of haematuria: A report of over 1,000 cases. Ann R Coll Surg Engl 2002;84:203–205.

Denkhaus H, Crone-Munzebrock W, Huland H: Noninvasive ultrasound in detecting and staging bladder carcinoma. Urol Radiol 1985;7:121–131.

Dinney CP, Ro JY, Babaian RJ, Johnson DE: Lymphoepithelioma of the bladder: A clinicopathological study of 3 cases. J Urol 1993;149:840–841.

Drew PA, Furman J, Civantos F, Murphy WM: (1996). The nested variant of transitional cell carcinoma: An aggressive neoplasm with innocuous histology. Mod Pathol 1996;9:989–994.

Eble JN, Young RH: (1997). Carcinoma of the urinary bladder: A review of its diverse morphology. Semin Diagn Pathol 1997;14:98–108.

Haleblian GE, Skinner EC, Dickinson MG, et al: Hydronephrosis as a prognostic indicator in bladder cancer patients. J Urol 1998;160:2011–2014.

Johansson SL, Borghede G, Holmang S: Micropapillary bladder carcinoma: A clinicopathological study of 20 cases. J Urol 1999;161:1798–1802.

Leroy X, Leteurtre E, De La Taille A, et al: Microcystic transitional cell carcinoma: A report of 2 cases arising in the renal pelvis. Arch Pathol Lab Med 2002;126:859–861.

Letocha H, Ahlstrom H, Malmstrom PU, et al: Positron emission tomography with L-methyl-11C-methionine in the monitoring of therapy response in muscle-invasive transitional cell carcinoma of the urinary bladder. Br J Urol 1994;74:767–774.

Lopez JI, Elorriaga K, Imaz I, Bilbao FJ: Micropapillary transitional cell carcinoma of the urinary bladder. Histopathology 1999;34:561–562.

Lopez-Beltran A, Croghan GA, Croghan I, et al: Prognostic factors in bladder cancer: A pathologic, immunohistochemical, and DNA flow-cytometric study. Am J Clin Pathol 1994;102:109–114.

Lopez-Beltran A, Martin J, Garcia J, Toro M: (1988). Squamous and glandular differentiation in urothelial bladder carcinomas: Histopathology, histochemistry and immunohistochemical expression of carcinoembryonic antigen. Histol Histopathol 1988;3:63–68.

Lopez-Beltran A, Pacelli A, Rothenberg HJ, et al: Carcinosarcoma and sarcomatoid carcinoma of the bladder: Clinicopathological study of 41 cases. J Urol 1998;159:1497–1503.

Messing EM, Vaillancourt A: Hematuria screening for bladder cancer. J Occup Med 1990;32:838–845.

Paik ML, Scolieri MJ, Brown SL, et al: Limitations of computerized tomography in staging invasive bladder cancer before radical cystectomy. J Urol 2000;163:1693–1696.

Reuter VE: Sarcomatoid lesions of the urogenital tract. Semin Diagn Pathol 1993;10:188–201.

Varkarakis MJ, Gaeta J, Moore RH, Murphy GP: Superficial bladder tumor: Aspects of clinical progression. Urology 1974;4:414–420.

Zukerberg LR, Harris NL, Young RH: Carcinomas of the urinary bladder simulating malignant lymphoma: A report of five cases. Am J Surg Pathol 1991;15:569–576.

Squamous Cell Carcinoma

Fortuny J, Kogevinas M, Chang-Claude J, et al: Tobacco, occupation and non-transitional-cell carcinoma of the bladder: an international case-control study. Int J Cancer 1999;80:44–46.

Ghoneim MA, Ashamallah AK, Awaad HK, Whitmore WF Jr: Randomized trial of cystectomy with or without preoperative radiotherapy for carcinoma of the bilharzial bladder. J Urol 1985;134:266–268.

Mostafa MH, Helmi S, Badawi AF, et al: Nitrate, nitrite and volatile N-nitroso compounds in the urine of Schistosoma haematobium and Schistosoma mansoni infected patients. Carcinogenesis 1994;15:619–625.

Parkin DM, Ferlay J, Hamdi-Cherif M, et al: Cancer in Africa: Epidemiology and Prevention. IARC Scientific Publication No. 153. Lyon, France, IARC Press, 2003.

Sarma KP: Squamous cell carcinoma of the bladder. Int Surg 1970;53:313–319.

Adenocarcinoma (Nonurachal) and Urachal Carcinoma

Gill HS, Dhillon HK, Woodhouse CR: Adenocarcinoma of the urinary bladder. Br J Urol 1989;64:138–142.

Grignon DJ, Ro JY, Ayala AG, et al: Primary adenocarcinoma of the urinary bladder: A clinicopathologic analysis of 72 cases. Cancer 1991;67:2165–2172.

Jacobo E, Loening S, Schmidt JD, Culp DA: Primary adenocarcinoma of the bladder: A retrospective study of 20 patients. J Urol 1977;117:54–56.

Johnson DE, Hodge GB, Abdul-Karim FW, Ayala AG: Urachal carcinoma. Urology 1985;26:218–221.

Kakizoe T, Matsumoto K, Andoh M, et al: Adenocarcinoma of urachus: Report of 7 cases and review of literature. Urology 1983;21:360–366.

Sheldon CA, Clayman RV, Gonzalez R, et al: Malignant urachal lesions. J Urol 1984;131:1–8.

Tamboli P, Mohsin SK, Hailemariam S, Amin MB: Colonic adenocarcinoma metastatic to the urinary tract versus primary tumors of the urinary tract with glandular differentiation: A report of 7 cases and investigation using a limited immunohistochemical panel. Arch Pathol Lab Med 2002;126:1057–1063.

Thomas DG, Ward AM, Williams JL: A study of 52 cases of adenocarcinoma of the bladder. Br J Urol 1971;43:4–15.

Torenbeek R, Lagendijk JH, Van Diest PJ, et al: Value of a panel of antibodies to identify the primary origin of adenocarcinomas presenting as bladder carcinoma. Histopathology 1998;32:20–27.

Wang HL, Lu DW, Yerian LM, et al: Immunohistochemical distinction between primary adenocarcinoma of the bladder and secondary colorectal adenocarcinoma. Am J Surg Pathol 2001;25:1380–1387.

Wheeler JD, Hill WT: Adenocarcinoma involving the urinary bladder. Cancer 1954;7:119–135.

Whitehead ED, Tessler AN: Carcinoma of the urachus. Br J Urol 1971;43:468–476.

Xiaoxu L, Jianhong L, Jinfeng W, Klotz LH: Bladder adenocarcinoma: 31 reported cases. Can J Urol 2001;8:1380–1383.

Small Cell Carcinoma

Abbas F, Civantos F, Benedetto P, Soloway MS: Small cell carcinoma of the bladder and prostate. Urology 1995;46:617–630.

Bastus R, Caballero JM, Gonzalez G, et al: Small cell carcinoma of the urinary bladder treated with chemotherapy and radiotherapy: Results in five cases. Eur Urol 1999;35:323–326.

Helpap B: Morphology and therapeutic strategies for neuroendocrine tumors of the genitourinary tract. Cancer 2002;95:1415–1420.

Mackey JR, Au HJ, Hugh J, Venner P: Genitourinary small cell carcinoma: Determination of clinical and therapeutic factors associated with survival. J Urol 1998;159:1624–1629.

Oesterling JE, Brendler CB, Burgers JK, et al: Advanced small cell carcinoma of the bladder: Successful treatment with combined radical cystoprostatectomy and adjuvant methotrexate, vinblastine, doxorubicin, and cisplatin chemotherapy. Cancer 1990;65:1928–1936.

Partanen S, Asikainen U: Oat cell carcinoma of the urinary bladder with ectopic adrenocorticotropic hormone production. Hum Pathol 1985;16:313–315.

Trias I, Algaba F, Condom E, et al: Small cell carcinoma of the urinary bladder: Presentation of 23 cases and review of 134 published cases. Eur Urol 2001;39:85–90.

Condyloma Acuminata and Squamous Papilloma

Cheng L, Leibovich BC, Cheville JC, et al: Squamous papilloma of the urinary tract is unrelated to condyloma acuminata. Cancer 2000;88:1679–1686.

Villous Adenoma

Cheng L, Montironi R, Bostwick DG: Villous adenoma of the urinary tract: A report of 23 cases, including 8 with coexistent adenocarcinoma. Am J Surg Pathol 1999;23:764–771.

Seibel JL, Prasad S, Weiss RE, et al: Villous adenoma of the urinary tract: A lesion frequently associated with malignancy. Hum Pathol 2002;33:236–241.

Tamboli P, Ro JY: Villous adenoma of urinary tract: A common tumor in an uncommon location. Adv Anat Pathol 2000;7:79–84.

Benign Mesenchymal Lesions

Bazeed MA, Aboulenien H: Leiomyoma of the bladder causing urethral and unilateral ureteral obstruction: A case report. J Urol 1988;140:143–144.

Bramwell SP, Pitts J, Goudie SE, Abel BJ: Giant leiomyoma of the bladder. Br J Urol 1987;60:178.

Kabalin JN, Freiha FS, Niebel JD: Leiomyoma of bladder: Report of 2 cases and demonstration of ultrasonic appearance. Urology 1990;35:210–212.

Knoll LD, Segura JW, Scheithauer BW: Leiomyoma of the bladder. J Urol 1986;136:906–908.

Lake MH, Kossow AS, Bokinsky G: Leiomyoma of the bladder and urethra. J Urol 1981;125:742–743.

Martin SA, Sears DL, Sebo TJ, et al: Smooth muscle neoplasms of the urinary bladder: A clinicopathologic comparison of leiomyoma and leiomyosarcoma. Am J Surg Pathol 2002;26:292–300.

Mutchler RW Jr, Gorder JL: Leiomyoma of the bladder in a child. Br J Radiol 1972;45:538–540.

Yusim IE, Neulander EZ, Eidelberg I, et al: Leiomyoma of the genitourinary tract. Scand J Urol Nephrol 2001;35:295–299.

Inflammatory Myofibroblastic Tumor

Cook JR, Dehner LP, Collins MH, et al: Anaplastic lymphoma kinase (ALK) expression in the inflammatory myofibroblastic tumor: A comparative immunohistochemical study. Am J Surg Pathol 2001;25:1364–1371.

Mahadevia PS, Alexander JE, Rojas-Corona R, Koss LG: Pseudosarcomatous stromal reaction in primary and metastatic urothelial carcinoma. A source of diagnostic difficulty. Am J Surg Pathol 1989;13:782–790.

Nochomovitz LE, Orenstein JM: Inflammatory pseudotumor of the urinary bladder—Possible relationship to nodular fasciitis: Two case reports, cytologic observations, and ultrastructural observations. Am J Surg Pathol 1985;9:366–373.

Ro JY, Ayala AG, Ordonez NG, et al: Pseudosarcomatous fibromyxoid tumor of the urinary bladder. Am J Clin Pathol 1986;86:583–590.

Tsuzuki T, Magi-Galluzzi C, Epstein JI: ALK-1 expression in inflammatory myofibroblastic tumor of the urinary bladder. Am J Surg Pathol 2004;28:1609–1614.

Wick MR, Brown BA, Young RH, Mills SE: Spindle-cell proliferations of the urinary tract: An immunohistochemical study. Am J Surg Pathol 1988;12:379–389.

Leiomyoma

Binsaleh S, Corcos J, Elhilali MM, Carrier S: Bladder leiomyoma: Report of two cases and literature review. Can J Urol 2004;11:2411–2413.

Martin SA, Sears DL, Sebo TJ, et al: Smooth muscle neoplasms of the urinary bladder: A clinicopathologic comparison of leiomyoma and leiomyosarcoma. Am J Surg Pathol 2002;26:292–300.

Neurofibroma

Cheng L, Scheithauer BW, Leibovich BC, et al: Neurofibroma of the urinary bladder. Cancer 1999;86:505–513.

Wilkinson LM, Manson D, Smith CR: Best cases from the AFIP: Plexiform neurofibroma of the bladder. Radiographics 2004;24(Suppl 1):S237–S242.

Hemangioma

Cheng L, Nascimento AG, Neumann RM, et al: Hemangioma of the urinary bladder. Cancer 1999;86:498–504.

Hall BD: Bladder hemangiomas in Klippel-Trenaunay-Weber syndrome. N Engl J Med 1971;285:1032–1033.

Hendry WF, Vinnicombe J: Haemangioma of bladder in children and young adults. Br J Urol 1971;43:309–316.

Jahn H, Nissen HM: Haemangioma of the urinary tract: Review of the literature. Br J Urol 1991;68:113–117.

Kato M, Chiba Y, Sakai K, Orikasa S: Endoscopic neodymium:yttrium aluminium garnet (Nd:YAG) laser irradiation of a bladder hemangioma associated with Klippel-Weber syndrome. Int J Urol 2000;7:145–148.

Leonard MP, Nickel JC, Morales A: Cavernous hemangiomas of the bladder in the pediatric age group. J Urol 1988;140:1503–1504.

Stroup RM, Chang YC: Angiosarcoma of the bladder: A case report. J Urol 1987;137:984–985.

Solitary Fibrous Tumor

Corti B, Carella R, Gabusi E, et al: Solitary fibrous tumour of the urinary bladder with expression of bcl-2, CD34, and insulin-like growth factor type II. Eur Urol 2001;39:484–488.

Kim SH, Cha KB, Choi YD, Cho NH: Solitary fibrous tumor of the urinary bladder. Yonsei Med J 2004;45:573–576.

Mentzel T, Bainbridge TC, Katenkamp D: Solitary fibrous tumour: Clinicopathological, immunohistochemical, and ultrastructural analysis of 12 cases arising in soft tissues, nasal cavity and nasopharynx, urinary bladder and prostate. Virchows Arch 1997;430:445–453.

Westra WH. Grenko RT, Epstein J. Solitary fibrous tumor of the lower urogenital tract: A report of five cases involving the seminal vesicles, urinary bladder, and prostate. Hum Pathol 2000;31:63–68.

Malignant Mesenchymal Tumors

Mackenzie AR, Whitmore WF Jr, Melamed MR: Myosarcomas of the bladder and prostate. Cancer 1968;22:833–844.

Mills SE, Bova GS, Wick MR, Young RH: Leiomyosarcoma of the urinary bladder: A clinicopathologic and immunohistochemical study of 15 cases. Am J Surg Pathol 1989;13:480–489.

Russo P, Brady MS, Conlon K, et al: Adult urological sarcoma. J Urol 1992;147:1032–1036; discussion 1036–1037.

Weitzner S: Leiomyosarcoma of urinary bladder in children. Urology 1978;12:450–452.

Rhabdomyosarcoma

Kumar S, Perlman E, Harris CA, et al: Myogenin is a specific marker for rhabdomyosarcoma: An immunohistochemical study in paraffin-embedded tissues. Mod Pathol 2000;13:988–993.

Leuschner I, Harms D, Mattke A, et al: Rhabdomyosarcoma of the urinary bladder and vagina: A clinicopathologic study with emphasis on recurrent disease. A report from the Kiel Pediatric Tumor Registry and the German CWS Study. Am J Surg Pathol 2001;25:856–864.

Scholtmeijer RJ, Tromp CG, Hazebroek FW: Embryonal rhabdomyosarcoma of the urogenital tract in childhood. Eur Urol 1983;9:69–74.

Leiomyosarcoma

Martin SA, Sears DL, Sebo TJ, et al: Smooth muscle neoplasms of the urinary bladder: A clinicopathologic comparison of leiomyoma and leiomyosarcoma. Am J Surg Pathol 2002;26:292–300.

Pedersen-Bjergaard J, Jonsson V, Pedersen M, Hou-Jensen K: Leiomyosarcoma of the urinary bladder after cyclophosphamide. J Clin Oncol 1995;13:532–533.

Rowland RG, Eble JN: Bladder leiomyosarcoma and pelvic fibroblastic tumor following cyclophosphamide therapy. J Urol 1983;130:344–346.

Germ Cell Tumors

Cauffield EW: Dermoid cysts of the bladder. J Urol 1956;75:801–804.

Lazebnik J, Kamhi D: A case of vesical teratoma associated with vesical stones and diverticulum. J Urol 1961;85:796–799.

Taylor G, Jordan M, Churchill B, Mancer K: Yolk sac tumor of the bladder. J Urol 1983;129:591–594.

Lymphoma

Abraham NZ Jr, Maher TJ, Hutchison RE: Extra-nodal monocytoid B-cell lymphoma of the urinary bladder. Mod Pathol 1993;6:145–149.

Kempton CL, Kurtin PJ, Inwards DJ, et al: Malignant lymphoma of the bladder: Evidence from 36 cases that low-grade lymphoma of the MALT-type is the most common primary bladder lymphoma. Am J Surg Pathol 1997;21:1324–1333.

Wazait HD, Chahal R, Sundurum SK, et al: MALT-type primary lymphoma of the urinary bladder: Clinicopathological study of 2 cases and review of the literature. Urol Int 2001;66:220–224.

Melanoma

Kerley SW, Blute ML, Keeney GL: Multifocal malignant melanoma arising in vesicovaginal melanosis. Arch Pathol Lab Med 1991;115:950–952.

Stein BS, Kendall AR: Malignant melanoma of the genitourinary tract. J Urol 1984;132:859–868.

Tainio HM, Kylmala TM, Haapasalo HK: Primary malignant melanoma of the urinary bladder associated with widespread metastases. Scand J Urol Nephrol 1999;33:406–407.

Paraganglioma

Cheng L, Leibovich BC, Cheville JC, et al: Paraganglioma of the urinary bladder: Can biologic potential be predicted? Cancer 2000;88:844–852.

Dow CJ, Palmer MK, O'Sullivan JP, Kirkham JS: Malignant phaeochromocytoma: Report of a case and a critical review. Br J Surg 1982;69:338–340.

Flanigan RC, Wittmann RP, Huhn RG, Davis CJ: Malignant pheochromocytoma of urinary bladder. Urology 1980;16:386–388.

Grignon DJ, Ro JY, Mackay B, et al: Paraganglioma of the urinary bladder: Immunohistochemical, ultrastructural, and DNA flow cytometric studies. Hum Pathol 1991;22:1162–1169.

Kato H, Suzuki M, Mukai M, Aizawa S: Clinicopathological study of pheochromocytoma of the urinary bladder: Immunohistochemical, flow cytometric and ultrastructural findings with review of the literature. Pathol Int 1999;49:1093–1099.

Leestma JE, Price EB Jr: Paraganglioma of the urinary bladder. Cancer 1971;28:1063–1073.

Linnoila RI, Keiser HR, Steinberg SM, Lack EE: Histopathology of benign versus malignant sympathoadrenal paragangliomas: Clinicopathologic study of 120 cases including unusual histologic features. Hum Pathol 1990;21:1168–1180.

Meyer JJ, Sane SM, Drake RM: Malignant paraganglioma (pheochromocytoma) of the urinary bladder: Report of a case and review of the literature. Pediatrics 1979;63:879–885.

Moyana TN, Kontozoglou T: Urinary bladder paragangliomas: An immunohistochemical study. Arch Pathol Lab Med 1988;112:70–72.

Carcinoid Tumors

Martignoni G, Eble JN: Carcinoid tumors of the urinary bladder:
    Immunohistochemical study of 2 cases and review of the literature.
    Arch Pathol Lab Med 2003;127:e22–e24.

Granular Cell Tumors

Fletcher MS, Aker M, Hill JT, et al: Granular cell myoblastoma of the
    bladder. Br J Urol 1985;57:109–110.
Yoshida T, Hirai S, Horii Y, Yamauchi T: Granular cell tumor of the urinary
    bladder. Int J Urol 2001;8:29–31.

Metastatic Tumors and Secondary Extension

Bates AW, Baithun SI: Secondary neoplasms of the bladder are
    histological mimics of nontransitional cell primary tumours:
    Clinicopathological and histological features of 282 cases.
    Histopathology 2000;36:32–40.
Silver SA, Epstein JI: Adenocarcinoma of the colon simulating primary
    urinary bladder neoplasia: A report of nine cases. Am J Surg Pathol
    1993;17:171–178.

5

Non-neoplastic Diseases of the Kidney

Stephen M. Bonsib

This chapter is divided into three sections: congenital anomalies and cystic diseases, vascular diseases, and tubulointerstitial diseases. Each category contains common or important entities that are encountered in the surgical pathology gross room and autopsy suite. Many lesions can be recognized by their gross appearance. Understanding of the normal macroscopic and microscopic features of the kidney is essential to enable recognition of the departures from normal, discussed in this chapter.

GROSS AND HISTOLOGIC FEATURES OF THE NORMAL KIDNEY

The kidneys are paired retroperitoneal organs that are covered by a fibrous capsule and insulated by adipose tissue within Gerota's fascia. Renal weight in newborns ranges from 13 to 44 g; this increases by adulthood to 125 to 170 g in men and 115 to 155 g in women. The average adult kidney is 11 to 12 cm long, 5 to 7 cm wide, and 2.5 to 3 cm thick. The kidney has a concave medial surface with a slit-like space called the hilum, through which pass the ureter, branches of the renal arteries and veins, nerves, and lymphatics within the renal sinus. The renal sinus is the central fat-containing compartment that invests the calyceal and pelvic portions of the collecting system (Fig. 5-1).

The subcapsular surface of the renal cortex may be smooth, or it may show the outlines of renal lobes; known as persistent fetal lobation, this is a normal anatomic variant without functional consequences. The kidney has 11 to 14 lobes. Each lobe is composed of a central conicomedullary pyramid surrounded by a cap of cortex. By the 28th week of gestation, the number of renal lobes is established; however, with the subsequent increase in renal mass, a process of lobar fusion ensues that reduces the number of renal pyramids to between 9 and 11. The renal parenchyma consists of the granular brown cortex and the paler striated medulla.

CORTEX

The cortex forms a 1.0 cm layer beneath the renal capsule and extends down between the renal pyramids, forming the columns of Bertin (Fig. 5-1). The cortex is organized into two architectural regions: the cortical labyrinth and the medullary rays (Fig. 5-2). The cortical labyrinth contains glomeruli, proximal and distal convoluted tubules, connecting tubules, and the initial portion of the collecting ducts, as well as interlobular arteries and veins, arterioles, venules, capillaries, and lymphatics. The principal components of the labyrinth are the proximal convoluted tubules. In the normal cortex, the tubules are closely packed, with basement

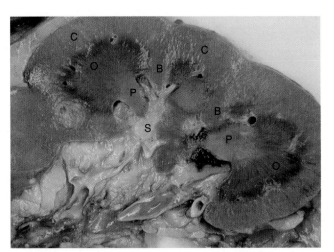

FIGURE 5-1

This bivalved kidney demonstrates the renal cortex (C) and columns of Bertin (B) situated between the renal pyramids. A renal pyramid consists of an outer medulla (O) and an inner medulla or papilla (P). The sinus fat (S) separates the renal parenchyma from the collecting system.

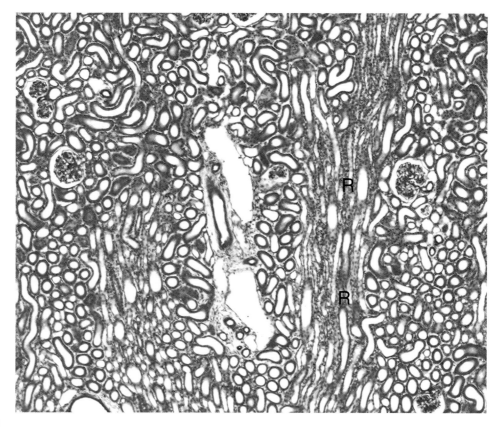

FIGURE 5-2

The cortical labyrinth contains the glomeruli, arteries, veins, and tubules; most tubules are proximal tubules. The medullary rays (R) contain the same tubular components as the outer medulla; note their longitudinal orientation relative to the convoluted tubules of the adjacent cortical labyrinth.

membranes in close apposition. The interstitial space is scant and contains the peritubular capillary plexus and interstitial cells. The base of the renal pyramid has faint perpendicular cortical extensions, the medullary rays. Medullary rays are so named because they contain the same tubular segments that are present in the outer strip of the outer medulla, the collecting ducts, and the proximal and distal straight tubules of the superficial and midcortical nephron.

MEDULLA

The medulla is divided into an outer medulla, composed of an outer stripe and an inner stripe, and the inner medulla or papilla (Fig. 5-1). The anatomic limits of each region are defined by their differing tubular composition (Table 5-1). The outer strip, the thinnest portion of the renal medulla, contains the straight portion of the proximal tubules, collecting ducts, and the distal straight tubules (also known as the thick ascending limbs of Henle). The inner strip is defined by transition of the straight portion of the proximal tubule into the thin descending limb of Henle. The inner medulla contains the thin descending and thin ascending limbs

TABLE 5-1
Tubular Segments within Each Zone of the Medulla

OUTER STRIP

Straight part of the proximal tubules

Straight distal tubules (thick ascending limb of Henle)

Collecting ducts

INNER STRIP

Thin descending limbs Henle

Thick ascending limbs of Henle

Collecting ducts

INNER MEDULLA

Thin descending limbs of Henle

Thin ascending limbs of Henle

Large collecting ducts (ducts of Bellini)

of Henle and the collecting ducts (ducts of Bellini). At the papillary tip, in the area cribrosa (cribriform appearance grossly), the epithelium of the ducts of Bellini transforms into the urothelium of the collecting ducts.

VASCULATURE

The main renal arteries arise from the aorta and give off a suprarenal artery to supply the adrenal glands, as well as a ureteric artery to each ureter. The most common pattern is division into anterior and posterior branches that give rise to five segmental renal arteries (Fig. 5-3). Most commonly, the anterior branch gives rise to four segmental arteries: the apical, upper, middle, and lower segmental arteries. Two segmental arteries supply the middle anterior portions of the kidney, and two polar segmental branches supply both the anterior and posterior polar aspects of the kidney. The posterior branch continues as a fifth segmental branch, the posterior segmental artery, to supply the middle posterior portions of the kidney. Deviation from this pattern is common.

A segmental artery branches within the renal sinus to form several interlobar arteries; these pierce the parenchyma between the pyramid surface and a column of Bertin to form a splay of six to eight arcuate arteries. The arcuate arteries curve along the corticomedullary junction to terminate at the midpoint of a renal lobe. Interlobular arteries arise from an arcuate artery. They extend to the renal capsule between medullary rays and are encircled by tiers of five to six glomeruli, which they supply with an afferent arteriole.

The microvascularization of the cortex begins with the glomerular afferent arteriole. It enters the renal corpuscle at the hilum and branches to form the capillary loops of the glomerular tuft, which then converge to become the efferent arteriole. The efferent arterioles of the superficial and midcortical nephrons transition into a peritubular capillary plexus that forms a uniformly distributed anastomosing vascular lattice amid the cortical tubules of the labyrinth. In the medullary rays, the capillary plexus assumes a more longitudinal orientation. The efferent arteriole of the deep or juxtamedullary glomeruli descend into the medulla, as discussed later.

The venous return of the cortex drains first from the medullary rays into the labyrinth and then enters small venules that converge to follow the arterial supply. The interlobular, arcuate, and interlobar veins run parallel to the arteries. The arcuate and interlobar veins are connected by abundant anastomoses and lateral tributaries that encircle the renal pyramids and calyces. The interlobar veins converge anterior to the pelvis to drain the three poles of the kidney and then unite to form the main renal vein. No veins are located within the medulla.

MEDULLA

The medullary blood supply has two sources. The principal blood supply is from efferent arterioles of the juxtamedullary glomeruli. The efferent arterioles begin as a splay of arterioles that descend toward the medulla. They converge as the descending arteriolar rectae, forming organized bundles in the inner strip of the outer medulla. At various points as they descend, branches supply the tubules with a rich capillary plexus. The bundle size diminishes as it descends into the inner medulla. Arterioles from spiral arterial branches of the interlobar arteries form the second blood supply, which is limited to the papillary tip. There are no arteries or veins within the renal medulla. The ascending arteriolar rectae form the venous return, which in general follows the descending arteriolar rectae, and empty into the arcuate veins.

RENAL LYMPHATIC SYSTEM

The kidneys have a dual lymphatic system. The major lymphatic drainage follows the vasculature and begins as small vessels in the adventitia of the peripheral interlobular arteries. These enlarge and become more numerous as they descend to the corticomedullary junction and enter the renal sinus. There are no lymphatic vessels amid the glomeruli and renal tubules or in the medulla. The second, separate lymphatic system exists within the renal capsule. It receives drainage from the most superficial cortex. Lymph courses along the

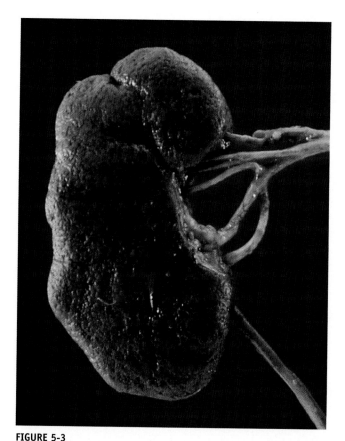

FIGURE 5-3

The main renal artery usually gives rise to five segmental branches. In this specimen, the first branch supplies the upper pole.

capsule and around to the hilum, to join the major lymphatic flow exiting the renal sinus.

COLLECTING SYSTEM

The renal collecting system consists of the calyces, the sac-like renal pelvis, and the ureter. The most proximal portions of the collecting system are the 9 to 11 funnel-shaped minor calyces that surround the individual papillary tips (Fig. 5-4). They have slender proximal extensions termed fornices. The major calyces represent the confluence of the minor calyces; they unite to form the renal pelvis, which represents the expanded upper portion of the ureter. There is no distinct delineation between the pelvis and the ureter; rather, a gradual transition occurs. A continuous layer of smooth muscle originates at the fornices and continues along the calyces and pelvis and down the ureter.

CONGENITAL ANOMALIES AND CYSTIC RENAL DISEASES

Abnormalities of genitourinary tract development occur in 10 % of the population and represent the most common cause of renal failure in children. There is no satisfactory classification of these anomalies. Although knowledge of embryologic development provides a tempting basis for explaining departures from normal, classification based on the underlying genetic defects will likely replace current schemes as knowledge increases about candidate genes and their products. A complicating factor may be the polygenetic nature of many disorders, in which multiple minor genetic defects affect susceptibility and influence the nature of the malformation expressed. Evolution in understanding of the genetic and molecular bases of urinary tract malformations will minimize the anatomic contribution of urinary tract obstruction, by placing it within a larger paradigm of sequential genetic and molecular misadventures that culminate in the malformed kidney.

CYSTIC RENAL DISEASES

There are many forms of renal cystic disease, but four are of greatest importance: adult or autosomal dominant polycystic kidney disease (AD-PKD), infantile or autosomal recessive polycystic kidney disease (AR-PKD), (Fig. 5-5) renal dysplasias, and acquired renal cystic disease (Ac-RCD). It is important to separate the two hereditary polycystic kidney diseases (AD-PKD and AR-PKD) (Fig. 5-6) from renal dysplasias, which are most often sporadic, and to distinguish the sporadic forms of dysplasia from those occurring in hereditary malformation syndromes (Tables 5-2 and 5-3).

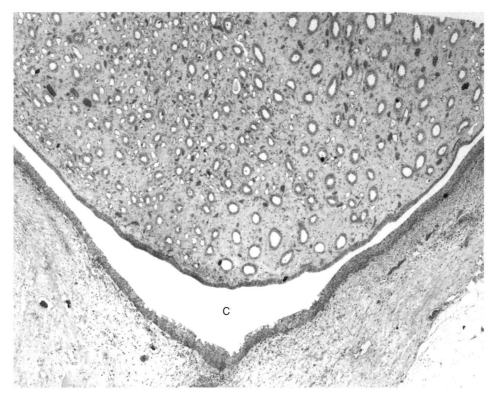

FIGURE 5-4

A renal papilla is tightly nestled within a minor calyx (C), the most proximal extension of the collecting system.

TABLE 5-2

Congenital Cystic Disease

	AD-PKD	AR-PKD	Dysplasia	Ac-RCD
Incidence	1:500-1:1,000	1:20-1:50,000	1:1,000-1:4,000	10-90% dialysis patients
Genetics/locus	Chromosome 16 or 4	Chromosome 6	Sporadic or hereditary	None
Size	Large	Large	Large or small	Small
Reniform shape	+	+	±	+
Bilateral	+	+	±	+
Segmental	−	−	±	−
Ureter abnormal	−	−	±	−
Uniform cysts	−	+	−	−
Liver abnormal	+	+	−	−
Other malformations	−	−	±	−

Ac-RCD, acquired renal cystic disease; AD-PKD, adult polycystic kidney disease; AR-PKD, infantile polycystic kidney disease.

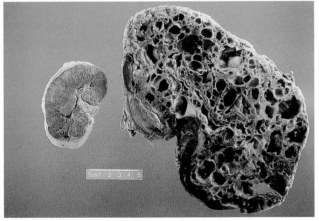

FIGURE 5-5

Autosomal recessive (AR) and autosomal dominant (AD) polycystic kidneys. Each kidney is massively enlarged, diffusely cystic, and reniform in shape.

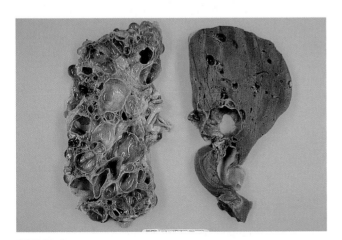

FIGURE 5-6

Liver and kidney in autosomal dominant polycystic kidney disease (AD-PKD). Notice the scattered hepatic cysts and diffuse renal cysts.

TABLE 5-3

Cystic Renal Disease Associated with Congenital Hepatic Fibrosis or Biliary Dysgenesis

Infantile polycystic kidney disease

Adult polycystic kidney disease

Juvenile nephronophthisis

Meckel-Gruber syndrome*

Zellweger syndrome*

Ivemark's syndrome*

Chondrodysplastic syndromes*

Trisomy C*

Trisomy D*

*Additional malformations are present.

ADULT (DOMINANT) POLYCYSTIC KIDNEY DISEASE

AD-PKD is the most common cystic renal disease and the most common genetic disease. It occurs with a frequency of 1:500 to 1:1000. It is the fourth leading cause of end-stage renal disease and accounts for 5% to 10% of dialysis patients. Patients vary in age at onset; most present in their 30s or 40s, and there is a 100% penetrance by age 80 years. Approximately 25% lack a family history, presumably representing a new mutation. Two principal genes have been identified, on chromosome 16 (90%) and chromosome 4 (10%), that encode for polycystin 1 and 2, respectively. These are membrane-associated glycoproteins that are expressed in the primary cilia of the distal nephron and collecting duct epithelial cells.

CLINICAL FEATURES

Patients with AD-PKD show variation in age at onset and profile of symptoms. Patients may present with chronic flank pain due to the massively enlarged kidneys, hematuria, or acute flank pain resulting from hemorrhage into a cyst. Hypertension develops early. Activation of the renin-angiotensin system secondary to intrarenal vascular occlusion by expanding cysts has been implicated. Urinary tract infection develops in 50% to 75% of cases and affects women more often than men. The infection may be confined to the collecting system or a cyst, or it may involve the parenchyma. Perinephric extension with abscess is a serious complication with a 60% mortality rate. Nephrolithiasis develops in 10% of patients, and renal cell carcinoma in 1% to 5%. An important extrarenal complication is berry aneurysms, which occur in 5% to 15% of the patients. Cysts are invariably present in the liver and often are present in the pancreas and spleen.

RADIOLOGIC FEATURES

Multiple and bilateral renal cysts and liver cysts are present. Cysts may also be identified in the pancreas and spleen.

PATHOLOGIC FEATURES

GROSS FINDINGS

Early in the disease, the kidney appears normal, with scattered small cysts in the cortex and medulla and normal intervening parenchyma. As the disease progresses, cysts enlarge and increase in number, resulting in massive renal enlargement of 2000 to 4000 g. The cysts are spherical and unilocular. Their contents vary from translucent to hemorrhagic. The collecting system and ureter are normal.

MICROSCOPIC FINDINGS

Cysts develop in all segments of the nephron, but only 1% of nephrons are affected. Most cysts are lined by a single layer of flattened to cuboidal epithelium (Fig. 5-7). Hyperplastic foci or polyp formation occurs in some cysts, and renal neoplasms, often of a papillary architecture, may be present. The cysts contain protein, red cells, or calcific deposits (Fig. 5-8). The intervening parenchyma in early cases appears normal (Fig. 5-7). In advanced cases, interstitial fibrosis with a lymphoid infiltrate, tubular atrophy, glomerulosclerosis, and vascular sclerosis develops.

ADULT (DOMINANT) POLYCYSTIC KIDNEY DISEASE—FACT SHEET

Definition
▶ Polycystic kidney disease caused by mutations in polycystin-1 or polycystin-2

Incidence and Location
▶ Incidence 1:500 to 1:1000

Morbidity and Mortality
▶ Renal failure, berry aneurysms, cardiovascular disease

Gender, Race, and Age Distribution
▶ No sex or race predominance
▶ Clinical onset in third to fourth decades

Clinical Features
▶ Flank pain, hematuria, hypertension, pyelonephritis

Radiologic Features
▶ Multiple and bilateral renal cysts
▶ Cysts in liver, often in pancreas and spleen

Prognosis and Treatment
▶ Fourth leading cause of end-stage renal disease
▶ Cardiovascular disease and cerebral vascular disease
▶ Close surveillance for renal and extrarenal complications

ADULT (DOMINANT) POLYCYSTIC KIDNEY DISEASE— PATHOLOGIC FEATURES

Gross Findings
▶ Initially kidneys appear normal
▶ Eventually kidneys become massively enlarged (2000-4000 g), with cysts in cortex and medulla

Microscopic Findings
▶ Cysts form in all segments of nephron
▶ Sclerosis of glomeruli, atrophy of tubules, calcification, inflammatory infiltrates
▶ Epithelial neoplasms, usually papillary in type

Differential Diagnosis
▶ Acquired renal cystic disease
▶ Multiple simple renal cysts

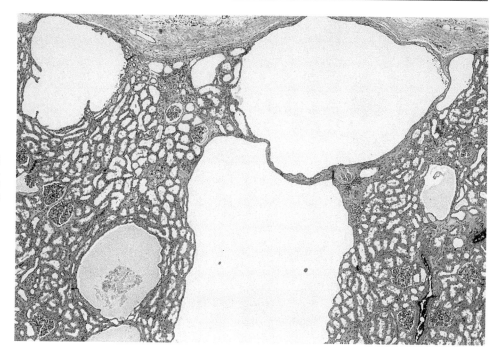

FIGURE 5-7

In the early stage of autosomal dominant polycystic kidney disease, large zones of normal-appearing cortex are interrupted by focal cyst formation.

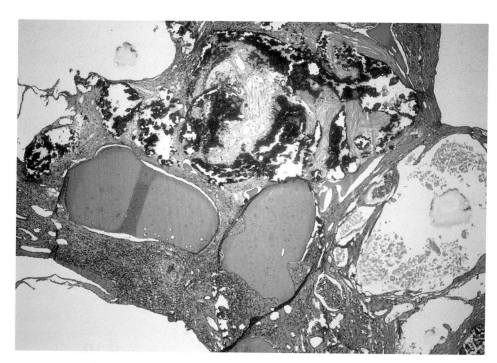

FIGURE 5-8

Typical appearance of autosomal dominant polycystic kidney disease at nephrectomy or autopsy, showing large cysts, diffuse nephron atrophy, interstitial fibrosis, and calcification.

DIFFERENTIAL DIAGNOSIS

Ac-RCD and multiple simple renal cortical cysts may be mistaken for AD-PKD. In Ac-RCD, the patient experiences renal failure from another cause unrelated to a cystic kidney disease, so the history is crucial. The kidney size in Ac-RCD is normal or small, not massively increased as in AD-PKD. Simple renal cysts occur in patients older than 40 years of age and may rarely be numerous enough to suggest AD-PKD on imaging studies. Grossly, the kidneys are not significantly enlarged and extrarenal cysts and symptoms of AD-PKD are absent. Histologic sections show a flattened to absent cell lining in simple cysts and do not reveal the parenchymal atrophy and proliferative lesions characteristic of AD-PKD (Fig. 5-9).

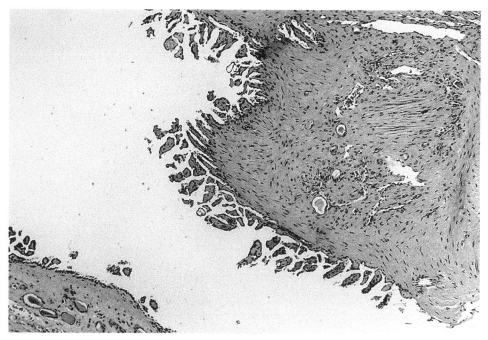

FIGURE 5-9
In autosomal dominant polycystic kidney disease, some cysts contain proliferative lesions; similar lesions occur in the parenchyma.

PROGNOSIS AND TREATMENT

Renal failure is common; extrarenal complications increase in importance with age. Infection and vascular disease represent the most common causes of death. There is no specific therapy, only careful surveillance.

INFANTILE (RECESSIVE) POLYCYSTIC KIDNEY DISEASE

AR-PKD is characterized by bilateral cystic kidney disease and congenital hepatic fibrosis, with or without dilation of intrahepatic bile ducts known as Caroli's disease. Parents lack the disease, and 25% of siblings will be affected. Genetic studies have identified a single gene, *PKHD1,* whose locus is 6p12. It encodes for the protein fibrocystin, a component of the primary cilia of collecting duct principal cells.

CLINICAL FEATURES

Severely affected patients with neonatal onset die from pulmonary hypoplasia resulting from thoracic compromise by the massively enlarged kidneys. Despite

---

INFANTILE (RECESSIVE) POLYCYSTIC KIDNEY DISEASE—FACT SHEET

Definition
▶ Polycystic kidney disease and congenital hepatic fibrosis resulting from *PKHD1* mutations

Incidence and Location
▶ Incidence 1:20 to 1:50,000

Morbidity and Mortality
▶ Neonatal death in severely affected cases
▶ Death from portal hypertension and esophageal varices in childhood

Gender, Race, and Age Distribution
▶ No gender or race predilection
▶ Manifest at birth or during childhood

Clinical Features
▶ Pulmonary failure in severely affected neonates
▶ Portal hypertension in less severely affected children

Radiologic Features
▶ Radial cysts in cortex and medulla in neonates
▶ Multiple rounded cortical to elongate medullary cysts in children

Prognosis and Treatment
▶ Neonatal death from pulmonary hypoplasia
▶ Childhood death from portal hypertension

impressive cystic alteration, renal function is usually preserved. If the kidneys are nonfunctional, maternal oligohydramnios develops, and a Potter's phenotype is present at birth. Patients who survive into childhood may develop respiratory insufficiency and pneumothoraces, or they may develop portal hypertension with resulting gastrointestinal hemorrhage from esophageal varices.

RADIOLOGIC FEATURES

Severely affected infants can be detected in utero by ultrasonography, which reveals massively enlarged, diffusely cystic kidneys.

PATHOLOGIC FEATURES

GROSS FINDINGS

The kidneys are massively enlarged to 200 to 600 g in neonatal presentations. The cysts extend radially from the medulla to the cortex, imparting a distinctive spongy appearance to the kidneys (Fig. 5-10). Despite the impressive gross appearance, organogenesis of the kidneys appears normal based on microdissection studies. In less severely affected kidneys of older children, the appearance is variable. The kidneys are smaller and the cortical cysts are variably distributed, larger, rounded, and fewer (Fig. 5-11). Medullary cysts are always present and tend to be elongated.

The collecting system and ureter are normal.

MICROSCOPIC FINDINGS

In the severely affected neonates, the cortex and medulla are expanded by elongated collecting duct cysts

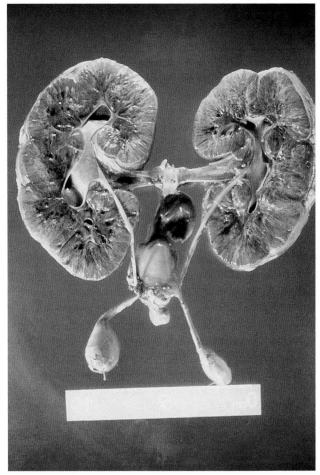

FIGURE 5-10

In the neonatal severe form of autosomal recessive polycystic kidney disease (AR-PKD), the massively enlarged kidneys have a diffuse, spongy quality due to cortical and medullary collecting duct cysts. Notice that the collecting system and ureter are normal.

INFANTILE (RECESSIVE) POLYCYSTIC KIDNEY DISEASE— PATHOLOGIC FEATURES

Gross Findings
► Neonatal onset: massively enlarged (200-600 g) kidneys, diffuse collecting duct cysts in cortex and medulla
► Childhood onset: minimally enlarged kidneys; rounded, variably distributed cysts in cortex and medulla

Microscopic Findings
► Cysts lined by cuboidal collecting duct cells
► Normal intervening nephron structures
► Liver shows a bile duct plate abnormality

Differential Diagnosis
► Adult (dominant) polycystic kidney disease
► Medullary sponge kidney

---

lined with uniform cuboidal cells. The intervening nephrons appear normal (Fig. 5-12). In kidneys of older patients, the number of collecting duct cysts are fewer and the parenchyma adjacent to the cysts develops atrophic changes with tubulointerstitial scarring and glomerulosclerosis, creating a resemblance to AD-PKD. In the liver, the portal bile ducts are dilated and have an irregular pattern of anastomosing channels at the periphery of portal areas (Fig. 5-13). There is a further expansion of the portal zones with increasing age, and congenital hepatic fibrosis eventually develops in infants and children.

DIFFERENTIAL DIAGNOSIS

The appearance of the kidneys is distinctive in severe neonatal cases. In childhood presentations, early-onset AD-PKD and medullary sponge kidney may be considered. The liver bile duct plate lesion of congenital

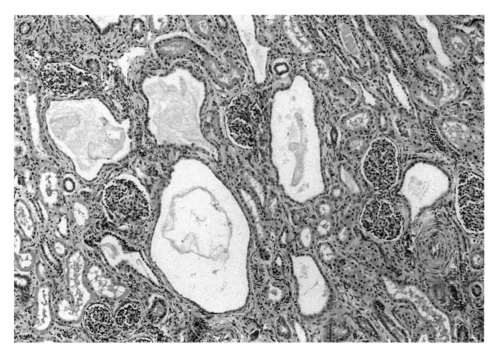

FIGURE 5-11

In those patients with autosomal recessive polycystic kidney disease who survive into childhood, the collecting duct cysts are smaller, fewer, and more rounded. Interstitial fibrosis is beginning to develop.

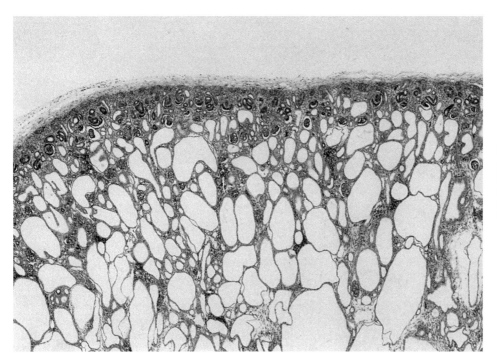

FIGURE 5-12

In autosomal recessive polycystic kidney disease, the cysts involve collecting ducts and the intervening nephrons are characteristically normal.

hepatic fibrosis is a useful diagnostic feature of AR-PKD if liver biopsy is performed. However, a number of other diseases may be associated with renal cysts and liver disease, including AD-PKD (Table 5-3). Awareness of any additional anomalies is important for proper classification. Medullary sponge kidney is usually detected in adults but may be encountered in children evaluated for nephrolithiasis. The medullary cysts cluster in the papillary tip, and cortical cysts and hepatic cysts are absent.

PROGNOSIS AND TREATMENT

Many cases of AR-PKD result in stillbirth or early neonatal death from pulmonary hypoplasia. Patients who survive into childhood have milder cystic renal disease, permitting better pulmonary development. However, with increasing age, the liver disease worsens, culminating in congenital hepatic fibrosis, portal hypertension, and death from bleeding esophageal varices.

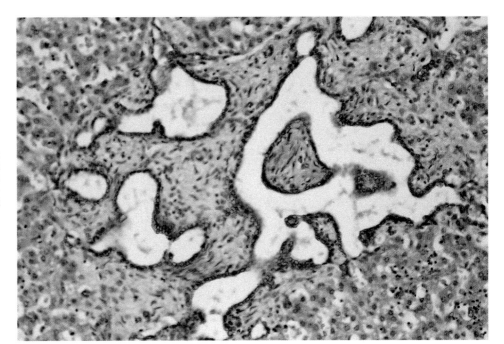

FIGURE 5-13
In autosomal recessive polycystic kidney disease, the liver bile duct plate developmental abnormality is characterized by a complex arrangement of interconnected bile duct structures.

RENAL DYSPLASIA

Renal dysplasia refers to the presence of a metanephric structure with aberrant nephronic differentiation. Dysplastic kidneys should not be confused with hypoplastic kidneys, which are small and extremely rare but otherwise normally developed, nor with polycystic kidney diseases, which, although cystic, do not contain dysplastic elements.

CLINICAL FEATURES

Multicystic renal dysplasia is the most common cause of unilateral renal enlargement in infants. Evaluation of the contralateral urinary tract is important, because abnormalities occur in 40% of cases. Bilateral involvement usually results in neonatal death from pulmonary hypoplasia.

Renal dysplasia is most often sporadic, but it may be syndromic and develop as part of a multiple malformation syndrome (Table 5-4) or chromosomal anomaly, some of which are hereditary. Rarely, renal agenesis or renal dysplasia is familial (usually autosomal dominant); this is known as hereditary renal adysplasia. There may also be concomitant malformation of müllerian structures, a condition referred to as hereditary urogenital adysplasia.

RENAL DYSPLASIA—FACT SHEET

Definition
▶ A dysplastic kidney is a metanephric structure with aberrant nephronic differentiation

Incidence and Location
▶ Incidence 1:1000 to 1:4000

Morbidity and Mortality
▶ Unilateral disease: flank mass
▶ Bilateral disease: neonatal death or chronic renal failure in children

Gender, Race, and Age Distribution
▶ Males > females
▶ No racial predilection
▶ Dysplasia detected at birth, in childhood, or incidentally in adulthood

Clinical Features
▶ Bilateral severe disease: maternal oligohydramnios, neonatal pulmonary and renal failure
▶ Unilateral renal mass in infants and children
▶ Chronic renal failure in childhood

Radiologic Features
▶ Multicystic, aplastic, diffusely cystic kidney
▶ May be unilateral, bilateral, or segmental
▶ Lower urinary tract abnormality

Prognosis and Treatment
▶ Determined by extent of disease and associated extrarenal malformations

TABLE 5-4

Multiple Malformation Syndromes in Which Renal Dysplasia May Occur

COMMON OCCURRENCE

VATER (VACTERL) association

MURC syndrome

Prune-belly syndrome

Caudal regression syndrome

Cloacal exstrophy

Urogenital sinus syndrome

Urorectal septum syndrome sequence

Meckel-Gruber syndrome*

Dandy-Walker syndrome*

Short rib-polydactyly syndrome*

Elejalde's syndrome*

OCCASIONAL OCCURRENCE

Trisomy C

Trisomy 13

Trisomy 18

Persisting mesonephric duct syndrome

Zellweger syndrome*

Jeune's syndrome*

Smith-Lemli-Opitz syndrome*

Beckwith-Wiedemann syndrome*

Laurence-Moon-Bardet-Biedl syndrome*

---

*Autosomal recessive inheritance.

RENAL DYSPLASIA—PATHOLOGIC FEATURES

Gross Findings

► Large and partially or completely cystic or small and solid

Microscopic Findings

► Aberrantly formed nephron components, cysts, dysplastic tubules, fetal cartilage
► Normal-appearing nephrons with abnormal architectural organization

Differential Diagnosis

► Sporadic forms
► Hereditary forms

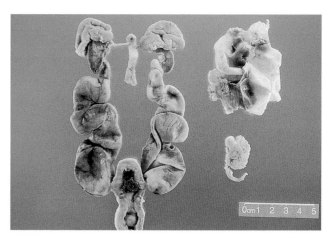

FIGURE 5-14

Bilateral hypodysplastic kidneys are shown on the left side with adrenal glands and with hydroureters secondary to a posterior urethral valve. On the right side are a neonatal multicystic dysplastic kidney and an aplastic kidney from a 35-year woman with vaginal ureteral ectopia.

RADIOLOGIC FEATURES

Multiple renal cysts are present, often in association with lower urinary tract abnormalities.

PATHOLOGIC FEATURES

GROSS FINDINGS

Dysplastic kidneys may be classified as multicystic and aplastic dysplasia, hypoplastic dysplasia, segmental dysplasia, and diffuse cystic dysplasia (Figs. 5-14, 5-15, and 5-16). Multicystic and aplastic dysplasias are associated with pelvocaliceal occlusion and ureteral atresia; they range from large irregular cystic masses to small rudimentary structures that lack lobar organization. The multicystic and aplastic forms differ only in the extent of cyst formation. Hypodysplastic kidneys have patent ureters, often have a reniform shape with

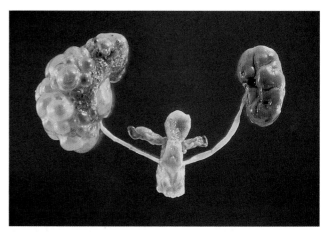

FIGURE 5-15

This example of unilateral multicystic renal dysplasia is from a newborn with multiple congenital anomalies. One kidney is normal, and the other is diffusely cystic.

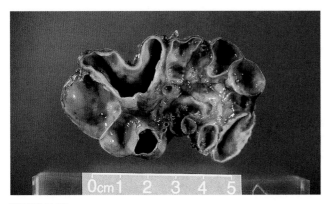

FIGURE 5-16

This bivalved multicystic dysplastic kidney shows diffuse round cysts of variable size with no intervening normal parenchyma and absent development of the collecting system. This was associated with ureteral atresia.

MICROSCOPIC FINDINGS

The various types of dysplastic kidneys vary greatly in histologic appearance (Figs. 5-17, 5-18, and 5-19). A lobar organization with rudimentary to well-developed corticomedullary organization may be present, and regions of fairly normal-appearing nephrons may be observed. Alternatively, the renal tissue may contain only large cysts and/or aberrant-appearing glomeruloid and tubular structures. The two most characteristic histologic features are islands of cartilage, believed to be derived from the fetal blastema, and dysplastic ducts lined with columnar epithelium and surrounded by collars of spindle cells, believed to be derived from the ampullary bud.

ANCILLARY STUDIES

If multiple malformations are encountered in a pediatric autopsy, it is important to obtain tissue for karyotype analysis.

DIFFERENTIAL DIAGNOSIS

The pathologist must distinguish sporadic forms of renal dysplasia, which are most common, from heredi-

corticomedullary differentiation, and may be partially functional. Segmental dysplasia usually occurs in the upper pole moiety of kidneys with duplication of the collecting system (duplex kidney). Diffuse cystic dysplasia refers to large reniform kidneys that often have a patent ureter and a recognizable collecting system. The parenchyma consists of poorly developed pyramids and diffuse, uniform, rounded cortical cysts.

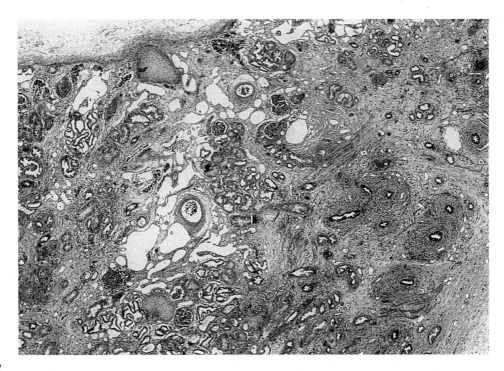

FIGURE 5-17

In this example of renal dysplasia, many nephron structures are present, but they lack proper organization and are associated with small, dysplastic ducts and cartilage. Cysts were present elsewhere.

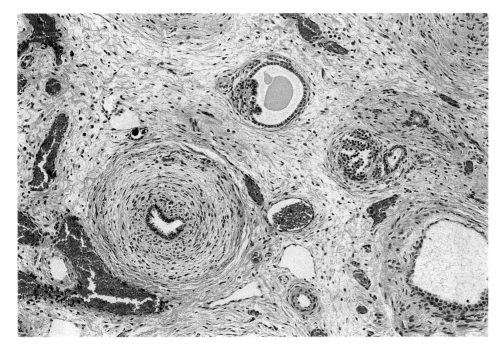

FIGURE 5-18

This example of renal dysplasia shows a few abnormally formed nephrons with abortive glomeruli, immature tubules, and a dysplastic duct.

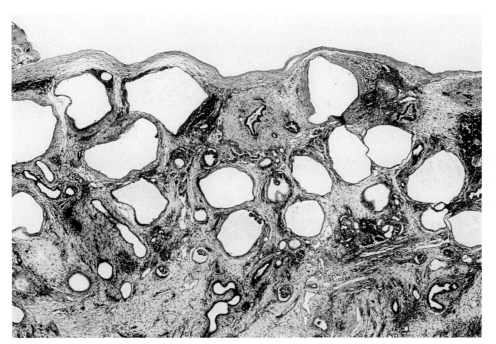

FIGURE 5-19

In this specimen of renal dysplasia, there is rudimentary corticomedullary development with numerous cortical cysts and a few abortive nephron structures. The medullary portion is at the bottom of the photograph.

tary forms, which have parental counseling implications. It is beyond the scope of this chapter to delve into the nuances of renal dysplasias associated with malformation syndromes and chromosomal anomalies. However, detailed assessment for extrarenal malformations, initiation of cytogenetic evaluation, consultation with clinicians well versed in malformation syndromes, and obtaining a pertinent family history are essential for classification of the process.

PROGNOSIS AND TREATMENT

Renal dysplasia is most often unilateral; if the contralateral kidney is normal, a benign prognosis is expected. If dysplasia is severe and bilateral, infants present with oligohydramnios and die of pulmonary hypoplasia. Renal dysplasias associated with extra-renal malformations have a prognosis influenced by the severity of their major organ abnormalities.

ACQUIRED RENAL CYSTIC DISEASE

The term Ac-RCD refers to the development of multiple and bilateral renal cysts in a patient whose chronic renal failure cannot be attributed to a hereditary cystic disease.

CLINICAL FEATURES

Cysts are present in 8% of patients at the time dialysis is initiated, and they increase in incidence, number, and size in proportion to the duration of dialysis. After 3 to 5 years of dialysis, approximately 50% of patients develop cysts, and by 10 years almost 90% have cysts. Ac-RCD is asymptomatic in its early stages. Latter complications include flank pain, intrarenal and retroperitoneal hemorrhage, cyst infection, and renal cortical neoplasms. Papillary renal adenomas develop in 10% to 20% of patients, and papillary renal cell carcinoma accounts for 3% to 4% of all deaths.

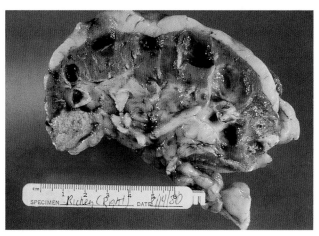

FIGURE 5-20
End-stage kidney with acquired renal cystic disease. The kidney size is reduced with a modest number of cysts. A papillary renal cell carcinoma is visible on the left.

RADIOLOGIC FEATURES

Imaging of the end-stage kidney may reveal multiple, 1- to 3-cm, cortical or medullary cysts (Fig. 5-20). The size and number of cysts increase with time in the affected patient. Solid neoplasms may be present.

PATHOLOGIC FEATURES

GROSS FINDINGS

The kidney size is rarely increased. It is usually normal or reduced in size, with weights of 80 to 100 g despite extensive cystic alteration. The cysts initially form in cortical tubules, but in advanced cases medullary cysts occur. Eventually, the kidney may

---

ACQUIRED RENAL CYSTIC DISEASE—FACT SHEET

Definition
▶ Bilateral renal cysts associated with chronic renal failure not from a hereditary renal cystic disease

Incidence and Location
▶ Bilateral
▶ Accounts for 8% of patients initiating dialysis
▶ 90% incidence of cysts by 10 years

Morbidity and Mortality
▶ Cyst hemorrhage and infection
▶ Renal cell carcinomas

Gender, Race, and Age Distribution
▶ No gender or racial predilection

Clinical Features
▶ Flank pain and hematuria

Radiologic Features
▶ Multiple bilateral cysts in a small to normal-sized kidney

Prognosis and Treatment
▶ Death from renal carcinoma in 3-4%
▶ Nephrectomy if symptomatic or if neoplasms are detected

ACQUIRED RENAL CYSTIC DISEASE—PATHLOGIC FEATURES

Gross Findings
▶ Normal-sized or small kidneys
▶ Multiple cortical and medullary cysts

Microscopic Findings
▶ End-stage parenchymal changes, epithelial-lined cysts
▶ Cortical neoplasms, most often of a papillary type

Differential Diagnosis
▶ Adult (dominant) polycystic kidney disease

be replaced by cysts, resembling a smaller version of AD-PKD. Most cysts are less than 0.5 cm, but cysts 2 to 3 cm in size can develop. If renal neoplasms are present, they are usually multiple and bilateral and range in size from microscopic to macroscopic.

MICROSCOPIC FINDINGS

The cortex is that of an end-stage kidney with widespread glomerulosclerosis, tubular atrophy, and interstitial fibrosis. The cysts are lined with flattened, cuboidal, or columnar epithelium with foci of epithelial hyperplasia. The cysts may contain proteinaceous to hemorrhagic fluid. Most tumors are of a papillary type (Fig. 5-21). However, other renal cortical neoplasms have been reported.

DIFFERENTIAL DIAGNOSIS

Grossly and histologically, the kidneys in Ac-RCD resemble those of AD-PKD, but they are dramatically smaller. The history of end-stage kidney disease makes the diagnosis obvious.

PROGNOSIS AND TREATMENT

The major concern is a renal cell carcinoma. Nephrectomy is performed if a solid tumor is detected.

ABNORMALITIES IN FORM AND POSITION

MALROTATION, RENAL ECTOPIA, AND RENAL FUSION

It is useful to group abnormalities of form and position, because they often occur in combination. For instance, fused kidneys are always ectopic, and most ectopic or fused kidneys also are abnormally rotated.

Rotation Anomaly

During ascent of the kidney to a lumbar location, the renal pelvis rotates 90 degrees from an anterior to a medial position. Failure of the pelvis to assume a medial orientation, reverse rotation, or over-rotation to a posterior or even lateral location results in a spectrum of orientation abnormalities known as rotation anomalies. The most common rotation anomaly is nonrotation or incomplete medial rotation with an anterior location of the pelvis and ureter. This may occur as an isolated abnormality in an otherwise normal kidney. It always accompanies renal ectopia or renal fusion.

Renal Ectopia

Failure of the kidney to assume its proper location in the renal fossa is known as renal ectopia. There are several varieties named according to location. The most common form is inferiorly located kidneys. The origin

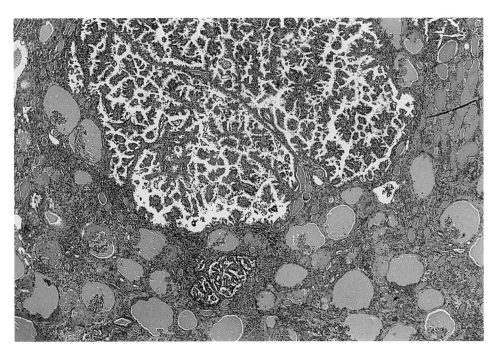

FIGURE 5-21

This field shows the atrophic cortex and a papillary renal cell carcinoma in an end-stage kidney with acquired renal cystic disease. Cysts were present elsewhere.

of the renal artery from a normal aortic location identifies a lower situated kidney as ptotic rather than ectopic. Cephalad ectopia is usually associated with an omphalocele, because the kidney continues its ascent when the abdominal organs herniate into the omphalocele sac. In crossed ectopia, the kidney is situated opposite the side of insertion of its ureter into the trigone. In 90% of cases, there is also fusion to the other kidney.

Renal Fusion

Renal fusion may involve all or only portions of each kidney. The fused kidneys may be midline or unilateral (crossed fused). Horseshoe kidney, the most common form of renal fusion, is a midline fusion of the renal masses, each with its own ureter and pelvis. The fusion is typically at the lower poles, with a variable quantity of fused parenchyma. The horseshoe kidney is always ectopic, with anterior ureters, and is usually situated anterior to the aorta and vena cava. Occasionally, the fusion is posterior to the vena cava or even posterior to both the aorta and the vena cava.

CLINICAL FEATURES

Each anomaly may occur in isolation or as one component of a more serious complex of malformations affecting other urologic sites or organ systems. Each type may be completely innocent and asymptomatic. However, although their ureters are normally located within the bladder, their pelves are nonrotated. In renal fusion, this is commonly coupled with high insertion of the ureter on the pelvis. If urinary tract symptoms develop, they result from impaired urinary drainage, which can cause hydronephrosis or pain and may be complicated by infection or nephrolithiasis.

RADIOLOGIC FEATURES

Ultrasound evaluation of a patient with urinary tract symptoms is a simple, noninvasive method to determine the type of anomaly and to identify the major complication, urinary tract obstruction.

PATHOLOGIC FEATURES

GROSS FINDINGS

Malrotation

The kidney shape may appear normal or abnormal. Its renal pelvis is not medial. It is most often anterior, and rarely may be lateral or posterior (Fig. 5-22).

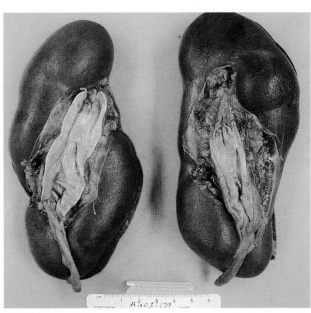

FIGURE 5-22

This is an example of the most common form of incompletely rotated kidneys, with anterior renal pelves and ureters. The kidneys appear grossly dysmorphic but were histologically and functionally normal.

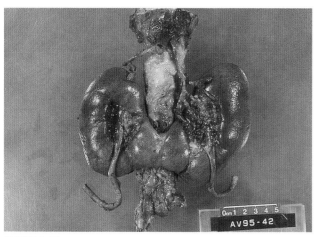

FIGURE 5-23

In horseshoe kidney, there is fusion of the lower poles with anterior pelves and high insertion of the ureters.

Renal Ectopia

The kidney shape may be normal, or it may be abnormal if associated with fusion.

Renal Fusion

The kidneys are nonreniform in shape if crossed fused, or they are horseshoe-shaped (Fig. 5-23). The pelves and ureters are anterior (nonrotated). The ureters are usually normally placed in the bladder, but they may have a high insertion on the pelvis, leading to obstruction.

MICROSCOPIC FINDINGS

The kidneys are histologically normal unless affected by urinary tract obstruction or associated with another developmental anomaly such as renal dysplasia.

MALROTATION, RENAL ECTOPIA, AND RENAL FUSION—PATHOLOGIC FEATURES

Gross Findings
▶ *Rotation abnormality:* renal pelvis is anterior, lateral, posterior
▶ *Renal ectopia:* location is pelvic, thoracic, crossed
▶ *Renal fusion:* lower pole (horseshoe) or complete and globular

Microscopic Findings
▶ Normal
▶ Complications from obstruction
▶ Developmental abnormality such as renal dysplasia

PROGNOSIS AND TREATMENT

Each of these malformations may have no clinical significance, or may develop complications due to urinary tract obstruction, or may be one component of a serious malformation complex.

RENAL AGENESIS

Absence of the kidney and its corresponding ureter due to a failure of differentiation is renal agenesis (Table 5-5).

CLINICAL FEATURES

Renal agenesis may be unilateral or bilateral, sporadic or syndromic and associated with serious developmental field defects affecting hindgut, cloacal-derived structures, and lower extremities. In unilateral agenesis, the overall renal function may be normal and the condition entirely asymptomatic. In 70% of patients, unilateral agenesis is associated with additional anomalies affecting the genital tract, reflecting an abnormality in development of both the mesonephric duct and structures derived from the müllerian duct.

TABLE 5-5
Renal Agenesis

SPORADIC FORMS
Unilateral renal agenesis
Bilateral renal agenesis (Potter's syndrome)
SYNDROMIC RENAL AGENESIS
Chromosomal anomalies (trisomy 13 and 18)
VATER association
Mullerian aplasia syndrome (MURCS)
Sirenomelia (caudal regression syndrome)
Cloacal exstrophy
Fasier syndrome
Williams syndrome
Hereditary renal adysplasia
Multiple malformation syndromes, NOS

NOS, not otherwise specified.

RENAL AGENESIS—FACT SHEET

Definition
▶ Absence of one or both kidneys due to failure of differentiation

Incidence and Location
▶ Incidence 1:3000 to 1:5000
▶ Bilateral disease is most common

Morbidity and Mortality
▶ Unilateral disease: symptomatic, associated with urogenital or other malformations
▶ Bilateral disease: fatal

Gender, Race, and Age Distribution
▶ No gender or racial predilection

Clinical Features
▶ Unilateral disease: asymptomatic
▶ Bilateral agenesis: oligohydramnios syndrome and pulmonary failure
▶ Additional anomalies may be present

Radiologic Features
▶ Absent kidney and enlarged adrenal
▶ Enlarged contralateral kidney with unilateral agenesis

Prognosis and Treatment
▶ Unilateral disease: prognosis is influenced by associated extrarenal malformations
▶ Bilateral disease: fatal

Bilateral renal agenesis is a uniformly fatal disorder known as Potter's syndrome. Approximately 40% of affected fetuses are stillbirths, and those born alive die of pulmonary failure within 48 hours. Mothers present with oligohydramnios, because fetal urine normally accounts for most of the amniotic fluid in the second half of gestation. Oligohydramnios impairs pulmonary development, resulting in pulmonary hypoplasia, and produces a variety of distinctive gross features known as the Potter's or oligohydramnios phenotype.

In syndromic renal agenesis, one or, rarely, both kidneys may be absent as a component of a constellation of congenital anomalies. This may also occur in a familial disorder with renal dysplasia, known as hereditary renal adysplasia. Extrarenal anomalies are responsible for many complications and the lethal nature of many syndromes.

RADIOLOGIC FEATURES

Ultrasound studies will reveal the absence of one or both kidneys. The ipsilateral adrenal gland and the contralateral kidney are usually enlarged in unilateral agenesis.

PATHOLOGIC FEATURES

GROSS FINDINGS

In unilateral renal agenesis, the renal fossa is empty and the corresponding adrenal gland is enlarged or more globular in shape. The contralateral kidney may be hypertrophic and up to twice the normal size. The corresponding bladder hemitrigone represents the distal continuation of the ureteral smooth muscle and therefore is absent. In bilateral agenesis, both adrenals are globular, and the bladder trigone is absent (Fig. 5-24). There are also abnormalities of the oligohydramnios state, including the characteristic Potter's facies, positional deformities of the lower extremities, and placental amnion nodosum (Fig. 5-25).

DIFFERENTIAL DIAGNOSIS

It is important to determine whether the agenesis is sporadic, syndromic, or hereditary. Identification of extrarenal anomalies, pertinent family history, cytogenetic evaluation, and consultation with knowledgeable clinicians are mandatory for appropriate genetic counseling.

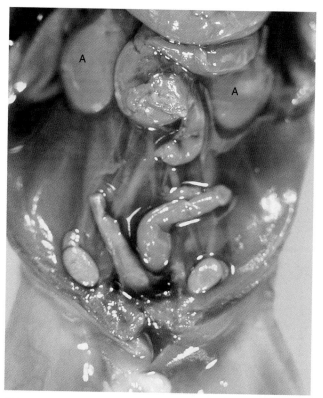

FIGURE 5-24

Potter's bilateral renal and ureteral agenesis. After removal of most of the gastrointestinal tract, the renal fossae contained adrenal glands (A) but no kidneys.

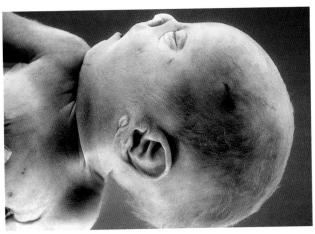

FIGURE 5-25
Potter's facies in Potter's syndrome. Notice the recessed chin, low posterior-rotated ears, beaked nose, and epicanthic folds.

sis; it occurred in younger patients with severe hypertension and renal failure (Table 5-6).

BENIGN NEPHROSCLEROSIS

Benign nephrosclerosis refers to renal damage resulting from essential hypertension, usually defined as a diastolic blood pressure in excess of 90 mm Hg. Its pathogenesis is multifactorial. Genetic factors appear to be important, although no specific genetic marker has been identified. It affects 24% of adults in the United States, with a higher incidence among African Americans. Although most patients (90% to 95%) have idiopathic disease, there are numerous secondary causes (Table 5-6).

CLINICAL FEATURES

PROGNOSIS AND TREATMENT

Unilateral disease may be benign and asymptomatic, or it may be serious if accompanied by other malformations. Bilateral disease is fatal.

Benign nephrosclerosis is usually asymptomatic. Hypertension characteristically first appears between the ages of 45 and 54 years. Renal damage takes years

VASCULAR DISEASES

Vascular diseases are the most common causes of renal injury, owing to the high incidence of atherosclerosis and hypertension. A cardiovascular contribution to renal injury was recognized more than 100 years ago by Volhard and Fahr, who first separated it from other forms of renal disease. They also recognized the existence of two types. The most common form they named benign nephrosclerosis; it occurred in older patients who had mild hypertension and mild renal impairment. The second form they named malignant nephrosclero-

---

TABLE 5-6
Types and Causes of Hypertension

PRIMARY

Benign (essential) hypertension

Malignant hypertension

SECONDARY

Renal artery stenosis

Acute glomerulonephritis

Chronic renal diseases

Neoplasms
   Renin-producing tumors
   Adrenal cortical tumors
   Pheochromocytoma

Endocrine abnormalities
   Thyrotoxicosis
   Adrenal cortical hyperplasia
   Hyperparathyroidism
   Oral contraceptives

Neurogenic causes

Miscellaneous vascular causes
   Preeclampsia
   Thrombotic microangiopathy
   Vasculitis
   Coarctation of aorta

RENAL AGENESIS—PATHOLOGIC FEATURES

Gross Findings
▶ Unilateral agenesis: empty renal fossa, enlarged adrenal gland, enlarged contralateral kidney
▶ Bilateral agenesis: empty renal fossas, enlarged adrenals, oligohydramnios phenotype

Differential Diagnosis
▶ Sporadic form
▶ Hereditary forms

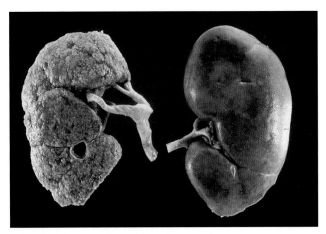

FIGURE 5-26

In arterial nephrosclerosis *(left)* secondary to a long history of essential hypertension, there is a diffuse, coarsely granular subcapsular surface. The normal kidney *(right)* has a smooth surface.

to develop and is manifested by a slowly rising serum creatinine concentration. Low-grade proteinuria is common, but nephrotic-range proteinuria may occasionally develop.

PATHOLOGIC FEATURES

GROSS FINDINGS

The kidneys are symmetrically reduced and weigh between 60 and 120 g. They have a uniform granular subcapsular surface and a thin cortex (Fig. 5-26). The magnitude of these changes is influenced by the severity and duration of the hypertension.

MICROSCOPIC FINDINGS

The subcapsular granularity corresponds to shallow scars that contain sclerotic glomeruli, atrophic tubules, and thick-walled arterioles (Figs. 5-27 and 5-28). The characteristic vascular lesion affects arterioles, which show either medial hyperplasia or, more often, hyalinosis with eosinophilic material expanding the intima and media and resultant luminal compromise. Glomeruli initially exhibit capillary loop wrinkling, with collagenous tissue filling Bowman's space (Fig. 5-29), beginning at the vascular pole, and progressing to global sclerosis. Arteries of interlobular size or greater show

myointimal thickening with duplication of the elastic lamina. Lipid and calcification are not usually present.

DIFFERENTIAL DIAGNOSIS

Small remote infarcts also produce subcapsular scars, and chronic glomerulonephritis results in a granular surface. Remote infarcts are usually larger. They are single or, more often, multiple. If multiple, they do not affect the entire kidney in a uniform manner; rather, they are irregularly distributed and vary in size. Microscopically, a periodic acid-Schiff (PAS) stain can distinguish the ischemic obsolescent glomerulus of benign nephrosclerosis from an infarcted glomerulus. In an infarcted glomerulus, the PAS stain shows a condensed, collapsed glomerular tuft without the collagenous tissue in Bowman's space that is observed in benign nephrosclerosis (Fig. 5-29). Chronic glomerulonephritis

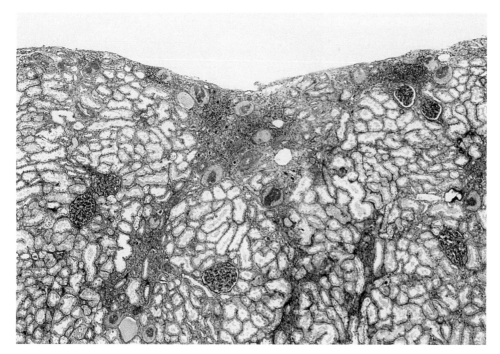

FIGURE 5-27

Benign nephrosclerosis (periodic acid-Schiff stain). The shallow subcapsular scars that result in the granular surface contain sclerotic glomeruli, atrophic tubules, and thickened arterioles.

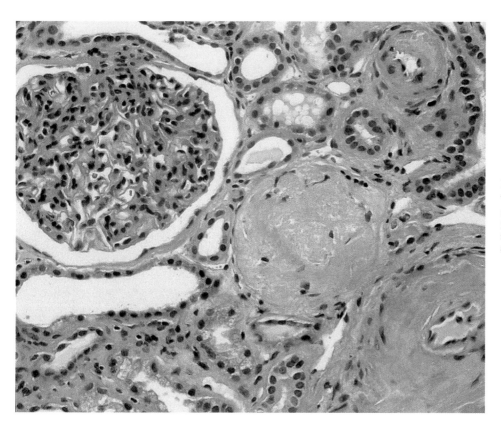

FIGURE 5-28

This scar in a kidney with benign nephrosclerosis contains a completely sclerotic glomerulus, a nonsclerotic glomerulus, and a thickened arteriole *(lower right)*.

affects glomeruli throughout the cortex rather than demonstrating the subcapsular accentuation of injury of benign nephrosclerosis. Chronic glomerulonephritis may also show residual distinctive glomerular changes corresponding to the type of glomerular disease, and patients have a history of proteinuria and/or hematuria.

PROGNOSIS AND TREATMENT

Prolonged untreated essential hypertension poses a risk for renal insufficiency and generalized atherosclerotic vascular disease (ASVD). Although it does not cause

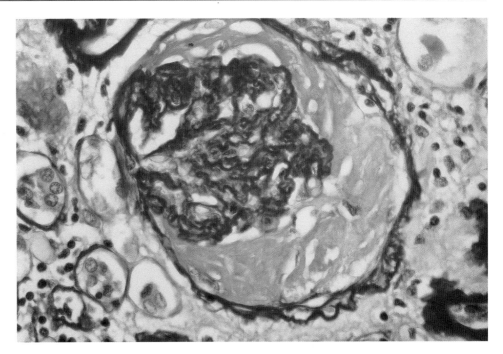

FIGURE 5-29

The ischemic glomerulus in benign nephrosclerosis has a uniformly collapsed tuft with collagenous tissue filling Bowman's space. (Periodic acid-Schiff stain.)

renal failure in most patients, hypertension is sufficiently prevalent to account for 15% to 30% of end-stage renal disease.

MALIGNANT NEPHROSCLEROSIS

Malignant nephrosclerosis develops as a consequence of malignant hypertension. It may arise in a patient with benign hypertension, or it may develop de novo.

CLINICAL FEATURES

Patients present with renal failure, headache, dizziness, and impaired vision, and their diastolic blood pressure exceeds 120 to 140 mm Hg. Retinal hemorrhages, exudates, and papilledema are present. Hematuria, proteinuria, and a microangiopathic hemolytic anemia develop.

PATHOLOGIC FEATURES

GROSS FINDINGS

The kidney in untreated malignant nephrosclerosis may have a normal or increased weight to 400 g. Petechial subcapsular hemorrhages are characteristic. The cortex may also be mottled red and yellow if infarcts develop.

MICROSCOPIC FINDINGS

A range of lesions is encountered, reflecting the sequence of injury and repair. Fibrinoid necrosis characterizes the acute lesion in untreated cases (also referred to in nephropathology as acute thrombotic microangiopathy). Glomeruli show capillary loop thrombosis (Fig. 5-30) and mesangiolysis resulting from necrosis of endothelial and mesangial cells. The

---

MALIGNANT NEPHROSCLEROSIS—FACT SHEET

Definition
▶ Renal damage produced by malignant hypertension

Incidence
▶ 1-2 cases/100,000 per year

Morbidity and Mortality
▶ Renal failure, stroke, myocardial infarction

Gender, Race, and Age Distribution
▶ Males > females
▶ African Americans > other races

Clinical Features
▶ Diastolic pressure 120-140 mm Hg, headache, ocular findings
▶ Hematuria, proteinuria, microangiopathic hemolytic anemia

Prognosis and Treatment
▶ Renal failure is usually irreversible

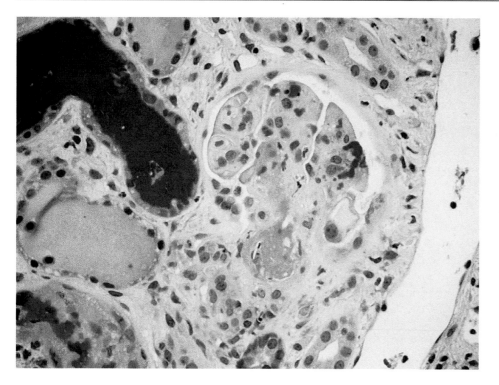

FIGURE 5-30

In thrombotic microangiopathy of malignant hypertension, there is arteriolar and glomerular capillary thrombosis with many red cells within renal tubules.

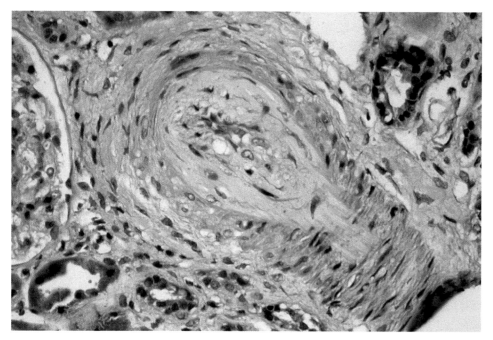

FIGURE 5-31

This artery from a patient with malignant hypertension shows mucoid intimal thickening resulting in marked luminal compromise and early myointimal proliferation.

arterioles develop a necrotizing arteriolitis with thrombosis, reflecting necrosis of endothelium and medial smooth muscle cells. The interlobular and arcuate arteries show mucoid intimal thickening and may also contain subendothelial fibrin and fragmented red blood cells (Fig. 5-31).

In treated cases, reparative and involutional changes may predominate or be superimposed on continuing acute changes. Glomeruli show ischemic wrinkling and collapse, or they may show an impressive lucent subendothelial expansion and capillary loop basement membrane reduplication. These are best demonstrated on a PAS or silver stain. The arterioles and arteries show concentric ("onion-skin") myointimal proliferation, known as proliferative endarteritis, which results in severe luminal occlusion (Fig. 5-32).

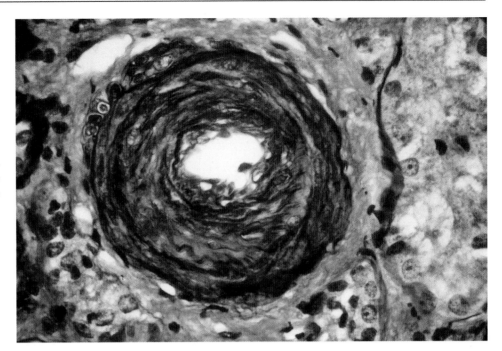

FIGURE 5-32
This artery shows the "onion-skin" concentric myointimal thickening of malignant hypertension. (Periodic acid-Schiff stain.)

MALIGNANT NEPHROSCLEROSIS—PATHOLOGIC FEATURES

Gross Findings

▶ Petechial subcapsular hemorrhages, infarcts, cortical necrosis

Microscopic Findings

▶ Acute changes: fibrinoid necrosis (acute thrombotic microangiopathy) of arterioles and glomeruli
▶ Chronic changes: glomerular collapse, glomerular basement membrane duplication, concentric myointimal proliferation of arteries (proliferative endarteritis)

Differential Diagnosis

▶ Hemolytic-uremic syndrome
▶ Systemic sclerosis

DIFFERENTIAL DIAGNOSIS

Hemolytic-uremic syndrome (HUS) and systemic sclerosis produce identical glomerular and vascular lesions. Renal failure developing before severe hypertension, or a preexisting condition that predisposes to a HUS syndrome (e.g., gastroenteritis in children, chemotherapy, radiation therapy) implicates HUS. Conversely, a presentation with severe hypertension that antedates renal failure implicates primary malignant hypertension. In many patients, however, both conditions are present at presentation, and the temporal sequence cannot be determined. Extrarenal and serologic features of systemic sclerosis should be sought. However, because 5% of patients with systemic sclerosis initially present with renal disease, these cases will be misclassified until the extrarenal components become manifest.

PROGNOSIS AND TREATMENT

Renal failure is usually irreversible. Hypertension must be controlled to avoid injury to other organs (e.g., cardiac, central nervous system). Without treatment, there is a 90% fatality rate at 1 year.

RENAL ARTERY STENOSIS

In 1934, Goldblatt and colleagues first established a role for decreased renal perfusion in hypertension by partially occluding one renal artery of a dog and demonstrating reversal of hypertension with restoration of the blood flow. This form of hypertension, known as renovascular hypertension, results from renal artery stenosis (RAS) and accounts for 1% to 5% of patients with hypertension. There are many causes of RAS, but two account for the majority of cases: ASVD (two thirds of cases) and fibromuscular dysplasia (FMD) (one third of cases). The remaining causes, although numerous, comprise fewer than 1% of cases (Table 5-7).

TABLE 5-7
Causes of Renal Artery Stenosis

Atherosclerosis (ASVD)

Fibromuscular dysplasia (FMD)

Rare other causes
  Renal artery dissection
  Renal artery aneurysm
  Renal artery thrombosis
  Renal artery emboli
  Arterial-venous malformation
  Arteritis
  Radiation injury
  Transplant artery stenosis
  Neurofibromatosis

CLINICAL FEATURES

Patients present with a severe, often resistant form of hypertension, usually of recent onset, or exacerbation of previously controlled hypertension. In the most common form of RAS, that related to ASVD, a male predominance is present. Patients usually present after 50 years of age and have significant atherosclerosis of the aorta and other major arteries. Bilateral disease occurs in 30% of cases and, if severe, causes ischemic chronic renal failure.

RENAL ARTERY STENOSIS—FACT SHEET

Definition
▶ Occlusion or narrowing of the main or a segmental renal artery

Incidence and Location
▶ 0.1-5% of hypertension cases
▶ Unilateral or bilateral

Morbidity and Mortality
▶ Hypertension and resultant complications

Gender, Race, and Age Distribution
▶ Atherosclerotic RAS: older patients, males > females
▶ FMD: middle-aged females

Radiologic Features
▶ Localized stenosis or a "string of beads" appearance on angiogram

Prognosis and Treatment
▶ Atherosclerotic: progression; angioplasty may not reverse hypertension or improve renal function
▶ FMD: progression if untreated; hypertension is reversible, renal damage preventable if treated early

---

FMD of the renal arteries affects young to middle-aged women and is the most common cause of RAS in children. There are five histologic subtypes; despite histologic differences, they have similar clinical presentations. They each involve the main renal artery and may extend into segmental branches. FMD is commonly bilateral.

RADIOLOGIC FEATURES

Angiographic studies in atherosclerotic RAS show stenosis at the ostia or in the proximal portions of the main renal artery. The most common appearance in FMD RAS is a "string of beads" appearance. The most modern evaluation modalities are duplex ultrasound and magnetic resonance angiography.

PATHOLOGIC FEATURES

GROSS FINDINGS

The kidney in chronic RAS has a distinctive smooth subcapsular surface and uniform cortical thinning. If the main renal artery is stenotic, the entire kidney becomes small (40 to 70 g) and uniformly contracted (Fig. 5-33). If a segmental artery is stenotic or, conversely, if a segmental artery is free of stenosis while the main renal artery is stenotic, a characteristic line of transition from thin cortex to thicker cortex will be apparent. Because atherosclerosis-related RAS develops over many years and is often a complication of essential hypertension, the kidney may also exhibit changes of benign nephrosclerosis, or it may contain remote infarcts from aortic atheroemboli.

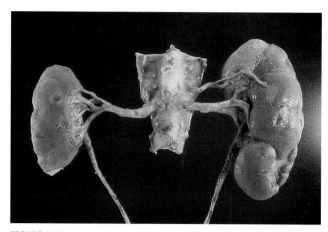

FIGURE 5-33
The kidney with atherosclerotic chronic renal artery stenosis on the left is uniformly contracted and has a smooth subcapsular surface. Notice that the kidney on the right is larger. Its renal artery is patent, but it has an upper polar artery that is stenotic, resulting in cortical atrophy limited to the upper pole. There is also a remote infarct in the lower pole.

RENAL ARTERY STENOSIS—PATHOLOGIC FEATURES

Gross Findings

▶ Uniformly contracted kidney in distribution of the occluded artery

Microscopic Findings

▶ Diffuse tubular atrophy, intact closely spaced glomeruli
▶ Atherosclerotic arterial changes
▶ Intimal, medial, or adventitial lesion of FMD

Differential Diagnosis

▶ Chronic tubulointerstitial nephritis

MICROSCOPIC FINDINGS

The kidney in RAS of recent onset develops enlargement of the juxtaglomerular apparatus (Fig. 5-34) and metaplasia of smooth muscle cells of the afferent arteriole to form contractile filament–poor, renin-synthesizing cells. After several weeks, the juxtaglomerular apparatus becomes inconspicuous and the parenchyma supplied by the stenotic artery shows distinctive alterations. The glomeruli appear normal or slightly contracted. The tubules, however, are diffusely affected. They are small and round, with mild tubular basement membrane thickening and a uniform pattern of interstitial fibrosis. The loss of tubular mass results in close approximation of glomeruli (Fig. 5-35). If there has

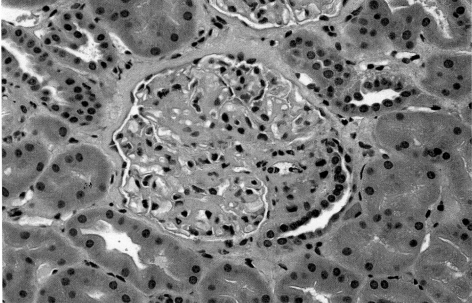

FIGURE 5-34

Acute renal artery stenosis in a renal transplantation patient. There is marked enlargement of the juxtaglomerular apparatus.

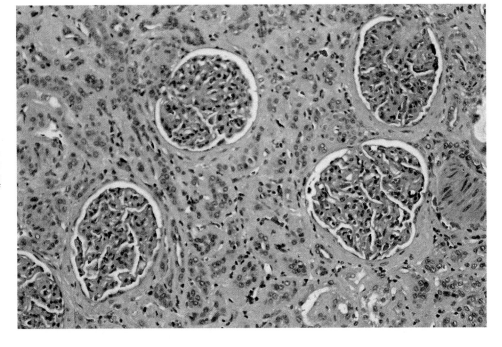

FIGURE 5-35

There is diffuse tubular atrophy with closely spaced glomeruli. The loss of tubular volume results in the small, uniformly contracted kidney of chronic renal artery stenosis.

been a long history of essential hypertension, subcapsular changes of benign nephrosclerosis also will be present.

In atherosclerotic RAS, the renal artery is occluded by thickened intima containing myointimal cells, lipid and foam cells, cholesterol clefts, and calcification. There is irregular duplication of elastica with sclerosis and atrophy of medial smooth muscle.

There are five histologic forms of FMD.

Intimal fibroplasia produces circumferential intimal thickening along the main renal artery and may also extend into its segmental branches (Fig. 5-36).

Medial hyperplasia consists of a localized segment of disorganized medial smooth muscle thickening. The intima is not thickened, and the internal elastic lamina is intact.

Medial fibroplasia with aneurysms, the most frequent and distinctive form, is characterized by ridges of medial thickening without fibrosis, alternating with areas of extreme medial thinning in which there is close approximation of the internal and external elastic lamina (Fig. 5-37).

Perimedial fibroplasia, the second most common form, is characterized by an irregular pattern of fibrosis

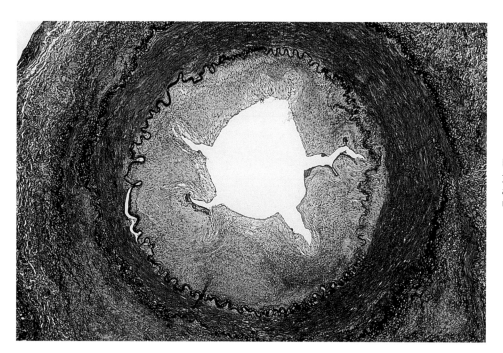

FIGURE 5-36
Intimal fibromuscular dysplasia has an intact elastic lamina and prominent occlusive intimal thickening.

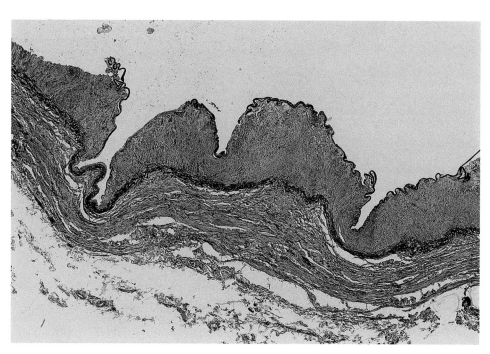

FIGURE 5-37
Medial fibromuscular dysplasia with aneurysms has alternating zones of attenuated and thickened media.

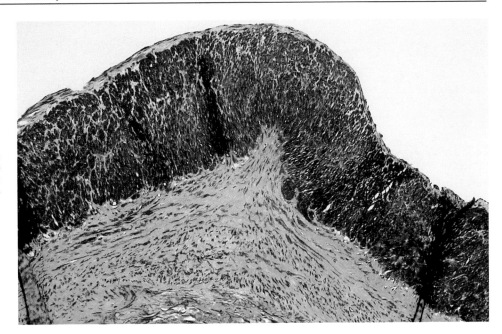

FIGURE 5-38
Perimedial fibromuscular dysplasia shows prominent fibrosis on the outer aspect of the media with variable degrees of medial thickening.

that replaces the outer one-half to two-thirds of the media with fibrous tissue (Fig. 5-38).

Periarterial fibroplasia, the rarest form, consists of dense collagenous tissue within the adventitia that restricts arterial expansion during systole.

DIFFERENTIAL DIAGNOSIS

The diffuse tubulointerstitial disease of chronic RAS may raise consideration of a chronic tubulointerstitial nephritis. The combination of a symmetrically contracted kidney in the presence of known RAS is distinctive, compared with the more granular surface and irregularly contracted appearance of the kidney in most other forms of chronic tubulointerstitial nephritis, which would not be associated with a stenotic artery. The uniformity of changes in RAS is also apparent histologically. The combination of small tubules without significant interstitial inflammation in RAS contrasts with the irregularly distributed fibrosing and often inflammatory components seen in other forms of chronic tubulointerstitial nephritis, which would also demonstrate advanced glomerulosclerosis rather than the glomerular sparing of chronic RAS.

PROGNOSIS AND TREATMENT

Treatment of atherosclerotic forms of RAS consists of medical control of the blood pressure. Restoration of blood flow is not usually performed. If medical treatment cannot control the blood pressure, nephrectomy may be indicated. Renal artery angioplasty or bypass is the usual treatment for FMD. The prognosis for FMD

is better than that for atherosclerosis-associated RAS because the patient is younger, hypertension is of more recent onset, and atherosclerosis-related complications are absent. Left untreated, all lesions tend to progress over several years.

CORTICAL AND MIXED CORTICAL AND MEDULLARY NECROSIS

Renal cortical and mixed renal cortical and medullary necrosis is a serious, usually bilateral, ischemic injury that arises as a complication of an extrarenal disease. Obstetric causes are most frequent in adults. Congenital heart disease, birth asphyxia, and sepsis account for most pediatric cases (Table 5-8).

TABLE 5-8
Causes of Renal Cortical Necrosis

Obstetric complications
  Abruptio placentae
  Septic abortion
  Intrauterine fetal demise
Infections
  Sepsis
  Peritonitis
Burns
Gastrointestinal hemorrhage
Transfusion reactions
Toxins
Hemolytic uremia syndrome

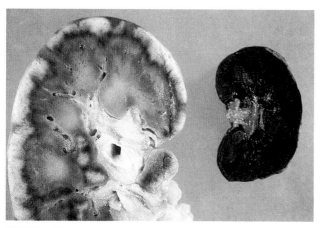

FIGURE 5-39

Adult kidney and pediatric kidney with cortical necrosis. The adult kidney shows the typical cortical pallor of arterial ischemic necrosis, whereas the pediatric kidney shows hemorrhagic necrosis.

CLINICAL FEATURES

Patients develop acute renal failure, flank pain, anuria, or hematuria, which may be gross.

PATHOLOGIC FEATURES

GROSS FINDINGS

The kidneys are soft and enlarged. The cortex is either pale with a thin subcapsular rim of sparing, or diffusely hemorrhagic if vascular perfusion has been reestablished (Fig. 5-39).

CORTICAL AND MIXED CORTICAL AND MEDULLARY NECROSIS— FACT SHEET

Definition
► Ischemic necrosis of cortex and medulla

Incidence and Location
► Usually bilateral

Morbidity and Mortality
► Renal failure with high fatality rate

Gender, Race, and Age Distribution
► Adults: females > males because of obstetric complications
► Pediatric: congenital heart disease, birth asphyxia, and sepsis

Clinical Features
► Anuria and gross hematuria

Prognosis and Treatment
► Renal and patient outcomes are poor
► Supportive therapy, must correct underlying cause

MICROSCOPIC FINDINGS

There is coagulation necrosis of all cortical and medullary structures, often with vascular thrombosis and interstitial hemorrhage (Figs. 5-40 and 5-41).

PROGNOSIS AND TREATMENT

Renal failure is irreversible, and the fatality rate is high because of the serious extrarenal causes.

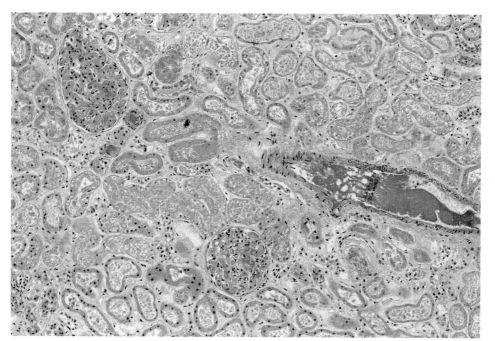

FIGURE 5-40

In this specimen of cortical necrosis, there is diffuse coagulation necrosis of glomeruli and tubules, as well as a thrombosed artery.

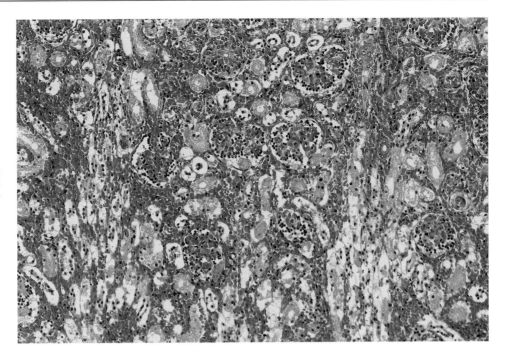

FIGURE 5-41

In this specimen of cortical necrosis in a newborn, necrotic nephrons and severe interstitial hemorrhage are observed.

CORTICAL AND MIXED CORTICAL AND MEDULLARY NECROSIS— PATHOLOGIC FEATURES

Gross Findings

▶ Diffusely pale or hemorrhagic cortex

Microscopic Findings

▶ Coagulation necrosis of cortical and medullary structures

EMBOLIC RENAL DISEASE AND INFARCTS

Deprivation of arterial perfusion of sufficient duration will cause renal infarction because of the end artery organization of the renal blood flow.

CLINICAL FEATURES

If a renal infarct is small, it may be clinically asymptomatic and functionally insignificant. Larger infarcts cause flank or abdominal pain, hematuria, and hypertension. If the infarcts are bilateral and widespread, renal failure may result. Embolic material originates from the aorta, or from the heart in patients with valvular disease or atrial fibrillation. Aortic atheroemboli are the most frequent. If an infected aortic valve vegetation is responsible, hematogenous pyelonephritis and microabscesses develop.

EMBOLIC DISEASE AND INFARCTS—FACT SHEET

Definition

▶ Ischemic necrosis secondary to acute arterial occlusion

Incidence and Location

▶ Unilateral or bilateral, any lobe

Morbidity and Mortality

▶ Small infarcts: minimal morbidity and mortality
▶ Large infarcts: flank symptoms, hematuria, impaired renal function

Gender, Race, and Age Distribution

▶ Elderly patients with ASVD
▶ Younger patients with endocarditis or mitral valve disease
▶ Males > females

Prognosis and Treatment

▶ Good prognosis unless lesions are large and bilateral

PATHOLOGIC FEATURES

GROSS FINDINGS

The acute infarct has a sharply demarcated zone of pallor with a hemorrhagic rim (Fig. 5-42). The remote infarct appears as a sharply delineated, wedge-shaped cortical depression (Fig. 5-43). The larger the artery occluded, the larger the infarct. Occlusion of an arcuate artery or one of its branches affects only the cortex. An interlobar artery or larger artery occlusion results in infarction of both cortex and medulla.

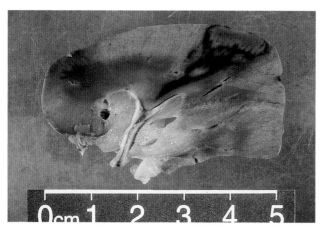

FIGURE 5-42

In acute infarct, there is a central pale, wedge-shaped zone with a hyperemic rim.

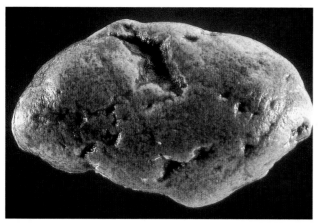

FIGURE 5-43

Remote infarcts appear as discrete depressed areas. The smaller infarcts represent occlusion of interlobular and arcuate arteries. The largest infarct is from occlusion of an interlobar artery.

EMBOLIC DISEASE AND INFARCTS—PATHOLOGIC FEATURES

Gross Findings

▶ Acute: pale, wedge-shaped lesion with hyperemic rim
▶ Chronic: depressed cortical scar

Microscopic Findings

▶ Acute: coagulation necrosis with a rim of granulocytes
▶ Chronic: fibrotic scar with ghosts of glomeruli and tubules

Differential Diagnosis

▶ Hypertensive nephrosclerosis
▶ Chronic glomerulonephritis

MICROSCOPIC FINDINGS

In the acute infarct, there is coagulation necrosis of glomeruli and tubules (Fig. 5-44). After several days, a peripheral rim of neutrophils and histiocytes develops. In the remote infarct, ghost-like remnants of glomeruli and tubules are present within fibrous tissue (Fig. 5-45). These are easily revealed by a PAS stain.

DIFFERENTIAL DIAGNOSIS

A PAS stain is helpful to distinguish a remote infarct from other chronic forms of injury, such as hypertensive nephrosclerosis or chronic glomerulonephritis. Infarcted glomeruli contain a uniformly condensed mass of capillary loop basement membranes, without the collagenous tissue in Bowman's space that forms with other causes of glomerulosclerosis (Fig. 5-46).

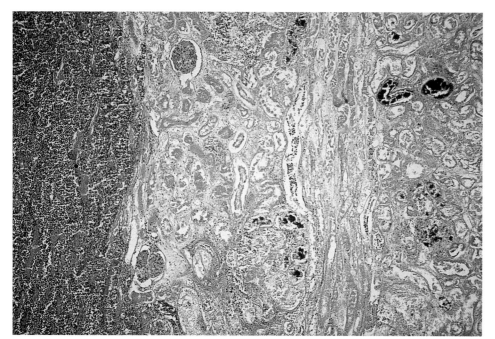

FIGURE 5-44

In acute infarct, there is coagulation necrosis with a broad rim of neutrophils and histiocytes.

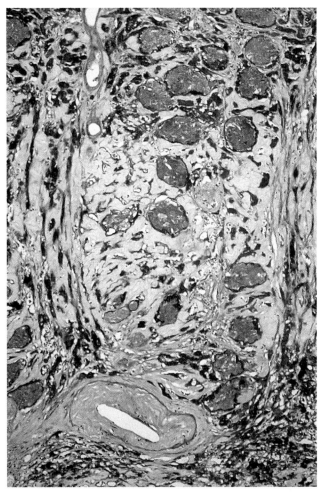

FIGURE 5-45
Remnants of glomerular and tubular basement membranes are revealed by periodic acid-Schiff stain in remote cortical infarct. Notice the cholesterol embolus in an arcuate artery. Although this artery is too small to account for the size of the infarct, it provides a clue to the underlying cause.

Most infarcts are small and without a significant effect on renal function. Renal insufficiency develops when the infarcts are large and bilateral.

PAPILLARY NECROSIS

Renal papillary necrosis refers to ischemic necrosis of all or portions of the renal pyramids. It develops as a complication of other diseases such as diabetes mellitus, sickle cell disease, analgesic abuse, urinary tract obstruction, and infection. Most patients have multiple risk factors. Diabetes is the most common cause today (Table 5-9). In the 1950s, papillary necrosis became a

TABLE 5-9

Causes of Renal Papillary Necrosis*

Diabetes mellitus
Urinary tract obstruction
Acute pyelonephritis
Analgesic abuse
Sickle cell disease
Hypoxia
Dehydration

*Combination of above = 55%.

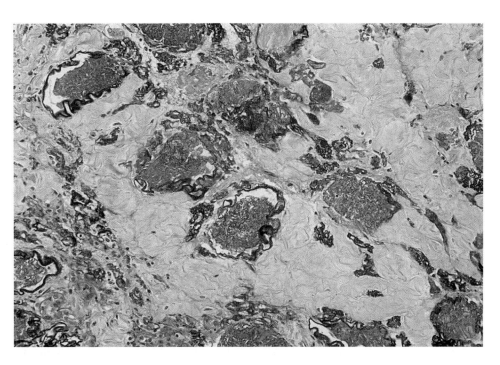

FIGURE 5-46
Infarcted glomeruli have a compacted glomerular tuft without the collagen in Bowman's space that is seen in ischemic obsolescence.

serious problem when phenacetin-containing analgesic combinations were in widespread use. Analgesic nephropathy, as it came to be known, was at that time the leading cause of chronic renal failure and renal papillary necrosis.

The dual blood supply to the renal medulla explains why the risk factors predispose to papillary necrosis. The major contribution is from the efferent arterioles of the juxtamedullary glomeruli. These drain into the outer medulla, forming the vasa recta. The second source arises from the interlobar artery. As it courses along a minor calyx, it gives rise to several spiral arteries that anastomose with arterioles from the opposite side, forming a plexus in the papilla.

CLINICAL FEATURES

Bilateral and diffuse renal papillary necrosis manifests as an acute devastating illness with renal failure, fever, chills, flank pain, and hematuria. When papillary necrosis is less extensive, it may be asymptomatic or associated with a concentrating defect. The patient may also develop flank pain and hematuria, or ureteral colic if a papilla sloughs and lodges in a ureter.

PATHOLOGIC FEATURES

GROSS FINDINGS

Papillary necrosis usually does not involve the entire renal pyramid. A medullary form and a papillary form have been described. In the papillary form, the necrosis is more extensive. The entire papillary tip, the most vulnerable portion of the pyramid, and the inner

---

PAPILLARY NECROSIS—PATHOLOGIC FEATURES

Gross Findings
▶ Pale dusky renal pyramid with a yellow rim

Microscopic Findings
▶ Coagulation necrosis with a rim of granulocytes

Differential Diagnosis
▶ Diabetes mellitus
▶ Sickle cell disease
▶ Urinary tract obstruction and infection
▶ Analgesic abuse

---

medulla are necrotic, whereas the outer medulla is often preserved. In the medullary form, the peripheral or forniceal portions of the pyramid are intact and the central portions are necrotic. The necrotic portion of the pyramid is pale or dusky with a rim of enhancement (Fig. 5-47). Alternatively, the infarcted pyramid may slough, leaving a jagged defect.

MICROSCOPIC FINDINGS

In the acute lesion, there is coagulation necrosis with a rim in neutrophils and histiocytes (Fig. 5-48). In chronic lesions, ghosts of tubules, hemosiderin, and even dystrophic calcification may be seen (Fig. 5-49).

DIFFERENTIAL DIAGNOSIS

Papillary necrosis is a complication of other diseases. Therefore, the history is essential. Specifically, infor-

---

PAPILLARY NECROSIS—FACT SHEET

Definition
▶ Coagulation necrosis of portions of the renal medulla

Incidence and Location
▶ Uncommon
▶ May involve one, multiple, or all pyramids

Morbidity and Mortality
▶ Asymptomatic to devastating irreversible renal failure

Gender, Race, and Age Distribution
▶ Children or adults
▶ African Americans with sickle cell anemia

Prognosis and Treatment
▶ Asymptomatic to irreversible renal failure

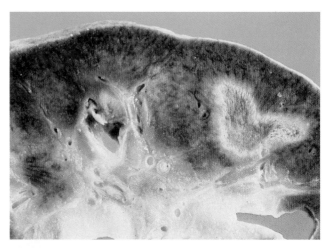

FIGURE 5-47
Papillary necrosis. Notice the pale infarcted pyramids and a sloughed pyramid in the center.

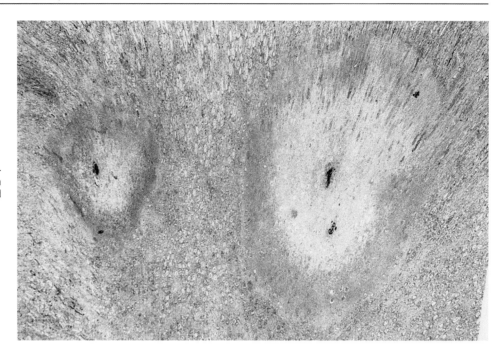

FIGURE 5-48

In this specimen of papillary necrosis, there is central coagulation necrosis and a rim of histiocytes and neutrophils.

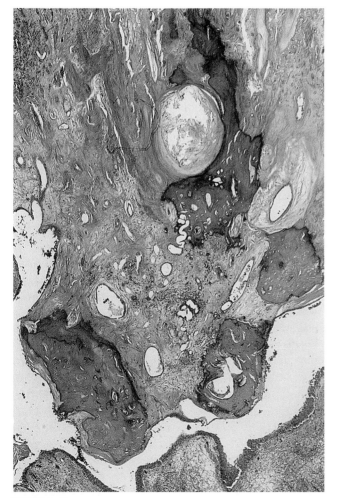

FIGURE 5-49

This specimen of remote papillary necrosis shows a fibrotic infarcted pyramid with dystrophic calcification.

mation regarding the presence of diabetes, sickle cell disease, urinary tract obstruction or infection, and analgesic use should be solicited.

PROGNOSIS AND TREATMENT

The lesion is not reversible. The prognosis depends on the extent of the process. Diabetics have the worst prognosis. If the condition is bilateral and diffuse, irreversible renal failure results.

RENAL ARTERY DISSECTION (DISSECTING ANEURYSM)

Renal artery dissection is a disruption of the intima that usually extends into the media with creation of a false lumen or a double channel. This may result in a complete vascular occlusion leading to renal infarction (Table 5-10).

CLINICAL FEATURES

A patient with dissection presents with hypertension, flank pain, and hematuria. The hypertension may or may not precede dissection, but it is invariably present after dissection. The most common cause is extension from an aortic dissection in ASVD. Primary renal artery dissection is rare, and in the past it was usually a

RENAL ARTERY DISSECTION (DISSECTING ANEURYSM)—FACT SHEET

Definition
▶ Creation of a false lumen after intimal disruption

Incidence and Location
▶ Rare
▶ Can affect either kidney

Morbidity and Mortality
▶ The kidney is usually not salvageable

Gender, Race, and Age Distribution
▶ Most common in elderly men with ASVD
▶ Second most common in young women with FMD

Clinical Features
▶ Hypertension, flank pain, and hematuria

Prognosis and Treatment
▶ Nephrectomy is curative unless dissection originates from the aorta

RENAL ARTERY DISSECTION (DISSECTING ANEURYSM)— PATHOLOGIC FEATURES

Gross Findings
▶ Thrombosed artery ± collapsed intima may be visible

Microscopic Findings
▶ Thrombosed artery and collapsed intima visible

Differential Diagnosis
▶ Identify predisposing arterial disease: ASVD, FMD, iatrogenic

MICROSCOPIC FINDINGS

The collapsed lumen is visible, with the dissection plane usually at the media-adventitia junction (Fig. 5-50). If the underlying cause is ASVD or FMD, arterial changes of these will be present.

PROGNOSIS AND TREATMENT

There is no treatment. Nephrectomy is usually performed.

RENAL ARTERY ANEURYSM

An aneurysm of the main renal artery or one of its tributaries may be a true aneurysm, either congenital or acquired, or it may be a false aneurysm, which usually results from trauma.

CLINICAL FEATURES

Most aneurysms are small and asymptomatic. If a large vessel is involved, it may be associated with thrombosis and vascular occlusion, leading to infarction or hypertension. Pain is an ominous symptom that usually indicates impending rupture or dissection. The risk of rupture is greatest during pregnancy and parturition.

TABLE 5-10

Causes of Renal Artery Dissection

Extension from aortic dissection
Fibromuscular dysplasia
Blunt abdominal trauma
Catheter injury
Spontaneous or idiopathic

---

complication of preexisting FMD. Catheter-related causes are increasing with the increasing frequency of procedures to correct RAS. Dissection due to blunt trauma is rare and is usually the consequence of an automobile accident. Spontaneous dissection without identifiable cause also occurs.

PATHOLOGIC FEATURES

GROSS FINDINGS

The renal artery may appear thrombosed, or the collapsed native lumen and false lumen may be visible. The dissection may be limited to the main renal artery, or it may propagate along its major arterial branches. Acute cortical infarcts may be associated.

PATHOLOGIC FEATURES

GROSS FINDINGS

Three types of aneurysms have been identified: saccular (70%), fusiform (22%), and intrarenal (8%). There is localized expansion of an artery with thinning of its wall. Changes of ASVD or FMD may be present.

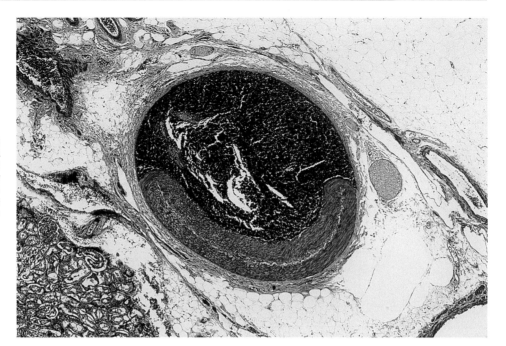

FIGURE 5-50
This segmental renal artery shows distal propagation from a main renal artery dissection that complicated angioplasty for main renal artery stenosis. Notice the collapsed intima and media with creation of a false lumen at the media-adventitia interface. (Elastichrome stain.)

RENAL ARTERY ANEURYSM—FACT SHEET

Definition
▶ Localized expansion of a renal artery

Incidence and Location
▶ Rare—0.01-0.1% of autopsies
▶ Right side > left side

Morbidity and Mortality
▶ Hypertension
▶ Death if artery ruptures

Gender, Race, and Age Distribution
▶ Variable age range and sex

Clinical Features
▶ Hypertension and pain

Prognosis and Treatment
▶ Small aneurysms <2 cm may remain stable or enlarge
▶ Lesions >4 cm and enlarging lesions require surgical treatment
▶ Rupture is usually fatal

MICROSCOPIC FINDINGS

The media is often thinned, and changes of ASVD or FMD may be present (Fig. 5-51).

PROGNOSIS AND TREATMENT

Small aneurysms (< 2 cm) are monitored; they may remain stable or enlarge. Size greater than 4 cm or an enlarging lesion requires surgical treatment. Rupture is usually fatal. Management of lesions in the range of 2 to 4 cm is unclear.

TUBULOINTERSTITIAL DISEASES

Disorders of tubules and interstitium are discussed together because alterations in one affect the other. Nephrons comprise most of the renal cortical volume; the renal interstitium consists of a slender zone separating the cortical tubules. Although normally scant, the interstitium can expand rapidly after an acute injury. Conversely, because tubules comprise 90% of the cortical mass, tubular atrophy is responsible for most of the cortical thinning in chronic renal disease.

It is important to distinguish acute tubulointerstitial diseases from chronic ones, because their prognoses differ substantially. Acute tubulointerstitial diseases have a rapid clinical onset and are associated with

---

RENAL ARTERY ANEURYSM—PATHOLOGIC FEATURES

Gross Findings
▶ Localized enlargement of artery
▶ May be associated with changes of ASVD or FMD

Microscopic Findings
▶ Medial thinning
▶ May be associated with changes of ASVD or FMD

Differential Diagnosis
▶ Identify predisposing arterial disease

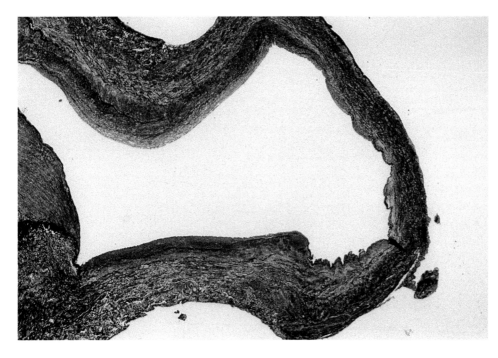

FIGURE 5-51

This renal artery aneurysm arose as a complication of medial fibromuscular dysplasia. The attenuated aneurysm wall consists of intima and adventitia without media.

interstitial edema and variable inflammation and are potentially reversible. The inflammation is usually neutrophilic in infectious etiologies (pyelonephritis), and is principally lymphohistiocytic in allergic and auto-immune forms. Chronic tubulointerstitial diseases have a gradual or insidious onset and are associated with irreversible tubular atrophy and interstitial fibrosis.

ACUTE TUBULOINTERSTITIAL DISEASES

ACUTE TUBULAR NECROSIS

Acute tubular necrosis, the most common renal parenchymal cause of acute renal failure, is divided into ischemic and toxic forms. Ischemic injury is more common. It results from decreased renal perfusion secondary to hemorrhage, hypotension, or dehydration (Table 5-11). In some patients these causes are not observed directly but are inferred based on the clinical setting. The causes of toxic acute tubular necrosis are diverse and exogenous in origin.

CLINICAL FEATURES

Patients first have decreased urine output (oliguria or rarely anuria) resulting in an elevated blood urea nitrogen (BUN) and serum creatinine concentration. Increased body weight, edema, and dyspnea may

TABLE 5-11
Causes of Acute Tubular Necrosis

Ischemia
Antibiotics
   Aminoglycosides
   Amphotericin B
   Polymyxin B
   Rifampicin
   Cephalosporin
   Colistin
Radiographic contrast agents
Nonsteroidal anti-inflammatory drugs
Chemotherapeutic agents
   Cisplatinum
Organic solvents
   Carbon tetrachloride
   Ethylene glycol
   Trichloroethylene
Insecticides and herbicides
Heavy metals
   Mercury
   Bismuth
   Lead
   Cadmium
   Uranium
   Arsenic
Rhabdomyolysis
Hemolysis
Cocaine
Toxins
   Insect stings
   Snake bites
   Mushroom poisoning

develop. The urine usually contains renal epithelial cells and muddy brown casts. The urine sodium level may be elevated because of loss of sodium conservation.

PATHOLOGIC FEATURES

GROSS FINDINGS

The kidneys may appear normal but more often are enlarged and swollen, with increased renal weight (usually > 200 g) due to interstitial edema. The cortex is pale, with hyperemia (Fig. 5-52) at the cortico-medullary junction.

MICROSCOPIC FINDINGS

There is cortical interstitial expansion due to edema without significant inflammation. A mononuclear cell infiltrate may be seen at the corticomedullary junction, or within the vessels in the vasa recta of the outer medulla. The tubules can show two patterns of injury. The first is coagulation necrosis of tubular cells, which is most commonly seen at autopsy (Fig. 5-53). The nuclei disappear, the cell membranes become indistinct, and cell debris may slough into the lumen. The proximal tubules are affected more than the distal tubules. The second pattern is more subtle, resulting from single cell necrosis and sloughing. It is characterized by attenuation or flattening of the tubular epithelium with widely spaced nuclei (Figs. 5-54 and 5-55). The remaining cells lose their brush border and spread out to cover the basement membrane. There may be short segments of denuded tubular basement membranes. Mitotic figures are present but usually infrequent. Distal tubules and collecting ducts contain granular casts of sloughed cells.

Most toxic causes of acute tubular necrosis produce no specific morphologic clues and appear identical to ischemia-related causes, although coexistent interstitial fibrosis may be present. There are a few that have diagnostically useful features. Isometric tubular vacuolization is seen in cases associated with intravenous immunoglobulin G (IgG). Numerous birefringent oxalate crystals are present in renal tubular oxalosis (Fig. 5-56). Pigmented casts are present in rhabdomyolysis-associated cases. Tubular intranuclear inclusions may be detected in lesions associated with heavy metal exposure. Chemotherapy-related causes may result in marked nuclear atypia.

DIFFERENTIAL DIAGNOSIS

Acute tubular necrosis must be distinguished from autolysis, especially in autopsy material. Autolysis is recognized when epithelial cells having intact cell membranes and preserved nuclei separate from tubular basement membranes and from each other. The renal weight is not increased in autolysis as it is in acute

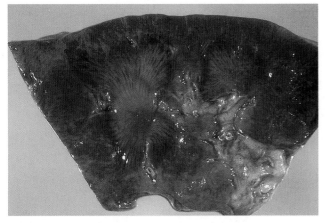

FIGURE 5-52
In this kidney with acute tubular necrosis, there is marked hyperemia of the outer strip of the outer medulla.

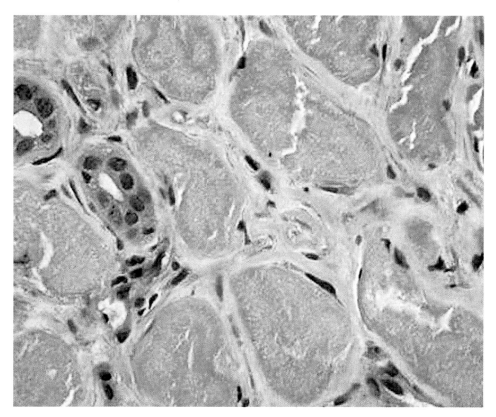

FIGURE 5-53

This autopsy kidney shows coagulation necrosis of proximal tubules with two preserved distal tubules.

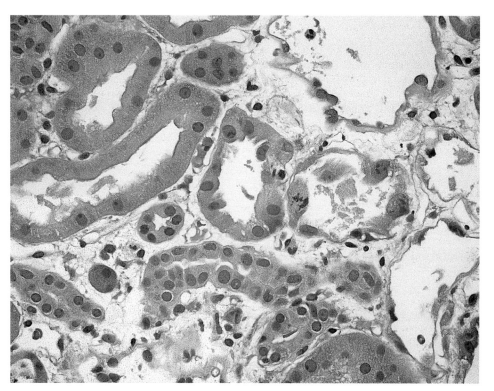

FIGURE 5-54

In this renal biopsy specimen of acute tubular necrosis, there is mild tubular epithelial cell attenuation at the upper left and severe attenuation at the upper right associated with interstitial edema. A tubular cell mitotic figure is present in the center.

tubular necrosis, in which renal weights of 200 g and more are typical.

It is difficult to identify toxic causes of acute tubular necrosis, because they often develop in the context of therapy for other illnesses or may result from difficult-to-identify exogenous agents. The isometric vacuoliza-

tion of intravenous IgG must be distinguished from that of other osmotic agents. History is crucial. In heavy metal lesions such as those caused by bismuth, cadmium, and lead, proximal tubular intranuclear inclusions may be present. The coexistence of interstitial fibrosis may suggest one of these more chronic

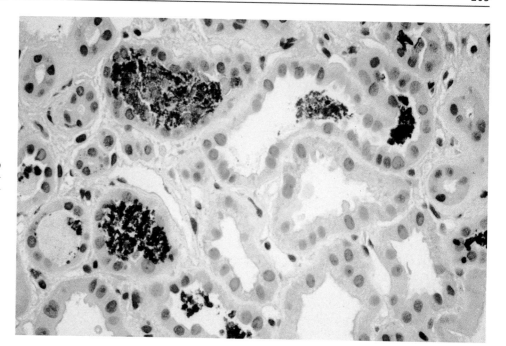

FIGURE 5-55

Acute tubular necrosis secondary to rhabdomyolysis. These casts are positive for myoglobin. (Immunoperoxidase stain for myoglobin.)

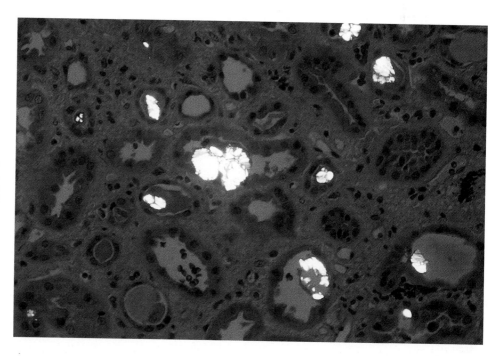

FIGURE 5-56

In this specimen of ethylene glycol–associated acute tubular necrosis, numerous tubular calcium oxalate crystals are easily demonstrated by polarization.

insults. Birefringent calcium oxalate crystals, if numerous, implicate an oxalate source, most often ethylene glycol. Pigmented casts in distal tubules are present in rhabdomyolysis-related cases and may be confirmed by immunoperoxidase stain for myoglobin (Fig. 5-55).

PROGNOSIS AND TREATMENT

Recovery of renal function in ischemia-related cases is possible, provided the medical condition responsible for

acute tubular necrosis is controlled. In toxic causes of acute tubular necrosis, irreversibility is more common.

ACUTE INTERSTITIAL NEPHRITIS

Acute interstitial nephritis is an inflammatory, immunologically mediated cause of acute renal failure first described in detail by Councilman in 1898. Before the use of antibiotics, acute interstitial nephritis was usually caused by a bacterial infection, most often scarlet fever or diphtheria. Today, acute transplant rejection and allergic drug reactions are the most common causes. However, other infections, both bacterial and viral, immune complex formation, and antitubular basement antibodies can also produce acute interstitial nephritis (Table 5-12).

CLINICAL FEATURES

Patients have decreased urine output and elevated concentrations of BUN and serum creatinine. They may have fever, flank pain, or a rash. The peripheral blood may have an elevated eosinophil count, and the urine frequently contains red blood cells and white blood cells that may include eosinophils.

PATHOLOGIC FEATURES

GROSS FINDINGS

The kidneys are enlarged, soft, and pale secondary to edema.

MICROSCOPIC FINDINGS

In acute interstitial nephritis there is interstitial expansion by edema and a variably distributed, mixed cell infiltrate (Fig. 5-57) consisting principally of lymphocytes and monocytes. Smaller numbers of plasma cells and eosinophils may be present. The lymphocytes infiltrate between tubular epithelial cells (tubulitis), which may themselves appear reactive or show individual cell necrosis. Endovasculitis, necrotizing vas-

culitis, or small granulomas may develop in cases of transplant rejection or allergic reactions. Small, non-caseating granulomas are also encountered occasionally in patients who have renal involvement with sarcoidosis. Cytomegalovirus, adenovirus, and polyomavirus-related causes produce intranuclear viral inclusions within tubular cells, and occasionally in endothelial and glomerular epithelial cells. Adenovirus appears as smudgy intranuclear inclusions; cytomegalovirus produces large eosinophilic intranuclear inclusions with halos; and polyoma BK virus causes nucleomegaly, karyolysis, and pale intranuclear inclusions.

ACUTE INTERSTITIAL NEPHRITIS—FACT SHEET

Definition
► Inflammatory tubulointerstitial cause of acute renal failure

Incidence and Location
► Second leading cause of acute renal failure

Morbidity and Mortality
► Renal failure

Clinical Features
► Decreased urine output, azotemia, hematuria, eosinophiluria, eosinophilia
► Rash, fever, flank pain

Prognosis and Treatment
► Reversible if offending agent eliminated

ACUTE INTERSTITIAL NEPHRITIS—PATHOLOGIC FEATURES

Gross Findings
► Increased renal weight

Microscopic Findings
► Interstitial mononuclear cell infiltrate, tubular injury, interstitial edema
► Viral inclusions in certain viral causes

Ultrastructural Features
► Tubular basement membrane immune complex deposits

Immunohistochemical Features
► Granular or linear fluorescence for IgG and C3
► Immunoperoxidase demonstration of BK polyoma virus, cytomegalovirus, adenovirus

Differential Diagnosis
► Allergic reaction
► Autoimmune condition
► Transplant rejection

TABLE 5-12

Infection-related Tubulointerstitial Nephritis

ACUTE INFECTION
Acute pyelonephritis
Pyonephrosis
Perinephric abscess
Emphysematous pyelonephritis
Fungal infections
Viral infections

CHRONIC INFECTION
Chronic pyelonephritis
Xanthogranulomatous pyelonephritis
Malakoplakia
Tuberculosis

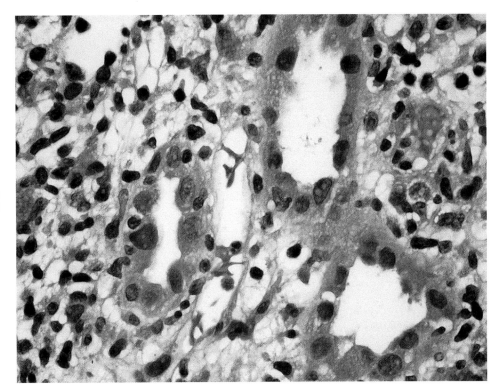

FIGURE 5-57

In acute interstitial nephritis, there is an interstitial mononuclear cell infiltrate, edema, and tubulitis.

ANCILLARY STUDIES

IMMUNOHISTOCHEMISTRY

In antibody-mediated cases, immune complex deposits may be identified within tubular basement membranes or in peritubular capillaries, or a linear tubular basement membrane reaction may be demonstrated if antitubular basement membrane antibody is present. Immunoperoxidase stains can confirm the presence of BK polyoma virus, cytomegalovirus, and adenovirus.

ULTRASTRUCTURAL FEATURES

Electron microscopy can demonstrate tubular basement membrane immune complex deposits and intranuclear viral particles. The size, location, and organization of the viral particles assist classification.

DIFFERENTIAL DIAGNOSIS

History and laboratory data are required to establish the cause, because there are few morphologically discriminatory features except for those cases in which an intranuclear viral inclusion or antibody deposition is detected. Before the use of antibiotics, acute interstitial nephritis was usually caused by infections. Today, acute transplant rejection and allergic drug reactions are the first consideration. It is not possible to identify a bacterial cause in a patient receiving antibiotics. The presence of a rash, fever, eosinophilia, or eosinophiluria implicates an allergic cause, but often they are absent. Almost any drug can cause an allergic reaction. The presence of significant proteinuria is commonly associated with reaction to nonsteroidal anti-inflammatory drugs (NSAIDs). In patients with a systemic autoimmune disease such as Sjögren's syndrome or sarcoidosis, the underlying disease is usually implicated.

PROGNOSIS AND TREATMENT

The condition is reversible if the offending agent can be eliminated or the underlying immunologic disease controlled.

ACUTE PYELONEPHRITIS

Acute pyelonephritis is a bacterial infection of the kidney. Males account for most pediatric cases, and females account for most adult cases. Two avenues of renal infection occur: ascending and hematogenous. Ascending acute pyelonephritis is most common and originates from a lower urinary tract infection. *Escherichia coli* is the most frequently implicated organism, followed by other enteric bacteria *Proteus*, *Klebsiella*, and *Enterobacter*. The voyage to the kidney begins with bacterial cystitis followed by vesicoureteral reflux. Vesicoureteral reflux may be a congenital, often hereditary, abnormality in the anatomy of the ureterovesical junction. Alternatively, reflux may develop in nonrefluxing systems with severe cystitis or if there is distal obstruction or a neurogenic bladder. The kidney is infected when intrarenal reflux occurs. The architecture of the renal pyramids influences their susceptibility to intrarenal reflux (see later discussion). The infection extends up the medullary rays before generalized cortical spread occurs. Hematogenous pyelonephritis is the second route of infection. It usually complicates prolonged sepsis or infectious endocarditis. The organisms responsible are more often gram-positive bacteria or fungi.

Several complications can result from prolonged infections.

Pyonephrosis refers to the near-total destruction of an obstructed kidney by acute pyelonephritis.

Perinephric abscess is the accumulation of infectious material and neutrophils within perinephric fat. It usually originates from rupture of a renal abscess or from pyonephrosis.

Emphysematous pyelonephritis is an uncommon but life-threatening complication. Gas bubbles develop within the renal parenchyma and may extend into perinephric and even retroperitoneal sites. Approximately 90 % of patients have diabetes mellitus, and urinary tract obstruction is present in approximately 40 %. *E. coli* is responsible in 68 % of cases and *Klebsiella* in 9 % of cases; a mixed infection occurs in 19 % of cases.

CLINICAL FEATURES

Patients present with fever, leukocytosis, and flank tenderness and may have a variety of complications. Pyuria and urinary white blood cell casts are present.

PATHOLOGIC FEATURES

GROSS FINDINGS

In ascending acute pyelonephritis, yellow-white suppurative foci or overt abscesses develop in the pyramids and may extend into the cortex. In hematogenous forms, the kidneys are peppered with abscesses, which are more numerous in the cortex than in the medulla. The kidney in emphysematous pyelonephritis shows widespread abscesses with papillary necrosis and cortical infarcts (Fig. 5-58) and may appear cystic due to gas bubbles.

MICROSCOPIC FINDINGS

There is an intense neutrophilic response within the tubules and interstitium (Fig. 5-59). In sites of early

---

ACUTE PYELONEPHRITIS—FACT SHEET

Definition
▶ Acute bacterial infection of the kidney

Incidence and Location
▶ Common
▶ Cortex and medulla

Morbidity and Mortality
▶ Renal insufficiency if bilateral

Gender, Race, and Age Distribution
▶ Ascending form: males > females in children, females > males in adults
▶ Hematogenous form: sepsis and infective endocarditis

Clinical Features
▶ Fever
▶ Leukocytosis; white blood cells and white blood cell casts in urine

Prognosis and Treatment
▶ Antibiotic treatment or surgical resection

---

involvement, neutrophils and, rarely, bacteria can be seen within tubules and collecting ducts of the cortex and medulla. Soon the suppurative inflammation spills into the interstitium. Glomeruli may be spared initially, but with increasing severity generalized parenchymal destruction occurs, resulting in abscess formation that may extend into the perinephric tissues. In emphysematous pyelonephritis, empty spaces lacking epithelial cell linings form, distorting the parenchyma. Adjacent areas show vascular thrombosis, ischemic necrosis, suppurative inflammation, and abscesses (Figs. 5-60 and 5-61).

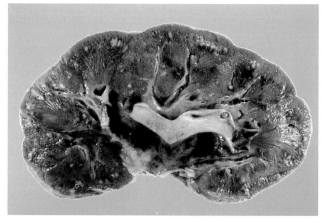

FIGURE 5-58

In hematogenous acute pyelonephritis, there is a miliary pattern of small cortical abscesses.

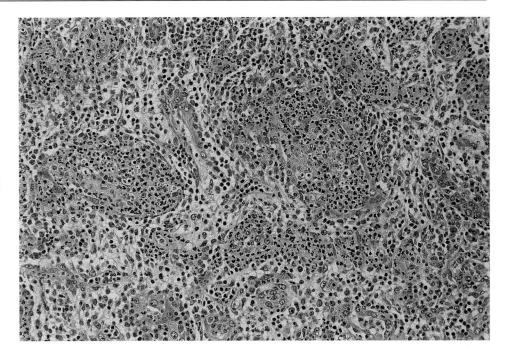

FIGURE 5-59

Ascending acute pyelonephritis. There is an intense intratubular and interstitial neutrophilic infiltrate.

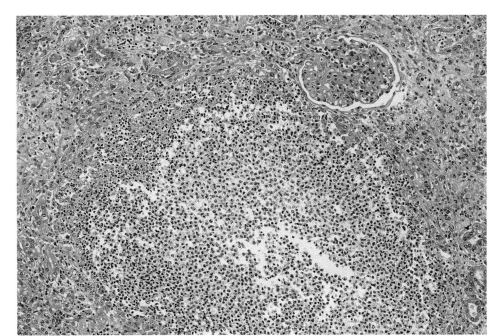

FIGURE 5-60

Hematogenous acute pyelonephritis. This microabscess was one of many that developed in a patient with prolonged sepsis.

ACUTE PYELONEPHRITIS—PATHOLOGIC FEATURES

Gross Findings
► Abscesses

Microscopic Findings
► Suppurative inflammation in tubules and interstitium

Differential Diagnosis
► Ascending forms
► Hematogenous forms
► Acute interstitial nephritis with numerous neutrophils

DIFFERENTIAL DIAGNOSIS

In acute pyelonephritis, ascending infection should be distinguished from hematogenous forms. The most important clinical information is the type of infection, urinary tract versus sepsis or endocarditis. A history of urosepsis makes the gross and histologic observations very important. The status of the lower urinary tract must be evaluated, because the presence of urethral obstruction or ureteral dilatation or stenosis is a risk factor for an ascending source. The pattern of the suppurative inflammation is also useful. More severe inflammation in papillary tissue implicates an ascending

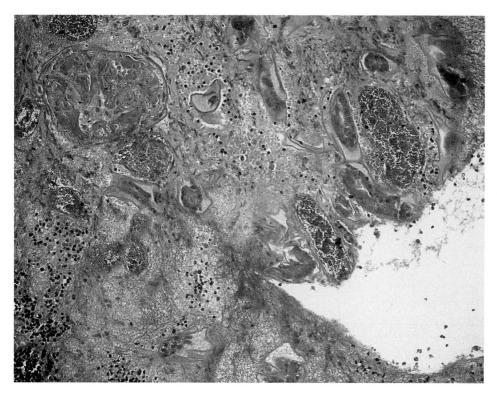

FIGURE 5-61

In emphysematous pyelonephritis, there is diffuse coagulation necrosis, hemorrhage, empty spaces formed by gas bubbles, and tubules packed with bacteria.

infection, whereas cortical microabscesses with little papillary collecting duct inflammation implicates a hematogenous route.

Neutrophils may be seen in severe forms of acute interstitial nephritis, such as those caused by allergic reaction or transplant rejection. However, in these situations a mononuclear infiltrate predominates; neutrophils are far less numerous and are preferentially interstitial rather than intratubular. The clinical history and results of cultures will help resolve the rare case in which uncertainty exists.

Acute pyelonephritis often responds to antibiotic therapy. Renal function may be compromised with repeated episodes, which can lead to the development of chronic pyelonephritis. Complications of nephric and perinephric abscess and pyonephrosis require nephrectomy and pose risk of sepsis. Emphysematous pyelonephritis does not respond to antibiotics; the risk of sepsis is high, and the prognosis is grave.

CHRONIC TUBULOINTERSTITIAL DISEASE

Chronic Pyelonephritis

Chronic pyelonephritis is the chronic tubulointerstitial sequela of one or more possible contributing factors: recurrent or smoldering bacterial infection, vesicoureteral reflux, or urinary tract obstruction. It is responsible for 5% to 15% of end-stage kidney disease. Chronic pyelonephritis is subdivided into reflux nephropathy (or chronic nonobstructive pyelonephritis) and obstructive pyelonephritis.

REFLUX NEPHROPATHY (CHRONIC NONOBSTRUCTIVE PYELONEPHRITIS)

Reflux nephropathy refers to chronic renal injury that develops in patients who have vesicoureteral reflux, a congenital disorder in which there is regurgitation of urine from the bladder into a ureter because of inadequate ureteral development. Often a familial disorder, it is typically detected after a urinary tract infection at an early age. The reflux often decreases with increasing age, but the renal scars are already present, possibly developing at the time of the first infection.

Not all urinary tract infections with vesicoureteral reflux lead to reflux nephropathy, because of the architecture of the renal pyramids. Renal pyramids are of two types, simple and compound. In a simple pyramid, the Bellini ducts open through a convex papilla at an oblique angle and close with an increase in intrapelvic pressure. Conversely, compound pyramids have concave surfaces, and Bellini's ducts fail to close with increased intrapelvic pressure, resulting in intrarenal reflux. Reflux nephropathy represents the combined effects of vesicoureteral reflux and intrarenal reflux, which transmits high pressures and permits infection to gain access to the renal parenchyma. Compound papillae are usually located in the polar regions of the kidney, the location of most scars in reflux nephropathy.

CHRONIC OBSTRUCTIVE PYELONEPHRITIS

In chronic obstructive pyelonephritis, the kidney is damaged by pressure-related atrophy that may or may not be accompanied by bacterial infection. The obstruction may be ureteral or urethral in origin.

CLINICAL FEATURES

Patients may be asymptomatic, or they may present with flank symptoms, hypertension, polydipsia and polyuria from a concentrating defect, or renal failure. Proteinuria may also occur, and it identifies patients who are at risk for renal failure from focal segmental glomerulosclerosis, which develops in 5% of patients with reflux nephropathy.

PATHOLOGIC FEATURES

GROSS FINDINGS

The kidneys are small and irregularly contracted, weighing from 30 to 50 g, and the renal pelves and ureters are usually dilated with thickened walls.

REFLUX NEPHROPATHY (CHRONIC NONOBSTRUCTIVE PYELONEPHRITIS)—FACT SHEET

Definition
▶ Chronic tubulointerstitial disease secondary to recurrent or smoldering infection, vesicoureteral reflux, or chronic urinary tract obstruction

Incidence and Location
▶ May be unilateral or bilateral

Morbidity and Mortality
▶ Represents 5-15% of end-stage kidney disease

Clinical Features
▶ Asymptomatic to flank pain
▶ Uremia, polyuria, polydipsia, concentrating defect

Prognosis and Treatment
▶ Scars are irreversible
▶ Renal function related to extent of disease and laterality

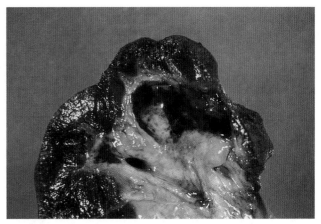

FIGURE 5-62

In this kidney with reflux nephropathy, there are two zones of cortical scarring, with effaced pyramids adjacent to nonscarred cortex.

In *reflux nephropathy,* there are depressed polar scars overlying damaged renal pyramids and dilated calyces. The cortex adjacent to the scars may be unaffected or hypertrophic (Fig. 5-62).

In *obstructive chronic pyelonephritis,* the kidney is hydronephrotic with diffuse calyceal dilation, blunting or effacement of all papillae, and cortical thinning (Fig. 5-63).

MICROSCOPIC FINDINGS

The cortical scars show periglomerular fibrosis, global glomerulosclerosis, extensive tubular atrophy, and an interstitial mononuclear cell infiltrate. The tubules contain eosinophilic casts (thyroidization) (Fig. 5-64), and arteries show striking intimal sclerosis. The renal pyramids may show mild blunting of papillary tips in mild cases or complete effacement of pyramids in advanced cases. The collecting system shows chronic pyelitis and ureteritis, with lymphoid aggregates

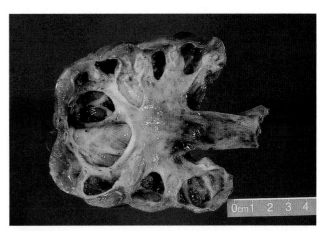

FIGURE 5-63

This kidney with chronic obstructive pyelonephritis shows severe hydronephrosis and ureteral dilatation with effacement of all renal pyramids and severe cortical attenuation.

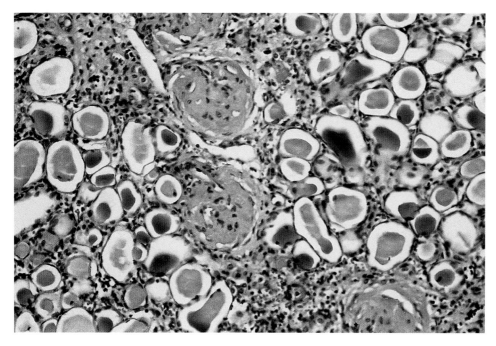

FIGURE 5-64
This is the "thyroidization" form of tubular atrophy, with colloid-like tubular casts characteristic of end-stage chronic pyelonephritis.

or germinal centers in the mucosa (Fig. 5-65). The uninvolved cortex in reflux nephropathy may appear normal, or it may exhibit compensatory nephron hypertrophy. Segmental sclerosing glomerular lesions characterize focal segmental glomerulosclerosis.

DIFFERENTIAL DIAGNOSIS

The gross appearance of the kidney usually distinguishes reflux nephropathy from obstructive pyelonephritis. Reflux nephropathy has polar scars, whereas obstructive pyelonephritis shows diffuse hydronephrosis, with cortical and medullary atrophy. Scars resulting from renal infarcts are grossly distinguished from pyelonephritic scars by the absence of pelvic and ureteral abnormalities. Furthermore, small infarcts involve only cortex and not the medulla. Histologically, the glomeruli in an infarct consist of a tight PAS-positive aggregate of glomerular basement membranes, whereas the glomeruli in a pyelonephritic scar contain collagen in and around the sclerotic glomerular tuft. Interstitial inflammation is much more severe in chronic pyelonephritis compared with other types of scar.

PROGNOSIS AND TREATMENT

The prognosis depends on the extent of disease, unilateral versus bilateral. If significant proteinuria is present, the course will be that of focal segmental glomerulosclerosis: 30% to 50% of patient will progress to end-stage renal disease over a protracted interval. Correction of reflux and prevention of recurrent infection does not prevent progression of this glomerular lesion.

REFLUX NEPHROPATHY (CHRONIC NONOBSTRUCTIVE PYELONEPHRITIS)—PATHOLOGIC FEATURES

Gross Findings
▶ Polar scars in reflux nephropathy
▶ Diffuse scarring in obstructive chronic pyelonephritis

Microscopic Findings
▶ Tubular atrophy, interstitial fibrosis, chronic inflammation, glomerulosclerosis

Differential Diagnosis
▶ Reflux nephropathy
▶ Obstructive nephropathy
▶ Infarcts

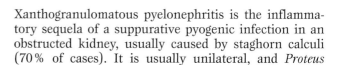

XANTHOGRANULOMATOUS PYELONEPHRITIS

Xanthogranulomatous pyelonephritis is the inflammatory sequela of a suppurative pyogenic infection in an obstructed kidney, usually caused by staghorn calculi (70% of cases). It is usually unilateral, and *Proteus* species and *E. coli* are the most common infective

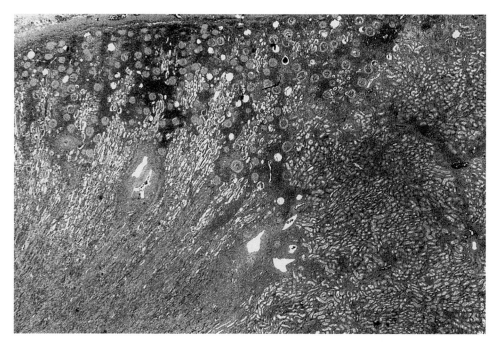

FIGURE 5-65

In reflux nephropathy, normal cortex *(right side)* is discretely delineated from the scarred zone of chronic pyelonephritis *(left side)*.

agents. It begins with suppurative inflammation and edema within pelvic mucosa and sinus fat, resulting in pelvicaliceal ulceration and fat necrosis, and then extends to the medulla, resulting in necrosis. The cortex, perinephric fat, and even retroperitoneal tissue may eventually be involved (Table 5-13).

CLINICAL FEATURES

Patients present with flank pain, fever, fatigue, and pyuria.

TABLE 5-13

Granulomatous Diseases of the Kidney

Xanthogranulomatous pyelonephritis

Malakoplakia

Mycobacterial infection

Fungal infection

Parasitic infection

Urate nephropathy

Sarcoidosis

Vasculitis

Drug hypersensitivity

XANTHOGRANULOMATOUS PYELONEPHRITIS—FACT SHEET

Definition
▶ Xanthogranulomatous sequela of a pyogenic infection in an obstructed urinary tract

Incidence and Location
▶ Usually unilateral
▶ Diffuse, segmental, or focal

Morbidity and Mortality
▶ Involved kidney is destroyed

Gender, Race, and Age Distribution
▶ 70% of patients are female

Clinical Features
▶ Renal mass and flank pain

Radiologic Features
▶ Lipid-rich mass and calculus

Prognosis and Treatment
▶ Nephrectomy is curative

PATHOLOGIC FEATURES

GROSS FINDINGS

The kidney has a dilated, thickened pelvis containing a staghorn calculus (Fig. 5-66). Yellow nodular tumor

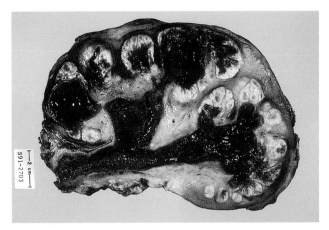

FIGURE 5-66

In this kidney with xanthogranulomatous pyelonephritis, there is xanthomatous transformation of renal pyramids with similar thickening of pelvic urothelium. A staghorn calculus was present.

XANTHOGRANULOMATOUS PYELONEPHRITIS— PATHOLOGIC FEATURES

Gross Findings

► Yellow masses in medulla and cortex
► Thickened yellow lining to the collecting system

Microscopic Findings

► Central zone of neutrophils rimmed by foam cells and a fibroblastic response

Differential Diagnosis

► Renal neoplasm
► Granulomatous infection

---

masses replace the renal pyramids, line the pelvis, and may involve the cortex or perinephric tissues. The masses may be diffuse, or they may involve portions of the kidney, giving rise to segmental and focal patterns. The diffuse form is most common. The segmental or focal forms are more difficult to diagnose and more likely to be mistaken for neoplasms. Segmental xanthogranulomatous pyelonephritis is polar and is more common in children. The focal (or tumefactive) form is a cortical variant that lacks communication with the pelvis and is not associated with pyelitis, calculi, or urinary tract obstruction.

MICROSCOPIC FINDINGS

The xanthogranulomatous nodules have a zonal pattern (Fig. 5-67). There is a central nidus of necrotic debris and neutrophils that is surrounded by the zone of foamy macrophages. The most peripheral tissue shows a fibroblastic response as the host attempts to confine or organize the inflammatory process (Fig. 5-68).

ANCILLARY STUDIES

IMMUNOHISTOCHEMISTRY

The xanthoma cells are CD68 positive and cytokeratin negative, and the reactive fibrous tissue is vimentin positive and cytokeratin negative.

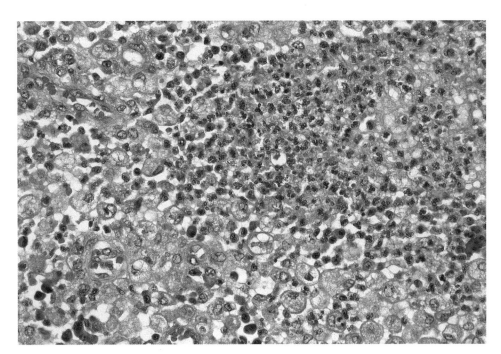

FIGURE 5-67

The mass lesions of xanthogranulomatous pyelonephritis have a central zone of neutrophils with a broad rim of foamy macrophages.

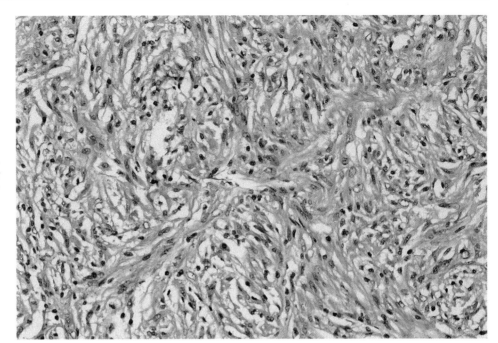

FIGURE 5-68
The peripheral regions of xantho-granulomatous pyelonephritis show exuberant fibroplasia with a stori-form growth pattern.

DIFFERENTIAL DIAGNOSIS

The mass lesions of xanthogranulomatous pyelonephritis may grossly elicit concern for a neoplasm. The presence of a large calculus and xanthomatous thickening of the pelvis mucosa should suggest the correct diagnosis, which is usually straightforward once the histologic findings are available. On occasion, histologic examination may also elicit consideration of a neoplasm. The foam cells of xanthogranulomatous pyelonephritis can resemble clear cell renal carcinoma, and the fibroblastic response can resemble a spindle-cell neoplasm. The bubbly microvesicular fat of the foam cells contrasts with the cleared-out cytoplasm that is characteristic of clear cell renal cell carcinoma. Although minimal cytologic atypia and lack of mitoses may be seen in both carcinoma and xanthogranulomatous pyelonephritis, the presence of atypia and mitoses is helpful to diagnose carcinoma. Exclusion of epithelial markers by immunohistochemistry should resolve any uncertainty. The spindle cells in xanthogranulomatous pyelonephritis usually have limited atypia and mitotic activity. This is helpful, because sarcomas and sarcomatoid carcinomas usually have marked nuclear atypia and frequent mitoses.

PROGNOSIS AND TREATMENT

The kidney is usually nonfunctional. Nephrectomy is indicated because of symptoms and, on occasion, because of neoplastic concerns.

MALAKOPLAKIA

Malakoplakia is an uncommon granulomatous disease that is most frequently observed in the urinary tracts of middle-aged women as a complication of recurrent infections. Bladder involvement is 4 to 10 times as common as upper tract involvement, and renal involvement is rare. *E. coli* is the most common agent.

CLINICAL FEATURES

Patients have fever, flank pain, and renal failure because bilateral disease is typical.

PATHOLOGIC FEATURES

GROSS FINDINGS

The kidneys show obstructive changes with dilated pelves and calyces. The typical mucosal lesion of malakoplakia is characterized by a yellow-brown soft (*malakos*) plaque (*plakos*) that often has central umbilication. The parenchymal lesions consist of similar soft, yellow-brown nodules.

MICROSCOPIC FINDINGS

There are masses of large eosinophilic histiocytes (von Hansemann histiocytes), and many contain

MALAKOPLAKIA—FACT SHEET

Definition
▶ A chronic granulomatous complication of recurrent urinary tract infections

Incidence and Location
▶ Bilateral

Morbidity and Mortality
▶ Renal failure

Gender, Race, and Age Distribution
▶ Young to middle-aged women

Clinical Features
▶ Fever, flank pain

Prognosis and Treatment
▶ Irreversible renal failure

DIFFERENTIAL DIAGNOSIS

A similar, possibly precursor lesion is megalocytic interstitial nephritis (MIN). In MIN, there is a similar massive histiocytic infiltrate with creation of a mass; however, Michaelis-Gutmann bodies are not demonstrable.

PROGNOSIS AND TREATMENT

Renal failure is usually irreversible.

MALAKOPLAKIA—PATHOLOGIC FEATURES

Gross Findings
▶ Dilated renal pelves and calyces
▶ Soft yellow-brown nodules, parenchymal or mucosal

Microscopic Findings
▶ Masses of large eosinophilic histiocytes, basophilic target-like inclusions

Differential Diagnosis
▶ Megalocytic interstitial nephritis
▶ Granulomatous infections

basophilic inclusions (Michaelis-Gutmann bodies) (Fig. 5-69). PAS, calcium, or iron staining enhance the target-like appearance of these cytoplasmic inclusions. The calcium and iron stains indicate their mineralized nature.

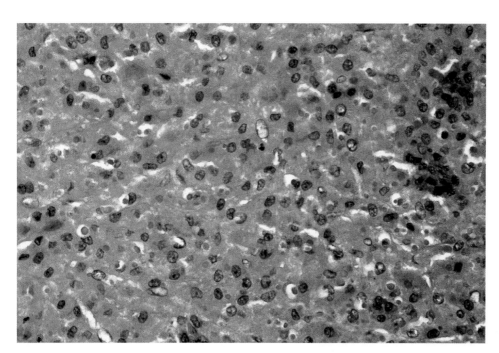

FIGURE 5-69

In malakoplakia, there are sheets of large eosinophilic Von Hansemann histiocytes. Notice the pale-appearing Michaelis-Gutmann bodies, which will appear targetoid on periodic acid-Schiff (PAS), calcium, or iron staining.

SUGGESTED READINGS

General Reading

Bonsib SM: Non-neoplastic diseases of the kidney. In Bostwick DG, Eble JN (eds): Urologic Surgical Pathology. St Louis, Mosby, 1997, pp 1–82.

Gross and Histologic Features of the Normal Kidney

Beeuwkes R 3rd: The vascular organization of the kidney. Annu Rev Physiol 1980;42:531–542.

Bonsib SM: Renal anatomy and histology. In: Jennette JC, Olson JL, Schwartz MM, Silva FG (eds): Heptinstall's Pathology of the Kidney. Philadelphia, Lippincott-Raven, 2006, Chapter 1.

Brodel M: The intrinsic blood vessels of the kidney and their significance in nephrotomy. Bull Johns Hopkins Hosp 1901;12:10–13.

Clapp WL: Adult kidney. In Sternberg SS (ed): Histology for Pathologists. New York, Raven Press, 1997, pp 677–708.

de C Baker SB: The blood supply of the renal papilla. Br J Urol 1959;31:53–59.

Fine H: The development of the lobes of the metanephros and fetal kidney. Acta Anat (Basel) 1982;113:93–107.

Hodson CJ: The renal parenchyma and its blood supply. Curr Probl Diagn Radiol 1978;7:1–32.

Holmes MJ, O'Morchoe PJ, O'Morchoe CC: Morphology of the intrarenal lymphatic system: Capsular and hilar communications. Am J Anat 1977;149:333–351.

Kriz W: Structural organization of the renal medulla: Comparative and functional aspects. Am J Physiol 1981;241:R3–R16.

Kriz W: Structural organization of renal medullary circulation. Nephron 1982;31:290–295.

Potter EL: Normal and abnormal development of the kidney. Chicago, Year Book Medical Publishers, 1972.

Sampaio FJ, Aragao AH: Anatomical relationship between the intrarenal arteries and the kidney collecting system. J Urol 1990;143:679–681.

Satyapal KS: Classification of the drainage patterns of the renal veins. J Anat 1995;186(Pt 2):329–333.

Cystic Renal Diseases

Grantham JJ: Polycystic kidney disease: From the bedside to the gene and back. Curr Opin Nephrol Hypertens 2001;10:533–542.

Igarashi P, Somlo S: Genetics and pathogenesis of polycystic kidney disease. J Am Soc Nephrol 2002;13:2384–2398.

Kaariainen H, Koskimies O, Norio R: Dominant and recessive polycystic kidney disease in children: Evaluation of clinical features and laboratory data. Pediatr Nephrol 1988;2:296–302.

Pohl M, Bhatnagar V, Mendoza SA, Nigam SK: Toward an etiological classification of developmental disorders of the kidney and upper urinary tract. Kidney Int 2002;61:10–19.

Woolf AS, Price KL, Scambler PJ, Winyard PJD: Evolving concepts in human renal dysplasia. J Am Soc Nephrol 2004;15:998–1007.

Woolf AS, Winyard PJ: Advances in the cell biology and genetics of human kidney malformations. J Am Soc Nephrol 1998;9:1114–1125.

Yoder BK, Hou X, Guay-Woodford LM: The polycystic kidney disease proteins, polycystin-1, polycystin-2, polaris, and cystin, are co-localized in renal cilia. J Am Soc Nephrol 2002;13:2508–2516.

Zerres K, Volpel MC, Weiss H: Cystic kidneys: Genetics, pathologic anatomy, clinical picture, and prenatal diagnosis. Hum Genet 1984;68:104–135.

Adult (Dominant) Polycystic Kidney Disease

Blyth H, Ockenden BG: Polycystic disease of the liver and kidneys in childhood. J Med Genet 1971;8:257–284.

Fick GM, Johnson AM, Strain JD, et al: Characteristics of very early onset autosomal dominant polycystic kidney disease. J Am Soc Nephrol 1993;3:1863–1870.

Gregoire JR, Torres VE, Holley KE, Farrow GM: Renal epithelial hyperplastic and neoplastic proliferation in autosomal dominant polycystic kidney disease. Am J Kidney Dis 1987;9:27–38.

Keith DS, Torres VE, King BF, et al: Renal cell carcinoma in autosomal dominant polycystic kidney disease. J Am Soc Nephrol 1994;4:1661–1669.

Perrone RD, Cohen J, Harrington J, Zusman C: Extrarenal manifestations of ADPKD. Kidney Int 1997;51:2022–2036.

Infantile (Recessive) Polycystic Kidney Disease

Capisonda R, Phan V, Traubuci J, et al: Autosomal recessive polycystic kidney disease: Outcomes from a single-center experience. Pediatr Nephrol 2003;18:119–126.

Gang DL, Herrin JT: Infantile polycystic disease of the liver and kidneys. Clin Nephrol 1986;25:28–36.

Helczynski L, Wells TR, Landing BH, Lipsey AI: The renal lesion of congenital hepatic fibrosis: Pathologic and morphometric analysis, with comparison to the renal lesion of infantile polycystic disease. Pediatr Pathol 1984;2:441–455.

Jorgensen MJ: The ductal plate malformation. Acta Pathol Microbiol Scand Suppl 1977;(257):1–87.

Lieberman E, Salinas-Madrigal L, Gwinn JL, et al: Infantile polycystic disease of the kidneys and liver: Clinical, pathological and radiological correlations and comparison with congenital hepatic fibrosis. Medicine (Baltimore) 1971;50:277–318.

Lonergan GJ, Rice RR, Suarez ES: Autosomal recessive polycystic kidney disease: Radiologic-pathologic correlation. Radiographics 2000;20:837–855.

McDonald RA, Avner ED: Inherited polycystic kidney disease in children. Semin Nephrol 1991;11:632–642.

Roy S, Dillon MJ, Trompeter RS, Barratt TM: Autosomal recessive polycystic kidney disease: Long-term outcome of neonatal survivors. Pediatr Nephrol 1997;11:302–306.

Wang S, Luo Y, Wilson PD, et al: The autosomal recessive polycystic kidney disease protein is localized to primary cilia, with concentration in the basal body area. J Am Soc Nephrol 2004;15:592–602.

Zerres K, Muecher G, Becker J, et al: Prenatal diagnosis of autosomal recessive polycystic kidney disease (ARPKD): Molecular genetics, clinical experience, and fetal morphology. Am J Med Genet 1998;76:137–144.

Renal Dysplasia

Atiyeh B, Husmann D, Baum M: Contralateral renal abnormalities in patients with renal agenesis and noncystic renal dysplasia. Pediatrics 1993;91:812–815.

Bernstein J: Developmental abnormalities of the renal parenchyma: Renal hypoplasia and dysplasia. Pathol Annu 1968;3:213–247.

Bonsib SM, Koontz P: Renal maldevelopment: A pediatric renal biopsy study. Mod Pathol 1997;10:1233–1238.

Glassberg KI, Stephens FD, Lebowitz RL, et al: Renal dysgenesis and cystic disease of the kidney: A report of the Committee on Terminology, Nomenclature and Classification, Section on Urology, American Academy of Pediatrics. J Urol 1987;138:1085–1092.

Ichikawa I, Kuwayama F, Pope IV JC, et al: Paradigm shift from classic anatomic theories to contemporary cell biological views of CAKUT. Kidney Int 2002;61:889–898.

Matsell DG: Renal dysplasia: New approaches to an old problem. Am J Kidney Dis 1998;32:535–543.

Murugasu B, Cole BR, Hawkins EP, et al: Familial renal adysplasia. Am J Kidney Dis 1991;18:490–494.

Roodhooft AM, Birnholz JC, Holmes LB: Familial nature of congenital absence and severe dysgenesis of both kidneys. N Eng J Med 1984;310:1341–1345.

Taxy JB: Renal dysplasia: A review. Pathol Annu 1985;20(Pt 2):139–159.

Acquired Renal Cystic Disease

Cheuk W, Lo ES, Chan AK, Chan JK: Atypical epithelial proliferations in acquired renal cystic disease harbor cytogenetic aberrations. Hum Pathol 2002;33:761–765.

Dunnill MS, Millard PR, Oliver D: Acquired cystic disease of the kidneys: A hazard of long-term intermittent maintenance haemodialysis. J Clin Pathol 1977;30:868–877.

Gronwald J, Baur AS, Holtgreve-Grez H, et al: Chromosomal abnormalities in renal cell neoplasms associated with acquired renal cystic disease: A series studied by comparative genomic hybridization and fluorescence in situ hybridization. J Pathol 1999;187:308–312.

Hughson MD, Hennigar GR, McManus JF: Atypical cysts, acquired renal cystic disease, and renal cell tumors in end stage dialysis kidneys. Lab Invest 1980;42:475–480.

Hughson MD, Meloni AM, Silva FG, Sandberg AA: Renal cell carcinoma in an end-stage kidney of a patient with a functional transplant: Cytogenetic and molecular genetic findings. Cancer Genet Cytogenet 1996;89:65–68.

Ishikawa I, Kovacs G: High incidence of papillary renal cell tumours in patients on chronic haemodialysis. Histopathology 1993;22:135–139.

Ishikawa I, Saito Y, Asaka M, et al: Twenty-year follow-up of acquired renal cystic disease. Clin Nephrol 2003;59:153–159.

Maisonneuve P, Agodoa L, Gellert R, et al: Cancer in patients on dialysis for end-stage renal disease: An international collaborative study. Lancet 1999;354:93–99.

Matson MA, Cohen EP: Acquired cystic kidney disease: Occurrence, prevalence, and renal cancers. Medicine (Baltimore) 1990;69:217–226.

Nadasdy T, Laszik Z, Lajoie G, et al. Proliferative activity of cyst epithelium in human renal cystic diseases. J Am Soc Nephrol 1995;5:1462–1468.

Noronha IL, Ritz E, Waldherr R, et al: Renal cell carcinoma in dialysis patients with acquired renal cysts. Nephrol Dial Transplant 1989;4:763–69.

Malrotation

Weyrauch HMJ: Anomalies of renal rotation. Surg Gynecol Obstet 1939;69:183–199.

Renal Ectopia

Aliotta PJ, Seidel FG, Karp M, Greenfield SP: Renal malposition in patients with omphalocele. J Urol 1987;137:942–944.

Hendren WH, Donahoe PK, Pfister RC: Crossed renal ectopia in children. Urology 1976;7:135–144.

Kelalis PP, Malek RS, Segura JW: Observations on renal ectopia and fusion in children. J Urol 1973;110:588–592.

Malter IJ, Stanley RJ: The intrathoracic kidney: with a review of the literature. J Urol 1972;107:538–541.

McDonald JH, McClellan DS: Crossed renal ectopia. Am J Surg 1957;93:995–1002.

Thompson GJ, Pace JM: Ectopic kidney: A review of 97 cases. Surg Gynecol Obstet 1939;69:935–943.

Renal Fusion

Boatman DL, Kolln CP, Flocks RH: Congenital anomalies associated with horseshoe kidney. J Urol 1972;107:205–207.

Zondek LH, Zondek T: Horseshoe kidney and associated congenital malformations. Urol Int 1964;18:347–356.

Renal Agenesis

Acien P, Ruiz JA, Hernandez JF, et al:. Renal agenesis in association with malformation of the female genital tract. Am J Obstet Gynecol 1991;165:1368–1370.

Candiani GB, Fedele L, Candiani M: Double uterus, blind hemivagina, and ipsilateral renal agenesis: 36 Cases and long-term follow-up. Obstet Gynecol 1997;90:26–32.

Cascio S, Paran S, Puri P: Associated urological anomalies in children with unilateral renal agenesis. J Urol 1999;162:1081–1083.

Curry CJ, Jensen K, Holland J, et al: The Potter sequence: A clinical analysis of 80 cases. Am J Med Genet 1984;19:679–702.

Emanual B, Nachman R, Aronson N, Hirshhorn K: Prenatal diagnosis of bilateral renal agenesis. Obstet Gynecol 1977;49:478–480.

Emanuel B, Nachman R, Aronson N, Weiss H: Congenital solitary kidney: A review of 74 cases. Am J Dis Child 1974;127:17–19.

Potter EL: Bilateral absence of ureters and kidneys: A report of 50 cases. Obstet Gynecol 1965;25:3–12.

Roodhooft AM, Birnholz JC, Holmes LB: Familial nature of congenital absence and severe dysgenesis of both kidneys. N Engl J Med 1984;310:1341–1345.

Rush WH Jr,Currie DP: Hemitrigone: Renal agenesis or single ureteral ectopia. Urology 1978;11:161–163.

Thompson DP, Lynn HB: Genital anomalies associated with solitary kidney. Mayo Clin Proc 1966;41:538–548.

Benign and Malignant Nephrosclerosis

Akikusa B, Kondo Y, Irabu N, Shigematsu H: Renal vascular lesions in severe hypertension: Transitional changes from benign to malignant nephrosclerosis. Acta Pathol Jpn 1983;33:323–331.

Kashgarian M: Pathology of small blood vessel disease in hypertension. Am J Kidney Dis 1985;5:A104–A110.

Katafuchi R, Takebayashi S: Morphometrical and functional correlations in benign nephrosclerosis. Clin Nephrol 1987;28:238–243.

MacMahon HE: Malignant nephrosclerosis: A reappraisal. Pathol Annu 1968;3:297–334.

Marcantoni C, Ma LJ, Federspiel C, Fogo AB: Hypertensive nephrosclerosis in African Americans versus Caucasians. Kidney Int 2002;62:172–180.

Ono H, Ono Y: Nephrosclerosis and hypertension. Med Clin North Am 1997;81:1273–1288.

Ruggenenti P, Remuzzi G: Malignant vascular disease of the kidney: Nature of the lesions, mediators of disease progression, and the case for bilateral nephrectomy. Am J Kidney Dis 1996;27:459–475.

Schwartz GL, Strong CG: Renal parenchymal involvement in essential hypertension. Med Clin North Am 1987;71:843–858.

Sommers SC, Melamed J: Renal pathology of essential hypertension. Am J Hypertens 1990;3:583–587.

Vikse BE, Aasarod K, Bostad L, Iversen BM: Clinical prognostic factors in biopsy-proven benign nephrosclerosis. Nephrol Dial Transplant 2003;18:517–23.

Renal Artery Stenosis

Harrison EG Jr, McCormack LJ: Pathologic classification of renal arterial disease in renovascular hypertension. Mayo Clin Proc 1971;46:161–167.

Luscher TF, Lie JT, Stanson AW, et al: Arterial fibromuscular dysplasia. Mayo Clin Proc 1987;62:931–952.

Marcussen N: Atubular glomeruli in renal artery stenosis. Lab Invest 1991;65:558–565.

Olin JW: Renal artery disease: Diagnosis and management. Mt Sinai J Med 2004;71:73–85.

Ratliff NB: Renal vascular disease: Pathology of large blood vessel disease. Am J Kidney Dis 1985;5:A93–A103.

Stimpel M, Groth H, Greminger P, et al: The spectrum of renovascular hypertension. Cardiology 1985;72(Suppl 1):1–9.

Youngberg SP, Sheps SG, Strong CG:. Fibromuscular disease of the renal arteries. Med Clin North Am 1977;61:623–641.

Cortical and Mixed Cortical and Medullary Necrosis

Chugh KS, Jha V, Sakhuja V, Joshi K: Acute renal cortical necrosis: A study of 113 patients. Ren Fail 1994;16:37–47.

Grunfeld JP, Ganeval D, Bournerias F: Acute renal failure in pregnancy. Kidney Int 1980;18:179–191.

Kleinknecht D, Grunfeld JP, Gomez PC, et al: Diagnostic procedures and long-term prognosis in bilateral renal cortical necrosis. Kidney Int 1973;4:390–400.

Lerner GR, Kurnetz R, Bernstein J: Renal cortical and medullary necrosis in the first 3 months of life. Ped Nephrol 1992;6:516–518.

Thurlbeck WM, Castleman B: Atheromatous emboli to the kidneys after aortic surgery. N Engl J Med 1957;257:442–447.

Embolic Renal Disease and Infarcts

Colt HG, Begg RJ, Saporito JJ, et al: Cholesterol emboli after cardiac catheterization: Eight cases and a review of the literature. Medicine (Baltimore) 1988;67:389–400.

Domanovits H, Paulis M, Nikfardjam M, et al: Acute renal infarction: Clinical characteristics of 17 patients. Medicine (Baltimore) 1999;78:386–394.

Fine MJ, Kapoor W, Falanga V: Cholesterol crystal embolization: A review of 221 cases in the English literature. Angiology 1987;38:769–784.

Gasparini M, Hofmann R, Stoller M: Renal artery embolism: Clinical features and therapeutic options. J Urol 1992;147:567–572.

Goldberg G: Renal infarction. Ann Emerg Med 1985;14:611–614.

Jones DB, Iannaccone PM: Atheromatous emboli in renal biopsies: An ultrastructural study. Am J Pathol 1975;78:261–276.

Richards AM, Eliot RS, Kanjuh VL, et al: Cholesterol embolism: A multiple-system disease masquerading as polyarteritis nodosa. Am J Cardiol 1965;15:696–707.

Papillary Necrosis

Eknoyan G, Qunibi WY, Grissom RT, et al: Renal papillary necrosis: An update. Medicine (Baltimore) 1982;61:55–73.

Eknoyan G, Sabatini S: Renal papillary necrosis reappraised. Semin Nephrol 1984;4:3–4.

Griffin MD, Bergstralhn EJ, Larson TS: Renal papillary necrosis: A sixteen-year clinical experience. J Am Soc Nephrol 1995;6:248–256.

Kincaid-Smith P: Pathogenesis of the renal lesion associated with the abuse of analgesics. Lancet 1967;1:859–862.

Zadeii G, Lohr JW: Renal papillary necrosis in a patient with sickle cell trait. J Am Soc Nephrol 1997;8:1034–1039.

Renal Artery Dissection (Dissecting Aneurysm)

Edwards BS, Stanson AW, Holley KE, Sheps SG: Isolated renal artery dissection, presentation, evaluation, management, and pathology. Mayo Clin Proc 1982;57:564–571.

Muller BT, Reiher L, Pfeiffer T, et al: Surgical treatment of renal artery dissection in 25 patients: Indications and results. J Vasc Surg 2003;37:761–768.

Slavis SA, Hodge EE, Novick AC, Maatman T: Surgical treatment for isolated dissection of the renal artery. J Urol 1990;144:233–237.

Renal Artery Aneurysm

Altebarmakian VK, Caldamone AA, Dachelet RJ, May AG: Renal artery aneurysm. Urology 1979;13:257–260.

Poutasse EF: Renal artery aneurysms. J Urol 1975;113:443–449.

Smith JN, Hinman F Jr: Intrarenal arterial aneurysms. J Urol 1967;97:990–996.

Acute Tubular Necrosis

Abuelo JG: Renal failure caused by chemicals, foods, plants, animal venoms, and misuse of drugs: An overview. Arch Intern Med 1990;150:505–510.

Bacchi CE, Rocha N, Carvalho M, et al: Immunohistochemical characterisation of probable intravascular haematopoiesis in the vasa rectae of the renal medulla in acute tubular necrosis. Pathol Res Pract 1994;190:1066–1070.

Bonventre JV: Dedifferentiation and proliferation of surviving epithelial cells in acute renal failure. J Am Soc Nephrol 2003;14(Suppl 1):S55–S61.

Cooper K, Bennett WM: Nephrotoxicity of common drugs used in clinical practice. Arch Intern Med 1987;147:1213–1218.

Haas M, Spargo BH, Wit EJ, Meehan SM: Etiologies and outcome of acute renal insufficiency in older adults: A renal biopsy study of 259 cases. Am J Kidney Dis 2000;35:433–447.

Jao W: Iatrogenic renal disease as revealed by renal biopsy. Semin Diagn Pathol 1988;5:63–79.

Mehta RL, Chertow GM: Acute renal failure definitions and classification: time for change? J Am Soc Nephrol 2003;14:2178–2187.

Nissenson AR: Acute renal failure: Definition and pathogenesis. Kidney Int Suppl 1998;66:S7–S10.

Wan L, Bellomo R, Di Giantomasso D, Ronco C: The pathogenesis of septic acute renal failure. Curr Opin Crit Care 2003;9:496–502.

Acute Interstitial Nephritis

Ito M, Hirabayashi N, Uno Y, et al: Necrotizing tubulointerstitial nephritis associated with adenovirus infection. Hum Pathol 1991;22:1225–1231.

Michel DM, Kelly CJ: Acute interstitial nephritis. J Am Soc Nephrol 1998;9:506–515.

Nasr SH, Koscica J, Markowitz GS, D'Agati VD: Granulomatous interstitial nephritis. Am J Kidney Dis 2003;41:714–719.

Platt JL, Sibley RK, Michael AF: Interstitial nephritis associated with cytomegalovirus infection. Kidney Int 1985;28:550–552.

Rastegar A, Kashgarian M: The clinical spectrum of tubulointerstitial nephritis. Kidney Int 1998;54:313–327.

Rossert J: Drug-induced acute interstitial nephritis. Kidney Int 2001;60:804–817.

Acute Pyelonephritis

Dembry LM, Andriole VT: Renal and perirenal abscesses. Infect Dis Clin North Am 1997;11:663–680.

Edelstein H, McCabe RE: Perinephric abscess: Modern diagnosis and treatment in 47 cases. Medicine (Baltimore) 1988;67:118–131.

Efstathiou SP, Pefanis AV, Tsioulos DI, et al: Acute pyelonephritis in adults: Prediction of mortality and failure of treatment. Arch Intern Med 2003;163:1206–1212.

Huang JJ, Tseng CC: Emphysematous pyelonephritis: Clinicoradiological classification, management, prognosis, and pathogenesis. Arch Intern Med 2000;160:797–805.

Ivanyi B, Rumpelt HJ, Thoenes W: Acute human pyelonephritis: Leukocytic infiltration of tubules and localization of bacteria. Virchows Arch A Pathol Anat Histopathol 1988;414:29–37.

Klein FA, Smith MJ, Vick CW 3rd, Schneider V: Emphysematous pyelonephritis: Diagnosis and treatment. South Med J 1986;79:41–46.

Lin KY, Chiu NT, Chen MJ, et al: Acute pyelonephritis and sequelae of renal scar in pediatric first febrile urinary tract infection. Pediatr Nephrol 2003;18:362–365.

Michaeli J, Mogle P, Perlberg S, et al: Emphysematous pyelonephritis. J Urol 1984;131:203–208.

Roberts JA: Pyelonephritis, cortical abscess, and perinephric abscess. Urol Clin North Am 1986;13:637–645.

Sheinfeld J, Erturk E, Spataro RF, Cockett AT: Perinephric abscess: Current concepts. J Urol 1987;137:191–194.

Shokeir AA, El-Azab M, Mohsen T, El-Diasty T: Emphysematous pyelonephritis: A 15-year experience with 20 cases. Urology 1997;49:343–346.

Thomsen OF, Ladefoged J: Pyelonephritis and interstitial nephritis: Clinical-pathological correlations. Clin Nephrol 2002;58:275–281.

Chronic Pyelonephritis

Arant BS Jr: Vesicoureteric reflux and renal injury. Am J Kidney Dis 1991;17:491–511.

Bailey RR: The relationship of vesico-ureteric reflux to urinary tract infection and chronic pyelonephritis-reflux nephropathy. Clin Nephrol 1973;1:132–141.

Cotran RS: Nephrology forum: Glomerulosclerosis in reflux nephropathy. Kidney Int 1982;21:528–534.

El-Khatib MT, Becker GJ, Kincaid-Smith PS: Reflux nephropathy and primary vesicoureteric reflux in adults. Q J Med 1990;77:1241–1253.

Hodson CJ, Cotran RS: Reflux nephropathy. Hosp Pract (Hosp Ed) 1982;17:133–1335, 138–41, 148–156.

Klahr S: Obstructive nephropathy. Kidney Int 1998;54:286–300.

Tamminen TE, Kaprio EA: The relation of the shape of renal papillae and of collecting duct openings to intrarenal reflux. Br J Urol 1977;49:345–354.

Wan J, Greenfield SP, Ng M, et al: Sibling reflux: A dual center retrospective study. J Urol 1996;156:677–679.

Zucchelli P, Gaggi R: Reflux nephropathy in adults. Nephron 1991;57:2–9.

Xanthogranulomatous Pyelonephritis

Abomelha MS, Shaaban AA, Haleem A, et al: Xanthogranulomatous pyelonephritis: Report of 14 cases. J Urol Pathol 1995;3:213–222.

Antonakopoulos GN, Chapple CR, Newman J, et al: Xanthogranulomatous pyelonephritis: A reappraisal and immunohistochemical study. Arch Pathol Lab Med 1988;112:275–281.

Bingol-Kologlu M, Ciftci AO, Senocak ME, et al: Xanthogranulomatous pyelonephritis in children: Diagnostic and therapeutic aspects. Eur J Pediatr Surg 2002;12:42–48.

Chuang CK, Lai MK, Chang PL, et al: Xanthogranulomatous pyelonephritis: Experience in 36 cases. J Urol 1992;147:333–336.

Cohen MS: Granulomatous nephritis. Urol Clin North Am 1986;13:647–659.

Parsons MA, Harris SC, Longstaff AJ, Grainger RG: Xanthogranulomatous pyelonephritis: A pathological, clinical and aetiological analysis of 87 cases. Diagn Histopathol 1983;6:203–219.

Wise GJ, Silver DA: Fungal infections of the genitourinary system. J Urol 1993;149:1377–1388.

Zorzos I, Moutzouris V, Korakianitis G, Katsou G: Analysis of 39 cases of xanthogranulomatous pyelonephritis with emphasis on CT findings. Scand J Urol Nephrol 2003;37:342–347.

Malakoplakia

al-Sulaiman MH, al-Khader AA, Mousa DH, et al: Renal parenchymal malakoplakia and megalocytic interstitial nephritis: Clinical and histological features. Report of two cases and review of the literature. Am J Nephrol 1993;13:483–488.

August C, Holzhausen HJ, Schroder S: Renal parenchymal malakoplakia: Ultrastructural findings in different stages of morphogenesis. Ultrastruct Pathol 1994;18:483–491.

Dobyan DC, Truong LD, Eknoyan G: Renal malakoplakia reappraised. Am J Kidney Dis 1993;22:243–252.

Esparza AR, McKay DB, Cronan JJ, Chazan JA: Renal parenchymal malakoplakia: Histologic spectrum and its relationship to megalocytic interstitial nephritis and xanthogranulomatous pyelonephritis. Am J Surg Pathol 1989;13:225–236.

Hill GS, Droz D, Nochy D: The woman who loved well but not too wisely, or the vicissitudes of immunosuppression. Am J Kidney Dis 2001;37:1324–1329.

Krupp G, Schneider W, Gobel U, et al: Tumefactive megalocytic interstitial nephritis in a patient with Escherichia coli bacteremia. Am J Kidney Dis 1995;25:928–933.

McClure J: Malakoplakia. J Pathol 1983;140:275–330.

Tam VK, Kung WH, Li R, Chan KW: Renal parenchymal malakoplakia: A rare cause of ARF with a review of recent literature. Am J Kidney Dis 2003;41:E13–E17.

6

Neoplasms of the Kidney

Eyas M. Hattab • Liang Cheng • John N. Eble

Renal Cell Carcinoma

Renal cell carcinomas are tumors that arise from the renal tubular epithelium. Before their origin in the tubules was confirmed, they were thought to arise from adrenal rests and were accordingly termed "hypernephromas." They are, by far, the most common renal cancers, accounting for more than 90% of all malignancies arising in the kidney. Renal cell carcinomas vary greatly in incidence from one region to another, but their significant male predominance is maintained throughout the world. Tobacco smoking, obesity, hypertension, and exposure to environmental chemicals such as arsenic compounds are but a few of the risk factors implicated in the development of renal cancer. Significant advances in ancillary studies, including electron microscopy, immunohistochemistry, molecular genetics, and cytogenetics, led to recognition of many types of renal cell carcinoma, each with its own clinical, histopathologic, and prognostic characteristics. This chapter follows the 2004 World Health Organization (WHO) classification of renal cancers.

CLEAR CELL RENAL CELL CARCINOMA

Clear cell renal cell carcinoma accounts for 60% to 70% of primary renal epithelial tumors.

CLINICAL FEATURES

Clear cell renal carcinoma increases steadily in incidence with age, reaching a plateau in the sixth and seventh decades of life. Men are more often affected than women, with a ratio of approximately 2 to 1. Due largely to improvements in imaging techniques, the classic triad of hematuria, pain, and flank mass is now seen much less frequently than in the past. In approximately 30% of patients, metastatic disease constitutes the initial presentation.

The majority of renal cell carcinomas, including those of the clear cell type, are sporadic; however, hered-

CLEAR CELL RENAL CELL CARCINOMA—FACT SHEET

Definition

▶ The most common variant of renal epithelial tumors, composed of cells with clear or granular-eosinophilic cytoplasm and a prominent but delicate capillary network

Incidence and Location

▶ 2% of all malignancies and about 70% of renal cell carcinomas
▶ Renal cortex, either kidney

Morbidity and Mortality

▶ Approximately 50% of patients die of the disease

Gender, Race, and Age Distribution

▶ Male predominance (M/F ratio, 2:1)
▶ Primarily in adults, sixth to seventh decades

Clinical Features

▶ Hematuria is the single most common presenting sign
▶ Fewer than 10% of patients present with the classic triad of flank mass, pain, and hematuria

Prognosis and Treatment

▶ Surgical excision offers the only hope for cure
▶ Systemic chemotherapy is not effective against advanced disease
▶ 15-20% advanced disease responds to immunotherapy
▶ About half of patients die of the disease

itary forms exist. As a general rule, inherited renal neoplasms manifest at a younger age and are much more likely to be multiple and bilateral. Von Hippel-Lindau (VHL) disease-associated clear cell renal cell carcinomas are the most common. The *VHL* tumor suppressor gene has been mapped to chromosome 3p25 and can be altered by various mutations and loss of heterozygosity. The most common genetic abnormalities encountered in sporadic clear cell renal cell carcinomas involve terminal deletion of the short arm of chromosome 3 (3p) and mutations in the *VHL* gene.

PATHOLOGIC FEATURES

GROSS FINDINGS

Clear cell renal cell carcinomas are ordinarily solitary and randomly distributed throughout the renal cortex. Both kidneys are affected equally. When multiple neoplasms occur, carcinoma is often accompanied by a papillary adenoma. Bilateral lesions are less common, accounting for 0.5% to 3.0% of cases. As mentioned earlier, multicentricity and/or bilaterality should raise suspicion of a familial condition.

The typical appearance of renal cell carcinoma of the clear cell type is that of a well-circumscribed, rounded, lobulated mass usually protruding from the renal cortex (Fig. 6-1). Cysts are very common. Foci of hemorrhage, necrosis, and calcification are often present. A golden-yellow appearance is usually imparted by a rich lipid content of tumor cells. Higher-grade tumors may not be as yellow, because they contain less lipid and glycogen.

MICROSCOPIC FINDINGS

Clear cell renal cell carcinoma is characterized by alveolar nests and sheets of carcinoma cells interspersed by a prominent network of delicate blood vessels (Fig. 6-2A and B). It can also grow in various other architectural patterns, including wide trabecular (Fig. 6-2C), tubular (Fig. 6-2D), microcystic filled with either eosinophilic proteinaceous fluid or fresh hemorrhage (Fig. 6-2E), and, infrequently, pseudopapillary (Fig. 6-2F). Using the usual histologic preparation methods, the lipid content of tumor cells is dissolved away, leaving behind an empty "clear cell" cytoplasm surrounded by a distinct cell membrane (Fig. 6-2B). Such neutral lipids can be identified in unfixed tissues using oil red O and Sudan IV reaction. Periodic acid-Schiff (PAS) stain demonstrates the abundant glycogen.

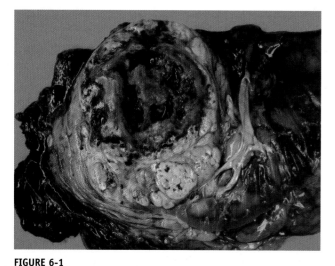

FIGURE 6-1

This clear cell renal cell carcinoma is well-circumscribed, with central necrosis and hemorrhage.

CLEAR CELL RENAL CELL CARCINOMA—PATHOLOGIC FEATURES

Gross Findings

► Solitary renal cortical mass
► Well-circumscribed, lobulated
► Golden yellow
► Necrosis and hemorrhage

Microscopic Findings

► Nests and sheets of clear cells
► Delicate vascular network
► Occasionally pseudopapillary, tubular, trabecular, microcystic, or sarcomatoid pattern

Ultrastructural Features

► Abundant cytoplasmic lipid and glycogen
► Tubular differentiation: microlumens, microvilli, and brush border

Fine-needle Aspiration Biopsy Findings

► Cohesive nests of clear cells with delicate capillaries

Immunohistochemical Findings

► Cam5.2, AE1-AE3, EMA, vimentin, RCC and CD10 positive
► Keratin 34βE12 negative, only rarely S-100 or CEA positive

Differential Diagnosis

► Chromophobe renal cell carcinoma
► Papillary renal cell carcinoma
► Adrenocortical carcinoma
► Epithelioid angiomyolipoma
► Metastatic carcinoma

Aggregates of cells with granular or eosinophilic cytoplasm are more frequent in higher-grade carcinomas. Brightly eosinophilic, PAS-positive hyalin globules, both intracytoplasmic and extracytoplasmic, may be seen. Sarcomatoid change is found in about 5% of the cases and universally implies a worse prognosis. Not to be confused with rhabdoid tumors of the kidney, rhabdoid cells with large eccentric nuclei, macronucleoli, and prominent acidophilic globular cytoplasm are also seen in a small proportion of clear cell renal cell carcinomas (Fig. 6-2G). These tumors tend to have a disproportionately higher frequency of sarcomatoid component.

GRADING

Nuclear grade is second only to stage as the most significant prognostic indicator in renal cell carcinoma. Although grading was originally devised for the clear cell variant, it has proved useful for papillary and chromophobe carcinomas as well. Three- and four-tiered grading systems exist. The four-tiered Fuhrman system employs nuclear size, nuclear shape, chromatin pattern, and nucleolar prominence. Under a 10× objective lens, grade 1 cells display small nuclei, dense chromatin, and inconspicuous nucleoli closely resembling those of lymphocytes (Fig. 6-3A). Grade 2 cells have finely granular chromatin but small nucleoli that are not discernible at

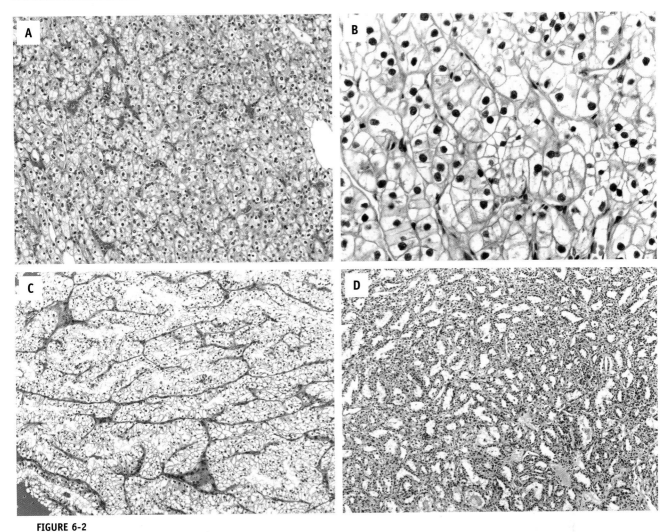

FIGURE 6-2

A, A typical clear cell renal cell carcinoma contains solid nests of clear cells separated by a prominent delicate vascular network. **B,** Tumor cells have water-clear cytoplasm surrounded by a distinct cell membrane. Other architectural patterns include wide trabecular (**C**) and tubular (**D**).

Continued

10× magnification (Fig. 6-3B). On the other hand, the nucleoli of grade 3 cells should be easily detected at this magnification (Fig. 6-3C). Grade 4 cells show prominent nuclear pleomorphism, hyperchromasia, and macronucleoli (Fig. 6-3D). Consensus is that grading should be based on the worst areas, not counting scattered cells. The large majority of clear cell carcinomas are Fuhrman grades 2 and 3. Renal cell carcinoma with sarcomatoid change is currently graded as grade 4.

ANCILLARY STUDIES

ULTRASTRUCTURAL FEATURES

Electron microscopic examination reveals abundant cytoplasmic glycogen and lipid droplets. Evidence of tubular differentiation, including microvilli and brush border, may also be identified.

IMMUNOHISTOCHEMISTRY

Clear cell renal cell carcinomas are commonly reactive for brush border antigens, low-molecular-weight cytokeratins (LMWCKs), and vimentin. High-molecular weight cytokeratins (HMWCKs) are rarely expressed. Most react with epithelial membrane antigen (EMA), RCC marker (RCC Ma), CD10, CD68, MUC1, and MUC3. Placental alkaline phosphatase (PLAP) is also frequently detected. Only rarely are tumors reactive for S-100, α-fetoprotein (AFP), or carcinoembryonic antigen (CEA).

FINE-NEEDLE ASPIRATION BIOPSY

Cohesive nests of fairly uniform cells with pale-staining cytoplasm in association with fine capillaries are characteristic. Tumor cells typically show well-defined cell membranes, round nuclei, and small nucleoli.

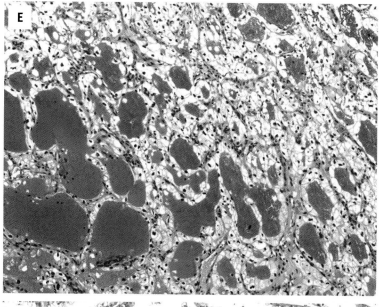

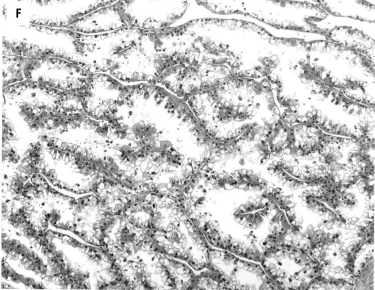

FIGURE 6-2, CONT'D

Microcysts filled with blood (**E**), and infrequently pseudo-papillae (**F**), can be present. **G,** Occasionally, tumor cells assume rhabdoid morphology with large eccentric nuclei, macronucleoli, and prominent acidophilic globular cytoplasm.

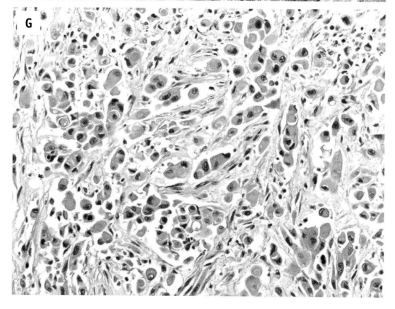

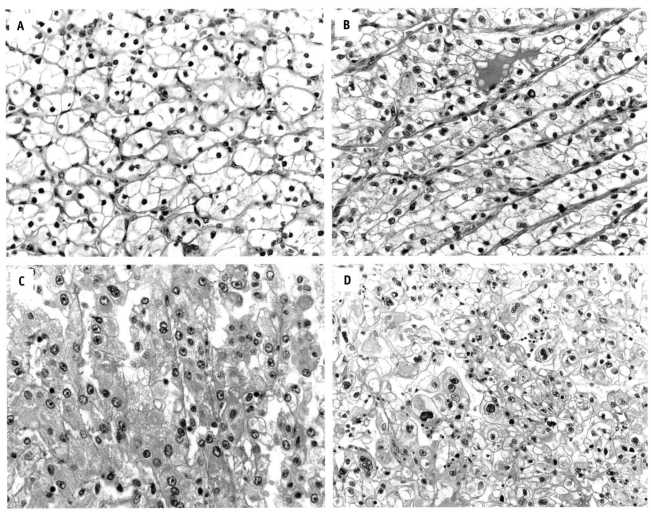

FIGURE 6-3
Fuhrman nuclear grading: **A**, grade 1; **B**, grade 2; **C**, grade 3; **D**, grade 4.

DIFFERENTIAL DIAGNOSIS

Some clear cell renal cell carcinomas demonstrate a focal "pseudopapillary" growth pattern secondary to tumor cell dropout sparing the cells at the periphery of blood vessels. Unlike papillary renal carcinoma, histiocytes and intracellular hemosiderin are usually absent from the papillae. Classic clear cell foci are usually evident elsewhere, but, if necessary, CK7 may be useful in some cases, because it often is expressed in papillary renal cell carcinoma but not in clear cell renal cell carcinoma.

Chromophobe renal cell carcinoma can be distinguished from clear cell renal cell carcinoma by its gross appearance and characteristic microscopic features. Chromophobe renal cell carcinoma manifests as a nonencapsulated mass with a homogeneous, light tan cut surface. The cytoplasm of tumor cells is not "clear" but rather translucent and reticulated. In most cases, the impression of chromophobe renal cell carcinoma can be confirmed by a positive Hale's colloidal iron stain. Electron microscopy is rarely necessary.

Adrenocortical carcinoma may enter into the differential diagnosis of clear cell renal cell carcinoma. Adrenocortical carcinomas do not stain for epithelial membrane antigen (EMA) and are negative for most cytokeratins, but their expression of inhibin, which is negative in renal cell carcinomas, is consistent.

Other potential entities include epithelioid angiomyolipoma and metastatic carcinoma. Ultimately, adequate sampling is paramount in all cases and should significantly reduce the need for ancillary studies. Should morphologic and immunohistochemical studies prove inconclusive, genetic analysis may provide some answers, because the various types of renal cell carcinomas exhibit their own sets of genetic abnormalities.

PROGNOSIS AND TREATMENT

Treatment options for renal cell carcinomas, including the clear cell type, are limited. Until now, early detection and surgical resection offered the best, and perhaps only, hope for cure. Given recent improvements in diagnostic techniques, tumors are increasingly detected in the early stages of disease, making conservative surgical excision (e.g., nephron-sparing surgeries) possible. Systemic treatment of metastatic clear cell renal cell carcinomas is not effective. Only 15-20% of advanced-stage disease responds to immunotherapy.

Tumor stage is the single most important criterion influencing prognosis in renal cell carcinoma. Other factors include nuclear grade, margin status, and histologic type. The overall survival rate for patients with the clear cell variant after nephrectomy is about 50%.

MULTILOCULAR CYSTIC RENAL CELL CARCINOMA

The diagnosis of multilocular cystic renal cell carcinoma is reserved for a rare subset of clear cell renal cell carcinomas which are entirely cystic and in which the septa between the cysts contain small clusters of clear cells that are indistinguishable from grade 1 clear cell carcinoma.

CLINICAL FEATURES

The presentation and demographic features of patients with multilocular cystic renal cell carcinoma are no different from those of patients with the clear cell type.

PATHOLOGIC FEATURES

GROSS FINDINGS

These tumors are well-circumscribed masses of variably sized cysts filled with serous or hemorrhagic fluid; they have fibrous septa and are surrounded by a fibrous pseudocapsule (Fig. 6-4). Solid expansile nodules of carcinoma are not present. Calcification, sometimes in the form of osseous metaplasia, is present in approximately 20% of the tumors.

MICROSCOPIC FINDINGS

The cysts are usually lined by a single layer of attenuated flat or plump epithelial cells with clear to pale cytoplasm (Fig. 6-5A). Occasionally, the lining is absent or is made up of several layers of cells. The nuclei almost always are small and spherical and have dense

chromatin (Fig. 6-5B). The fibrotic and often densely collagenous septa contain occasional small aggregates of epithelial cells with clear cytoplasm closely resembling those cells lining the cysts. The small collections of clear cells are accompanied by increased vascularity and are never in the form of solid expansile nodules.

ANCILLARY STUDIES

IMMUNOHISTOCHEMISTRY

The clusters of epithelial cells within the septa react with antibodies to cytokeratins and EMA but not histiocytic markers.

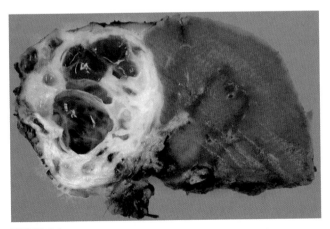

FIGURE 6-4

Multilocular cystic renal cell carcinoma, showing a well-circumscribed mass with variably sized cysts containing serous fluid.

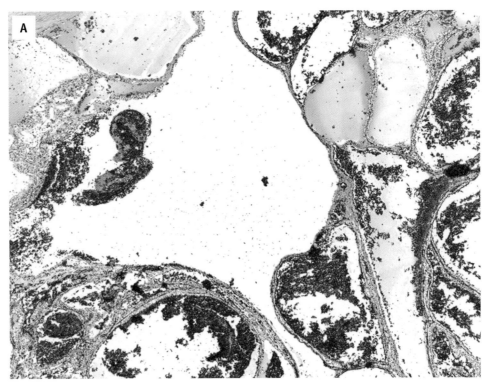

FIGURE 6-5
This multilocular cystic renal cell carcinoma is multicystic with thin, fibrous septae (**A**) which are lined with clear cells with grade 1 nuclei (**B**).

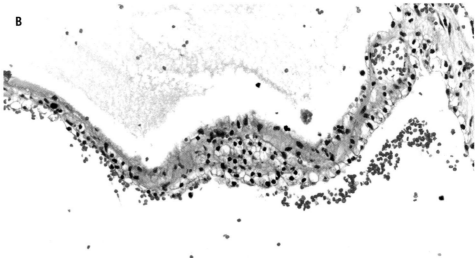

DIFFERENTIAL DIAGNOSIS

Multilocular cystic renal cell carcinomas are distinguished from multilocular renal cysts (cystic nephromas) by the presence of clusters of clear cells within the fibrous septa. The lining epithelium is not a reliable feature to separate the two. Immunostains for cytokeratin and EMA may be useful in highlighting the cancerous cells.

Because of their excellent outcome, multilocular cystic renal cell carcinomas must be distinguished from other clear cell renal cell carcinomas. Although cystic change is common in clear cell renal cell carcinoma, such tumors almost always contain expansive nodules of carcinoma. The presence of solid tumor nodules of any size should automatically disqualify any given cystic renal neoplasm from the diagnosis of multilocular cystic renal cell carcinoma.

PROGNOSIS AND TREATMENT

This type of renal cell carcinoma is so far always cured by surgical excision.

MULTILOCULAR CYSTIC RENAL CELL CARCINOMA—PATHOLOGIC FEATURES

Gross Findings
- ▶ Well-circumscribed mass of small and large cysts
- ▶ Serous or hemorrhagic content
- ▶ Occasionally calcified

Microscopic Findings
- ▶ Cysts lined by single layer of cells
- ▶ Small collections of clear epithelial cells within fibrous septa
- ▶ No expansive nodules of tumor cells

Immunohistochemical Findings
- ▶ Identical to clear cell variant of renal cell carcinoma

Differential Diagnosis
- ▶ Cystic nephroma
- ▶ Renal cell caracinoma with extensive cystic change

PAPILLARY RENAL CELL CARCINOMA—FACT SHEET

Definition
- ▶ Renal carcinoma with papillary or tubulopapillary architecture, at least 0.5 cm in greatest dimension

Incidence and Location
- ▶ Comprises approximately 10-15% of all renal cell carcinomas

Morbidity and Mortality
- ▶ 5-year survival ranges between 49% and 84% for both types
- ▶ Longer survival rates for type 1 tumors

Gender, Race, and Age Distribution
- ▶ Similar to clear cell renal cell carcinoma

Clinical Features
- ▶ More likely to be bilateral or multiple than other renal cell carcinomas

Prognosis and Treatment
- ▶ Significantly better outcome than that of the clear cell type
- ▶ Type 1 tumors behave less aggressively than type 2

PAPILLARY RENAL CELL CARCINOMA

Only papillary renal tumors larger than 0.5 cm are classified as carcinoma. Smaller lesions are best classified as papillary adenomas.

CLINICAL FEATURES

Papillary renal cell carcinomas show age and sex distributions similar to those for clear cell renal cell carcinoma. The majority of patients present with unilateral lesions, although, compared with other types of renal cell carcinomas, papillary renal cell carcinoma is more likely to be bilateral or multifocal. An autosomal dominant hereditary form of papillary renal cancer, characterized by late onset with bilateral and multiple tumors, has been identified. In sporadic papillary renal cell carcinoma, trisomy of chromosomes 7 and 17 and loss of chromosome Y are the most common genetic alterations. Hereditary papillary renal cell carcinoma manifests a germline mutation of the *c-met* gene.

PATHOLOGIC FEATURES

GROSS FINDINGS

Most papillary renal cell carcinomas manifest as well-circumscribed, discrete renal cortical masses containing foci of hemorrhage and necrosis. A surrounding fibrous pseudocapsule often is present (Fig. 6-6). The tumors vary greatly in size, and in one series more than

50% were larger than 6 cm in diameter. The number of foamy macrophages and the extent of hemosiderin deposition and hemorrhage influence the color of these tumors. As mentioned earlier, multifocality is more common in papillary renal cell carcinoma than in other types.

MICROSCOPIC FINDINGS

Papillary renal cell carcinoma comprises variable proportions of papillae and tubulopapillary structures

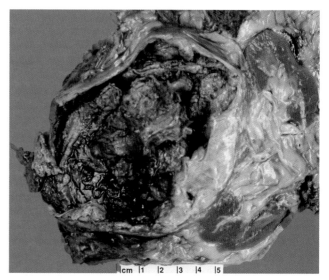

FIGURE 6-6
A fibrous pseudocapsule is a frequent finding in the papillary variant of renal cell carcinoma. Note the extensive hemorrhage and necrosis.

PAPILLARY RENAL CELL CARCINOMA—PATHOLOGIC FEATURES

Gross Findings

▶ Solitary, well-circumscribed cortical mass
▶ Fibrous pseudocapsule
▶ Necrosis and hemorrhage

Microscopic Findings

▶ Papillae with true fibrovascular cores
▶ Type 1: single layer of cells, usually low-grade nuclear features
▶ Type 2: pseudostratified nuclei, usually high-grade nuclear features

Ultrastructural Features

▶ Not helpful

Fine-needle Aspiration Biopsy Findings

▶ Papillary clusters in a background of necrosis

Immunohistochemical Findings

▶ Pancytokeratin and LMWCK positive
▶ HMWCK (34βE12) usually negative
▶ CK7 expressed in 87% of type 1 and 20% of type 2 tumors

Differential Diagnosis

▶ Papillary adenoma
▶ Clear cell renal cell carcinoma with pseudopapillary growth pattern
▶ Collecting duct carcinoma

(Fig. 6-7A,B). Identification of fibrovascular cores is the key to the diagnosis, because other variants of renal cell carcinoma may contain "pseudopapillary" areas. Tightly compact growth of papillae may impart a solid appearance (Fig. 6-7C). Collections of foamy macrophages expanding papillary cores are characteristic (Fig. 6-7B). Psammoma bodies are common (Fig. 6-7D). Sarcomatoid change occurs in approximately 5% of papillary renal cell carcinomas.

Two types of papillary renal cell carcinoma (type 1 and type 2) are recognized and have been shown to have slightly different prognoses. Papillary renal cell carcinoma, type 1, accounts for approximately two thirds of all papillary renal cell carcinomas and is composed of papillae covered by a single layer of small cells and scanty, pale cytoplasm and nuclei rather uniformly lying near the basement membrane (Fig. 6-7A,B). Papillary renal cell carcinoma, type 2, is composed of papillae covered by single layers of cells with more abundant, typically eosinophilic cytoplasm and pseudostratified nuclei (Fig. 6-7E). The Fuhrman nuclear grading system appears to stratify papillary renal cell carcinoma usefully.

ANCILLARY STUDIES

ULTRASTRUCTURAL FEATURES

Electron microscopic examination is not particularly useful.

IMMUNOHISTOCHEMISTRY

Papillary renal cell carcinomas are usually strongly reactive with antibodies to pancytokeratins and LMWCKs but only rarely with antibodies to HMWCKs. CK7 expression is more frequent in type 1 (87%) than in type 2 (20%). Reactivity for vimentin and EMA is variable and inconsistent. CD9 and CD10 are both expressed in papillary renal cell carcinoma.

FINE-NEEDLE ASPIRATION BIOPSY

In the proper clinical setting, papillary clusters in a background of necrosis are diagnostic. Foamy macrophages and intracellular hemosiderin are commonly found. Cellular features are largely dependent on the subtype.

DIFFERENTIAL DIAGNOSIS

Lesions smaller than 5 mm have been designated papillary adenomas, whereas 5 mm or larger are classified as carcinomas. Papillary renal cell carcinoma can be confused with clear cell renal cell carcinoma exhibiting a pseudopapillary growth pattern. Such pseudopapillae are typically devoid of the fibrovascular cores of papillary carcinomas. Clear cell renal cell carcinoma is also much less likely to show calcification, cytoplasmic hemosiderin, and islands of foamy macrophages expanding papillae. Additionally, CK7 expression is virtually lacking in clear cell renal cell carcinoma but is frequently seen in the papillary variant, especially type 1.

Collecting duct carcinoma with papillary features can be distinguished from papillary renal cell carcinoma by its medullary location in the kidney, its high-grade features, and intracytoplasmic and luminal mucin. In contrast to collecting duct carcinoma, papillary renal cell carcinoma rarely demonstrates a desmoplastic stroma. Immunohistochemically, unlike most papillary renal cell carcinomas, collecting duct carcinoma reacts with CEA and HMWCKs.

PROGNOSIS AND TREATMENT

The prognosis for papillary renal cell carcinoma is significantly better than that for the clear cell type and similar to that of chromophobe renal cell carcinoma.

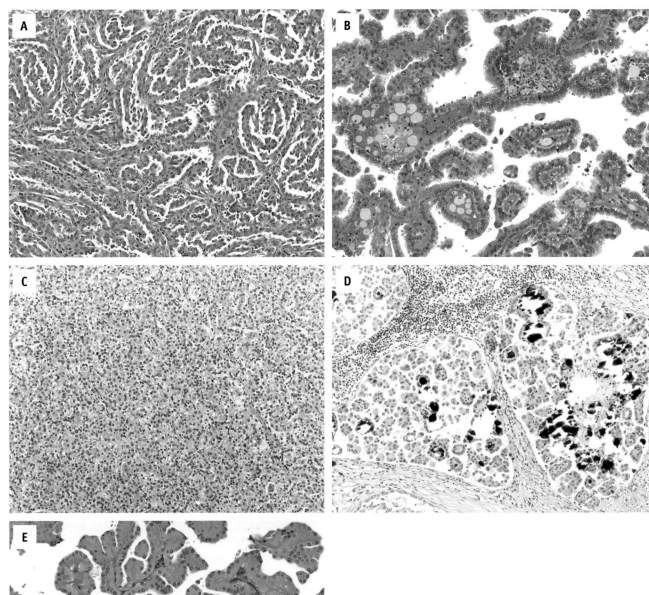

FIGURE 6-7

A, Tightly packed tubulopapillary structures characterize this papillary renal cell carcinoma, type 1. **B,** Note the aggregates of macrophages and prominent papillary structures in a type 1 papillary renal cell carcinoma showing grade 3 nuclei. **C,** Tightly compact growth of papillae may impart a solid appearance. **D,** Psammomatous calcification is also common. **E,** Type 2 papillary renal cell carcinoma showing prominent fibrovascular cores.

Tubulo cystic Carcinoma of Kidney
rare ... comprised of tubules & cysts
lined by eosinophilic / hob nail/
focally clear cells.

Extensive necrosis and abundance of foamy macrophages have been linked to improved outcome. Longer survival times have been demonstrated for type 1 tumors compared with type 2 papillary renal cell carcinoma.

CHROMOPHOBE RENAL CELL CARCINOMA

Chromophobe renal cell carcinomas make up approximately 5% of renal cell neoplasms in surgical series. The intercalated cells of the renal collecting ducts, which are also believed to give rise to oncocytoma, have been proposed as the cells from which chromophobe renal cell carcinoma arises.

CLINICAL FEATURES

There are no signs or symptoms specific to chromophobe renal cell carcinoma, and the demographic characteristics of patients with chromophobe renal cell carcinoma are similar to those of patients with clear cell renal cell carcinoma. Familial chromophobe renal cell carcinoma has been reported in the Birt-Hogg-Dubé syndrome. Chromophobe renal cell carcinomas typically have losses of multiple whole chromosomes, most frequently from among 1, 2, 6, 10, 13, 17, and 21.

CHROMOPHOBE RENAL CELL CARCINOMA—FACT SHEET

Definition
▶ A malignant renal parenchymal tumor with large pale cells and prominent cell membranes, thought to arise from the intercalated cells of renal collecting ducts

Incidence and Location
▶ 5% of all renal cell carcinomas
▶ Lower pole of kidney

Morbidity and Mortality
▶ Fewer than 10% of patients die of the disease

Gender, Race, and Age Distribution
▶ Similar to clear cell renal cell carcinoma

Clinical Features
▶ Indistinguishable from clear cell renal cell carcinoma

Prognosis and Treatment
▶ Most patients are cured by nephrectomy
▶ Sarcomatoid phenotype associated with aggressive behavior

PATHOLOGIC FEATURES

GROSS FINDINGS

Chromophobe renal cell carcinomas are often spherical, well-circumscribed, pseudoencapsulated masses with homogeneous tan or light brown cut surfaces (Fig. 6-8).

MICROSCOPIC FINDINGS

A solid growth pattern predominates, but a focal glandular component may be present. The nuclear contours may be spherical or irregular, are slightly pleomorphic, and are often wrinkled. Most chromophobe renal cell carcinomas are nuclear grade 2, but some are grade 3 or 4. We have never seen a chromophobe renal cell carcinoma of nuclear grade 1. Unlike clear cell renal cell carcinoma, the blood vessels often are thick-walled and hyalinized. Irregular aggregates of finely granular calcium deposits and small numbers of psammoma bodies are common. Two forms of chromophobe renal cell carcinoma are recognized: classic and eosinophilic. The cells of the classic type range from very large round to medium size and are polygonal with prominent cell borders and pale cytoplasm, which often has clumps of pink material in it (Fig. 6-9A). Frequently, there is also a population of smaller cells with granular, eosinophilic cytoplasm. When the tumor is entirely composed of eosinophilic cells, it is diagnosed as the eosinophilic variant of chromophobe renal cell carcinoma (Fig. 6-9B). Hale's colloidal iron stain diffusely colors the cytoplasm of the carcinoma cells blue (Fig. 6-9C). Chromophobe renal cell carcinoma undergoes sarcomatoid change in approximately 5% of cases (Fig. 6-9D).

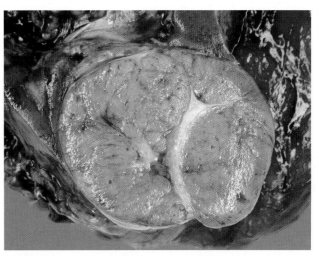

FIGURE 6-8
Chromophobe renal cell carcinoma, showing a well-circumscribed spherical mass with tan, homogenous, fleshy consistency and a central scar.

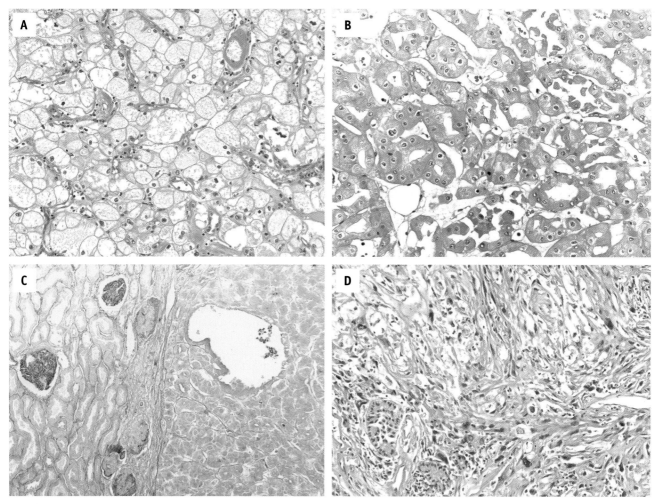

FIGURE 6-9

A, The classic form of chromophobe renal cell carcinoma is made up of large round cells with well defined borders and a finely reticulated cytoplasm. Often, there is also a population of smaller cells with granular, eosinophilic cytoplasm. **B,** The eosinophilic variant is composed entirely of eosinophilic cells. **C,** Hale's colloidal iron stain diffusely colors the cytoplasm of the carcinoma cells blue. Glomeruli in the same figure serve as a positive internal control, and renal tubules as negative internal control. **D,** A sarcomatoid component may be seen in approximately 5% of chromophobe renal cell carcinoma.

ANCILLARY STUDIES

ULTRASTRUCTURAL FEATURES

Abundant round to oval cytoplasmic microvesicles, 150 to 300 nm in diameter, are characteristic. Tissue processing for paraffin embedding dissolves the vesicles, so ultrastructural examination must be done on glutaraldehyde-fixed samples. The eosinophilic cells show abundant mitochondria and fewer microvesicles.

IMMUNOHISTOCHEMISTRY

Antibody to CK7 is useful in diagnosing chromophobe renal cell carcinoma. It typically reacts strongly with the great majority of cells, and the reaction is accentuated at the cell membrane (Fig. 6-10).

FINE-NEEDLE ASPIRATION BIOPSY

Cytologically, clusters and individual cells characterized by reticular or granular cytoplasm and thick cell membranes are typical. The nuclei are variable in size, have irregular contours, and may be binucleated. Hale's colloidal iron stain may be applied to cytology specimens.

DIFFERENTIAL DIAGNOSIS

Classic chromophobe renal cell carcinoma often can be diagnosed with confidence on sections stained with hematoxylin and eosin. Clear cell renal cell carcinoma occasionally enters into the differential diagnosis of

CHROMOPHOBE RENAL CELL CARCINOMA—PATHOLOGIC FEATURES

Gross Findings

▶ Solitary, spherical, well-circumscribed mass
▶ Pseudocapsule
▶ Homogenous, tan or light brown cut surface

Microscopic Findings

▶ Classic: finely reticulated pale cytoplasm with prominent cell membrane
▶ Eosinophilic: smaller cells with granular eosinophilic cytoplasm
▶ Thick hyalinized blood vessels
▶ Calcification, including psammoma bodies are common
▶ Positive Hale's colloidal iron stain

Ultrastructural Features

▶ Abundant cytoplasmic microvesicles
▶ Eosinophilic variant: abundant mitochondria, few microvesicles
▶ Not useful in paraffin-embedded tissue

Fine-needle Aspiration Biopsy Findings

▶ Cells with reticulated/granular cytoplasm and thick cell borders
▶ Irregular, variable-size nuclei, sometimes binucleate
▶ Positive Hale's colloidal iron stain

Immunohistochemical Findings

▶ Positive CK7, accentuated at the cell membrane

Differential Diagnosis

▶ Clear cell renal cell carcinoma
▶ Oncocytoma

chromophobe renal cell carcinoma, and the correct diagnosis is usually achieved by adequate sampling, the use of Hale's colloidal iron stain, or electron microscopy.

Eosinophilic chromophobe renal cell carcinoma closely resembles renal oncocytoma. Hale's colloidal iron stain is negative in oncocytomas, and in oncocytoma only scattered cells or small clumps of cells react with antibody to CK7.

PROGNOSIS AND TREATMENT

Most patients with chromophobe renal cell carcinoma are cured by nephrectomy. The majority of patients who do poorly have a sarcomatoid component. However, cases have been recorded in which metastases had occurred but sarcomatoid change was absent. There are no clinical differences between the classic and eosinophilic variants.

CARCINOMA OF THE COLLECTING DUCTS OF BELLINI

Thought to originate from the principal cells of the collecting ducts of Bellini in the renal medulla, collecting duct carcinoma comprises 0.1% of renal cell neoplasms in surgical series.

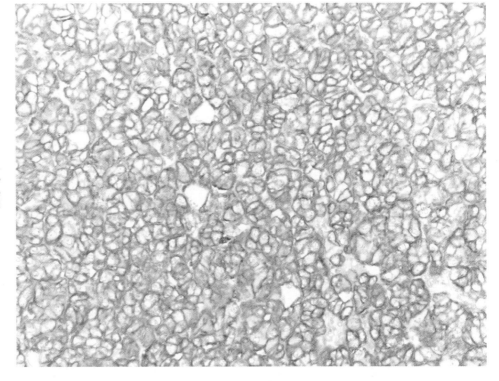

FIGURE 6-10

In chromophobe renal cell carcinoma, cytokeratin 7 stain typically reacts strongly with most of the cells, and the reaction is accentuated at the cell membrane.

CLINICAL FEATURES

A wide age range at presentation (13 to 83 years) has been described. Some authors believe that these tumors tend to afflict younger patients, with a mean age of 34 years. Because of the high-grade nature of collecting duct carcinoma, presentation with the classic triad of flank mass, pain, and hematuria is not uncommon. One third to one half of all patients have metastatic disease at the time of detection. Genetic data on collecting duct carcinoma are sparse; however, initial reports show deletions involving chromosomes 1, 6, 8, 14, 15, 21, and 22. Amplifications of *ERBB2* (*Her2/neu*) have been detected.

PATHOLOGIC FEATURES

GROSS FINDINGS

Small collecting duct carcinomas can be seen to arise in a medullary pyramid. However, most collecting duct carcinomas are large, infiltrative masses involving both the cortex and medulla. On cut surface, the tumor is firm and light gray to tan-white, with invasive borders. Hemorrhage, necrosis, and cystic changes are common.

MICROSCOPIC FINDINGS

Collecting duct carcinoma is composed of complex, highly infiltrative cords or tubular structures embedded in inflamed desmoplastic stroma (Fig. 6-11). Small cysts

---

CARCINOMA OF THE COLLECTING DUCTS OF BELLINI—FACT SHEET

Definition
► A rare malignant renal epithelial tumor arising from the cells of the collecting ducts of renal medulla

Incidence and Location
► Comprises approximately 0.1% of renal cell carcinomas

Morbidity and Mortality
► One half to two thirds of patients die within the first 2 years

Gender, Race, and Age Distribution
► Wide age range (13-83 years), possibly younger patients

Clinical Features
► Flank mass, pain, and hematuria

Prognosis and Treatment
► Poor prognosis; worse than clear cell variant

---

form from dilation of the tubular structures. A single layer of cuboidal to columnar cells with predominantly eosinophilic cytoplasm and often with hobnail morphology lines the tubules and cysts. The nuclei are large and pleomorphic, with prominent nucleoli and coarse chromatin. Mitotic figures often are numerous. Sometimes, the epithelium lining collecting ducts elsewhere in the kidney appears dysplastic. Sarcomatoid change is common in collecting duct carcinomas.

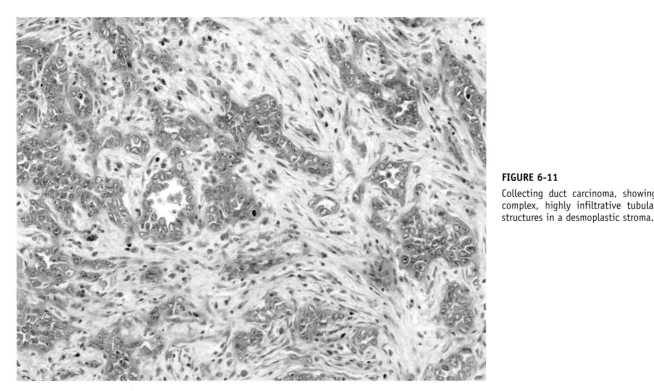

FIGURE 6-11
Collecting duct carcinoma, showing complex, highly infiltrative tubular structures in a desmoplastic stroma.

CARCINOMA OF THE COLLECTING DUCTS OF BELLINI— PATHOLOGIC FEATURES

Gross Findings

▶ Medullary location
▶ Light gray to white cut surface, with invasive borders
▶ Necrosis, hemorrhage and cystic changes

Microscopic Findings

▶ Tubular/tubulopapillary structure with tapered ends
▶ Desmoplastic stroma
▶ High-grade nuclear features, brisk mitosis
▶ Cytoplasmic mucin

Ultrastructural Features

▶ Well-formed cell junctions, short apical microvilli, and prominent basal lamina

Fine-needle Aspiration Biopsy Findings

▶ Cohesive nests of cells with glandular features and high-grade nuclear morphology resembling metastatic carcinoma

Immunohistochemical Findings

▶ LMWCK and HMWCK, CK7, CEA, PNA, and UEA positive
▶ CD10 negative

Differential Diagnosis

▶ Papillary renal cell carcinoma
▶ Urothelial carcinoma with glandular features
▶ Renal medullary carcinoma
▶ Metastatic carcinoma

ANCILLARY STUDIES

ULTRASTRUCTURAL FEATURES

The tumor cells feature short apical microvilli and a prominent basal lamina. They contain well-formed cell junctions.

IMMUNOHISTOCHEMISTRY

There is no specific immunoprofile for collecting duct carcinomas. Most stain for LMWCK and broad-spectrum cytokeratins, CEA, peanut lectin agglutinin (PNA), and *Ulex europaeus* agglutinin (UEA). The majority expresses the HMWCKs 34βE12 and CK7. CD10 is negative.

FINE-NEEDLE ASPIRATION BIOPSY

Cohesive nests of tumor cells with glandular features and individual cells characterized by large, irregular, hyperchromatic nuclei with vesicular chromatin and macronucleoli are seen in aspirate samples. The cytoplasm is usually eosinophilic and finely vacuolated. Intracytoplasmic mucin may also be seen.

DIFFERENTIAL DIAGNOSIS

The differential diagnosis includes papillary renal cell carcinoma (discussed earlier), urothelial carcinoma with glandular differentiation, medullary carcinoma, and metastatic carcinoma. Urothelial carcinoma presents the most difficult challenge, because it shares many features with collecting duct carcinoma, such as the propensity to form tubular glands, desmoplastic stroma, tumor cells in adjacent collecting tubules, and intra-cytoplasmic mucin. Additionally, the immunohisto-chemical profiles are similar. The finding of in situ urothelial carcinoma within adjacent calyces or in the renal pelvis is supportive of the diagnosis of urothelial carcinoma.

PROGNOSIS AND TREATMENT

The majority of collecting duct carcinomas are high-grade neoplasms that carry a significantly higher mortality rate than most types of renal cell carcinoma. One half to two thirds of patients die within the first 2 years after diagnosis. Lymph node and visceral metastases are common, and bony metastasis is usually osteoblastic.

RENAL MEDULLARY CARCINOMA

This is a rapidly growing, highly aggressive renal cell carcinoma involving the medulla. It has a strong association with sickle cell trait and possibly arises from the distal portions of the collecting ducts.

CLINICAL FEATURES

Affected individuals are children and young adults with sickle cell trait. Patients have a reported age range of 11 to 39 years and a mean of 22 years. There is male predilection at a ratio of 2:1. Most patients present with advanced disease.

PATHOLOGIC FEATURES

GROSS FINDINGS

Renal medullary carcinoma appears as a solitary, poorly circumscribed mass with infiltrative borders centered in the medulla. The reported size varies from 4 to 12cm (mean, 7 cm). The cut surface is gray-white with extensive foci of hemorrhage and necrosis.

MICROSCOPIC FINDINGS

This is a poorly differentiated neoplasm made up of cells with eosinophilic or amphophilic cytoplasm arranged in solid sheets often punctuated by circular holes, giving a lace-like appearance. The nests of carcinoma cells are embedded in a desmoplastic stroma (Fig. 6-12), which is infiltrated by polymorphonuclear granulocytes and lymphocytes. The neoplastic nuclei are large and have prominent nucleoli. Occasionally, cells have a rhabdoid or squamoid appearance. Sickled erythrocytes may be recognizable within the blood vessels.

ANCILLARY STUDIES

IMMUNOHISTOCHEMISTRY

The tumor cells are positive for keratin AE1-AE3 and variably reactive for EMA and CEA. They are negative for HMWCK.

DIFFERENTIAL DIAGNOSIS

The distinctive clinical features of renal medullary carcinoma are extremely important in distinguishing it from morphologically similar renal tumors; namely collecting duct carcinoma and certain types of urothelial carcinoma. Immunohistochemical and ultrastructural features are rarely helpful.

PROGNOSIS AND TREATMENT

Regarded by many as a more aggressive variant of collecting duct carcinoma, renal medullary carcinoma

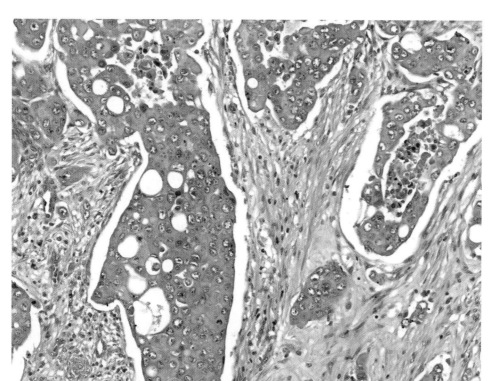

FIGURE 6-12

Nests and islands of high-grade eosinophilic cells embedded in a desmoplastic stroma characterize renal medullary carcinoma.

RENAL MEDULLARY CARCINOMA—PATHOLOGIC FEATURES

Gross Findings

▶ Solitary, poorly circumscribed mass
▶ Infiltrative borders
▶ Hemorrhage and necrosis

Microscopic Findings

▶ Lace-like appearance
▶ Desmoplastic stroma
▶ Inflammatory infiltrate

Immunohistochemical Findings

▶ LMWCK and usually EMA and CEA positive
▶ HMWCK negative

Differential Diagnosis

▶ Collecting duct carcinoma
▶ High-grade urothelial carcinoma

RENAL CARCINOMAS ASSOCIATED WITH XP11.2 TRANSLOCATIONS/*TFE3* GENE FUSIONS—FACT SHEET

Definition

▶ A distinctive group of renal cell carcinomas characterized by translocations involving the *TFE3* gene at chromosome Xp11.2

Incidence and Location

▶ 26-41% of all pediatric renal cell carcinomas

Morbidity and Mortality

▶ Advanced stage and potential for late recurrence, but indolent behavior

Gender, Race, and Age Distribution

▶ Children and young adults

Clinical Features

▶ t(X;1): *PRCC-TFE3* gene fusion
▶ t(X;17): *ASPSCR1-TFE3* gene fusion

Prognosis and Treatment

▶ t(X;17): advanced stage, but indolent behavior
▶ t(X;1): late lymph node metastasis

---

carries a very high mortality rate. Most patients are dead within the first year after discovery. Chemotherapy prolongs life by a few months but does not alter the course of the disease.

RENAL CARCINOMAS ASSOCIATED WITH XP11.2 TRANSLOCATIONS/*TFE3* GENE FUSIONS

A subset of renal cell carcinomas preferentially affect young patients and are characterized by various mutations involving chromosome Xp11.2 that result in gene fusions involving the *TFE3* transcription factor gene.

CLINICAL FEATURES

The majority of patients are children and young adults. Several different mutations have been identified, the most common of which is t(X;1), which results in *PRCC-TFE3* gene fusion. The t(X;17) translocation results in *ASPSCR1 (ASPL)-TFE3* gene fusion identical to that seen in alveolar soft part sarcoma. The *ASPSCR1-TFE3* carcinomas consistently present at advanced stage with lymph node metastasis.

PATHOLOGIC FEATURES

GROSS FINDINGS

Xp11.2 carcinomas share many similarities with clear cell renal cell carcinoma. They manifest as solitary cortical masses characterized by tan-yellow cut surfaces with foci of hemorrhage and necrosis.

MICROSCOPIC FINDINGS

Unlike other types of renal cell carcinoma, Xp11.2 renal cell carcinomas are not defined by their histologic features. However, a papillary architecture combining clear cell features is perhaps the most distinctive characteristic (Fig. 6-13A). Alternatively, a nested pattern made up of cells with ample acidophilic cytoplasm may be seen (Fig. 6-13B). The t(X;17) carcinomas differ from their t(X;1) counterpart by having (1) less compact, alveolar or pseudopapillary architecture with hyalin nodules; (2) voluminous cytoplasm and prominent cell borders; and (3) abundant psammoma bodies.

ANCILLARY STUDIES

ULTRASTRUCTURAL FEATURES

Not surprisingly, the ultrastructural features of Xp11.2 carcinomas are very similar to those of the clear cell variant of renal cell carcinoma. The uncommon t(X;17) subtype may show membrane-bound cytoplasmic granules or rhomboidal crystals identical to those of alveolar soft part sarcoma.

IMMUNOHISTOCHEMISTRY

Nuclear immunoreactivity for the *TFE3* gene product is the only consistent and most reliable

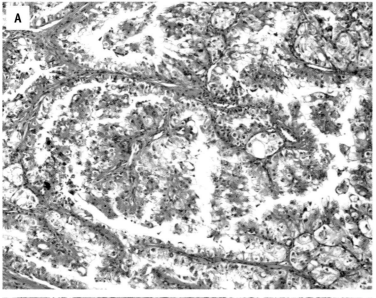

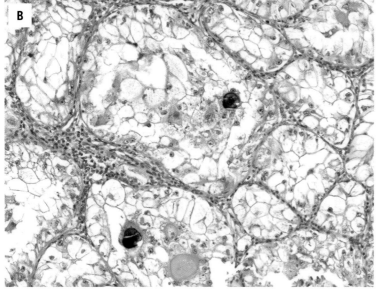

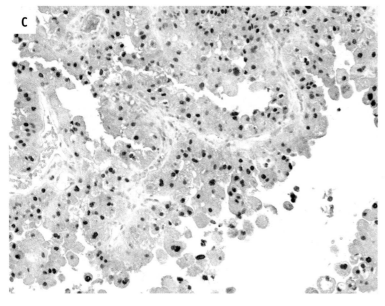

FIGURE 6-13

Renal carcinomas associated with Xp11.2 translocations/*TFE3* gene fusions. **A,** This example of translocation t(X;17) carcinoma shows papillary architectures lined with clear cells, the most distinctive feature. **B,** Tumor cells can also have clear cytoplasm with calcification in a nested pattern. **C,** Positive reaction to antibodies against *TFE3* gene product is characteristic.

RENAL CARCINOMAS ASSOCIATED WITH XP11.2 TRANSLOCATIONS/*TFE3* GENE FUSIONS—PATHOLOGIC FEATURES

Gross Findings
- ▶ Solitary cortical mass
- ▶ Tan-yellow cut surface
- ▶ Hemorrhage and necrosis

Microscopic Findings
- ▶ Not particularly distinctive
- ▶ Papillary architecture lined with clear cells
- ▶ Tumor cells with voluminous clear or amphophilic cytoplasm
- ▶ t(X;17): psammoma bodies

Ultrastructural Features
- ▶ Similar to clear cell renal cell carcinoma
- ▶ t(X;17): membrane-bound cytoplasmic granules

Immunohistochemical Findings
- ▶ Nuclear labeling for TFE3 protein
- ▶ EMA and keratins underexpressed, CD10 positive

Differential Diagnosis
- ▶ Clear cell renal cell carcinoma
- ▶ Chromophobe renal cell carcinoma
- ▶ Oncocytic renal neoplasms

---

immunohistochemical stain (Fig. 6-13C). Focal or no staining for EMA, Cam5.2, and vimentin is common.

DIFFERENTIAL DIAGNOSIS

Although this group of tumors is characterized by Xp11.2 translocations, these alterations are not specific to renal cell carcinoma and may be seen in other neoplasms, most notably alveolar soft part sarcoma. The relationship, if any, between these tumors is not clear. Although Xp11.2 carcinomas show clear cell features mimicking the clear cell variant of renal cell carcinoma, the latter entity is exceedingly rare in patients younger than 25 years of age.

PROGNOSIS AND TREATMENT

Information on this relatively new entity is still emerging. Early indications are that the t(X;17) carcinomas are in an advanced stage at presentation, with lymph node involvement, but nevertheless appear indolent, paralleling the behavior of their genetic counterpart, alveolar soft tissue part sarcoma. On the other hand, the t(X;1) carcinomas show a propensity to late recurrences

decades after the initial diagnosis, usually in the form of lymph node metastasis.

POSTNEUROBLASTOMA RENAL CELL CARCINOMA

Fewer than two dozen cases of a renal cell carcinoma with oncocytic features have been reported in children who survived neuroblastoma. Not all of the patients were treated for the neuroblastoma, suggesting that the pathogenesis of this group of neoplasms is probably more closely related to neuroblastoma than to an effect of therapy. Additionally, the genetic alterations detected in these tumors did not conform to those seen in other renal cell carcinomas, supporting the view that they may indeed be a distinctive entity. All affected children were diagnosed with neuroblastoma at 2 years of age or younger, and the majority had advanced-stage neuroblastoma. In a well-characterized group of patients, renal cell carcinoma was detected at ages ranging from 5 to 14 years and occurred 3 to 12 years (average, 9 years) after the neuroblastoma diagnosis. Morphologically, many of these tumors were described as having a typical clear cell appearance; however, the best-documented postneuroblastoma carcinomas were characterized as oncocytic with solid and papillary architecture and abundant eosinophilic cytoplasm. At least one patient experienced metastatic disease to lymph nodes and liver.

MUCINOUS TUBULAR AND SPINDLE CELL RENAL CARCINOMA

This is an uncommon, recently described renal cell carcinoma that has occurred in patients from a wide range of ages (17 to 82 years, mean 53 years), predominantly in women. Most tumors are single and asymptomatic, although flank pain and hematuria have been reported. Macroscopically, they appear as large, well-circumscribed, homogeneous, tan-white-pinkish lesions, sometimes centered in the renal medulla. The name is descriptive of their most common histologic appearance: a mixture of tubules and spindle-shaped epithelial cells in a background of extracellular mucinous material (Fig. 6-14). The mucinous component is highlighted by Alcian blue. The nuclei are bland, spherical or oval, with inconspicuous nucleoli. These low-grade nuclear features are the same in both the tubular and the spindle cell elements. The immunohistochemical profile of mucinous tubular and spindle cell carcinoma is not well characterized. Positive reactivity for vimentin and EMA is a consistent finding. A few cases showed characteristic chromosomal losses involving chromosomes 1, 4, 6, 8, 13, and 14, with gains at 7, 11, 16, and 17. However, 3p alteration, trisomy 7 and/or

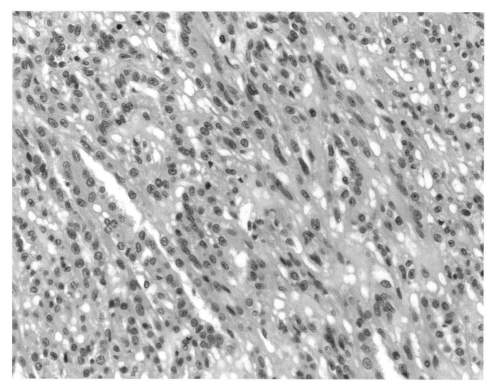

FIGURE 6-14
Tubules and smelting of spindle cells in a mucinous background comprise this mucinous tubular and spindle cell carcinoma.

17 have not been reported. The prognosis seems favorable with majority of the patients free of disease after surgical resection.

PAPILLARY ADENOMA OF THE KIDNEY

Papillary adenomas of the kidney are renal cortical tumors with papillary or tubulopapillary architecture, low-grade nuclear features, and a size of 5 mm or less. They are the most common renal epithelial neoplasms, with an incidence as high as 22% in some autopsy studies.

CLINICAL FEATURES

Most papillary adenomas are found incidentally, either in nephrectomy specimens or at autopsy. They are more frequently detected in kidneys with chronic pyelonephritis, long-term dialysis, acquired cystic renal disease, or renal vascular disease. They may also be a manifestation of von Hippel-Lindau syndrome, especially in children. They have a wide age range at presentation and their incidence steadily increases with age.

PAPILLARY ADENOMA OF THE KIDNEY—FACT SHEET

Definition
▶ Low-grade papillary/tubulopapillary tumors of the renal cortex, no larger than 5 mm in diameter

Incidence and Location
▶ Most common tumor of renal tubular epithelium
▶ Renal cortex

Gender, Race, and Age Distribution
▶ Wide age range
▶ Incidence increases with age

Clinical Features
▶ Incidental finding
▶ More common in diseased kidneys (chronic pyelonephritis, acquired renal cystic disease, and renal vascular disease)
▶ May be part of VHL syndrome

Prognosis and Treatment
▶ Benign
▶ No additional therapy required

PATHOLOGIC FEATURES

GROSS FINDINGS

Papillary adenomas appear as well-circumscribed but nonencapsulated, yellow-gray cortical nodules. By definition, they are 5 mm or less in greatest dimension, and small lesions may easily escape macroscopic examination. The majority of adenomas are solitary, but multiple and bilateral lesions do occur. When they are very numerous, this has been called "renal adenomatosis."

MICROSCOPIC FINDINGS

Papillary adenomas are characterized by papillary, tubular, or tubulopapillary architecture (Fig. 6-15). The lining cells are round to oval with uniform small nuclei and inconspicuous nucleoli similar to Fuhrman grades 1 and 2 nuclei. Mitotic figures are absent or very rare. Psammoma bodies and foamy macrophages are commonly present.

DIFFERENTIAL DIAGNOSIS

These neoplasms may be indistinguishable histologically from low-grade papillary renal cell carcinoma, so that size becomes the sole criterion that separates the two.

PAPILLARY ADENOMA OF THE KIDNEY—PATHOLOGIC FEATURES

Gross Findings
► Well-circumscribed yellow-gray nodules
► ≤5 mm in greatest dimension

Microscopic Findings
► Papillary, tubular, or tubulopapillary architecture
► Low-grade nuclear features

Differential Diagnosis
► Low-grade papillary renal cell carcinoma

PROGNOSIS AND TREATMENT

These neoplasms are benign and do not warrant additional therapy or follow-up.

ONCOCYTOMA

Oncocytomas are benign renal epithelial neoplasms composed entirely of cells with abundant granular eosinophilic cytoplasm rich in mitochondria and have been postulated to arise from the intercalated cells of collecting ducts. They account for approximately 5% to 10% of all surgically resected renal epithelial tumors.

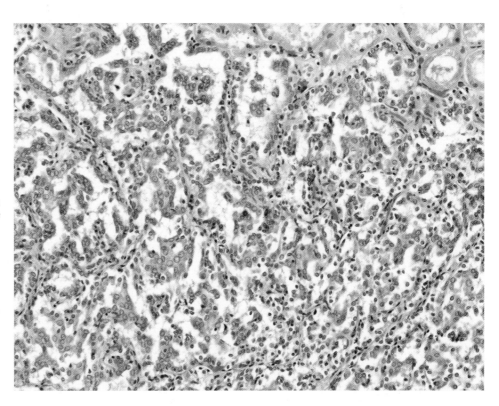

FIGURE 6-15
A papillary adenoma, showing a tubular architecture and low-grade nuclei.

CLINICAL FEATURES

Oncocytomas are tumors of adults, with a peak incidence in the seventh decade of life. There is a 2:1 male predominance. The majority are discovered incidentally during workup for unrelated conditions. A minority manifest with hematuria, pain, or palpable mass.

Most cases are sporadic, although familial cases have been reported in association with Birt-Hogg-Dubé syndrome. Unlike most other renal epithelial tumors, no one genetic abnormality characterizes oncocytomas. However, losses involving chromosomes 1 and Y are most frequently seen. Most importantly, oncocytomas consistently lack abnormalities in chromosome 3, which are so frequent in clear cell renal cell carcinomas.

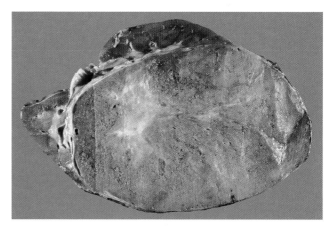

FIGURE 6-16

Oncocytoma, showing a well-circumscribed mass with a light-brown homogenous cut surface and a central scar.

PATHOLOGIC FEATURES

GROSS FINDINGS

Oncocytomas are typically solitary, well-circumscribed, nonencapsulated renal neoplasms that vary greatly in size. They have a fairly homogeneous cut surface with a characteristic appearance that is mahogany-brown or, less frequently, tan to pale yellow (Fig. 6-16). A central zone of stroma is present in one third of the tumors and appears to correlate with size, because it is more common in larger tumors. Hemorrhage and necrosis are seen in a small subset of oncocytomas.

MICROSCOPIC FINDINGS

Oncocytoma is composed of cells with abundant, finely granular eosinophilic cytoplasm growing in sheets with inconspicuous vasculature or as nests of cells growing in an edematous hypocellular stroma (Fig. 6-17A,B). Microcystic formation is frequent. Occasionally, the cystic changes are extensive (Fig. 6-17C). The neoplastic cells are round to polygonal and

---

ONCOCYTOMA—FACT SHEET

Definition

▶ Benign renal epithelial neoplasm composed entirely of cells with abundant granular eosinophilic cytoplasm rich in mitochondria

Incidence and Location

▶ 5-10% of all surgically resected renal epithelial tumors

Morbidity and Mortality

▶ Completely benign neoplasm

Gender, Race, and Age Distribution

▶ Adults, peak in seventh decade
▶ M/F ratio, 2:1

Clinical Features

▶ Majority asymptomatic
▶ Occasionally hematuria, pain, or flank mass

Prognosis and Treatment

▶ Benign
▶ Surgical excision is not necessary

ONCOCYTOMA—PATHOLOGIC FEATURES

Gross Findings

▶ Well-circumscribed, nonencapsulated mass
▶ Homogeneous, mahogany-brown cut surface
▶ One third with central scar

Microscopic Findings

▶ Solid nests of uniform tumor cells
▶ Loose, hyalinized, fibrous stroma
▶ Abundant granular eosinophilic cytoplasm
▶ Round uniform nuclei

Ultrastructural Features

▶ Abundant mitochondria

Fine-needle Aspiration Biopsy Findings

▶ Cohesive nests or single cells with abundant granular eosinophilic cytoplasm

Immunohistochemical Findings

▶ Positive for EMA and most keratins
▶ Vimentin negative

Differential Diagnosis

▶ Chromophobe renal cell carcinoma; eosinophilic variant
▶ Clear cell renal cell carcinoma, rich in eosinophilic and granular cells
▶ Papillary renal cell carcinoma

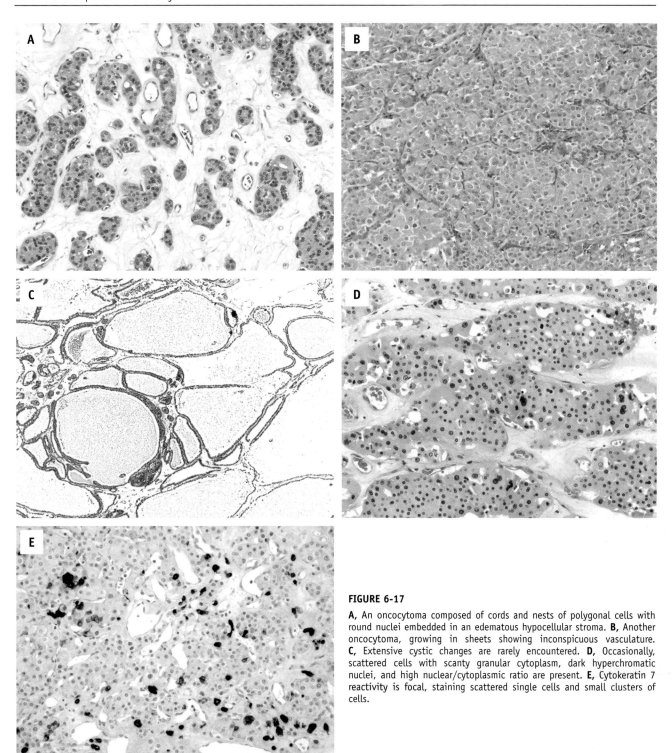

FIGURE 6-17

A, An oncocytoma composed of cords and nests of polygonal cells with round nuclei embedded in an edematous hypocellular stroma. **B,** Another oncocytoma, growing in sheets showing inconspicuous vasculature. **C,** Extensive cystic changes are rarely encountered. **D,** Occasionally, scattered cells with scanty granular cytoplasm, dark hyperchromatic nuclei, and high nuclear/cytoplasmic ratio are present. **E,** Cytokeratin 7 reactivity is focal, staining scattered single cells and small clusters of cells.

have regular round nuclei with nucleoli that frequently are visible with the 10× objective. Mitotic figures are absent or very rare. Occasionally, scattered cells with scanty granular cytoplasm, dark hyperchromatic nuclei, and high nuclear/cytoplasmic ratio are present (Fig. 6-17D). Microscopic invasion of perirenal fat occasionally is present and has no adverse prognostic significance.

ANCILLARY STUDIES

ULTRASTRUCTURAL FEATURES

Ultrastructurally, the cytoplasm of oncocytes is filled with mitochondria. Cytokeratin-containing globular filamentous bodies have also been reported.

IMMUNOHISTOCHEMISTRY

Oncocytomas are immunoreactive with antibodies to EMA and most keratins. Their CK7 reactivity is focal, decorating scattered single cells and small clusters of cells (Fig. 6-17E). Oncocytoma is invariably negative for vimentin.

FINE-NEEDLE ASPIRATION BIOPSY

Fine-needle biopsy reveals cohesive nests and individual cells characterized by abundant granular and eosinophilic cytoplasm and uniform round nuclei with or without nucleoli. Because other renal neoplasms may contain foci of oncocytic change, unequivocal diagnosis of oncocytoma by this method alone is discouraged.

DIFFERENTIAL DIAGNOSIS

Although oncocytomas have a characteristic macroscopic appearance, occasionally they may be confused with renal cell carcinomas of the chromophobe or clear cell type. The most problematic differential diagnosis of oncocytoma is that involving the eosinophilic variant of chromophobe renal cell carcinoma. Oncocytomas are negative with Hale's colloidal iron stain, whereas diffuse positive blue cytoplasmic staining is typical of chromophobe renal cell carcinoma. Although both oncocytoma and chromophobe renal cell carcinoma react with antibodies to CK7, the reaction of oncocytoma is typically limited to scattered single cells or small clusters of cells, whereas the reaction of chromophobe is typically positive in the great majority of cells.

Clear cell renal cell carcinoma composed predominantly of granular eosinophilic cells is a less common diagnostic possibility; it often can be distinguished from oncocytoma by higher nuclear grade and mitotic activity. A positive reaction with antibody to vimentin is common in clear cell renal cell carcinoma and excludes oncocytoma.

PROGNOSIS AND TREATMENT

Oncocytomas are benign neoplasms that show no progression or metastasis.

RENAL CELL CARCINOMA, UNCLASSIFIED

The category of unclassified renal cell carcinoma was created out of necessity to serve as a "catch-all" for those cases of renal cell carcinoma that do not fit into one of the currently defined entities under the 2004 WHO classification system. Additionally, the creation of the unclassified renal cell carcinoma category facilitated recognition of several new entities, such as the mucinous tubular and spindle cell carcinoma and the Xp11.2 carcinoma. A prime example of renal cell carcinoma that should be assigned to this category is renal cell carcinoma with extensive sarcomatoid morphology lacking a recognizable epithelial component. Further supporting the placement of "sarcomatoid carcinoma" into the unclassified group is the lack of evidence that such tumors arise de novo. A more plausible explanation is that the sarcomatoid component overgrows the original antecedent element to such a degree that it becomes unrecognizable. Because unclassified renal cell carcinoma comprises a heterogeneous group of tumors with little in common, they share no defined clinical, morphologic, immunohistochemical, ultrastructural, or genetic characteristics. Suffice it to say that approximately 5% of renal cell carcinomas fall into this category.

Metanephric Tumors

Metanephric renal tumors are a group of recently described benign neoplasms characterized by a wide morphologic spectrum. Tumors composed exclusively of epithelial nephroblastic cells are termed "metanephric adenomas," and those made up exclusively of stromal cells are called "metanephric stromal tumors." The term "metanephric adenofibroma" is applied to a subset of tumors with a mixture of both components.

METANEPHRIC ADENOMA

Metanephric adenoma is the most common of the metanephric tumors.

CLINICAL FEATURES

Metanephric adenoma has a wide age range of presentation and is the most common renal epithelial neoplasm of children and young adults; however, most metanephric adenomas occur in adults (mean age, 41 years). There is a 2:1 female predominance. The clinical findings are generally not specific to metanephric adenoma, but 10% to 15% of patients have polycythemia, which usually is cured by resection of the tumor.

PATHOLOGIC FEATURES

GROSS FINDINGS

Metanephric adenomas are well-circumscribed, non-encapsulated masses that vary greatly in diameter.

Their cut surfaces are gray to tan to yellow and often show foci of hemorrhage and necrosis. Calcification may be present.

MICROSCOPIC FINDINGS

More than 75% of metanephric adenomas lack pseudocapsules. Typically, metanephric adenomas are densely cellular neoplasms composed of tightly packed small round acini or small branching tubules (Fig. 6-18A). Foci of papillary architecture are common, often consisting of stubby papillae reminiscent of immature glomeruli. Often, the stroma is inconspicuous, but sometimes it is hyalinized or edematous. Psammoma bodies are common. The epithelial tumor cells are uniform, small, and cytologically bland, with oval, hyperchromatic nuclei without visible nucleoli. Mitotic figures are absent or rare.

ANCILLARY STUDIES

IMMUNOHISTOCHEMISTRY

WT1 is frequently detectable in the nuclei of metanephric adenomas. The cells of metanephric adenoma are frequently negative for EMA, CK7, and cytokeratin AE1-AE3.

DIFFERENTIAL DIAGNOSIS

Metanephric adenomas are distinguished from papillary renal cell carcinomas by their lack of encapsulation, the sharp interface between the tumor and the kidney (Fig. 6-18B), the absence of nucleoli, and the relative lack of mitotic activity. Papillary adenoma and papillary renal cell carcinoma do not react with antibody to WT1. Additionally, CK7 is largely absent in metanephric adenoma but frequently present in papillary renal cell carcinoma.

PROGNOSIS AND TREATMENT

Metanephric adenoma is almost always cured by excision. A few case reports suggest that metanephric adenomas can rarely metastasize, but this is not completely clear.

METANEPHRIC ADENOFIBROMA

CLINICAL FEATURES

Only a small number of cases of metanephric adenofibroma have been studied. Patients have ranged in age from 5 months to 36 years (mean, 82 months). So far, there is a male predominance. Presenting symptoms include polycythemia, hematuria, and hypertension.

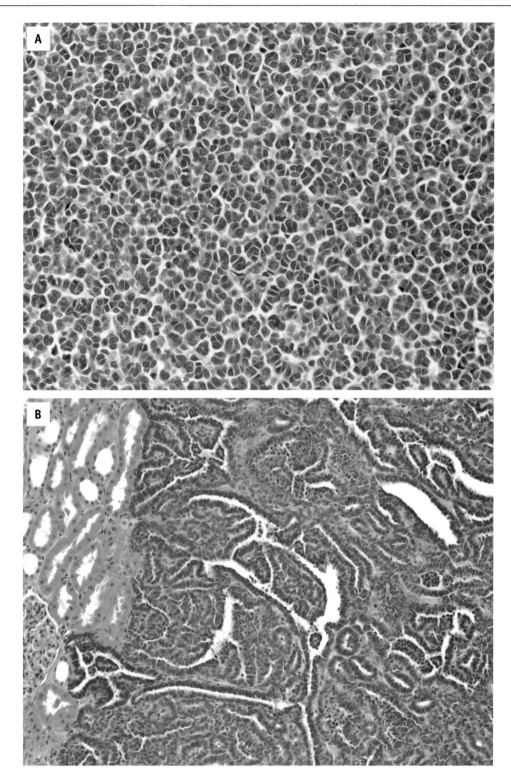

FIGURE 6-18

Metanephric adenomas may be composed of sheets of back-to-back cells (**A**) or, more frequently, tightly packed branching tubules (**B**). Note the sharp border with kidney.

PATHOLOGIC FEATURES

GROSS FINDINGS

Metanephric adenofibromas tend to be centered in the medulla and often are at least partially cystic.

MICROSCOPIC FINDINGS

Metanephric adenofibroma is composed of variable proportions of epithelial nodules and a moderately cellular stromal component. The epithelial nodules are identical to metanephric adenoma. The stroma is made up of fibroblast-like bland spindle cells with pale eosinophilic cytoplasm, oval nuclei, and inconspicuous

cytoplasm. Mitotic figures are rare. The stromal component shows a tendency toward infiltrative growth and as a result has irregular borders with the adjacent renal parenchyma. Angiodysplasia and heterologous elements occasionally are present.

ANCILLARY STUDIES

IMMUNOHISTOCHEMISTRY

The stromal component of metanephric adenofibroma is immunoreactive for CD34. The epithelial component reacts in a similar fashion to metanephric adenoma.

PROGNOSIS AND TREATMENT

This is a benign lesion that is cured by excision. A single case of metanephric adenosarcoma has been reported.

METANEPHRIC STROMAL TUMOR

CLINICAL FEATURES

Metanephric stromal tumor is primarily a pediatric renal neoplasm occurring in infants and the very young. The mean age at presentation is 24 months. The majority of patients present with an abdominal mass, though hematuria and hypertension are not infrequent.

PATHOLOGIC FEATURES

GROSS FINDINGS

Metanephric stromal tumors appear as well-circumscribed, nonencapsulated solid or cystic masses centered in the renal medulla. They have an average diameter of approximately 5cm and display a tan, lobulated cut surface.

MICROSCOPIC FINDINGS

Metanephric stromal tumors lack a fibrous capsule and have a tendency toward infiltrative borders. They are composed of spindled to stellate cells characterized by elongated hyperchromatic nuclei and indistinct cytoplasmic processes. Mitoses are infrequent. The degree of cellularity varies from paucicellular to highly cellular. The most distinctive histologic finding is the presence of concentric laminations (onion-skin) of spindle tumor cells around entrapped renal tubules and vessels (Fig. 6-19). These laminations may be hypocellular or hypercellular compared with the surrounding stroma, imparting a characteristically nodular appearance. Angiodysplasia involving intratumoral arterioles is an almost constant feature represented by epithelioid transformation of the medial smooth muscle cells and myxoid change. Another unique, but infrequent, feature is the presence of juxtaglomerular cell hyperplasia within entrapped glomeruli. Heterologous elements in the form of glia, cartilage, or fat are seen in about one fifth of metanephric stromal tumors.

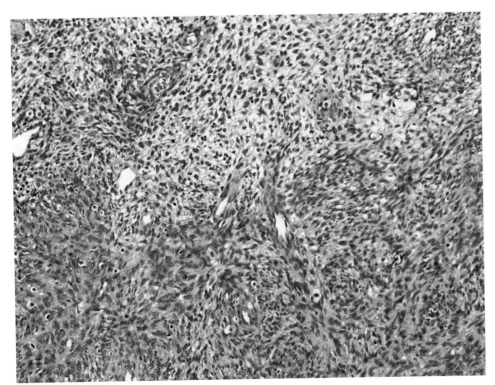

FIGURE 6-19

In metanephric stromal tumor, fascicles of spindle cells wrap around blood vessels.

ANCILLARY STUDIES

IMMUNOHISTOCHEMISTRY

The spindle tumor cells are immunoreactive for CD34. They are negative for desmin, cytokeratins, and S-100, although glial heterologous elements may stain for S-100 and gliofibrillary acidic protein (GFAP).

DIFFERENTIAL DIAGNOSIS

Most metanephric stromal tumors were previously classified as congenital mesoblastic nephromas; however, the latter show an invasive growth pattern and lack the characteristic features of metanephric stromal tumors, namely the angiodysplasia, the concentric laminations, the juxtaglomerular cell hyperplasia, and the heterologous elements.

The multitude of architectural patterns seen in metanephric stromal tumors (palisading, storiform, and hemangiopericytic patterns) draws resemblance to primary renal sarcomas such as clear cell sarcoma of the kidney. In contrast to renal sarcomas, necrosis is usually absent in metanephric stromal tumors, and so is vascular invasion. CD34 immunoreactivity is also helpful.

PROGNOSIS AND TREATMENT

Metanephric stromal tumors are benign neoplasms that appear incapable of local recurrence or distant metastasis. Surgical excision is therefore adequate. A small number of patients may suffer the consequences of extrarenal angiodysplasia resulting in significant morbidity and mortality.

Nephroblastic Tumors

NEPHROBLASTOMA

Also known as Wilms' tumor, nephroblastoma is the most common neoplasm of the kidneys in children. It has a reported incidence of approximately 1 per 8000 children.

CLINICAL FEATURES

Nephroblastoma has a peak incidence between 2 and 5 years of age. More than 90% of patients are younger

---

NEPHROBLASTOMA—FACT SHEET

Definition

▶ A malignant embryonal neoplasm derived from nephrogenic blastemal cells

Incidence and Location

▶ 1 in 8000 children
▶ Equal frequency in both kidneys

Morbidity and Mortality

▶ Favorable histology: 4-year survival rate (any stage) approximately 90%
▶ Unfavorable histology: 4-year survival rate 17-70% depending on stage

Gender, Race, and Age Distribution

▶ No significant sex predilection
▶ Higher incidence among African Americans
▶ Peak incidence, age 2-5 years

Clinical Features

▶ Abdominal mass
▶ Pain, hematuria, and hypertension
▶ 10% associated with dysmorphic syndromes

Prognosis and Treatment

▶ Prognosis depends on stage and histology
▶ Unfavorable outcome: high stage, anaplastic histology

---

than 6 years of age, with only rare cases occurring in patients 10 years or older. There is not a significant sex predilection, and geography does not seem to be a factor. A higher incidence is observed among African Americans. Most patients come to medical attention because of a palpable abdominal mass. Other presentations may include abdominal pain, hematuria, and hypertension.

Approximately 10% of nephroblastomas can be linked to a specific dysmorphic syndrome. Among those, WAGR syndrome (Wilms' tumor, aniridia, genitourinary malformation, mental retardation) is the best characterized. Patients with WAGR syndrome show consistent deletion of chromosome 11p13. The relevant gene in chromosome 11p13 has been isolated and is designated *WT1*. Other *WT1* mutations have been found in patients with Denys-Drash syndrome (severe glomerulopathy, pseudohermaphroditism, nephroblastoma) as well as a number of sporadic nephroblastomas. Genes other than *WT1* have also been implicated in the pathogenesis of Wilms' tumor, emphasizing the genetic heterogeneity of this entity.

Most nephroblastomas are solitary; however, synchronous and bilateral lesions may occur, especially in familial cases. These patients typically have a younger age at presentation and are more prone to develop renal failure.

Circulating serum mucin and elevated levels of hyaluronic acid have been detected in association with nephroblastoma.

PATHOLOGIC FEATURES

GROSS FINDINGS

Nephroblastomas usually are large, well-circumscribed, rounded, solitary renal masses that push against and distort the adjacent renal parenchyma. A surrounding fibrous pseudocapsule is often present. The cut surface is usually tan, pale and mucoid and may display foci of hemorrhage and cystic change. Depending on the stromal content of the tumor, a lobulated appearance may be seen.

MICROSCOPIC FINDINGS

Nephroblastomas are a group of very heterogeneous neoplasms, to the degree that one nephroblastoma may have little in common with another, depending on the cell composition and architectural patterns observed. The three most recognized patterns are the *blastemal,* the *epithelial,* and the *stromal.* Triphasic tumors are most distinctive (Fig. 6-20), but biphasic and monophasic tumors are not uncommon.

The cells of the *blastemal* pattern are small, round to oval, and have high nuclear/cytoplasmic ratios. They are characterized by a brisk mitotic activity, and, like small cell carcinoma of the lung, they show prominent nuclear overlapping. Several blastemal patterns have been described. The *diffuse blastemal* pattern is characterized by a fairly uniform population of noncohesive cells and uniquely infiltrative margins. In contrast, the

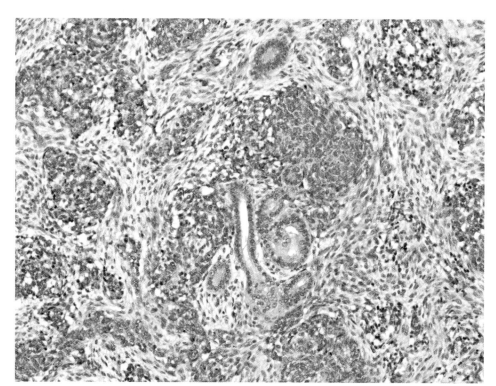

FIGURE 6-20
A triphasic nephroblastoma combining blastemal, epithelial, and stromal elements.

cells of other blastemal patterns tend to be more cohesive and their borders less infiltrative and more sharply defined. The *organized blastemal* pattern may be seen in the form of nodules (*nodular blastema*), anastomosing cords (*serpentine blastema*), or even palisaded arrangements (*basaloid blastema*) embedded in loose, myxoid, or fibromyxoid stroma (Fig. 6-21A). Such distinctive patterns are more common than the diffuse blastemal pattern, making the diagnosis of nephroblastoma less challenging.

Most nephroblastomas have some degree of *epithelial* differentiation, manifested either as homologous cell types, resembling normal nephrogenesis (Fig. 6-21B), or as heterologous (mucinous and squamous) cell types.

A variety of *stromal* patterns may be observed. In most cases, this is composed of immature myxoid and spindled mesenchymal cells; however, essentially any type of stromal differentiation, including smooth muscle, skeletal muscle, and neuroglial tissue, may be observed (Fig. 6-21C).

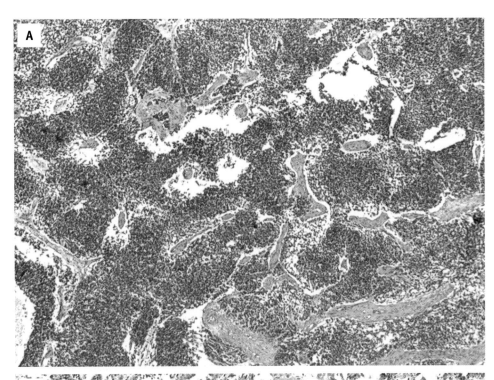

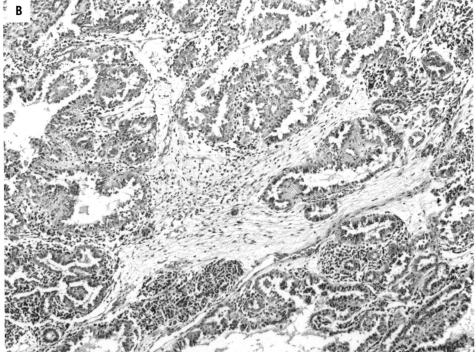

FIGURE 6-21

Nephroblastoma. **A,** Blastemal cells form anastomosing cords embedded in fibromyxoid stroma, termed serpentine blastema. **B,** Epithelial differentiation manifests as tubulopapillary structures.

Continued

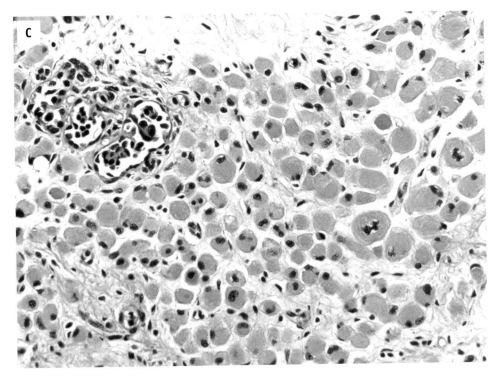

FIGURE 6-21, CONT'D
C, Skeletal muscle differentiation in stromal cells is evident.

Anaplasia

For therapeutic and prognostic purposes, nephroblastomas are histologically divided into two major categories. Those nephroblastomas that are highly responsive to current therapeutic modalities are said to have "favorable" histology, and those that do not respond well to chemotherapy are considered "unfavorable." The latter make up about 5% of nephroblastomas and are defined by nuclear anaplasia. Anaplasia is rare in patients younger than 2 years of age but increases in incidence thereafter. Recognition of anaplasia requires the presence of marked nucleomegaly and hyperchromasia with atypical multipolar polyploid mitotic figures. Anaplasia may be diffuse or focal. Anaplasia per se is not an indicator of the aggressiveness of a nephroblastoma but rather predictive of its resistance to adjuvant therapy.

Postchemotherapy changes

Necrosis, xanthogranulomatous reaction, and hemosiderin deposition are among the most common manifestations of chemotherapy. Less frequently, chemotherapy may induce maturation of blastemal, epithelial, and stromal elements.

ANCILLARY STUDIES

ULTRASTRUCTURAL FEATURES

Electron microscopy is rarely necessary for the diagnosis of nephroblastoma; however, the ultrastructural features of nephroblastoma cells are very similar to those of developing metanephrons.

IMMUNOHISTOCHEMISTRY

There is no single marker or panel of immunostains that is diagnostic of nephroblastoma; however, WT1 is the most useful single test. WT1 is expressed in primitive blastemal and epithelial cell types but absent in the differentiated epithelial and stromal elements (Fig. 6-22). Although it is safe to assume that most primitive-appearing tumors expressing WT1 are probably nephroblastomas, exceptions include desmoplastic small round cell tumor. The blastemal cells frequently express vimentin. Most nephroblastomas with anaplasia overexpress p53 protein, indicating a correlation between anaplasia and *TP53* gene mutations.

DIFFERENTIAL DIAGNOSIS

Diffuse blastemal nephroblastomas share morphologic resemblance with other small blue cell tumors, including primitive neuroectodermal tumors (PNET or Ewing's sarcoma), neuroblastomas, rhabdomyosarcomas, clear cell sarcomas, synovial sarcomas, and lymphomas. All of these tumors are much less common than nephroblastoma.

Patients with *neuroblastoma* tend to present with advanced disease, including metastases to unusual sites (other than regional lymph nodes, lungs, and liver). Grossly, these tumors lack the circumscription that is characteristic of most nephroblastomas, and they are

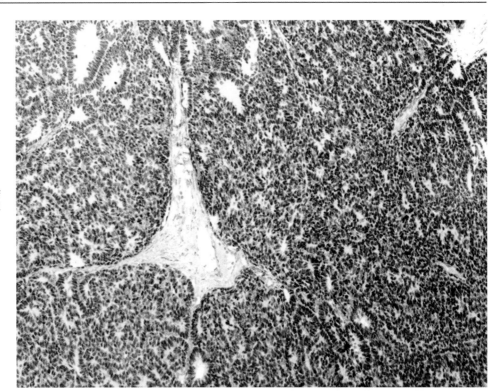

FIGURE 6-22
WT1 is expressed in the nuclei of primitive epithelial and blastemal cells of nephroblastomas.

usually hemorrhagic. Microscopically, neuroblastomas lack a fibrous pseudocapsule and have infiltrative borders. They show the characteristic Homer-Wright rosettes, and their nuclei are nonoverlapping and display a "salt and pepper" chromatin pattern. Unlike nephroblastomas, PNETs are immunoreactive for CD99 and FLI-1 and negative for WT1.

Should a nephroblastoma be primarily composed of a mixture of stromal elements including adipose tissue, cartilage, and mature neuroglial tissue, it may be confused with other mixed neoplasms, primarily teratoma. Historically, teratoid nephroblastomas have been frequently mischaracterized as immature teratoma.

Rarely, in adult patients, epithelial predominant nephroblastomas may resemble papillary renal cell carcinoma.

PROGNOSIS AND TREATMENT

Treatment of nephroblastoma is largely dependent on clinical stage and histology but includes surgical excision and adjuvant therapy, with radiotherapy usually reserved for advanced-stage disease. The large majority of nephroblastomas are low-stage tumors, have favorable histology, and therefore carry a favorable outcome and excellent prognosis. High-stage examples and those that display anaplastic features (unfavorable histology) do worse. Potential metastatic sites include regional lymph nodes, lungs, and liver.

Despite the invasive growth pattern that characterizes the diffuse blastemal pattern, this variant responds well to chemotherapeutic regimens. However, the finding of a significant blastemal population of cells after therapy is a poor prognostic indicator.

NEPHROGENIC RESTS AND NEPHROBLASTOMATOSIS

Nephrogenic rests are persistent foci of embryonal renal tissue that are believed to give rise to nephroblastomas. If diffuse or multiple nephrogenic rests are identified, the term "nephroblastomatosis" is applied.

CLINICAL FEATURES

Nephrogenic rests are present in the nephrectomy specimens of patients with nephroblastoma in 25% to 40% of cases.

PATHOLOGIC FEATURES

Depending of their topographic relationship to the renal lobe, nephrogenic rests are divided into perilobar and intralobar types. Perilobar nephrogenic rests are typically multiple, well-demarcated structures located at the periphery of the renal lobe (Fig. 6-23). Histologically, they are composed of blastemal or tubular patterns and very little stroma. In contrast, intralobar nephrogenic

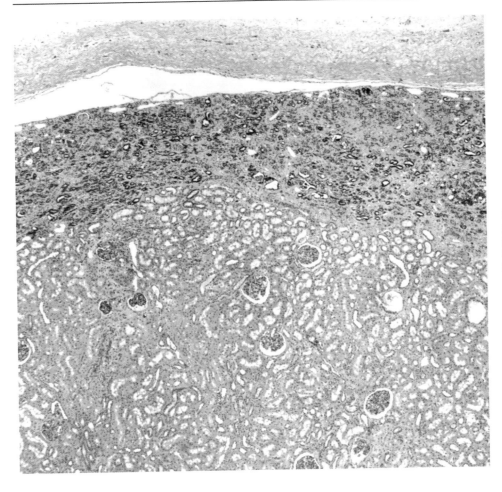

FIGURE 6-23
Perilobar nephrogenic rests are comprised of blastemal and primitive tubular structures located at the periphery of the renal lobe.

rests are usually solitary, ill-defined, stroma-rich lesions placed randomly within the renal lobe.

Either type of nephrogenic rest may pursue one or more of the following fates: (1) stay dormant (incipient or dormant nephrogenic rest); (2) mature, undergo peritubular scarring, and eventually disappear (sclerosing or obsolescent nephrogenic rests); (3) undergo active proliferation and growth to resemble nephroblastoma (hyperplastic nephrogenic rests) or occasionally to form a continuous band of embryonal cells at the lobar surface, leading to massive renal enlargement (diffuse hyperplastic nephroblastomatosis); and (4) grow rapidly, forming spherical, expansile nodules surrounded by peritumoral fibrous pseudocapsule and compressing rest remnants and normal kidney (nephroblastoma).

DIFFERENTIAL DIAGNOSIS

Actively hyperplastic nephrogenic rests can be distinguished from full-blown nephroblastomas by the usual absence of a fibrous pseudocapsule between the hyperplastic rest and normal kidney.

Because intralobar nephrogenic rests are most commonly found at the interface between the nephro-

blastoma and adjacent renal parenchyma, they may be easily misinterpreted as part of the infiltrating tumor. To avoid such confusion, it is helpful to remember that most nephroblastomas have a sharply demarcated pushing border with the kidney, as opposed to the ill-defined, irregular border of intralobar rests.

PROGNOSIS AND TREATMENT

The finding of nephrogenic rests increases the likelihood of subsequent development of nephroblastoma in the opposite kidney. If a patient is found to have nephroblastomatosis, serial imaging studies should be regularly performed to maximize the chances of early detection and treatment of nephroblastoma. Diffuse hyperplastic nephroblastomatosis requires chemotherapy.

CYSTIC PARTIALLY DIFFERENTIATED NEPHROBLASTOMA

Cysts are common in nephroblastomas, and in rare instances a tumor is composed entirely of cysts with delicate septa, without expansile nodules. Such tumors are called cystic partially differentiated nephroblastoma.

CLINICAL FEATURES

Cystic partially differentiated nephroblastoma occurs with greater frequency in boys than in girls; almost all patients are younger than 24 months of age. A palpable abdominal mass is the most common presentation.

PATHOLOGIC FEATURES

GROSS FINDINGS

The tumor often is large, measuring up to 18 cm in diameter. It is well circumscribed from the remaining kidney by a fibrous pseudocapsule. The lesion consists of cysts of variable size separated by thin septa lacking an expansile solid component. Septal elements protruding as gross polyps may be focally identified in the papillonodular variant of cystic partially differentiated nephroblastoma.

MICROSCOPIC FINDINGS

The cysts in cystic partially differentiated nephroblastoma are lined with flattened, cuboidal, or hobnail epithelium, or they may lack lining epithelium (Fig. 6-24A). The septa are variably cellular and contain undifferentiated and differentiated mesenchyme, blastema, and nephroblastomatous epithelial elements (Fig. 6-24B).

Focally, the septal elements may protrude into the cysts in microscopic papillary folds. The epithelial components consist mainly of mature and immature microscopic cysts resembling cross-sections of tubules and stubby papillae resembling immature glomeruli.

DIFFERENTIAL DIAGNOSIS

Cystic nephroblastoma can be distinguished from cystic partially differentiated nephroblastoma by the presence of solid expansile components. When no nephroblastoma elements are found, the term "cystic nephroma" has been applied, although it is recognized that these lesions are not the same as the morphologically similar ones that occur in adults.

Occasionally, a localized (segmental) variant of polycystic renal disease produces a grossly multicystic mass. It can be distinguished from a cystic partially differentiated nephroblastoma by the presence of intervening renal cortical and medullary elements. Furthermore, a distinct fibrous pseudocapsule is characteristically missing from localized polycystic kidney disease.

PROGNOSIS AND TREATMENT

Surgery is almost always curative, with only one recurrence reported.

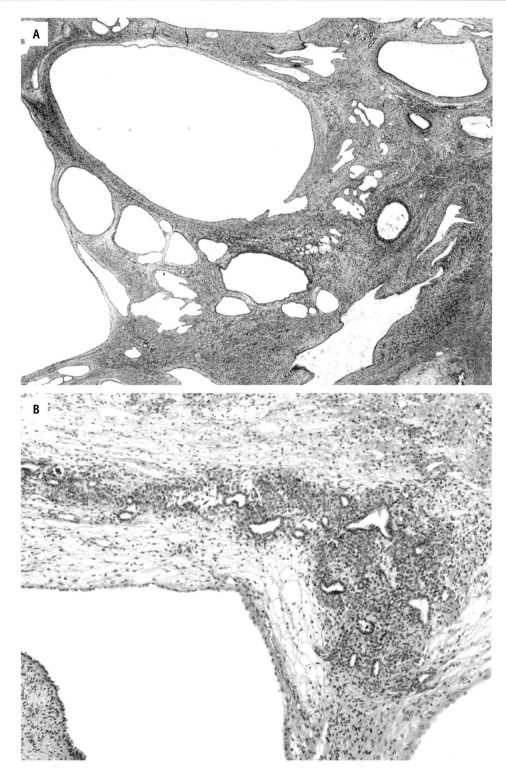

FIGURE 6-24

Cystic partially differentiated nephroblastoma. **A,** The multilocular cysts are lined with flattened, cuboidal or hobnail epithelium. **B,** The septa are variably cellular and contain undifferentiated and differentiated mesenchyme and blastema.

Soft Tissue Tumors

CLEAR CELL SARCOMA

Clear cell sarcoma of the kidney is a rare renal malignant mesenchymal neoplasm of children that has a striking propensity for metastasis to bone. Clear cell sarcoma accounts for approximately 3% to 5% of all childhood renal neoplasms.

CLINICAL FEATURES

The majority of patients affected by clear cell sarcoma of the kidney are clustered in the second and third years of life. The ratio of boys to girls is 2:1. The cell of origin for clear cell sarcoma is unknown.

PATHOLOGIC FEATURES

GROSS FINDINGS

Clear cell sarcomas of the kidney are unicentric, unilateral, irregularly shaped masses with light brown, homogeneous cut surfaces. Cysts are common.

MICROSCOPIC FINDINGS

Clear cell sarcoma of the kidney is characterized by cords of cells with pale cytoplasm and pale, vesicular nuclei separated by septa composed of small blood vessels and spindle cells with dark nuclei (Fig. 6-25A,B). Cells with clear cytoplasm are not typical of clear cell sarcoma of the kidney. Mitotic figures are less common than in nephroblastoma. The border with the kidney is not as sharp as in nephroblastoma, and there often is superficial patchy infiltration of the adjacent renal parenchyma.

A number of histologic variants have been described for clear cell sarcoma of the kidney, including myxoid, sclerosing, cellular, epithelioid, spindle cell, and palisading patterns. Recurrent or metastatic lesions may be deceptively bland-appearing, resembling fibromatosis and other benign myxoid lesions.

ANCILLARY STUDIES

ULTRASTRUCTURAL FEATURES

The cells of clear cell sarcoma of the kidney feature elongated cytoplasmic processes, scattered intermediate filaments, and abundant extracellular matrix.

CLEAR CELL SARCOMA—FACT SHEET

Definition
► A rare pediatric malignant mesenchymal neoplasm of the kidney with propensity for late recurrence and metastasis

Incidence and Location
► 3-5% of all renal pediatric neoplasms
► Renal medulla

Gender, Race, and Age Distribution
► No racial or geographic predilection
► Children; mean age, 36 months
► M/F ratio, 2:1

Clinical Features
► Most are stage 1 or 2 at presentation
► 5% present with hematogenous metastases
► No association with Wilms' tumor

Prognosis and Treatment
► Nephrectomy followed by chemotherapy
► 50-97% survival
► Late relapses: bone metastasis

CLEAR CELL SARCOMA—PATHOLOGIC FEATURES

Gross Findings
► Renal medulla
► Solitary, irregularly shaped mass
► Homogenous, light brown cut surface
► Often cystic

Microscopic Findings
► Several variants; classic is most common
► Classic: cords and nests of polygonal cells separated by delicate fibrovascular network and spindle cells
► Pale vesicular nuclei
► Clear cells infrequent
► Irregular, superficially infiltrative borders
► Other variants: myxoid, cellular, epithelioid, spindle, and palisading

Ultrastructural Features
► Elongated cytoplasmic processes
► Scattered intermediate filaments
► Abundant extracellular matrix

Immunohistochemical Findings
► Vimentin positive
► Negative for all other markers

Differential Diagnosis
► Nephroblastoma
► Congenital mesoblastic nephroma
► Metanephric stromal tumor
► PNET/Ewing's sarcoma
► Synovial sarcoma

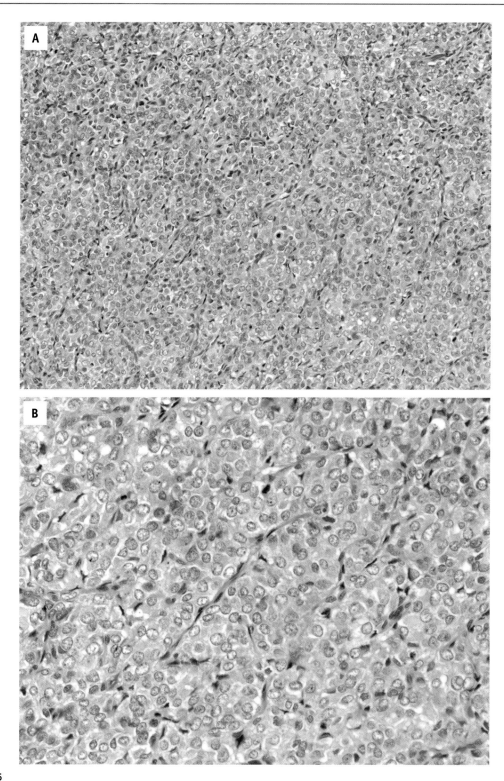

FIGURE 6-25

A, In clear cell sarcoma, sheets and nests of tumor cells are separated by thin vascular septa. **B,** Higher magnification shows the pale vesicular nuclei characteristic of this lesion.

IMMUNOHISTOCHEMISTRY

Clear cell sarcoma of the kidney is characterized by generalized failure to react with essentially all the widely used antibodies, with the exception of vimentin.

DIFFERENTIAL DIAGNOSIS

Perhaps the most challenging differential diagnosis of clear cell sarcoma of the kidney is nephroblastoma. Bilateral and multicentric tumors strongly favor nephroblastoma, and so do heterologous elements. Immunohistochemistry is also helpful, because nephroblastomas are usually reactive for WT1, whereas clear cell sarcoma of the kidney hardly reacts for any marker, except vimentin. Congenital mesoblastic nephroma may resemble spindle cell variants of clear cell sarcoma of the kidney but tends to occur at a younger age and demonstrates desmin immunoreactivity.

PROGNOSIS AND TREATMENT

Approximately one third of patients have metastases to regional lymph nodes at presentation, but only 5 % have distant metastasis. Treatment of clear cell sarcoma of the kidney requires nephrectomy followed by chemotherapy regimens that include Adriamycin (doxorubicin). The latter has resulted in significant improvement in survival rates, which vary from 50 % to 97 % depending on stage. Late relapses, especially in the form of metastasis to bone, are particularly characteristic.

RHABDOID TUMOR

Rhabdoid tumor of the kidney is a rare, highly malignant renal neoplasm of very young children. It is composed of cells with vesicular nuclei, prominent nucleoli, and eosinophilic cytoplasmic inclusions. Rhabdoid tumors account for approximately 2 % of all pediatric renal neoplasms.

CLINICAL FEATURES

Most patients are younger than 24 months of age (mean, 13 months). There is a 1.5:1 male predominance. Hematuria is the most common presentation, and hypercalcemia is a frequent finding. Tumors are rarely confined to the kidney; most patients are found to have disseminated disease at presentation. Reportedly, 15 % of infants with rhabdoid tumor of

---

RHABDOID TUMOR—FACT SHEET

Definition
► A rare, highly malignant renal neoplasm of young children composed of large cells with vesicular nuclei, prominent nucleoli and eosinophilic cytoplasmic inclusions

Incidence and Location
► 2% of all pediatric renal neoplasms

Gender, Race, and Age Distribution
► M/F ratio, 1.5:1
► <24 months of age; mean, 13 months

Clinical Features
► Hematuria
► Hypercalcemia
► Metastases at presentation
► 15% associated with posterior fossa PNET

Prognosis and Treatment
► Highly lethal; 75% die within 1 year after diagnosis
► Widespread hematogenous and lymphatic metastases
► No effective therapy

---

the kidney have an associated PNET of the posterior fossa midline.

Inactivation of the *SMARCB1* (*hSNF5/INI1*) gene on chromosome 22 constitutes a molecular hallmark of rhabdoid tumor of the kidney.

PATHOLOGIC FEATURES

GROSS FINDINGS

Rhabdoid tumors are poorly circumscribed, nonencapsulated masses characterized by a pale cut surface with extensive foci of hemorrhage and necrosis.

MICROSCOPIC FINDINGS

Tumors are composed of sheets of large cells exhibiting a vesicular chromatin pattern, prominent nucleoli, and eosinophilic cytoplasmic inclusions (Fig. 6-26A,B). The tumor borders are highly infiltrative, and lymphovascular space invasion is often widespread. Several other patterns exist, including sclerosing, epithelioid, spindled, and lymphomatoid.

ANCILLARY STUDIES

ULTRASTRUCTURAL FEATURES

The cytoplasmic inclusions are made up of intermediate filaments tightly whorled in a juxtanuclear position.

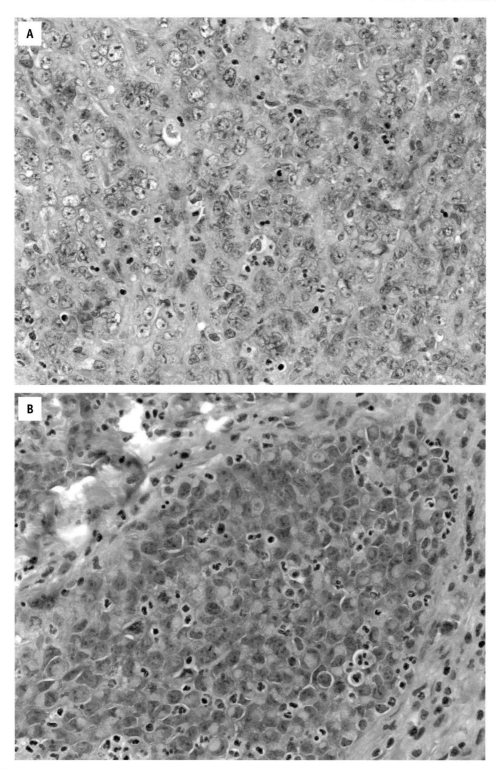

FIGURE 6-26

A, Sheets of large cells with vesicular nuclei and prominent nucleoli are evident in rhabdoid tumor. **B,** Note the characteristic eosinophilic cytoplasm (rhabdoid) inclusions.

RHABDOID TUMOR—PATHOLOGIC FEATURES

Gross Findings
- ▶ Poorly circumscribed, nonencapsulated mass
- ▶ Necrosis and hemorrhage common

Microscopic Findings
- ▶ Sheets of uniform cells with (1) large vesicular nuclei, (2) prominent nucleoli, (3) cytoplasmic inclusions

Ultrastructural Features
- ▶ Intermediate filaments adjacent to nucleus

Immunohistochemical Findings
- ▶ Vimentin positive
- ▶ Cytokeratin and EMA focally positive

Differential Diagnosis
- ▶ Nephroblastoma
- ▶ Neuroblastoma
- ▶ Mesoblastic nephroma
- ▶ Clear cell carcinoma of the kidney
- ▶ Renal medullary carcinoma
- ▶ Metastasis

IMMUNOHISTOCHEMISTRY

The tumor cells are diffusely and intensely reactive for vimentin but only focally reactive for cytokeratin and EMA.

DIFFERENTIAL DIAGNOSIS

The finding of rhabdoid features in other pediatric renal neoplasms may confront the examiner with diagnostic dilemmas. Such tumors include nephroblastoma, neuroblastoma, renal medullary carcinoma, mesoblastic nephroma, and clear cell sarcoma of the kidney. However, these rhabdoid features, when present, are focal, and careful examination of the entire tumor is necessary to arrive at the correct diagnosis. Renal medullary carcinoma occurs at a more advanced age than rhabdoid tumor and is almost exclusively found in patients with sickle cell disease.

PROGNOSIS AND TREATMENT

The diagnosis of rhabdoid tumor of the kidney carries a dismal prognosis, and effective therapy is lacking. Metastases to bone and brain are particularly common, causing death within 1 year after diagnosis in more than 75% of patients.

CONGENITAL MESOBLASTIC NEPHROMA

Congenital mesoblastic nephroma is a rare, low-grade spindle cell neoplasm of the kidney occurring in infants. It is the most common congenital renal neoplasm and comprises approximately 2% of all pediatric renal neoplasms.

CLINICAL FEATURES

More than 90% of affected patients are younger than 1 year of age, and about two thirds are diagnosed in the first 3 months of life. Most patients present with a palpable abdominal mass, although an increasing number of tumors are being detected sonographically in utero. The cellular type of mesoblastic nephroma shares many molecular and cytogenetic features with infantile fibrosarcoma.

PATHOLOGIC FEATURES

GROSS FINDINGS

Tumors are centered in the renal sinus. Classic mesoblastic nephroma is typically small and characterized by a firm, whorled cut surface resembling leiomyoma. Cellular examples are larger and more frequently soft and cystic, with foci of hemorrhage and necrosis.

CONGENITAL MESOBLASTIC NEPHROMA—FACT SHEET

Definition
- ▶ A rare, low-grade spindle cell neoplasm of infant's kidney

Incidence and Location
- ▶ Most common congenital renal neoplasm
- ▶ 2% of all pediatric renal neoplasms

Gender, Race, and Age Distribution
- ▶ Most common in first 3 months of life
- ▶ No patients in National Wilms' Tumor Study were older than 24 months at diagnosis

Clinical Features
- ▶ Abdominal mass
- ▶ Detected in utero by sonography

Prognosis and Treatment
- ▶ Benign course
- ▶ Cured by complete excision
- ▶ Recurrences are rare

CONGENITAL MESOBLASTIC NEPHROMA—PATHOLOGIC FEATURES

Gross Findings
- ▶ Renal sinus involvement
- ▶ Classic type: small, firm
- ▶ Cellular type: large, soft with hemorrhage and necrosis

Microscopic Findings
- ▶ Classic type: locally invasive; interlacing fascicles of bland fibroblastic cells with infrequent mitoses
- ▶ Cellular type: less invasive; ill-defined fascicles of densely packed, plump cells with high mitotic activity

Ultrastructural Features
- ▶ Fibroblastic and myofibroblastic ultrastructural features

Immunohistochemical Findings
- ▶ Vimentin and SMA positive

Differential Diagnosis
- ▶ Clear cell sarcoma
- ▶ Nephroblastoma
- ▶ Rhabdoid tumor

MICROSCOPIC FINDINGS

Congenital mesoblastic nephroma is categorized into two major histologic types: the "classic" variant resembles benign fibromatosis, (Fig. 6-27A,B) and the more common "cellular" variant is essentially identical to infantile fibrosarcoma (Fig. 6-27C). A "mixed" pattern is recognized when features of both variants are present in a single tumor.

Accordingly, the classic congenital mesoblastic nephroma comprises interlacing fascicles of bland fibroblastic cells with infrequent mitoses (Fig. 6-27A,B). The tumor is locally invasive, usually extending into adjacent renal fat. The cellular pattern, on the other hand, is made up of sheets or ill-defined fascicles of densely packed plump cells with high mitotic activity (Fig. 6-27C). Unlike the classic variant, the borders of cellular mesoblastic nephroma are less invasive and tend to form pushing margins. Necrosis and hemorrhage are naturally more frequent in cellular variants.

ANCILLARY STUDIES

ULTRASTRUCTURAL FEATURES

The cells of congenital mesoblastic nephroma have obvious fibroblastic and myofibroblastic features.

IMMUNOHISTOCHEMISTRY

The tumor cells are reactive for vimentin and usually for smooth muscle actin.

DIFFERENTIAL DIAGNOSIS

Clear cell sarcoma of the kidney may resemble congenital mesoblastic nephroma. Congenital mesoblastic nephroma occurs at a younger age than clear cell sarcoma of the kidney (which is exceptional in the first 6 months of life), and congenital mesoblastic nephroma seldom metastasizes. The latter frequently expresses vimentin and smooth muscle actin, both of which are absent from clear cell sarcoma of the kidney.

PROGNOSIS AND TREATMENT

Most patients are cured by simple nephrectomy alone, although recurrence and metastases may occur in a small minority of cases. Recurrence is thought to be a function of incomplete resection, and special attention should be directed toward obtaining a negative medial (renal sinus) margin.

OSSIFYING RENAL TUMOR OF INFANCY

Ossifying renal tumor of infancy is an exceedingly rare, benign neoplasm of the pelvicaliceal system. It shows male predominance and manifests clinically as a calcified mass mimicking a staghorn calculus. Gross examination reveals its intimate attachment to the renal parenchyma. Microscopically, this tumor is composed of bland spindle cells and osteoblast-like cells accompanied by variable osteoid matrix deposition. Mitotic figures are absent. To date, no instance of recurrence has been reported.

ANGIOMYOLIPOMA

Angiomyolipoma is a benign mesenchymal neoplasm composed of variable proportions of adipose tissue, smooth muscle, and abnormal vasculature. The perivascular epithelioid cell is thought to be the cell of origin. Although the kidney is the most frequent location for angiomyolipomas, they have been reported in other sites, including liver, lungs, lymph nodes, and retroperitoneum.

CLINICAL FEATURES

Angiomyolipoma occurs in two clinical settings: as a component of the tuberous sclerosis complex, and sporadically. In both settings, the ratio of female to male

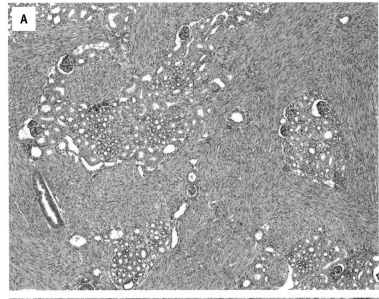

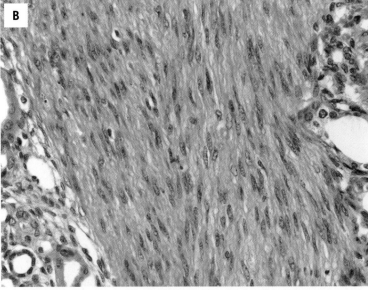

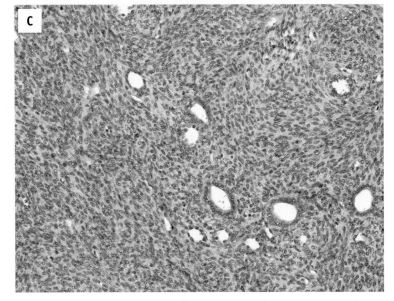

FIGURE 6-27

A and **B**, A benign fibromatosis-like pattern is seen in the classic variant of congenital mesoblastic nephroma. **C,** Cellular variant of congenital mesoblastic nephroma.

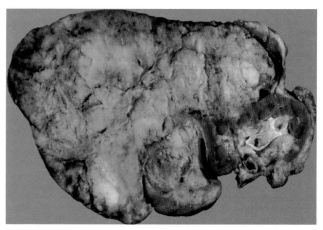

FIGURE 6-28
Angiomyolipoma. A very large, irregular, lobulated mass compressing the kidney.

patients is approximately 3:1. Angiomyolipomas occur from early childhood through adulthood in patients with tuberous sclerosis, and sporadic cases occur in adults with the majority of patients in their fifth and sixth decades. Approximately 70% of tuberous sclerosis patients develop angiomyolipoma, but fewer than half of those with angiomyolipoma manifest tuberous sclerosis. The most important complication of angiomyolipoma is hemorrhage, but this is uncommon in tumors smaller than 4 cm in diameter.

PATHOLOGIC FEATURES

GROSS FINDINGS

Most angiomyolipomas are solitary lesions, but about one fifth are multiple. The presence of multiple angiomyolipomas is strong evidence that the patient has tuberous sclerosis. Angiomyolipomas are well-circumscribed, nonencapsulated masses with yellow to pink lobulated cut surfaces (Fig. 6-28). The color and consistency of a given angiomyolipoma varies according to the relative proportions of fat and smooth muscle in it.

MICROSCOPIC FINDINGS

Angiomyolipomas are composed of a mixture of adipose tissue, smooth muscle, and thick-walled blood

vessels in variable proportions (Fig. 6-29A). Although adipose tissue usually predominates, predominance of smooth muscle is not rare. The smooth muscle cells are spindle-shaped or rounded. They may have substantial nuclear atypia and occasional mitotic figures (Fig. 6-29B). Small angiomyolipomas often are composed entirely of smooth muscle. The blood vessels can be diagnostically helpful; they have unusually thick walls, often hyalinized and lacking the muscular tissue and internal elastic lamina of normal arteries (Fig. 6-29C).

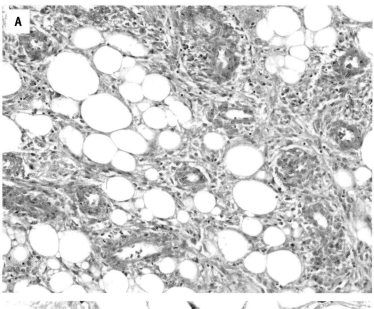

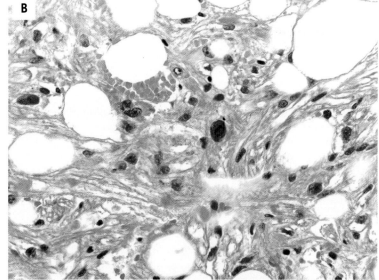

FIGURE 6-29

A, Angiomyolipoma comprised of fat, thick-walled blood vessels and smooth muscle. **B,** Nuclear atypia is not uncommonly observed. **C,** The blood vessels have unusually thick walls, often hyalinized and lacking the muscular tissue and internal elastic lamina of normal arteries.

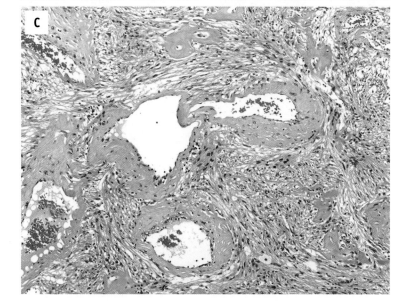

ANCILLARY STUDIES

ULTRASTRUCTURAL FEATURES

The spindle cells show typical smooth muscle morphology. Transitional cells with features of smooth muscle and adipocytes are sometimes identified. Structures resembling melanosomes and premelanosomes, as well as rhomboid structures, are also seen.

IMMUNOHISTOCHEMISTRY

The tumor cells characteristically coexpress smooth muscle markers (actins and desmin) and melanocytic markers (HMB-45, melan A, tyrosinase, and microphthalmia transcription factor) (Fig. 6-30). C-kit (CD117) is also positive. Epithelial markers including cytokeratins are negative.

DIFFERENTIAL DIAGNOSIS

Tumors predominantly composed of adipose tissue may be confused with well-differentiated liposarcoma, and those primarily composed of smooth muscle may be difficult to distinguish from leiomyoma, leiomyosarcoma, or sarcomatoid renal cell carcinoma. The presence of thick-walled blood vessels is an important clue to the diagnosis of angiomyolipoma in both categories. Angiomyolipoma typically lacks the degree of anaplasia and mitotic figures seen in sarcomatoid renal cell carcinoma and leiomyosarcoma.

PROGNOSIS AND TREATMENT

Angiomyolipomas are benign. However, extension into the renal vein and even vena cava may be misinterpreted as evidence of malignancy. Angiomyolipoma is occasionally found in lymph nodes draining a kidney bearing an angiomyolipoma. Neither this nor venous extension has any adverse prognostic significance. Angiomyolipoma should be distinguished from epithelioid angiomyolipoma, which is malignant.

EPITHELIOID ANGIOMYOLIPOMA

Epithelioid angiomyolipoma must be distinguished from ordinary angiomyolipoma, because it is capable of invasion and metastasis and has caused the deaths of a substantial percentage of the patients who have these tumors.

CLINICAL FEATURES

Some patients are symptomatic, presenting with flank pain, whereas in others the tumor is found incidentally in imaging studies. The lack of fat in these tumors makes their radiographic appearance resemble that of renal cell carcinoma.

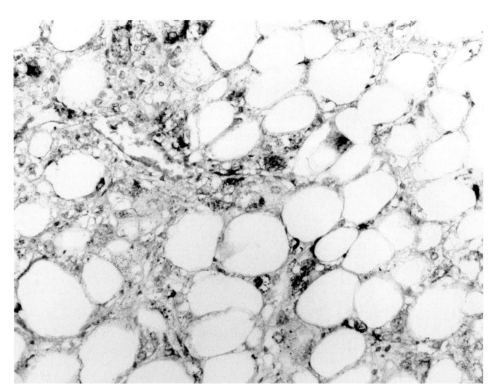

FIGURE 6-30

Melanocytic markers in angiomyolipoma. The tumor cells, especially those with epithelioid morphology, express HMB-45, one of the melanocytic markers.

EPITHELIOID ANGIOMYOLIPOMA—FACT SHEET

Definition
► Angiomyolipoma composed either entirely or predominantly of large epithelioid cells

Morbidity and Mortality
► Up to 50% of patients die of disease

Gender, Race, and Age Distribution
► Wide age range
► Affects men and women equally

Clinical Features
► >50% of patients have a history of tuberous sclerosis
► Frequently symptomatic with pain

Prognosis and Treatment
► Malignant neoplasm with the capacity to be locally aggressive and metastasize

---

EPITHELIOID ANGIOMYOLIPOMA—PATHOLOGIC FEATURES

Gross Findings
► Large solid tumor with infiltratiave growth
► Hemorrhage and necrosis may be extensive
► Extrarenal extension may occur

Microscopic Findings
► Mixture of polygonal cells with eosinophilic, granular cytoplasm and short spindle cells

Immunohistochemical Findings
► Positive for melanocytic markers
► Frequently positive for smooth muscle markers
► Negative for epithelial markers

Differential Diagnosis
► High-grade renal cell caracinoma
► Metastatic melanoma
► Adrenocortical carcinoma

PATHOLOGIC FEATURES

GROSS FINDINGS

Epithelioid angiomyolipomas are solid tumors that often are extensively hemorrhagic and may be necrotic.

MICROSCOPIC FINDINGS

Epithelioid angiomyolipoma has been mistaken for a high-grade renal cell carcinoma in frozen sections, in permanent sections, and by cytology. The tumors are composed either completely or predominantly of stubby spindle cells and polygonal cells with eosinophilic cytoplasm (Fig. 6-31). The hemorrhage and edema prevalent in these tumors can give an appearance of incipient necrosis. Puddles of hemorrhage in areas of polygonal cells closely resemble cysts filled with blood. A minority population of large round cells with amphophilic cytoplasm and eccentrically located nuclei and prominent nucleoli, resembling ganglion cells, is diagnostically helpful. Nuclear atypia and mitotic figures may be prominent.

ANCILLARY STUDIES

IMMUNOHISTOCHEMISTRY

Epithelioid angiomyolipomas invariably express melanocytic markers (e.g., HMB-45, melan A), particularly in the stubby spindle cells. Reactions with actins and desmin are frequently positive, whereas reactions for epithelial markers are negative.

DIFFERENTIAL DIAGNOSIS

High-grade carcinoma is the principal differential diagnostic consideration. Immunohistochemistry easily resolves this question, so the major obstacle to diagnosis is recognizing the possibility that the tumor is an epithelioid angiomyolipoma. Small foci of tissue similar to that of epithelioid angiomyolipoma are present occasionally in otherwise ordinary angiomyolipomas; these comprise in aggregate less than 5% of the tumor. The question of how much of the epithelioid angiomyolipoma pattern must be present for malignant behavior to be possible is not yet answered. The tumors with fatal outcomes appear all to have been entirely or almost entirely composed of epithelioid angiomyolipoma tissue.

PROGNOSIS AND TREATMENT

Epithelioid angiomyolipomas are malignant, and almost 50% of the patients have died of disease. Metastases to lung and liver are particularly common.

JUXTAGLOMERULAR CELL TUMOR

Juxtaglomerular cell tumor is a rare, benign, renin-secreting renal cortical neoplasm.

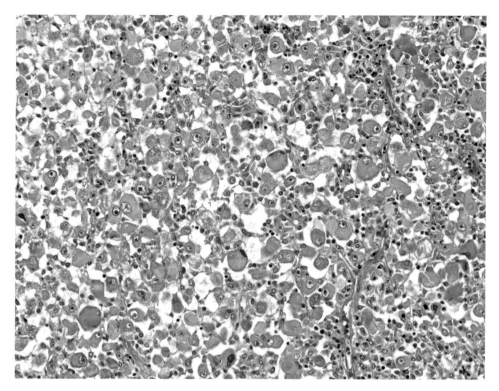

FIGURE 6-31
Sheets of polygonal cells with granular cytoplasm characterize epithelioid angiomyolipoma.

CLINICAL FEATURES

This tumor occurs primarily in young adults, with a mean age of 27 years. The ratio of female to male patients is approximately 2:1. Poorly controlled hypertension, associated with increased renin levels and hypokalemia, and a renal mass constitute the clinical hallmark of this neoplasm.

PATHOLOGIC FEATURES

GROSS FINDINGS

Juxtaglomerular cell tumor typically is a small, well-circumscribed, solitary mass in the renal cortex. Its cut surface is largely solid and light tan to yellow.

MICROSCOPIC FINDINGS

The tumor is composed of fairly uniform polygonal cells with granular eosinophilic cytoplasm and distinct

---

JUXTAGLOMERULAR CELL TUMOR—FACT SHEET

Definition
► A rare, benign, renin-secreting renal cortical neoplasm

Incidence and Location
► Rare
► Renal cortex

Gender, Race, and Age Distribution
► Female predominance (M/F ratio, 1:2)
► Young adults in second and third decades

Clinical Features
► Triad of poorly controlled hypertension, elevated renin levels, and renal mass

Prognosis and Treatment
► Simple excision is curative, including hypertension
► No reported recurrence or metastases

JUXTAGLOMERULAR CELL TUMOR—PATHOLOGIC FEATURES

Gross Findings
► Solitary, well-circumscribed, cortical mass
► Firm, light tan to yellow cut surface

Microscopic Findings
► Sheets, papillae, or trabeculae of uniform polygonal cells
► Granular eosinophilic cytoplasm
► Distinct cytoplasmic borders
► PAS and Bowie stain positive

Ultrastructural Features
► Rhomboid, renin-specific crystals

Immunohistochemical Findings
► Vimentin, actin, renin, CD31, and CD34 positive
► Desmin, cytokeratins, S-100, and HMB-45 negative

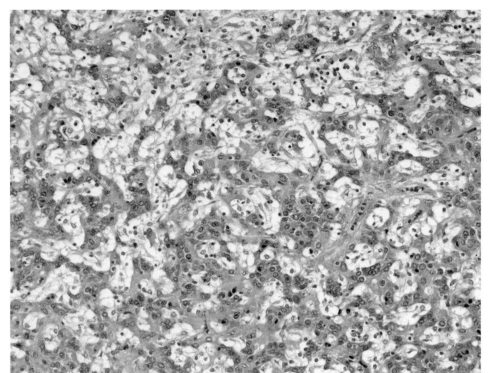

FIGURE 6-32

A hemangiopericytic vascular arrangement decorates juxtaglomerular cell tumor.

cell borders. The tumor cells may grow in sheets or leaf-like papillae or assume a trabecular pattern. A hemangiopericytic vascular arrangement and scant myxoid stroma are characteristic (Fig. 6-32). The cytoplasmic granules react with PAS and Bowie preparations. The nuclei lack atypia, and mitoses are uncommon.

ANCILLARY STUDIES

ULTRASTRUCTURAL FEATURES

Membrane-bound, rhomboid, renin-specific crystals are characteristic.

IMMUNOHISTOCHEMISTRY

The tumor cells react with renin, vimentin, actin, CD31, and CD34. They are negative for desmin, cytokeratins, S-100, HMB-45, and neuroendocrine markers.

PROGNOSIS AND TREATMENT

Simple excision is curative and results in resolution of hypertension in most cases. No incidents of recurrence or metastases have been reported.

RENOMEDULLARY INTERSTITIAL CELL TUMOR

Renomedullary interstitial cell tumors are common lesions that arise from the specialized interstitial cells of the renal medulla, which are believed to play a role in regulation of blood pressure.

CLINICAL FEATURES

These asymptomatic tumors are encountered at autopsy in approximately 50% of the adult population. In half of those cases, more than one lesion is detected. In spite of the role of the interstitial cells of renal medulla in regulating blood pressure, hypertension is not a feature of this group of neoplasms.

PATHOLOGIC FEATURES

GROSS FINDINGS

Renomedullary interstitial cell tumors are usually small (1 to 5 mm), white or pale gray nodules within a renal medullary pyramid.

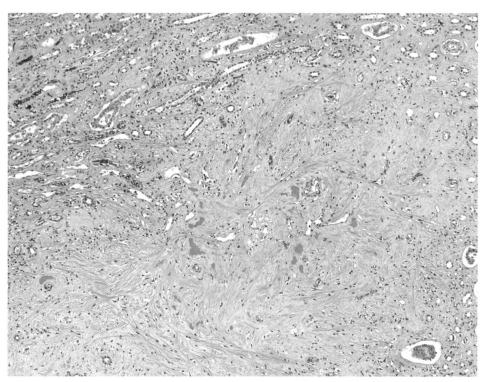

FIGURE 6-33

Amyloid deposits may be seen in renomedullary interstitial cell tumor.

MICROSCOPIC FINDINGS

Renomedullary interstitial cell tumors are composed of poorly formed fascicles of small stellate or polygonal cells in a background of loose, faintly basophilic stroma reminiscent of renal medullary stroma. Entrapped medullary tubules may be found at the periphery of these lesions. Some tumors are hyalinized, and others contain deposits of amyloid (Fig. 6-33).

DIFFERENTIAL DIAGNOSIS

Microscopically, these tumors may resemble metanephric stromal tumors. The latter, however, is rarely found in adults and has the characteristic collars of condensed stromal cells around entrapped renal tubules.

PROGNOSIS AND TREATMENT

Renomedullary interstitial cell tumors are benign lesions of no clinical significance.

CYSTIC NEPHROMA

Cystic nephroma is a benign cystic neoplasm of adults.

CLINICAL FEATURES

Primarily a neoplasm of middle-aged adults, cystic nephromas show a striking predilection toward women, with an 8:1 ratio. They are solitary, multilocular, cystic structures. Patients are usually asymptomatic, and most lesions are found incidentally.

CYSTIC NEPHROMA—FACT SHEET

Definition
▶ A benign cystic neoplasm comprised of epithelial and stromal elements

Gender, Race, and Age Distribution
▶ Striking female predominance (M/F ratio, 1:8)
▶ Middle-aged adults

Clinical Features
▶ Usually asymptomatic

Prognosis and Treatment
▶ Benign
▶ Excision is curative

PATHOLOGIC FEATURES

GROSS FINDINGS

Cystic nephroma is an encapsulated mass of cysts that is sharply demarcated from the adjacent renal parenchyma. The cysts range from small to large, and the septa are typically 1 to 2 mm thick. The inner surfaces of the cysts are smooth, and the content is typically clear yellow fluid. Expansile nodules of solid growth are not found in cystic nephromas.

MICROSCOPIC FINDINGS

The cysts are lined by a single layer of flattened, cuboidal or low columnar epithelial cells (Fig. 6-34A). These cells may display an acidophilic or clear cytoplasm and hobnail features (Fig. 6-34B). The septa may be densely fibrotic or more cellular and resemble ovarian stroma (Fig. 6-34C). Structures resembling cross-sections of renal tubules may be present in the septa.

ANCILLARY STUDIES

IMMUNOHISTOCHEMISTRY

The nuclei of the cellular stroma of cystic nephroma frequently react with antibodies to estrogen receptor and progesterone receptor, whereas the cytoplasm of the stroma often reacts with antibody to inhibin.

CYSTIC NEPHROMA—PATHOLOGIC FEATURES

Gross Findings
- ► Solitary, encapsulated, and well-demarcated
- ► Multilocular cystic mass
- ► Expansile nodules of solid growth absent

Microscopic Findings
- ► Cysts lined by single layer of epithelium
- ► Lining epithelial cells are flat, cuboidal, or low columnar
- ► Hyalinized or cellular stroma resembling ovarian stroma

Immunohistochemical Findings
- ► Stroma reactive to antibodies to estrogen receptor, progesterone receptor, and inhibin

Differential Diagnosis
- ► Multilocular cystic renal cell carcinoma
- ► Non-neoplastic multilocular renal cysts

DIFFERENTIAL DIAGNOSIS

As discussed previously, multilocular cystic renal cell carcinoma is distinguished from cystic nephroma by the presence of intraseptal clusters of clear cells in the former. Non-neoplastic cystic conditions are typically accompanied by abnormal renal architecture and remnants of nephrons in the fibrous septa.

PROGNOSIS AND TREATMENT

This is a benign lesion that is cured by excision.

MIXED EPITHELIAL AND STROMAL TUMOR

Mixed epithelial and stromal tumor is a rare complex renal neoplasm composed of a mixture of stromal and epithelial elements. In the literature, these tumors have been discussed with a variety of names: cystic hamartoma of renal pelvis, leiomyomatous renal hamartoma, adult mesoblastic nephroma, and solid and cystic biphasic tumors. Despite the previous designation as "adult mesoblastic nephroma," these tumors have no association with pediatric mesoblastic nephromas.

CLINICAL FEATURES

This is a tumor of adults with a striking female predominance (6:1). The mean age is perimenopausal (46 years). Presenting signs and symptoms include flank mass, flank pain, hematuria, or symptoms of urinary tract infection; 25% of tumors are found incidentally. An estrogenic influence is suspected.

PATHOLOGIC FEATURES

GROSS FINDINGS

The tumors often arise centrally in the kidney and grow as expansile masses, frequently herniating into the renal pelvis cavity (Fig. 6-35). The tumors are typically well-circumscribed and encapsulated and show a mixed solid and cystic growth pattern. They vary greatly in size, ranging from 2 to 24 cm in diameter.

MICROSCOPIC FINDINGS

Mixed epithelial and stromal tumors are complex tumors composed of a mixture of cysts and tubules (Fig. 6-36A). Some cysts and tubules are lined by colum-

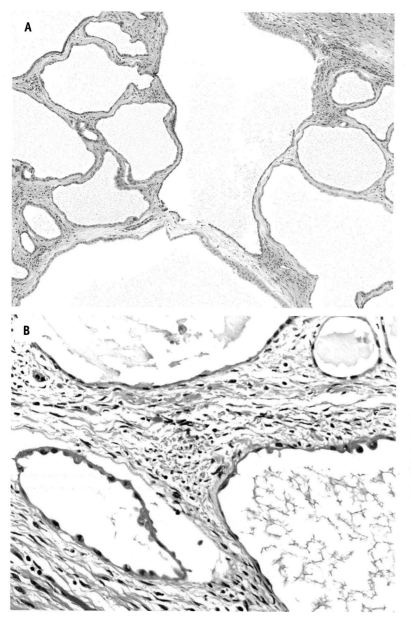

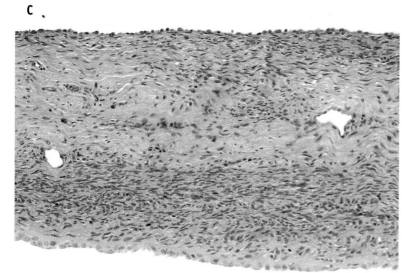

FIGURE 6-34

A, Cystic nephroma is characterized by a mixture of small and medium cysts lined by a one-cell layer of epithelial cells. **B,** The cysts are lined by a single layer of flattened, cuboidal, or low columnar epithelial cells. **C,** Structures resembling cross-sections of renal tubules may be present in the septa, and there may be dense, ovarian-like stroma.

MIXED EPITHELIAL AND STROMAL TUMOR—FACT SHEET

Definition

▶ A rare, complex adult renal neoplasm composed of a mixture of stromal and epithelial elements

Incidence and Location

▶ Rare
▶ Center of kidney

Gender, Race, and Age Distribution

▶ Striking female predominance (M/F ratio, 1:6)
▶ Perimenopausal women

Clinical Features

▶ Flank mass or pain
▶ Hematuria
▶ Urinary tract infections
▶ Incidental findings

Prognosis and Treatment

▶ Benign
▶ Excision is curative

---

them, to densely packed clusters of microcysts, to complex branching channels that may be dilated. These varied elements often are intermingled in the same area of the tumor. The stroma consists of a variably cellular population of spindle cells with plump nuclei and abundant cytoplasm (Fig. 6-36D). Areas of myxoid stroma and fascicles of smooth muscle cells may be present. Densely collagenous stroma is common, and fat is occasionally present. Mitotic figures and atypical nuclei are very uncommon.

ANCILLARY STUDIES

IMMUNOHISTOCHEMISTRY

The spindle cells react for vimentin, actins, and desmin. Their nuclei frequently express estrogen and progesterone receptors. The epithelial elements react with cytokeratins and often with vimentin.

DIFFERENTIAL DIAGNOSIS

Mixed epithelial and stromal tumor may have areas that can be confused with cystic nephroma or multilocular cystic renal cell carcinoma. Examination of multiple blocks will show the characteristic complex mixture of varied epithelial elements and varied stromal elements, which is typical of mixed epithelial and stromal tumor in almost all cases.

---

nar and cuboidal epithelium, which sometimes forms small papillary tufts (Fig. 6-36B). Other cysts are lined by flattened, cuboidal, or columnar cells (Fig. 6-36C). Their cytoplasm ranges from clear to pale, eosinophilic, or vacuolated. The architecture of cysts is varied and ranges from simple cysts with abundant stroma between

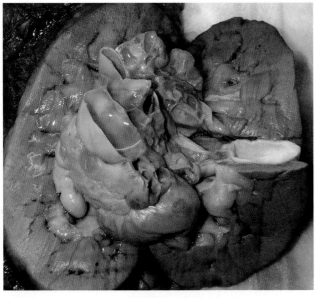

FIGURE 6-35

Mixed epithelial and stromal tumor of the kidney arises centrally in the kidney and grows as an expansile, cystic mass.

MIXED EPITHELIAL AND STROMAL TUMOR—PATHOLOGIC FEATURES

Gross Findings

▶ Central mass
▶ Well-circumscribed, encapsulated
▶ Complex solid and cystic architecture

Microscopic Findings

▶ Biphasic: epithelial and stromal elements
▶ Epithelial elements: varied cysts, and tubules
▶ Stromal elements: variably cellular, bland plump cells

Immunohistochemical Findings

▶ Epithelial elements: cytokeratins, vimentin positive
▶ Stromal elements: vimentin, actins, desmin, estrogen receptor, and progesterone receptor positive

Differential Diagnosis

▶ Cystic nephroma
▶ Multilocular cystic renal cell carcinoma

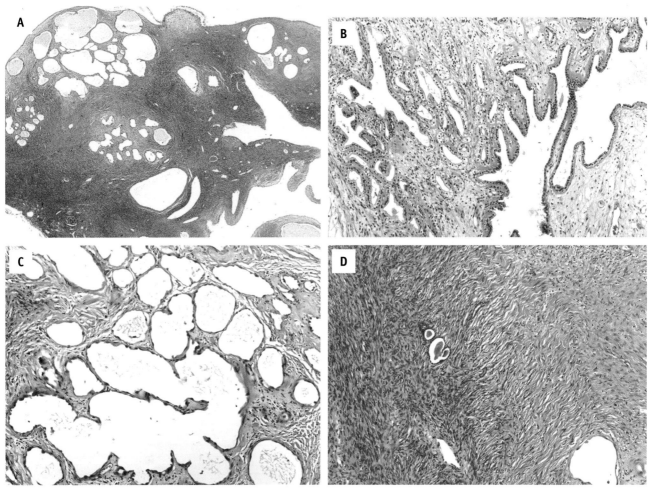

FIGURE 6-36

A, Mixed epithelial and stromal tumor of the kidney is composed of a mixture of cysts, tubules, and stromal components. **B,** Some cysts and tubules are lined by columnar and cuboidal epithelium. **C,** Other cysts are lined by flattened or cuboidal cells. **D,** The stroma consists of a variably cellular population of spindle cells.

PROGNOSIS AND TREATMENT

To date, all of these tumors appear to have been cured by surgical resection, with no recurrence or metastases.

Miscellaneous Mesenchymal Tumors

Other mesenchymal tumors involve the kidney but are not covered in this chapter, including leiomyoma, leiomyosarcoma, schwannoma, neurofibroma, solitary fibrous tumor, hemangiopericytoma, osteosarcoma, lymphangioma, hemangioma, angiosarcoma, rhabdomyosarcoma, malignant fibrous histiocytoma, and synovial sarcoma. Morphologically, these tumors are no different from their counterparts in other organs.

Neural/Neuroendocrine Tumors

RENAL CARCINOID TUMOR

Renal carcinoid tumor is a rare, low-grade neuroendocrine neoplasm arising in the kidney.

CLINICAL FEATURES

Most patients are adults in their fifth decade of life or older, although a wide age range has been reported. Both sexes are affected equally. Signs and symptoms are nonspecific and endocrine disturbances are very infrequent.

PATHOLOGIC FEATURES

GROSS FINDINGS

Renal carcinoid tumors are solitary, well-circumscribed, and usually encapsulated masses that are characterized by tan-yellow, fleshy cut surfaces. Foci of hemorrhage, calcification, and cystic degeneration may be present. Necrosis is uncommon.

MICROSCOPIC FINDINGS

Histologically, these tumors are similar to carcinoid tumors in other organs (Fig. 6-37A,B). The presence of nuclear atypia or mitotic figures may prompt the designation "atypical" carcinoid or "neuroendocrine/small cell" carcinoma if extreme anaplasia and numerous mitotic figures are present.

ANCILLARY STUDIES

ULTRASTRUCTURAL FEATURES

Like other neuroendocrine tumors, dense core granules are plentiful in renal carcinoid tumors.

IMMUNOHISTOCHEMISTRY

The neoplastic cells express neuroendocrine markers such as synaptophysin and chromogranin (Fig. 6-37C).

DIFFERENTIAL DIAGNOSIS

Before a diagnosis of renal carcinoid tumor is rendered, the possibility of metastases must be excluded.

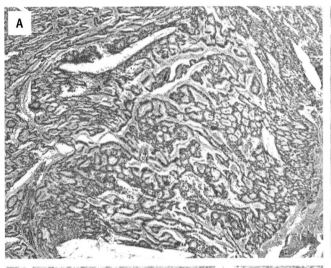

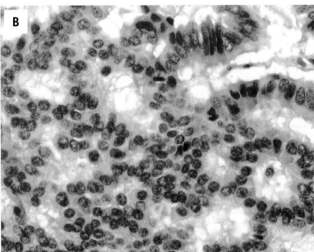

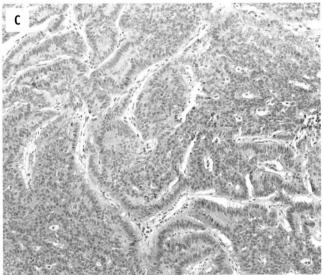

FIGURE 6-37

Carcinoid tumor of the kidney. Tumor cells form ribbons and cribriform structures (**A**) and have uniform nuclei with smooth chromatin and inconspicuous nucleoli (**B**). **C,** Neuroendocrine markers, such as synaptophysin, are positive in the tumor cells.

PROGNOSIS AND TREATMENT

Although histology is not predictive of long-term outcome, about one third of carcinoid tumors with typical histology metastasize, and a reportedly higher percentage of atypical carcinoids develop metastases.

NEUROENDOCRINE CARCINOMA OF THE KIDNEY

This is a poorly differentiated neuroendocrine epithelial neoplasm that is considered the high-grade end of a continuum with renal carcinoid tumor. It primarily affects older adults and tends to be large and locally invasive. The prognosis is poor.

PRIMITIVE NEUROECTODERMAL TUMOR (EWING'S SARCOMA)

PNET (Ewing's sarcoma) of the kidney is a rare malignant, small round blue cell neoplasm characterized by the translocation t(11:22)(q24;q12), which results in fusion of the EWSR1 and the EWSR2 (FLI1) oncogene.

CLINICAL FEATURES

A wide age range (4 to 69 years) has been recorded, with the majority of patients in their second or third decade of life. Presenting signs and symptoms are non-specific and include flank pain, hematuria, and palpable abdominal mass. Approximately 10% of patients have metastases at the time of presentation.

PATHOLOGIC FEATURES

GROSS FINDINGS

Macroscopically, these tumors are large, with a mean of 16 cm, and locally invasive, commonly overgrowing and replacing the host kidney. On cut surface, they appear as lobulated, tan-white masses with areas of hemorrhage and necrosis.

MICROSCOPIC FINDINGS

Similar to PNET in other locations, PNET of the kidney is composed of small round cells with scant cytoplasm, hyperchromatic nuclei, and finely dispersed chromatin (Fig. 6-38A). Pyknotic cells and mitotic figures may be prominent. The cells are arranged primarily in sheets with perivascular pseudorosettes (Fig. 6-38B).

ANCILLARY STUDIES

IMMUNOHISTOCHEMISTRY

The tumor cells characteristically express the CD99 (MIC2) gene product, CD99 (O13), or HBA71 and vimentin. FLI-1 immunoreactivity is seen in more than 50% of the cases. A minority of tumors react with cytokeratin and S-100.

PROGNOSIS AND TREATMENT

The prognosis depends largely on pathologic stage. Surgery followed by aggressive chemotherapy improves survival.

NEUROBLASTOMA

Primary neuroblastoma of the kidney is exceedingly rare. Morphologically, these tumors are indistinguishable from their adrenal counterparts.

LYMPHOID TUMORS

Primary renal lymphoma is rare, but renal involvement by a generalized lymphoma is common. Currently, post-transplantation lymphoproliferative disorders are among the most frequently diagnosed hematologic renal malignancies. Plasmacytoma of the kidney is usually a manifestation of systemic disease and only exceptionally a primary renal disease. Leukemic infiltration is diffuse and bilateral.

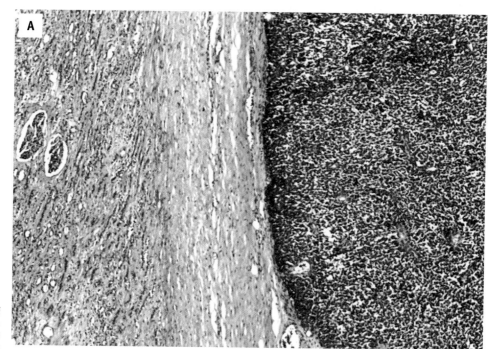

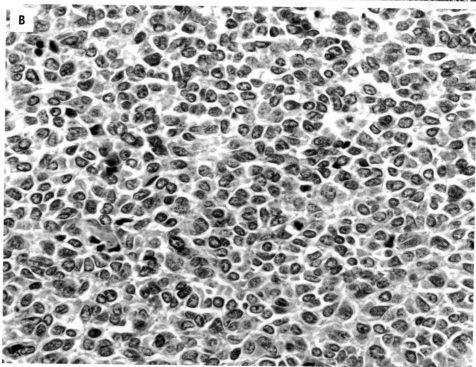

FIGURE 6-38

Primitive neuroectodermal tumor of the kidney. Lying directly adjacent to the renal parenchyma, the tumor is composed of small round cells with scant cytoplasm, hyperchromatic nuclei, and finely dispersed chromatin (**A**). Pyknotic cells and mitotic figures may be prominent. The cells are arranged primarily in sheets with pseudorosettes (**B**).

SUGGESTED READINGS

Clear Cell Renal Cell Carcinoma

Amin MB, Amin MB, Tamboli P, et al: Prognostic impact of histologic subtyping of adult renal epithelial neoplasms: An experience of 405 cases. Am J Surg Pathol 2002;26:281–291.

Cheville JC, Lohse CM, Zincke H, et al: Comparisons of outcome and prognostic features among histologic subtypes of renal cell carcinoma. Am J Surg Pathol 2003;27:612–624.

Eble JN, Sauter G, Epstein JI, et al: World Health Organization classification of tumors: Pathology and genetics of tumors of the urinary system and male genital organs. Lyons, IARC Press, 2004.

Fuhrman SA, Lasky LC, Limas C: Prognostic significance of morphologic parameters in renal cell carcinoma. Am J Surg Pathol 1982;6:655–663.

Moch H, Gasser T, Amin MB, et al: Prognostic utility of the recently recommended histologic classification and revised TNM staging system of renal cell carcinoma: A Swiss experience with 588 tumors. Cancer 2000;89:604–614.

Murphy WM, Grignon DJ, Perlman EJ: Tumors of the Kidney, Bladder, and Related Urinary Structures. Atlas of Tumor Pathology, 4th series,

Fascicle 1. Washington, DC, Armed Forces Institute of Pathology, 2004.

Störkel S, Eble JN, Adlakha K, et al: Classification of renal cell carcinoma: Workgroup No. 1. Union Internationale Contre le Cancer (UICC) and the American Joint Committee on Cancer (AJCC). Cancer 1997;80:987–989.

Multilocular Cystic Renal Cell Carcinoma

Eble JN, Bonsib SM: Extensively cystic renal neoplasms: Cystic nephroma, cystic partially differentiated nephroblastoma, multilocular cystic renal cell carcinoma, and cystic hamartoma of renal pelvis [review]. Semin Diagn Pathol 1998;15:2–20.

Hartman DS, Davis CJ Jr, Johns T, Goldman SM: Cystic renal cell carcinoma. Urology 1986;28:145–153.

Koga S, Yamasaki A, Nishikido M, et al: Multiloculated renal cell carcinoma. Int Urol Nephrol 1991;23:423–428.

Murad T, Komaiko W, Oyasu R, Bauer K: Multilocular cystic renal cell carcinoma. Am J Clin Pathol 1991;95:633–637.

Nassir A, Jollimore J, Gupta R, et al: Multilocular cystic renal cell carcinoma: A series of 12 cases and review of the literature [review]. Urology 2002;60:421–427.

Papillary Renal Cell Carcinoma

Amin MB, Corless CL, Renshaw AA, et al: Papillary (chromophil) renal cell carcinoma: Histomorphologic characteristics and evaluation of conventional pathologic prognostic parameters in 62 cases. Am J Surg Pathol 1997;21:621–635.

Brunelli M, Eble JN, Zhang S, et al: Gains of chromosomes 7, 17, 12, 16, and 20 and loss of Y occur early in the evolution of papillary renal cell neoplasia: A fluorescent in situ hybridization study. Mod Pathol 2003;16:1053–1059.

Delahunt B, Eble JN: Papillary renal cell carcinoma: A clinicopathologic and immunohistochemical study of 105 tumors. Mod Pathol 1997;10:537–544.

Delahunt B, Eble JN, McCredie MR, et al: Morphologic typing of papillary renal cell carcinoma: Comparison of growth kinetics and patient survival in 66 cases. Hum Pathol 2001;32:590–595.

Lager DJ, Huston BJ, Timmerman TG, Bonsib SM: Papillary renal tumors: Morphologic, cytochemical, and genotypic features. Cancer 1995;76:669–673.

Onishi T, Ohishi Y, Goto H, et al: Papillary renal cell carcinoma: Clinicopathological characteristics and evaluation of prognosis in 42 patients. BJU Int 1999;83:937–943.

Chromophobe Renal Cell Carcinoma

Abrahams NA, Maclennan GT, Khoury JD, et al: Chromophobe renal cell carcinoma: A comparative study of histological, immunohistochemical and ultrastructural features using high throughput tissue microarray. Histopathology 2004;45:593–602.

Crotty TB, Farrow GM, Lieber MM: Chromophobe cell renal carcinoma: Clinicopathological features of 50 cases. J Urol 1995;154:964–967.

Latham B, Dickersin GR, Oliva E: Subtypes of chromophobe cell renal carcinoma: An ultrastructural and histochemical study of 13 cases. Am J Surg Pathol 1999;23:530–535.

Thoenes W, Storkel S, Rumpelt HJ, et al: Chromophobe cell renal carcinoma and its variants: A report on 32 cases. J Pathol 1988;155:277–287.

Tickoo SK, Amin MB, Zarbo RJ: Colloidal iron staining in renal epithelial neoplasms, including chromophobe renal cell carcinoma: Emphasis on technique and patterns of staining. Am J Surg Pathol 1998;22:419–424.

Carcinoma of the Collecting Ducts of Bellini

Chao D, Zisman A, Pantuck AJ, et al: Collecting duct renal cell carcinoma: Clinical study of a rare tumor. J Urol 2002;167:71–74.

Fleming S, Lewi HJ: Collecting duct carcinoma of the kidney. Histopathology 1986;10:1131–1141.

Kennedy SM, Merino MJ, Linehan WM, et al: Collecting duct carcinoma of the kidney. Hum Pathol 1990;21:449–456.

Peyromaure M, Thiounn N, Scotte F, et al: Collecting duct carcinoma of the kidney: A clinicopathological study of 9 cases. J Urol 2003;170(4 Pt 1):1138–1140.

Srigley JR, Eble JN: Collecting duct carcinoma of kidney [review]. Semin Diagn Pathol 1998;15:54–67.

Renal Medullary Carcinoma

Avery RA, Harris JE, Davis CJ Jr, et al:. Renal medullary carcinoma: Clinical and therapeutic aspects of a newly described tumor. Cancer 1996;78:128–132.

Davis CJ Jr, Mostofi FK, Sesterhenn IA: Renal medullary carcinoma: The seventh sickle cell nephropathy. Am J Surg Pathol 1995;19:1–11.

Figenshau RS, Basler JW, Ritter JH, et al: Renal medullary carcinoma. J Urol 1998;159:711–713.

Rodriquez-Jurado R, Gonzalez-Crussi F: Renal medullary carcinoma: Immunohistochemical and ultrastructural observations. J Urol Pathol 1996;4:191–203.

Swartz MA, Karth J, Schneider DT, et al: Renal medullary carcinoma: Clinical, pathologic, immunohistochemical, and genetic analysis with pathogenetic implications. Urology 2002;60:1083–1089.

Renal Carcinomas Associated with Xp11.2 Translocations/*TFE3* Gene Fusions

Argani P, Antonescu CR, Illei PB, et al: Primary renal neoplasms with the ASPL-*TFE3* gene fusion of alveolar soft part carcinoma: A distinctive tumor entity previously included among renal cell carcinomas of children and adolescents. Am J Pathol 2001;159:179–192.

Argani P, Ladanyi M: Distinctive neoplasms characterised by specific chromosomal translocations comprise a significant proportion of pediatric renal cell carcinomas [review]. Pathology 2003;35:492–498.

Bruder E, Passera O, Harms D, et al: Morphologic and molecular characterization of renal cell carcinoma in children and young adults. Am J Surg Pathol 2004;28:1117–1132.

Perot C, Boccon-Gibod L, Bouvier R, et al: Five new cases of juvenile renal cell carcinoma with translocations involving Xp11.2: a cytogenetic and morphologic study. Cancer Genet Cytogenet 2003;143:93–99.

Postneuroblastoma Renal Cell Carcinoma

Eble JN: Mucinous tubular and spindle cell carcinoma and post-neuroblastoma carcinoma: Newly recognised entities in the renal cell carcinoma family [review]. Pathology 2003;35:499–504.

Fleitz JM, Wootton-Gorges SL, Wyatt-Ashmead J, et al: Renal cell carcinoma in long-term survivors of advanced stage neuroblastoma in early childhood. Pediatr Radiol 2003;33:540–545.

Koyle MA, Hatch DA, Furness PD 3rd, et al: Long-term urological complications in survivors younger than 15 months of advanced stage abdominal neuroblastoma. J Urol 2001;166:1455–1458.

Medeiros LJ, Palmedo G, Krigman HR, et al: Oncocytoid renal cell carcinoma after neuroblastoma: A report of four cases of a distinct clinicopathologic entity. Am J Surg Pathol 1999;23:772–780.

Vogelzang NJ, Yang X, Goldman S, et al: Radiation induced renal cell cancer: A report of 4 cases and review of the literature [review]. J Urol 1998;160(6 Pt 1):1987–1990.

Mucinous Tubular and Spindle Cell Carcinoma

Eble JN: Mucinous tubular and spindle cell carcinoma and post-neuroblastoma carcinoma: Newly recognised entities in the renal cell carcinoma family [review]. Pathology 2003;35:499–504.

Hes O, Hora M, Perez-Montiel DM, et al: Spindle and cuboidal renal cell carcinoma, a tumour having frequent association with nephrolithiasis: Report of 11 cases including a case with hybrid conventional renal cell carcinoma/spindle and cuboidal renal cell carcinoma components. Histopathology 2002;41:549–555.

Kuroda N, Toi M, Hiroi M, et al: Review of mucinous tubular and spindle-cell carcinoma of the kidney with a focus on clinical and pathobiological aspects. Histol Histopathol 2005;20:221–224.

Parwani AV, Husain AN, Epstein JI, et al: Low-grade myxoid renal epithelial neoplasms with distal nephron differentiation. Hum Pathol 2001;32:506–512.

Rakozy C, Schmahl GE, Bogner S, Storkel S: Low-grade tubular-mucinous renal neoplasms: Morphologic, immunohistochemical, and genetic features. Mod Pathol 2002;15:1162–1171.

Papillary Adenoma of the Kidney

Eble JN, Warfel K: Early human renal cortical epithelial neoplasia. Mod Pathol 1991;4:45A.

Faria V, Reis M, Trigueiros D: Renal adenoma: Identification of two histologic types. Eur Urol 1994;26:170–175.

Grignon DJ, Eble JN: Papillary and metanephric adenomas of the kidney [review]. Semin Diagn Pathol 1998;15:41–53.

Hughson MD, Buchwald D, Fox M: Renal neoplasia and acquired cystic kidney disease in patients receiving long-term dialysis. Arch Pathol Lab Med 1986;110:592–601.

Reis M, Faria V, Lindoro J, Adolfo A: The small cystic and noncystic noninflammatory renal nodules: A postmortem study. J Urol 1988;140:721–724.

Oncocytoma

Amin MB, Crotty TB, Tickoo SK, Farrow GM: Renal oncocytoma: A reappraisal of morphologic features with clinicopathologic findings in 80 cases. Am J Surg Pathol 1997;21:1–12. Erratum, Am J Surg Pathol 1997;21:742.

Cochand-Priollet B, Molinie V, Bougaran J, et al: Renal chromophobe cell carcinoma and oncocytoma: A comparative morphologic, histochemical, and immunohistochemical study of 124 cases. Arch Pathol Lab Med 1997;121:1081–1086.

Eble JN, Hull MT: Morphologic features of renal oncocytoma: A light and electron microscopic study. Hum Pathol 1984;15:1054–1061.

Perez-Ordonez B, Hamed G, Campbell S, et al: Renal oncocytoma: A clinicopathologic study of 70 cases. Am J Surg Pathol 1997;21:871–883.

Tickoo SK, Lee MW, Eble JN, et al: Ultrastructural observations on mitochondria and microvesicles in renal oncocytoma, chromophobe renal cell carcinoma, and eosinophilic variant of conventional (clear cell) renal cell carcinoma. Am J Surg Pathol 2000;24:1247–1256.

Renal Cell Carcinoma, Unclassified

Amin MB, Amin MB, Tamboli P, et al: Prognostic impact of histologic subtyping of adult renal epithelial neoplasms: An experience of 405 cases. Am J Surg Pathol 2002;26:281–291.

Kovacs G, Akhtar M, Beckwith BJ, et al: The Heidelberg classification of renal cell tumors [review]. J Pathol 1997;183:131–133.

Storkel S, Eble JN, Adlakha K, et al: Classification of renal cell carcinoma. Workgroup No. 1. Union Internationale Contre le Cancer (UICC) and the American Joint Committee on Cancer (AJCC). Cancer 1997;80:987–989.

Zisman A, Chao DH, Pantuck AJ, et al: Unclassified renal cell carcinoma: Clinical features and prognostic impact of a new histological subtype. J Urol 2002;168:950–955.

Metanephric Adenoma and Metanephric Adenofibroma

Arroyo MR, Green DM, Perlman EJ, et al.: The spectrum of metanephric adenofibroma and related lesions: Clinicopathologic study of 25 cases from the National Wilms' Tumor Study Group Pathology Center. Am J Surg Pathol 2001;25:433–444.

Brunelli M, Eble JN, Zhang S, et al: Metanephric adenoma lacks the gains of chromosomes 7 and 17 and loss of Y that are typical of papillary renal cell carcinoma and papillary adenoma. Mod Pathol 2003;16:1060–1063.

Davis CJ Jr, Barton JH, Sesterhenn IA, Mostofi FK: Metanephric adenoma: Clinicopathological study of fifty patients. Am J Surg Pathol 1995;19:1101–1114.

Gatalica Z, Grujic S, Kovatich A, Petersen RO: Metanephric adenoma: Histology, immunophenotype, cytogenetics, ultrastructure. Mod Pathol 1996;9:329–333.

Jones EC, Pins M, Dickersin GR, Young RH: Metanephric adenoma of the kidney: A clinicopathological, immunohistochemical, flow cytometric, cytogenetic, and electron microscopic study of seven cases. Am J Surg Pathol 1995;19:615–626.

Muir TE, Cheville JC, Lager DJ: Metanephric adenoma, nephrogenic rests, and Wilms' tumor: A histologic and immunophenotypic comparison. Am J Surg Pathol 2001;25:1290–1296.

Metanephric Stromal Tumor

Argani P, Beckwith JB: Metanephric stromal tumor: Report of 31 cases of a distinctive pediatric renal neoplasm. Am J Surg Pathol 2000;24:917–926.

Palese MA, Ferrer F, Perlman E, Gearhart JP: Metanephric stromal tumor: A rare benign pediatric renal mass. Urology 2001;58:462.

Nephroblastoma

Beckwith JB: National Wilms' Tumor Study: An update for pathologists. Pediatr Dev Pathol 1998;1:79–84.

Beckwith JB: New developments in the pathology of Wilms' tumor. Cancer Invest 1997;15:153–162.

Beckwith JB, Zuppan CE, Browning NG, et al: Histological analysis of aggressiveness and responsiveness in Wilms' tumor. Med Pediatr Oncol 1996;27:422–428.

Charles AK, Mall S, Watson J, Berry PJ: Expression of the Wilms' tumor gene WT1 in the developing human and in pediatric renal tumors: An immunohistochemical study. Mol Pathol 1997;50:138–144.

Parham DM, Roloson GJ, Feely M, et al: Primary malignant neuroepithelial tumors of the kidney: A clinicopathologic analysis of 146 adult and pediatric cases from the National Wilms' Tumor Study Group Pathology Center. Am J Surg Pathol 2001;25:133–146.

Nephrogenic Rests and Nephroblastomatosis

Beckwith JB: Nephrogenic rests and the pathogenesis of Wilms' tumor: Developmental and clinical considerations. Am J Med Genet 1998;79:268–273.

Beckwith JB: Precursor lesions of Wilms' tumor: Clinical and biological implications. Med Pediatr Oncol 1993;21:158–168.

Beckwith JB, Kiviat NB, Bonadio JF: Nephrogenic rests, nephroblastomatosis, and the pathogenesis of Wilms' tumor. Pediatr Pathol 1990;10:1–36.

Bove KE, McAdams AJ: The nephroblastomatosis complex and its relationship to Wilms' tumor: A clinicopathologic treatise. Perspect Pediatr Pathol 1976;3:185–223.

Hennigar RA, O'Shea PA, Grattan-Smith JD: Clinicopathologic features of nephrogenic rests and nephroblastomatosis. Adv Anat Pathol 2001;8:276–289.

Cystic Partially Differentiated Nephroblastoma

Brown JM: Cystic partially differentiated nephroblastoma. J Pathol 1975;115:175–178.

Eble JN: Cystic nephroma and cystic partially differentiated nephroblastoma: Two entities or one? Adv Anat Pathol 1994;1:99–102.

Eble JN, Bonsib SM: Extensively cystic renal neoplasms: Cystic nephroma, cystic partially differentiated nephroblastoma, multilocular cystic renal cell carcinoma, and cystic hamartoma of renal pelvis. Semin Diagn Pathol 1998;15:2–20.

Joshi VV, Banerjee AK, Yadav K, Pathak IC: Cystic partially differentiated nephroblastoma: A clinicopathologic entity in the spectrum of infantile renal neoplasia. Cancer 1977;40:789–795.

Joshi VV, Beckwith JB: Multilocular cyst of the kidney (cystic nephroma) and cystic, partially differentiated nephroblastoma: Terminology and criteria for diagnosis. Cancer 1989;64:466–479.

Clear Cell Sarcoma

Argani P, Perlman EJ, Breslow NE, et al: Clear cell sarcoma of the kidney: A review of 351 cases from the National Wilms' Tumor Study Group Pathology Center. Am J Surg Pathol 2000;24:4–18.

Marsden HB, Lawler W: Bone metastasizing renal tumor of childhood:

Histopathological and clinical review of 38 cases. Virchows Arch A Pathol Anat Histol 1980;387:341–351.

Schuster AE, Schneider DT, Fritsch MK, et al: Genetic and genetic expression analyses of clear cell sarcoma of the kidney. Lab Invest 2003;83:1293–1299.

Sotelo-Avila C, Gonzalez-Crussi F, Sadowinski S, et al: Clear cell sarcoma of the kidney: A clinicopathologic study of 21 patients with long-term follow-up evaluation. Hum Pathol 1985;16:1219–1230.

Rhabdoid Tumor

Douglass EC, Valentine M, Rowe ST, et al: Malignant rhabdoid tumor: A highly malignant childhood tumor with minimal karyotypic changes. Genes Chromosomes Cancer 1990;2:210–216.

Sotelo-Avila C, Gonzalez-Crussi F, deMello D, et al: Renal and extrarenal rhabdoid tumors in children: A clinicopathologic study of 14 patients. Semin Diagn Pathol 1986;3:151–163.

Vujanic GM, Sandstedt B, Harms D, et al: Rhabdoid tumour of the kidney: A clinicopathological study of 22 patients from the International Society of Pediatric Oncology (SIOP) nephroblastoma file. Histopathology 1996;28:333–340.

White FV, Dehner LP, Belchis DA, et al: Congenital disseminated malignant rhabdoid tumor: A distinct clinicopathologic entity demonstrating abnormalities of chromosome 22q11. Am J Surg Pathol 1999;23:249–256.

Congenital Mesoblastic Nephroma

Bolande RP, Brough AJ, Izant RJ Jr: Congenital mesoblastic nephroma of infancy: A report of eight cases and the relationship to Wilms' tumor. Pediatrics 1967;40:272–278.

Fitchev P, Beckwith JB, Perlman EJ: Congenital mesoblastic nephroma: Prognosis and outcome. Lab Invest 2003;83:2P.

Pettinato G, Manivel JC, Wick MR, Dehner LP: Classical and cellular (atypical) congenital mesoblastic nephroma: A clinicopathologic, ultrastructural, immunohistochemical, and flow cytometric study. Hum Pathol 1989;20:682–690.

Ossifying Renal Tumor of Infancy

Chatten J, Cromie WJ, Duckett JW: Ossifying tumor of infantile kidney: Report of two cases. Cancer 1980;45:609–612.

Glick RD, Hicks MJ, Nuchtern JG, et al: Renal tumors in infants less than 6 months of age. J Pediatr Surg 2004;39:522–525.

Sotelo-Avila C, Beckwith JB, Johnson JE: Ossifying renal tumor of infancy: A clinicopathologic study of nine cases. Pediatr Pathol Lab Med 1995;15:745–762.

Angiomyolipoma

Barnard M, Lajoie G: Angiomyolipoma: Immunohistochemical and ultrastructural study of 14 cases. Ultrastruct Pathol 2001;25:21–29.

Cheng L, Gu J, Eble JN, et al: Molecular genetic evidence for different clonal origin of components of human renal angiomyolipomas. Am J Surg Pathol 2001;25:1231–1236.

Eble JN: Angiomyolipoma of kidney. Semin Diagn Pathol 1998;15:21–40.

Farrow GM, Harrison EG Jr, Utz DC, Jones DR: Renal angiomyolipoma: A clinicopathologic study of 32 cases. Cancer 1968;22:564–570.

L'Hostis H, Deminiere C, Ferriere JM, Coindre JM: Renal angiomyolipoma: A clinicopathologic, immunohistochemical, and follow-up study of 46 cases. Am J Surg Pathol 1999;23:1011–1020.

Epithelioid Angiomyolipoma

Cibas ES, Goss GA, Kulke MH, et al: Malignant epithelioid angiomyolipoma ("sarcoma ex angiomyolipoma") of the kidney: A case report and review of the literature. Am J Surg Pathol 2001;25:121–126.

Eble JN, Amin MB, Young RH: Epithelioid angiomyolipoma of the kidney: A report of five cases with a prominent and diagnostically confusing epithelioid smooth muscle component. Am J Surg Pathol 1997;21:1123–1130.

Mai KT, Perkins DG, Collins JP: Epithelioid cell variant of renal angiomyolipoma. Histopathology 1996;28:277–280.

Pea M, Bonetti F, Martignoni G, et al: Apparent renal cell carcinomas in tuberous sclerosis are heterogeneous: The identification of malignant epithelioid angiomyolipoma. Am J Surg Pathol 1998;22:180–187.

Juxtaglomerular Cell Tumor

Duan X, Bruneval P, Hammadeh R, et al: Metastatic juxtaglomerular cell tumor in a 52-year-old man. Am J Surg Pathol 2004;28:1098–1102.

Martin SA, Mynderse LA, Lager DJ, Cheville JC: Juxtaglomerular cell tumor: A clinicopathologic study of four cases and review of the literature. Am J Clin Pathol 2001;116:854–863.

Squires JP, Ulbright TM, DeSchryver-Kecskemeti K, Engleman W: Juxtaglomerular cell tumor of the kidney. Cancer 1984;53:516–523.

Tamboli P, Ro JY, Amin MB, et al: Benign tumors and tumor-like lesions of the adult kidney. Part II: Benign mesenchymal and mixed neoplasms, and tumor-like lesions. Adv Anat Pathol 2000;7:47–66.

Renomedullary Interstitial Cell Tumor

Dall'Era M, Das S: Benign medullary fibroma of the kidney. J Urol 2000;164:2018.

Lerman RJ, Pitcock JA, Stephenson P, Muirhead EE: Renomedullary interstitial cell tumor (formerly fibroma of renal medulla). Hum Pathol 1972;3:559–568.

Tamboli P, Ro JY, Amin MB, et al: Benign tumors and tumor-like lesions of the adult kidney. Part II: Benign mesenchymal and mixed neoplasms, and tumor-like lesions. Adv Anat Pathol 2000;7:47–66.

Cystic Nephroma

Delahunt B, Thomson KJ, Ferguson AF, et al: Familial cystic nephroma and pleuropulmonary blastoma. Cancer 1993;71:1338–1342.

Eble JN, Bonsib SM: Extensively cystic renal neoplasms: Cystic nephroma, cystic partially differentiated nephroblastoma, multilocular cystic renal cell carcinoma, and cystic hamartoma of renal pelvis [review]. Semin Diagn Pathol 1998;15:2–20.

Joshi VV, Beckwith JB: Multilocular cyst of the kidney (cystic nephroma) and cystic, partially differentiated nephroblastoma: Terminology and criteria for diagnosis. Cancer 1989;64:466–479.

Mixed Epithelial and Stromal Tumor

Adsay NV, Eble JN, Srigley JR, et al: Mixed epithelial and stromal tumor of the kidney. Am J Surg Pathol 2000;24:958–970.

Michal M, Hes O, Bisceglia M, et al: Mixed epithelial and stromal tumors of the kidney: A report of 22 cases. Virchows Arch 2004;445:359–367.

Pierson CR, Schober MS, Wallis T, et al: Mixed epithelial and stromal tumor of the kidney lacks the genetic alterations of cellular congenital mesoblastic nephroma. Hum Pathol 2001;32:513–520.

Renal Carcinoid Tumor

Begin LR, Guy L, Jacobson SA, Aprikian AG: Renal carcinoid and horseshoe kidney: A frequent association of two rare entities. Case report and review of the literature. J Surg Oncol 1998;68:113–119.

Goldblum JR, Lloyd RV: Primary renal carcinoid. Case report and literature review. Arch Pathol Lab Med 1993;117:855–858.

Raslan WF, Ro JY, Ordonez NG, et al: Primary carcinoid of the kidney: Immunohistochemical and ultrastructural studies of five patients. Cancer 1993;72:2660–2666.

Primitive Neuroectodermal Tumor (Ewing's Sarcoma)

Antoneli CB, Costa CM, de Camargo B, et al: Primitive neuroectodermal tumor (PNET)/extraosseous Ewing sarcoma of the kidney. Med Pediatr Oncol 1998;30:303–307.

Marley EF, Liapis H, Humphrey PA, et al: Primitive neuroectodermal tumor of the kidney—another enigma: A pathologic, immunohistochemical, and molecular diagnostic study. Am J Surg Pathol 1997;21:354–359.

7

Introduction to Renal Biopsy

Laura Barisoni • Shane Meehan • Lois J. Arend

THE RENAL BIOPSY

INDICATION FOR RENAL BIOPSY

A full understanding of the clinical question and clinicopathologic correlation is important to guide the entire process of the renal biopsy, from triage of the tissue to the final diagnosis.

PREBIOPSY STUDIES

Complete clinical forms should accompany the biopsy (Table 7-1 for examples). The patient's medical history, family history, physical examination results, laboratory data concerning renal function, and appropriate serologic findings provide important information, not only for the nephrologists but also for the pathologist interpreting the kidney biopsy (Table 7-2).

CLINICAL SETTINGS IN WHICH KIDNEY BIOPSY IS EMPLOYED

The kidney reacts to injury in a limited number of ways: proteinuria, hematuria, and increased serum creatinine (acute or chronic). Table 7-3 lists the clinical indications for renal biopsy.

PROTEINURIA

One of the major clinical manifestations of glomerular disease is proteinuria, which is defined as the loss of greater than 150 mg protein in 24 hours. Proteinuria may result from an increase in plasma protein (e.g., Bence Jones proteins), from altered tubular reabsorption with addition of protein to tubular fluid (Tamm-Horsfall protein), or from altered glomerular permeability.

Proteinuria can be nephrotic (> 3 g/day) or subnephrotic (< 3 g/day). Nephrotic-range proteinuria may be associated with nephrotic syndrome (NS). See Tables 7-4, 7-5, and 7-6 for approaches to diagnosis of the cause of proteinuria. Isolated subnephrotic proteinuria is a common clinical problem. However, some of these patients have been diagnosed with membranous glomerulopathy (MGN); early idiopathic, familial, or secondary focal segmental glomerulosclerosis (FSGS); IgA nephropathy; metabolic disorders (e.g., diabetes); or hereditary disorders (e.g., Fabry's disease or Alport disease) (Table 7-6).

NEPHROTIC SYNDROME

NS is a constellation of clinical signs that may be seen in a number of different renal diseases and is characterized by proteinuria greater than 3 g/day, hypercholesterolemia, hypoalbuminemia, lipiduria, and peripheral edema (Tables 7-4 and 7-5). Children with NS usually are first treated for minimal change disease (MCD) and undergo renal biopsy if they fail to respond to steroid therapy. Most nephrologists believe that adult patients with NS should undergo kidney biopsy, because most of them will have renal disease other than minimal change disease, and a correct diagnosis is required for an appropriate therapeutic approach and as an indicator for prognosis (Table 7-4).

HEMATURIA

Hematuria can originate from any segment of the urinary tract. Glomerular hematuria is usually accompanied by red blood cell (RBC) casts. It may be isolated or associated with nephritic syndrome (Tables 7-7 and 7-8). Hematuria can be detected with or without proteinuria. If causes of nonglomerular hematuria have been excluded, a renal biopsy is needed to evaluate the possibility of glomerulopathies (Table 7-7).

NEPHRITIC SYNDROME

Nephritic syndrome is characterized by hematuria, RBC casts, azotemia, hypertension, and oliguria (Table 7-8). Patients with proliferative glomerulonephritis (GN) usually present with nephritic syndrome, and, considering the vast differential diagnosis, a biopsy is necessary. The rationale for a biopsy in these cases is not only diagnosis and management but also evaluation of morphologic features of progression of the disease (activity and chronicity indices) to guide the therapeutic approach (Table 7-8).

TABLE 7-1

Clinical Form

Date	Pt name ....
Nephrologist	Address ....
Office	....
Beeper	Hospital ID ....
Fax	Insurance ....
Fellow .... beeper	DOB................. Sex .... Race ....
	(age)

HISTORY (brief summary) and CLINICAL IMPRESSION   **RUSH**   **ROUTINE**

PAST MEDICAL HISTORY		FAMILY HISTORY
Proteinuria	HTN	Diabetes
Hematuria	Arthritis	Kidney disease
UT infection	Rash	HTN
Diabetes	Deafness	Allergy
Kidney pain	Edema	Deafness
PHYSICAL		
BP	Effusion	Rash
Fundi	Hepatomegaly	Edema
Arthritis	Splenomegaly	Others
LABORATORY DATA (at the time of biopsy)		
Hgb	BUN	VDRL
Hct	S. creatinine	Hep B
WBC	Glucose	Hep C
Platelets	Cholesterol	Cryoglobulin
Coagulation profile	Albumin	p-ANCA
Electrophoresis	Globulin	c-ANCA
- SPEP	Complement	Anti-GBM Ab
- UPEP	- C3	ASO titer
- SIEPEP	- C4	ANA
- UIEP		Anti ds DNA

URINE ANALYSIS	RENAL FUNCTION	SEDIMENT
pH	24h u. protein	RBC
Albumin	Creat. Clear.	WBC
Bence Jones		Epithelial cells
Glucose		Granular casts
Acetone		RBC casts
		WBC casts

THERAPY	FOR RENAL TRANSPLANT ONLY	
Antibiotics	Living related	Original disease
Steroids	Living unrelated	Previous bx
Analgesics	Cadaveric	Therapy
Immunosup.	X-match	Drug levels

TABLE 7-2

Algorithmic Approach to Serology in the Diagnosis of Renal Diseases

NORMAL COMPLEMENT	Perinuclear antineutrophil antibodies (p-ANCA/MPO)	No extrarenal disease	ANCA-associated crescentic and necrotizing glomerulonephritis
		Systemic necrotizing arteritis	Microscopic polyarteritis
		Respiratory necrotizing vasculitis without granulomas	Microscopic polyangiitis
	Cytoplasmic antineutrophil antibodies (c-ANCA/PR3)	Respiratory necrotizing vasculitis with granulomas	Wegener's granulomatosis
	Antiglomerular basement membrane autoantibodies (anti-GBM)	No lung hemorrhage	Anti-GBM glomerulonephritis
		Lung hemorrhage	Goodpasture syndrome
	Antihepatitis B antibodies	Hepatitis	Membranous glomerulopathy
	Antitreponemal antibodies	Syphilis	
	Carcinoembryonic antigen (CEA)	Tumor	
	Antithyroid antibodies	Thyroid disorders	
	HIV		Collapsing glomerulopathy
	Parvovirus B19		
	IgA fibronectin aggregates		IgA nephropathy
	κ or λ monoclonal spikes		Myeloma cast nephropathy AL amyloidosis (λ) Light-chain deposition disease (κ)
LOW COMPLEMENT	Cryoglobulins		Cryoglobulinemic glomerulonephritis
	ANA and anti-dsDNA		Lupus glomerulonephritis
	ANA, anti Scl-70, and anticentromere		Scleroderma
	Antiphospholipid antibodies		Antiphospholipid syndrome nephropathy ± lupus
	Verotoxin from *E. coli* O157:H7		Hemolytic-uremic syndrome (HUS)
	Antipathogen antibodies (e.g., ASO)		Postinfectious glomerulonephritis
	Hepatitis C		Hepatitis C-associated MPGN
	C3 nephritic factor		Idiopathic MPGN

ANA, antinuclear antibodies; ANCA, antineutrophil cytoplasmic autoantibodies; ASO, antistreptolysin O; dsDNA, double-stranded DNA; *E. coli, Escherichia coli;* HIV, human immunodeficiency virus; IgA, immunoglobulin A; MPGN, membranoproliferative glomerulonephritis; MPO, myeloperoxidase; PR3, proteinase 3.

Table 7-3

Indications for Renal Biopsy

Acute renal failure
Nephrotic syndrome
Nephritic syndrome
Proteinuria
Hematuria

Table 7-4
Differential Diagnosis of Nephrotic Syndrome

PODOCYTOPATHIES

Minimal change disease (MCD)
  Idiopathic
  Genetically determined
  Secondary
Focal segmental glomerulosclerosis (FSGS)
  Idiopathic
  Genetically determined
  Secondary
Mesangial sclerosis
  Idiopathic
  Genetically determined
Collapsing glomerulopathy (CG)
  Idiopathic
  Genetically determined
  Secondary

IMMUNE COMPLEX GLOMERULAR DISEASES

Membranous glomerulopathy (MGN)
  Idiopathic
  Secondary (autoimmune, infection, cancer)
C1q nephropathy
Others

GENERALIZED SYSTEMIC DISEASES

Diabetes
Amyloid
Systemic lupus erythematosus
Schönlein-Henoch purpura

ACUTE RENAL FAILURE

Acute renal failure (ARF) is defined as a rapidly increasing serum creatinine concentration. It can be accompanied by abnormal urine sediment (RBCs, white blood cells [WBCs], RBC casts, WBC casts, or epithelial casts) (Table 7-9). Approximately 25% of inpatients develop ARF, and morphologic evaluation is necessary to discriminate among acute tubular injury/acute tubular necrosis (ATN), interstitial nephritis, vasculitic processes, thrombotic microangiopathy (TMA), and proliferative and crescentic GN (Table 7-9).

CHRONIC RENAL FAILURE

Chronic renal failure is defined as a progressive increase in serum creatinine and decrease in glomerular filtration rate. It may reflect progression from any of the glomerular or tubulointerstitial forms of damage. Chronic renal failure is rarely an indication for renal biopsy.

EVALUATION OF FRESH TISSUE FOR TRIAGE

Fresh tissue should be placed in a Petri dish, immersed in saline, and examined under light microscopy (LM) with a 4× objective lens to evaluate for the presence of diagnostic tissue (cortex) (Fig. 7-1). Several different situations may occur.

One or two cores of renal cortex at least 1 cm in length each may have been received. In this case, a small fragment of cortex, measuring 0.3 to 0.4 cm in length, should be placed in optimum cutting temperature medium (OCT) and snap-frozen in liquid nitrogen for immunofluorescence (IF) studies. One to three fragments of cortex, approximately 0.1 cm each, should be fixed in glutaraldehyde for electron microscopy (EM) studies, and the remaining tissue should be fixed in 10% buffered formalin or other appropriate fixative and processed for LM.

Only a small portion of renal cortex may have been received. In this case, the clinical history should guide the pathologist. In general, in cases of suspected GN, LM and IF should be the priorities. EM can always be performed by reprocessing the frozen tissue or the formalin-fixed tissue after completion of the LM and IF studies. If necessary, the entire tissue can be fixed in formalin, and IF can be performed on paraffin sections after pronase digestion (see later discussion).

Early *transplant biopsies* usually do not need EM, unless it is specified or suggested in the requisition form (e.g., presence of proteinuria). IF and EM studies are advised if the patient received the transplant 6 months to 1 year before the time of the biopsy, to exclude recurrent or de novo GN. In cases of suspected antibody-mediated rejection, IF can be performed with antibodies against complement C4d on cortex or on a small portion of medulla (see section on kidney transplants).

PROCESSING AND STANDARD TECHNIQUES

LIGHT MICROSCOPY

Paraffin-embedded biopsy specimens are sectioned, obtaining 10 to 12 levels. Each slide or level should contain two to three serial sections, each 2 to 3 μm thick. One sectioning protocol is to stain levels 1, 6, and 12 with hematoxylin and eosin (H&E), levels 2 and 11 with Jones' silver stain, level 7 with periodic acid-Schiff stain (PAS), and 8 with trichrome. The intervening unstained slides can be used for additional studies as needed.

IMMUNOFLUORESCENCE

Tissue for IF studies should contain renal cortex and should be received in the renal laboratory in saline or in transport medium. IF can be performed on frozen sections, which is ideal, or on paraffin sections.

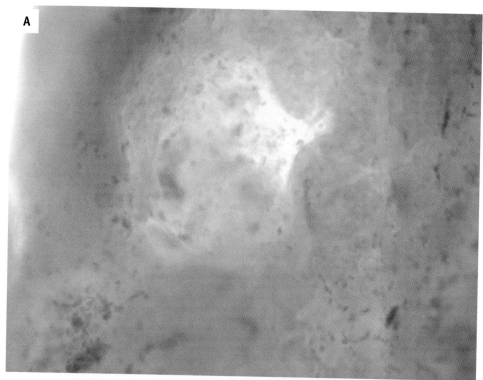

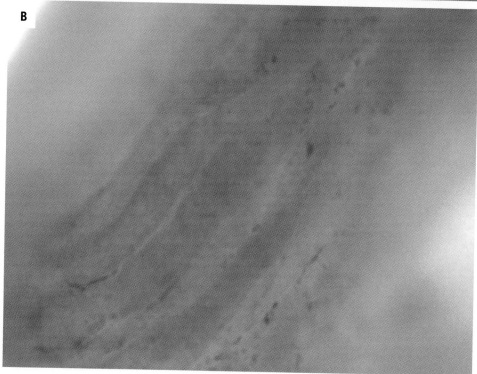

FIGURE 7-1

Fresh tissue. **A,** Cortex can be discriminated from medulla by the presence of round structures representing the glomeruli. **B,** The medulla appears composed of pink and pale stripes, representing tubules and vessels.

STANDARD IMMUNOFLUORESCENCE PANEL

The standard IF panel is performed on frozen tissue from native kidney biopsies and on transplant biopsy specimens (if recurrent or de novo glomerular disease is suspected). The most commonly used panel includes IgG, IgA, IgM, C3, C1q, fibrinogen, albumin, and kappa (κ) and lambda (λ) light chains. Staining with antibodies against κ and λ light chains are recommended;

not only are they useful internal controls, but they also allow early diagnosis of monoclonal gammopathies or primary amyloidosis.

IMMUNOFLUORESCENCE ON PARAFFIN SECTIONS

Immunofluorescence studies are performed on paraffin sections if no frozen tissue is available or in the

Table 7-5

Algorithmic Approach to Nephrotic Syndrome (NS)

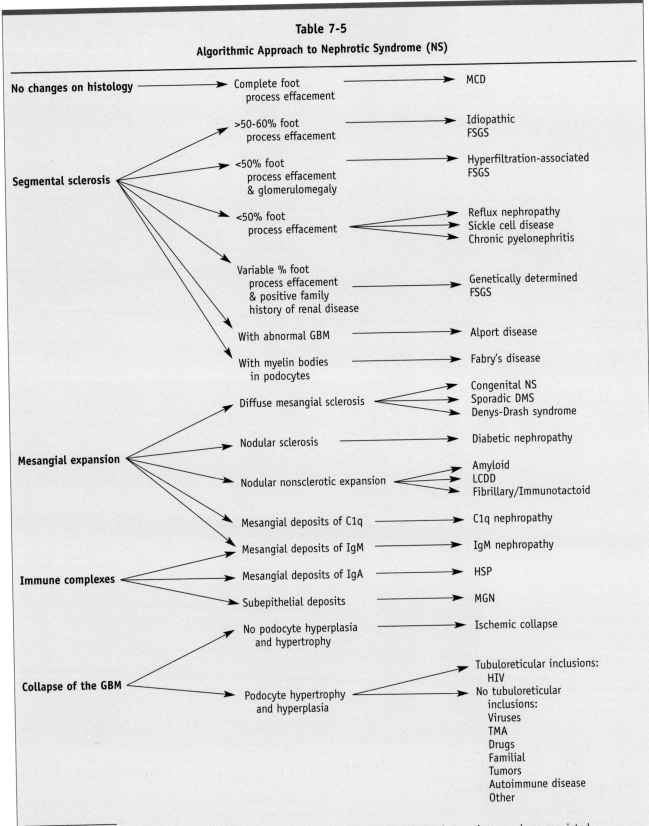

FSGS, focal segmental glomerulosclerosis; GBM, glomerular basement membrane; HIVAN, human immunovirus-associated nephropathy; HSP, Henoch-Schönlein purpura; Ig, immunoglobulin; LCDD, light-chain deposition disease; MCD, minimal change disease; MGN, membranous glomerulonephritis.

Table 7-6

Differential Diagnosis in Patients with Proteinuria without NS

FOCAL SEGMENTAL GLOMERULOSCLEROSIS

Early idiopathic
Some of the genetically determined forms
Secondary

IMMUNE COMPLEX-MEDIATED DISEASES

IgA nephropathy
Glomerulonephritis with membranoproliferative pattern
   Idiopathic
   Secondary (lupus, hepatitis C, hepatitis B, postinfectious,
   cryoglobulinemia)

GENERALIZED SYSTEMIC DISEASES

Pre-eclampsia
Diabetes
Amyloid
Systemic lupus erythematosus
Schönlein-Henoch purpura

TUBULAR DAMAGE

---

absence of glomeruli in the frozen or proteinase k tissue. Paraffin sections are first treated with pronase and then incubated with antibodies against IgG, IgA, IgM, C3, and C1q.

AMYLOID PANEL

The amyloid panel is performed in cases with positive Congo red and/or crystal violet staining. If IF findings for κ and λ light chain are negative, secondary amyloidosis should be suspected, and IF should be performed with antibodies against amyloid fibril protein (AA) and amyloid transthyretin (ATTR). Amyloid P component staining may confirm the diagnosis of amyloidosis.

ALPORT PANEL

The Alport panel is performed if thin basement membranes are present or an irregular texture of the glomerular basement membranes (GBM) is found on EM in specimens from patients with hematuria or hematuria and proteinuria. It includes IF staining with antibodies against collagen type IV α-1, -3, and -5 chains. A positive control (normal kidney) should be stained simultaneously to compare the intensity of the staining.

SUSPECTED ANTIBODY-MEDIATED REJECTION

If antibody mediated rejection is suspected, C4d staining can be performed on frozen tissue—preferably medulla, to preserve the cortex for microscopic evaluation. A positive control should be stained simultaneously. As positive control, tissue from a transplant nephrectomy with acute rejection or a lupus MGN can be used. C4d staining can also be performed on paraffin sections if frozen tissue is not available.

IMMUNOHISTOCHEMISTRY ON PARAFFIN SECTIONS

AMYLOID PANEL

The amyloid panel is indicated for primary (AL) amyloidosis with antibodies against κ and λ light chains and for secondary amyloidosis (AA) with antibodies against AA protein or ATTR. It is generally more expensive and time-consuming than studies on frozen tissue.

EVALUATION OF TUBULAR CASTS

Evaluation of tubular casts is performed in cases of suspected myeloma cast nephropathy (κ and λ light chains) and suspected ARF secondary to hemolysis or rhabdomyolysis (using antibodies against hemoglobin or myoglobin).

ALPORT PANEL

The Alport panel can be performed on paraffin sections if no frozen tissue is available and a diagnosis of thin basement membrane disease or Alport disease is suspected. It is the second choice after IF studies on frozen tissue.

SUSPECTED VIRAL INFECTION

BK virus. Investigation is indicated in transplant biopsies with atypical tubular epithelial nuclei. False-negative results may be caused by lack of medulla, where generally the BK virus infection is more prominent.

Epstein-Barr virus (EBV). Investigation is indicated in post-transplantation proliferative disorders.

Cytomegalovirus (CMV). Investigation is indicated in transplant biopsies and in cases of collapsing glomerulopathy (CGP) not associated with human immunodeficiency virus (HIV), which are very rare.

Parvovirus B19. Investigation is indicated in cases of non-HIV-associated CGP.

SUSPECTED ANTIBODY-MEDIATED REJECTION

C4d staining can also be performed on paraffin tissue, with results comparable to IF on frozen sections.

Table 7-7

Algorithmic Approach to Hematuria*

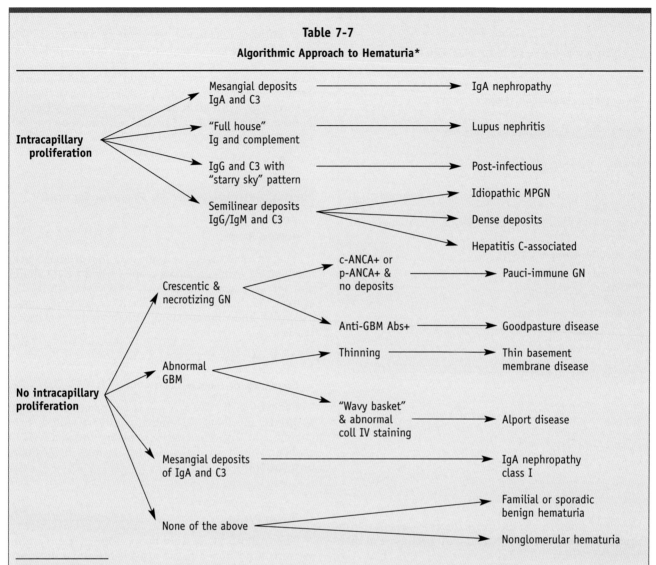

Abs, antibodies; ANCA, antineutrophil cytoplasmic autoantibodies; COL4, collagen type IV; GBM, glomerular basement membrane; GN, glomerulonephritis; Ig, immunoglobulin; MPGN, membranoproliferative glomerulopathy.
*Note: hematuria may or may not be associated with proteinuria, nephritic syndrome or acute renal failure.

UNUSUAL INTERSTITIAL INFLAMMATORY INFILTRATE

Unusual interstitial inflammatory infiltrate containing atypical lymphocytes or sheets of plasma cell should be investigated to rule out hematologic disorders.

ELECTRON MICROSCOPY

Whether EM should be performed in all cases of glomerular disease is controversial. In most cases EM studies provide confirmation of the diagnosis derived from LM and IF, but in approximately one third of the cases the diagnosis is modified by the ultrastructural findings. Ideally, fresh tissue should be fixed in glutaraldehyde. If cortex is not available to be fixed in glutaraldehyde or does not contain glomeruli, frozen tissue or formalin-fixed tissue can be reprocessed for EM. Of note, tissue received in transport medium is not well preserved and therefore is suboptimal for EM studies.

ALGORITHMIC APPROACH TO THE RENAL BIOPSY

Tables 7-4 through 7-9 summarize the algorithmic approach to renal biopsy.

Table 7-8
Algorithmic Approach to Acute Renal Failure

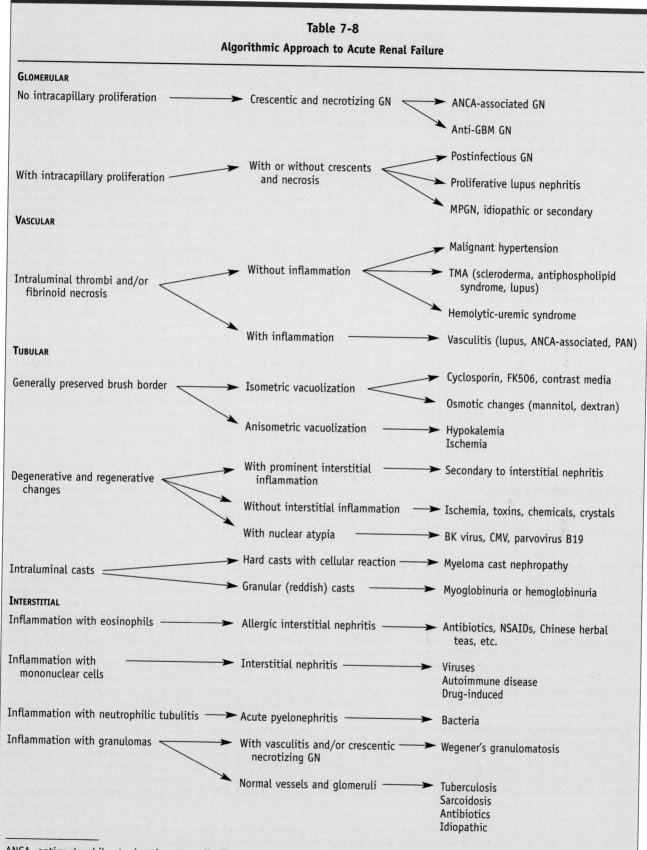

ANCA, antineutrophil cytoplasmic autoantibodies; CMV, cytomegalovirus; GBM, glomerular basement membrane; GN, glomerulonephritis; MPGN, membranoproliferative glomerulopathy; NSAIDs, nonsteroidal anti-inflammatory drugs; PAN, polyarteritis nodosa; TMA, thrombotic microangiopathy.

Table 7-9

Algorithmic Approach to Nephritic Syndrome

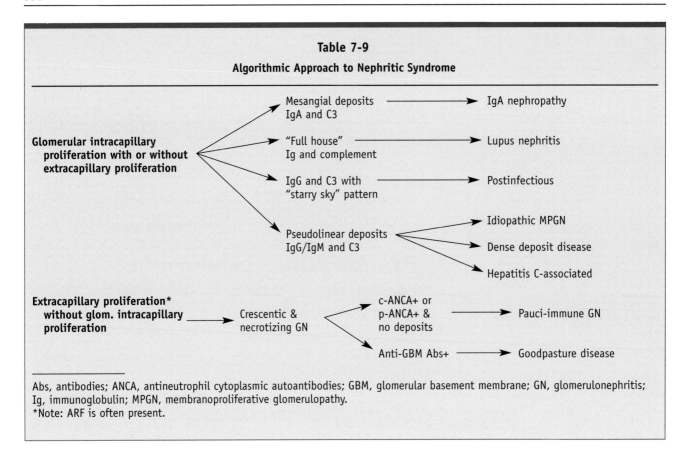

Abs, antibodies; ANCA, antineutrophil cytoplasmic autoantibodies; GBM, glomerular basement membrane; GN, glomerulonephritis; Ig, immunoglobulin; MPGN, membranoproliferative glomerulopathy.

*Note: ARF is often present.

GLOMERULAR DISEASES

Normal Anatomy of the Glomerulus

The glomerular tuft is composed of (1) extracellular matrix—the mesangial tree and the GBM, (2) mesangial cells, (3) fenestrated endothelial cells, and (4) podocytes. Glomeruli sit in the middle of the urinary space, surrounded by Bowman's capsule. The inner side of Bowman's capsule is lined by parietal epithelial cells.

Filtration Barrier

The filtration barrier is composed of fenestrated endothelium, GBM, and podocytes (on the outer surface) (Fig. 7-2). Normally, the glomerular capillary wall forms an effective barrier to filtration of albumin and other plasma constituents, based primarily on their size and charge.

PODOCYTOPATHIES

The most uniform pathologic finding in podocytopathies is alteration of structure and function of podocytes, which leads to foot process effacement and proteinuria (Table 7-10).

Podocytes

Podocytes are postmitotic cells whose function is based on their complex cytoarchitecture. They contain an actin-based cytoskeleton that is connected to the GBM by α3β1-integrin and dystroglycan. Moreover, they express a variety of unique proteins, which are part of the slit diaphragm or of the cell membrane. Although each protein has a specific function, they work in a synergistic manner to maintain the integrity of the filtration barrier.

Classification

The classification of podocytopathies is based on morphologic features, podocyte genotype and phenotype, and etiology (Table 7-11). Morphologically, four categories of diseases can be identified: (1) normal histology and extensive foot process effacement: MCD (Fig. 7-3), (2) diffuse mesangial sclerosis (rare), (3) segmental solidification of the glomerular tuft: FSGS (Fig. 7-4), and (4) segmental or global collapse of the glomerular

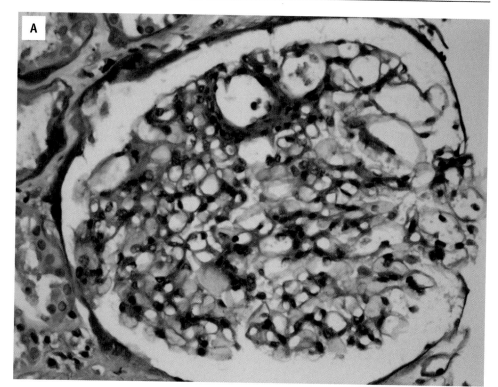

FIGURE 7-2

A, Light microscopic image of a normal glomerulus (hematoxylin and eosin stain, 40×). **B,** Electron microscopically, the filtration barrier is composed of the fenestrated endothelium *(arrows)*, glomerular basement membrane (GBM), and podocyte foot processes connected to each other by slit diaphragms *(arrowheads)*.

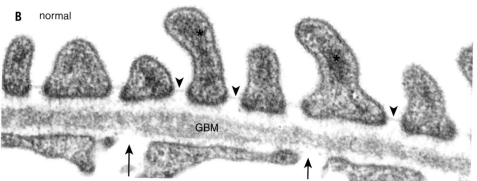

tuft with podocyte hypertrophy and hyperplasia: CGP (Fig. 7-5). Each category is further subclassified based on etiology and podocyte phenotype (Table 7-11). The three most common forms of podocytopathies, MCD, FSGS, and CGP, are discussed here.

MINIMAL CHANGE DISEASE AND VARIANTS

This condition is sometimes referred to as lipoid nephrosis (for the lipid in the urine and tubules) or nil disease. Several subgroups have been identified:
1. Idiopathic MCD
2. MCD associated with ARF
   a. Hemodynamic effect on renal parenchyma
   b. Toxic effect of proteinuria on tubular cells
   c. Associated with use of nonsteroidal anti-inflammatory drugs (NSAIDs)

3. MCD associated with malignancy (Hodgkin's lymphoma)
4. Diffuse mesangial hypercellularity
5. IgM nephropathy (mesangial expansion and deposits)
6. MCD with "tip lesions" (some authors classify this form within the subgroups of FSGS; others consider it an entity in between MCD and FSGS.)
7. Congenital

EPIDEMIOLOGY

MCD is the most common form of NS in children, although it may also occur in adults. In children, peak occurrence is between 2 and 6 years of age, and there is a male predominance. It may occur in association with ARF after the intake of NSAIDs or secondary to hemodynamic effects of the NS.

Table 7-10
Causes of Foot Process Effacement

Impaired formation of the slit-diaphragm complex (CNS and familial FSGS)

Abnormalities of the adhesive interaction between podocytes and GBM (MCD)

Alterations of transcription factors (mesangial sclerosis)

Abnormalities of the actin-based cytoskeleton (familial FSGS)

Alterations of the apical domain of podocytes

Mitochondrial dysfunction (DMS, FSGS and CGP)

Mechanical stress (secondary FSGS)

Viral infection (CG)

Acute ischemic injury (CG)

Toxic/metabolic effect (FSGS and CG)

CGP, collapsing glomerulopathy; CNS, congenital nephrotic syndrome; FSGS, focal segmental glomerulosclerosis; GBM, glomerular basement membrane; MCD, minimal change disease; TMA, thrombotic microangiopathy.

PATHOLOGIC FEATURES

MICROSCOPIC FINDINGS

In classic idiopathic MCD, the renal parenchyma is unremarkable. In elderly patients, occasional obsolescent glomeruli may be present. They may be accompanied by small foci of interstitial fibrosis and tubular atrophy. Approximately 2% to 8% of patients with idiopathic NS have diffuse mesangial hypercellularity. Although most authors consider this form to be a variant of MCD, the response to therapy and prognosis are less favorable compared with classic MCD. In rare cases, mild mesangial expansion and IgM mesangial deposits may be present (IgM nephropathy). These findings represent a variant of MCD of unknown significance. MCD with "tip lesions" is characterized by solidification of the tuft at the tubular pole of the glomerulus, accompanied by hypertrophy and bridging of podocytes toward the base of the proximal tubule. If associated with ARF, MCD is accompanied by acute tubular injury (sloughing and large vacuolization of the apical portion of the tubular cells, flattening or focal necrosis) and interstitial edema.

CLINICAL FEATURES

The classic presentation is rapid development of NS with selective proteinuria (albumin and low-molecular-weight proteins). Renal function and serum complement levels are usually normal (if not associated with ARF). Serology is negative.

ANCILLARY STUDIES

IMMUNOFLUORESCENCE

In classic forms of MCD, IF findings are negative. IgM and C3 deposits may be present in the mesangium in cases of IgM nephropathy, or at the tip of the glomerulus in cases with "tip lesions."

Table 7-11
Classification of Podocytopathies

	Idiopathic	Genetic	Reactive
MCD	Idiopathic *Steroid-sensitive* *Steroid-resistant*	Non-syndromic NPHS1 NPHS2 Syndromic DYSF	Clinical association *(Immunologic stimuli, Tumors)* Medications *(NSAID, gold, penicillamine, lithium, IF, pamidronate)*
FSGS	Idiopathic *Steroid-sensitive* *Steroid-resistant*	Non-syndromic ITGB4, NPSH2, NPHS3, NPHS1, NPHS2, COQ2, ACTN4, CD2AP, TRCP6, WT-1 Syndromic MtDNA, WT1, PAX2, COL4, GLA, LMX1B, COQ2	Post-adaptive nephron mass Initially normal nephron mass Medications *(tacrolimus, lithium, IF, pamidronate)*
DMS	Idiopathic	Non-syndromic WT1, NPHS1, NPSH2, NPHS3 Syndromic WT1, LAMB2	
CGP	Idiopathic	Non-syndromic COQ2 Syndromic *Action myoclonus renal failure*	Infections *(viruses, TB, others)* Clinical association *(Autoimmune diseases, TMA, tumors)* Medications *(IF, pamidronate)*

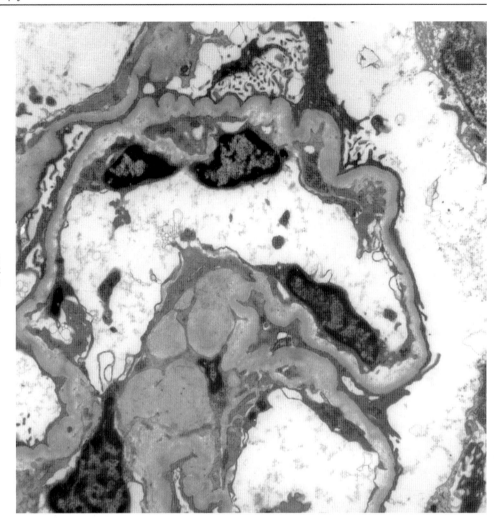

FIGURE 7-3

Minimal change disease. Electron microscopic image of complete foot process effacement with microvillous transformation.

ELECTRON MICROSCOPY

The only characteristic feature of MCD is complete foot process effacement, usually accompanied by reorganization of the actin-based cytoskeleton, which is found condensed at the "sole" of the effaced foot processes. In addition, microvillous transformation (cytoplasmic projections) of the luminal side of the foot processes and intracytoplasmic lipid droplets are a frequent finding (Fig. 7-3).

rather than MCD should be suggested, with the caveat that segmental sclerosis may have been missed by sampling error. The only exception to this rule is if the patient has been already treated with steroid before the renal biopsy, in which case partial foot process effacement may represent partial response to therapy. Experimental data show that MCD may be discriminated from FSGS based on marked reduction of podocyte dystroglycan expression in MCD, compared with normal positive staining in FSGS.

DIFFERENTIAL DIAGNOSIS

The main clinical problem is to discriminate between MCD and FSGS. Morphologically, the distinction is not difficult if a segmental solidification of the tuft is present; however, in some cases, the segmental sclerosis is very focal and may not be present in the first set of slides examined. It is a good practice to section the entire paraffin block to completely exclude FSGS. If foot process effacement is only focal, a diagnosis of FSGS

PROGNOSIS AND TREATMENT

The disease is often very responsive to steroid therapy; however, adults tend to respond more slowly to treatment than children. Some patients will be steroid dependent. If a patient is steroid resistant, FSGS should be suspected, and often on follow-up biopsy segmental sclerosis is present. Children with steroid-resistant NS often progress to chronic renal failure. In some of these

Table 7-12

Differences between Subgroups of Podocytopathies

Category	Minimal Change Disease	Mesangial Sclerosis	Focal Segmental Glomerulosclerosis	Collapsing Glomerulopathy
Definition	Acquired disease	Generally congenital	Varied etiology: Genetically transmitted Acquired idiopathic Secondary to hyperfiltration	Severe disease with wide etiology: Viral (HIV, CMV) Drug Ischemia
Incidence	50% of cases of NS in children	Rare	Most common cause of idiopathic NS	Frequency varies among regions within USA; rare in Europe
Gender, race, and age distribution	Male predominance Age: 2-6 years	0-6 years	Slight male predominance More frequent in AA adults	Slight male predominance More frequent in AA adults
Clinical presentation	NS	NS	NS or nephrotic-range proteinuria	Severe NS and increase in serum creatinine
Pathologic features	Normal morphology on LM; extensive foot process effacement and condensation of the actin-based cytoskeleton	Immature glomeruli, proliferating podocytes	Segmental sclerosis with adhesions and hyalinosis Variable degree of foot process effacement (> 60% in idiopathic forms)	Wrinkling and folding of the GBM with pseudocrescent formation (proliferating podocytes). Severe tubulointerstitial damage with microcysts.
Prognosis and therapy	Generally good response to steroid therapy	Poor	Dialysis in 6-10 years Few cases respond to steroid therapy	Dialysis in 6 months to 1 year Partial response to steroid or cyclosporine

AA, amyloid A; CMV, cytomegalovirus; GBM, glomerular basement membrane; HIV, human immunodeficiency virus; LM, light microscopy; NS, nephrotic syndrome.

patients, mutation for the gene encoding for podocin (a specific podocyte protein linked to familial FSGS) has been demonstrated.

FOCAL SEGMENTAL GLOMERULOSCLEROSIS

Segmental sclerosis by itself is a nonspecific pattern of injury. Several forms are identified, and a careful clinical-pathologic correlation is critical to discriminate between the different variants (Table 7-11). In particular, idiopathic FSGS should be discriminated from FSGS secondary to hyperfiltration or genetically determined forms because of therapeutic implications.

EPIDEMIOLOGY

FSGS is the most common cause of nephrotic proteinuria in the United States (versus IgA nephropathy in Europe and Asia), and it is one of the glomerular lesions that most frequently lead to chronic renal failure. African Americans are at higher risk than Caucasian Americans.

CLINICAL FEATURES

Between 70% and 80% of patients have NS; the remaining 20% to 30% have subnephrotic- or nephrotic-range proteinuria. Proteinuria tends to be nonselective. Occasionally, microhematuria is present; in these cases, thin basement membrane disease or Alport disease should be excluded.

PATHOLOGIC FEATURES

MICROSCOPIC FINDINGS

By definition, the lesions are focal, involving only some of the glomeruli, and segmental, involving only a

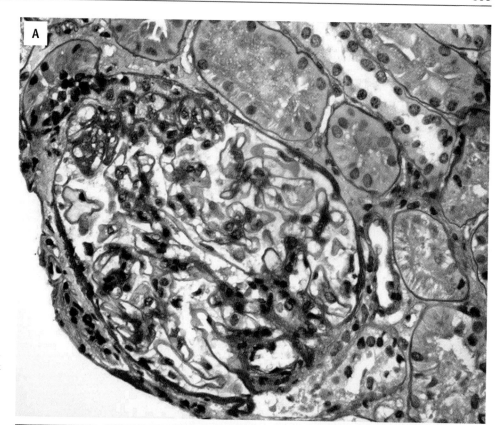

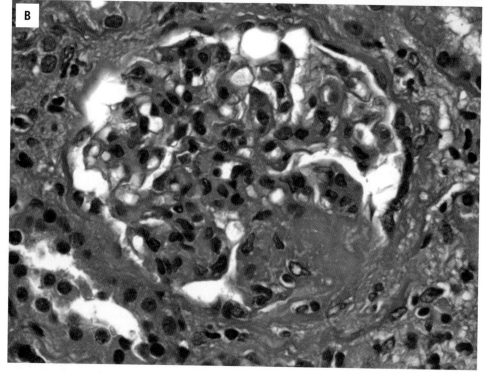

FIGURE 7-4

A, Tip lesion. Tip lesion is characterized by solidification of the tuft at the tubular pole (upper left corner). Foam cells or hyalinosis can be seen. Podocytes are hypertrophic and form bridges with parietal cells. **B,** FSGS. H&E showing a segmental solidification of the glomerular tuft with adhesion to the Bowman's capsule (40×) (right lower corner).

portion of the glomerular tuft. The classic FSGS lesion is characterized by segmental solidification of the glomerular tuft, accompanied by hyalinosis (protein insudation between the endothelial cells and the GBM) and occasional foam cells. Moreover, adhesion (synechia) of the tuft to the Bowman's capsule is typical. Podocytes are generally hypertrophic but not hyperplastic (Fig. 7-4). In the early phases, the segment of glomerular tuft involved may appear mildly hypercellular. Idiopathic FSGS may also present in association with tip lesions (tip lesion FSGS). Cellular lesion FSGS is a third variant of the disease, although rare. In FSGS secondary to hyperfiltration, such as that associated with long-standing history of hypertension and obesity or in the presence of a single kidney, glomerulomegaly may be appreciated. FSGS is usually accompanied by foci of interstitial fibrosis and tubular atrophy. In these areas, a sparse inflammatory infiltrate of mononuclear cells (MNCs) may be present, but it is generally restricted to the areas of fibrosis.

ANCILLARY STUDIES

IMMUNOFLUORESCENCE

Nonspecific staining for IgM and C3 is frequently noted in the areas of sclerosis and hyalinosis. This phenomenon does not represent an immune-mediated disease but rather nonspecific entrapment.

ELECTRON MICROSCOPY

The characteristic feature of FSGS is foot process effacement, which can vary from very focal in secondary forms (hyperfiltration mediated) to almost complete in idiopathic forms. Whereas the degree of foot process effacement is not an absolute criterion, it is sometimes helpful to discriminate between idiopathic and hyperfiltration-associated FSGS. There are no morphologic criteria for the genetically determined forms, but the clinical and family history suggests the diagnosis.

DIFFERENTIAL DIAGNOSIS

The differential diagnosis between FSGS and MCD was discussed in the MCD section. It is important to discriminate between FSGS and segmental solidification of the tuft secondary to other GN or healed necrotizing lesions. In cases of segmental sclerosis/scar secondary to GN, deposits may be present. Moreover, these patients do not present clinically with new onset of pure NS but tend to have a history of nephritic syndrome or hematuria and subnephrotic proteinuria. Idiopathic FSGS is a diagnosis of exclusion after secondary and familial FSGS are ruled out. In cases of suspected autosomal dominant or recessive FSGS, genetic studies are recommended to identify specific podocyte molecular defects (Table 7-11).

PROGNOSIS AND TREATMENT

FSGS is a progressive disease. Patients reach end-stage renal disease within few years. Negative prognostic factors are widespread glomerular and tubulointerstitial damage, high serum creatinine, severe proteinuria, steroid resistance, and African American race. FSGS recurs in approximately 30% of patients undergoing transplantation.

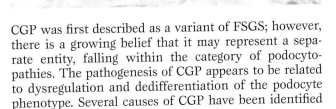

COLLAPSING GLOMERULOPATHY

CGP was first described as a variant of FSGS; however, there is a growing belief that it may represent a separate entity, falling within the category of podocytopathies. The pathogenesis of CGP appears to be related to dysregulation and dedifferentiation of the podocyte phenotype. Several causes of CGP have been identified (Table 7-11).

EPIDEMIOLOGY

CGP was first described in association with HIV infection (called HIV-associated nephropathy, or HIVAN); in 1986, Weiss described the first few cases of non-HIV-associated CGP (idiopathic CGP). Virus-associated and idiopathic CGP are generally more frequent in African Americans, with a slight male predilection. Other forms of CGP can also occur in Asians and Caucasians and are associated with use of medications such as pamidronate and interferon, vascular damage (severe hyalinosis and TMA), myeloma, or other causes. Idiopathic and virus-associated forms are frequent in young and middle-aged adults. Other forms have no predilection for any age.

CLINICAL FEATURES

CGP is characterized by severe NS with rapid increase of serum creatinine.

PATHOLOGIC FEATURES

MICROSCOPIC FINDINGS

The hallmark of the disease is segmental or global wrinkling and folding of the GBM (collapse) with obliteration of the capillary lumina. Overlying podocytes are hypertrophic and hyperplastic (podocytes express Ki-67), and form "pseudocrescents." They often contain

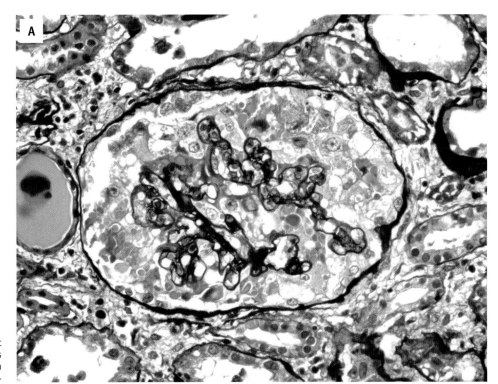

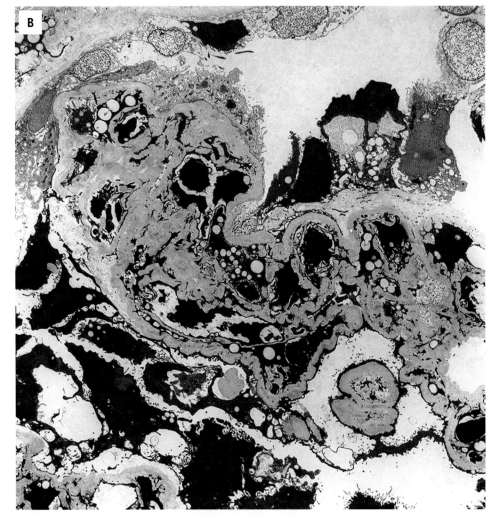

FIGURE 7-5

Collapsing glomerulopathy. **A,** Light microscopy with silver staining shows global collapse of the tuft, with wrinkling and folding of the glomerular basement membrane (GBM). The urinary space is occupied by proliferating podocytes that form pseudocrescents. Numerous protein reabsorption droplets are noted in the podocyte cytoplasm (40×). **B,** Podocytes lose foot processes and primary processes and reveal large cell bodies, directly "sitting" on the outer surface of the GBM, as seen in this electron microphotograph. Occasional detachment of podocytes from the underlying GBM is also noted, with interposition of new extracellular matrix. Microvillous transformation and pseudocysts are present. The GBM is wrinkled and folded.

protein reabsorption droplets, which stain red with trichrome staining. Rarely, mitosis can be seen. The tubulointerstitial compartment is also severely acutely and chronically damaged. Acute tubular injury, microcysts (dilated tubules with a scalloped outline containing eosinophilic casts), and interstitial inflammation of lymphocytes, monocytes, and plasma cells are noted throughout the entire parenchyma. Interstitial fibrosis and tubular atrophy are also prominent (Fig. 7-5A).

ANCILLARY STUDIES

IMMUNOFLUORESCENCE

IF findings are generally negative, but nonspecific positive staining of IgM and C3 can be present in the areas of collapse. Albumin and immunoglobulin often stain protein reabsorption droplets in podocytes and proximal tubular cells.

ELECTRON MICROSCOPY

In addition to the extensive foot process effacement, podocytes often acquire a cuboidal shape (resembling very immature precursors) and lose their primary processes. Rather than reorganization and condensation of the actin-based cytoskeleton, cells have a very pale cytoplasm, which may also contain numerous protein reabsorption droplets. The major distinction between HIVAN and all the other forms of CGP is the presence of tubuloreticular inclusions in endothelial cytoplasm (Fig. 7-5B).

DIFFERENTIAL DIAGNOSIS

The CGP lesions are often accompanied by segmental and global sclerosis, resembling FSGS. Regardless of the amount of sclerosis, the diagnosis of CGP over FSGS is made if at least one glomerulus contains a segmental collapse with pseudocrescents. Pseudocrescents can be difficult to discriminate from real crescents. In general, pseudocrescents are formed by podocytes only, are located around the collapsed glomerular tuft, and are separated from parietal cells and Bowman's capsule by the urinary space; real crescents contain epithelial cells but also inflammatory cells, fibrin, and occasional fibroblasts, and they tend to grow from the Bowman's capsule toward the glomerular tuft, from which they are separated by the urinary space.

PROGNOSIS AND TREATMENT

Idiopathic and virus-associated CGP generally have a poor prognosis. Idiopathic and HIV-associated forms

may respond to steroids and cyclosporin. For other forms of CGP, therapy should target the cause of the disease.

OTHER GLOMERULOPATHIES

MEMBRANOUS GLOMERULOPATHY

MGN can be idiopathic or associated with other diseases, including autoimmune disorders such as systemic lupus erythematosus (SLE), thyroiditis, rheumatoid arthritis, inflammatory bowel disease, hepatitis B infection, syphilis, occult cancer, toxins and medications (gold, mercury, and D-penicillamine). MGN is the most common de novo glomerulopathy in transplanted kidneys.

EPIDEMIOLOGY

MGN is one of the most common causes of NS in adults and elderly individuals without diabetes. It is rare in children.

CLINICAL FEATURES

Patients typically present with severe proteinuria and NS.

PATHOLOGIC FEATURES

MICROSCOPIC FINDINGS

In early stages of the disease, the glomeruli may appear unremarkable on LM. The most characteristic feature is uniform thickening of the glomerular capillary walls, which is caused by the deposition of immune complexes in the subepithelium. The trichrome stain may sometimes reveal fuchsinophilic subepithelial deposits. In intermediate stages of the disease, the silver stain (which stains extracellular matrix black) reveals spikes and holes in the GBM. The spikes represent the interposition of newly formed extracellular matrix between the deposits (optically clear on silver staining). As the disease progresses, holes in the GBM, which represent the deposits fully immersed in the extracellular matrix, become more prominent. In later stages, the deposits are reabsorbed and the GBM is remodeled. If there is concomitant mesangial expansion or hypercellularity, the possibility of secondary MGN should be investigated (Fig. 7-6A).

MEMBRANOUS GLOMERULOPATHY—FACT SHEET

Definition
▶ Idiopathic or secondary to other disease (hepatitis B, autoimmune, syphilis, tumor)
▶ Characterized by IgG and C3 granular deposits in the subepithelial region, thick GBM on LM, and subepithelial electron-dense deposits

Incidence
▶ Most common cause of NS in Caucasian-American adults and elderly

Gender, Race, and Age Distribution
▶ Middle-aged Caucasian-American adults

Clinical Features
▶ NS

Prognosis and Treatment
▶ 25% of the patients have spontaneous remission
▶ 50% of the patients have persistent proteinuria
▶ 25% of the patients have renal failure
▶ The treatment is controversial

ANCILLARY STUDIES

IMMUNOFLUORESCENCE

The classic picture of MGN is global and diffuse granular deposits along the GBM that stain for IgG and C3 (see Fig. 7-6B).

MEMBRANOUS GLOMERULOPATHY—PATHOLOGIC FEATURES

Microscopic Findings
▶ Diffusely thick GBM
▶ Spikes and holes on silver stain
▶ Mesangial expansion possible in secondary forms

Immunofluorescence
▶ Granular global deposition of IgG and C3 in the GBM

Ultrastructural Features
▶ Electron-dense granular deposits in the subepithelium
▶ As the disease progresses, deposits are partially and later completely immersed in basement membrane
▶ Reabsorption of the deposits and remodeling of the GBM in late stages
▶ Mesangial expansion and occasional mesangial deposits in secondary forms

Differential Diagnosis
▶ The most important discrimination is between idiopathic and secondary forms

ELECTRON MICROSCOPY

Pathognomonic of MGN is the presence of numerous subepithelial electron-dense deposits. In early stages, they can be very small, and EM is the most reliable technique to diagnose MGN. In later stages of the disease, electron-dense deposits are separated from one another by protrusion of newly formed basement membrane (spikes) or are completely immersed in the GBM (see Fig. 7-6C,D).

DIFFERENTIAL DIAGNOSIS

The most important differential diagnosis for idiopathic MGN is with secondary MGN. The presence of mesangial expansion and deposits suggests secondary MGN; however, idiopathic MGN can be diagnosed if all other conditions are clinically excluded.

PROGNOSIS AND TREATMENT

MGN is a slowly progressive disease. Bad prognostic features include high blood pressure, severe proteinuria, and the presence of associated segmental sclerosis and interstitial fibrosis. MGN can recur in renal transplants.

DIABETIC NEPHROPATHY

Type I diabetes is a metabolic disorder that affects the microvasculature. It affects children and adolescents and is caused by autoimmune destruction of the beta cells in the islets of Langerhans. Type II diabetes is caused by failure of the beta cells to meet the increasing demand for insulin in the blood. This form has a late onset in life and is more common in obese patients.

EPIDEMIOLOGY

Diabetes is the most common cause of end-stage renal disease in the United States.

CLINICAL FEATURES

Patients start developing microalbuminuria, and with time proteinuria becomes more severe, up to nephrotic range. The disease is often accompanied by the presence of hypertension. Evaluation of the retina is a good indi-

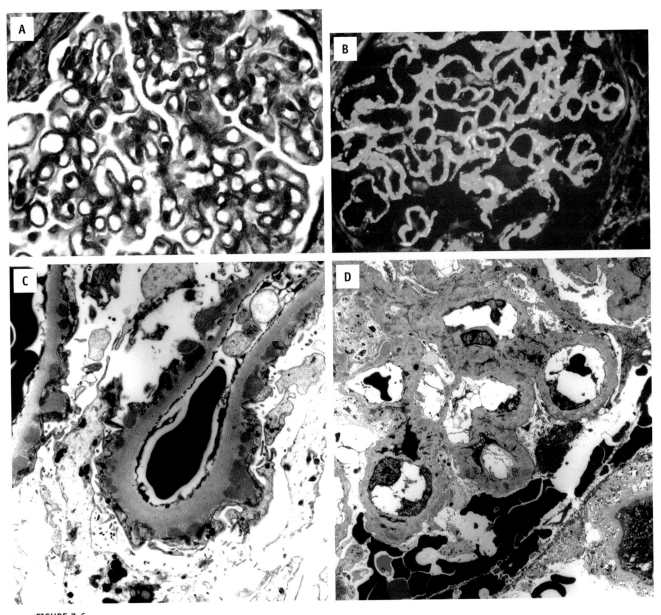

FIGURE 7-6

Membranous glomerulopathy. **A,** Light microscopy with silver staining shows thick glomerular basement membrane (GBM) with spikes and holes indicating the presence of numerous subepithelial deposits (40×). **B,** Granular global staining in the capillary loops for immunoglobulin G. **C,** Electron microscopy reveals numerous electron-dense deposits in the subepithelial space. Occasionally, deposits are partially embedded in the extracellular matrix, corresponding to the spikes noted on light microscopy. **D,** In more advanced disease, deposits are partially reabsorbed and fully embedded in the GBM. GBM remodeling also occurs late in the disease.

cator of progression of the disease at the level of the microvasculature. In the absence of retinopathy and presence of proteinuria, renal biopsy is indicated to rule out other causes of glomerular disease.

PATHOLOGIC FEATURES

MICROSCOPIC FINDINGS

Mesangial sclerosis is the most prominent feature, and it can be diffuse or nodular (classic Kimmelstiel-

Wilson nodular sclerosis). The nodules are initially mildly hypercellular, but with time they tend to become hypocellular and have a laminated appearance. Nodules are composed of collagen and therefore stain black with silver stain (Fig. 7-7A). The capillary walls are thickened, and occasional microaneurysms are also noted. Lesions are also accompanied by the accumulation of hyaline material, which can be found in the glomerular tuft (fibrin caps) or in Bowman's capsule (capsular drops). Other characteristic features include severe arteriolar hyalinosis, which involves both afferent and efferent arterioles. As in all diseases with proteinuria, proximal tubules may contain protein reabsorption

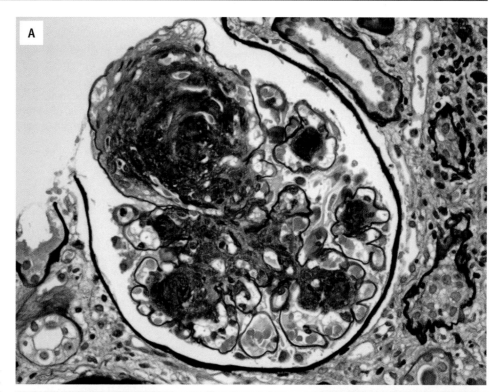

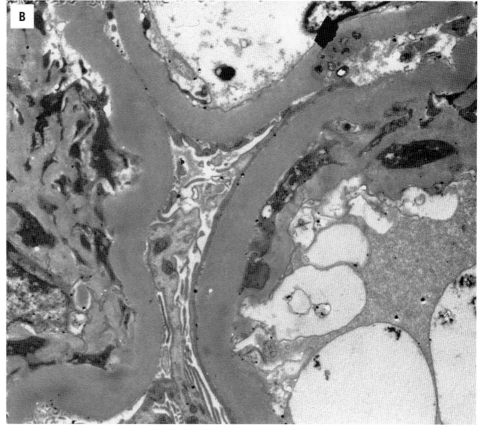

FIGURE 7-7

Diabetic nephropathy. **A,** Silver staining shows nodular mesangial expansion. The nodules are hypocellular and silver positive. Occasionally, microaneurysms of the glomerular capillaries are observed (40×). **B,** On ultrastructural analysis the glomerular basement membranes are markedly thickened. Podocytes reveal foot process effacement.

DIABETES MELLITUS—FACT SHEET

Definition
▶ Metabolic disorder affecting microvasculature due to high levels of glucose

Incidence
▶ Major cause of renal morbidity and mortality
▶ One of the leading causes of chronic renal failure in the United States

Gender, Race, and Age Distribution
▶ Type 1 diabetes is common in adolescents and young adults of northern European descent
▶ Type 2 diabetes is more common in adults and elderly, especially Native Americans

Clinical Features
▶ The disease first manifests with increased glomerular filtration rate and microalbuminuria; later, nephrotic-range proteinuria appears
▶ Slow progression to renal failure
▶ Hypertension is a common feature

Prognosis and Treatment
▶ Control of the blood glucose and angiotensin-converting enzyme (ACE) inhibitors retards progression
▶ Hypertension and severe proteinuria are negative prognostic factors
▶ End-stage renal disease occurs in 30% of patients with type 1 diabetes mellitus and in 20% of patients with type 2
▶ Type 1 diabetes accounts for 20% of deaths in patients younger than 40 years
▶ Most patients with end-stage renal disease are maintained on dialysis, and only few receive a renal transplant
▶ Diabetic nephropathy may recur after transplantation

ELECTRON MICROSCOPY

The earliest sign of diabetic nephropathy is thickening of the GBM up to 1000 to 3000 nm (normal thickness in adults varies between 300 and 350 nm). Mesangial sclerosis is also a common feature. When prominent nodules are present, they may appear formed by fibrillary material consistent with collagen (Fig. 7-7B).

DIFFERENTIAL DIAGNOSIS

Histologically, diabetic nodules must be differentiated from idiopathic nodular sclerosis, light-chain deposition disease (LCDD), amyloidosis, fibrillary or immunotactoid GN, and resolving membranoproliferative glomerulonephritis (MPGN). Differently from diabetic nephropathy, in idiopathic nodular glomerulosclerosis (common in nondiabetic heavy smokers), there is no significant hyalinosis in glomeruli and arterioles. Nodules caused by deposition of material other than collagen do not stain black on silver staining; moreover, in LCDD and primary amyloidosis, IF studies show positive staining for only one of the light chains. In secondary amyloidosis, not only are the nodules silver negative but they stain positive for AA amyloid or other amyloid proteins. Diabetic nodules are Congo red negative. Fibrillary and immunotactoid nodules are also Congo red negative, but they generally do not stain strongly positive with silver. In addition, on EM, the nodules are composed of fibrils measuring 12 to 30 nm in diameter (fibrillary) which are positive for IgG, or organized microtubular structures measuring 10 to 90 nm in diameter (immunotactoid) which are positive for IgG and either κ or λ light chains (Table 7-13).

droplets. Interstitial fibrosis and tubular atrophy is also a common feature. Tubular basement membranes (TBMs) of nonatrophic tubules are generally thickened and have a laminated appearance. A nonspecific inflammatory infiltrate accompanies the areas of fibrosis. If the inflammation is dense or rich in neutrophils or eosinophils, other diagnoses should be considered in addition to diabetic nephropathy, such as superimposed pyelonephritis or allergic interstitial nephritis (AIN).

ANCILLARY STUDIES

IMMUNOFLUORESCENCE

IF findings are generally negative or nonspecific. The most common and consistent finding is linear positive staining in the GBM and TBM for albumin and IgG. Nonspecific deposition of IgM and C3 can be seen in the areas of hyalinosis.

DIABETES MELLITUS—PATHOLOGIC FEATURES

Microscopic Findings
▶ Diffuse thickening of the GBM
▶ Nodular glomerulosclerosis
▶ Glomerular microaneurysms
▶ Hyalinosis (fibrin caps and capsular drops)
▶ Interstitial fibrosis
▶ Tubular atrophy
▶ Mild interstitial inflammation
▶ Hyalinosis of both afferent and efferent arterioles

Immunofluorescence Findings
▶ Linear staining in GBM and TBM for IgG and albumin

Ultrastructural Findings
▶ Diffuse thickening of the GBM
▶ Mesangial sclerosis
▶ Variable degree of foot process effacement
▶ Hyalinosis

Table 7-13

Differential Diagnosis in Diseases with Organized Deposits and/or Nodular Mesangial Expansion

Disease	Light Microscopy	Congo Red Staining	Immunofluorescence Studies	Ultrastructural Features
Diabetes	Acellular nodules Silver +	–	Linear staining for albumin in GBM and TBM	Mesangial sclerosis Thick GBM Foot process effacement
Primary amyloidosis	Acellular nodules Silver –	+ (+ after pretreatment with KMnO$_4$)	Mesangium, GBM, TBM, interstitium, arteries for one of the light chains (λ)	Nonbranching randomly arranged fibrils (8-11 nm)
Secondary amyloidosis	Acellular nodules Silver –	+ (– after pretreatment with KMnO$_4$)	Mesangium, GBM, TBM, interstitium, arteries for AA or other proteins	Nonbranching randomly arranged fibrils (8-11 nm)
Fibrillary glomerulonephritis	Mesangial expansion, mildly hypercellular, thick irregular GBM		IgG (IgG$_4$ isotype) and C3 in mesangium and GBM	Nonbranching randomly arranged fibrils (12-30 nm)
Immunotactoid glomerulonephritis	Mesangial expansion, mildly hypercellular, thick irregular GBM	–	IgG and κ and/or λ C3 in 50% of cases, GBM and mesangium	Nonbranching parallel arranged microtubules in subepithelium, mesangium, and subendothelium (10-90 nm)
Cryoglobulinemia	MPGN with hyaline thrombi	–	IgG and/or IgM and C3 In type I, only κ or λ	Microtubules in mesangium, subendothelium, and subepithelium (25-35 nm)
Light-chain deposition disease	Acellular nodules with glassy thick GBM and TBM	–	κ and, more rarely, λ, linear staining in GBM and TBM	Granular electron densities in the inner side of the GBM

AA, amyloid A; GBM, glomerular basement membrane; Ig, immunoglobulin; KMnO$_4$, potassium permanganate; MPGN, membranoproliferative glomerulonephritis; TBM, tubular basement membrane.

PROGNOSIS AND TREATMENT

Diabetic nephropathy is a slowly progressive disease. Presence of hypertension and severe proteinuria are negative prognostic factors.

GLOMERULONEPHRITIS CHARACTERIZED BY INTRACAPILLARY PROLIFERATION

IgA NEPHROPATHY AND HENOCH-SCHÖNLEIN PURPURA

IgA nephropathy (Berger's disease) and Henoch-Schönlein purpura (HSP) are two very similar diseases that are characterized by mesangial deposition of IgA and complement. In addition to mesangial proliferation and deposits, HSP is also characterized by systemic vasculitis. Some authors consider IgA nephropathy to be a variant of HSP limited to the kidney.

EPIDEMIOLOGY

IgA nephropathy is the most common glomerular disease in the world, especially in Asia and Europe; it is very rare among African Americans.

CLINICAL FEATURES

Hematuria (microscopic and occasionally macroscopic) is always present, sometimes accompanied by nephritic syndrome. In some cases, proteinuria (subnephrotic

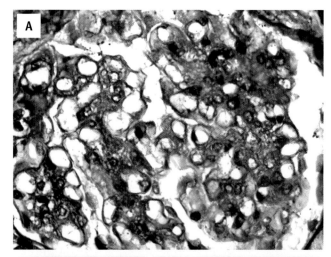

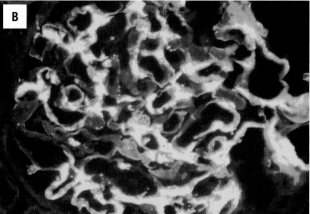

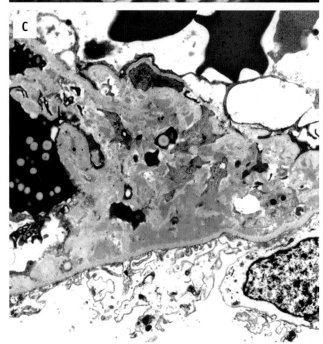

or nephrotic in 10%) is the presentation. Patients with HSP have also symptoms related to the vasculitis: abdominal pain, purpura, and joint pain. The renal disease is often exacerbated by infections of the respiratory or gastrointestinal tract.

PATHOLOGIC FEATURES

MICROSCOPIC FINDINGS

Mesangial expansion and mesangial cell proliferation are the most characteristic findings. However, the morphologic presentation is variable, and glomeruli may appear normal on LM or may have lesions resembling FSGS, mesangial expansion and proliferation, segmental to diffuse endocapillary proliferation with double contours, and, occasionally, extracapillary proliferation and necrosis. These last features reflect high activity of the disease (Fig. 7-8A).

ANCILLARY STUDIES

IMMUNOFLUORESCENCE

Invariably IgA and C3 are present, usually with a mesangial distribution but occasionally in the capillary walls with a pseudolinear pattern. In approximately one third of the cases, C1q is also present (Fig. 7-8B).

FIGURE 7-8

IgA nephropathy. **A,** Periodic acid-Schiff stain showing global mesangial expansion with mesangial cell proliferation (60×). **B,** On immunofluorescence, large mesangial deposits are positive for IgA. **C,** Electron microscopy shows mesangial and perimesangial electron-dense deposits.

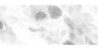

IgA NEPHROPATHY—PATHOLOGIC FEATURES

Microscopic Findings
▶ Mesangial proliferation (classic form)
▶ Occasional double contours
▶ May have extracellular proliferation (rare)—more common in HSP
▶ Five classes have been described: no histologic changes, mesangial proliferation, mesangial and intracapillary proliferation, extracapillary and mesangial and intracapillary proliferation, and sclerosing glomerulopathy

Immunofluorescence
▶ Mesangial IgA and C3

Ultrastructural Features
▶ Mesangial and perimesangial electron-dense deposits

Differential Diagnosis
▶ Class II lupus nephritis
▶ Focal and proliferative GN

ELECTRON MICROSCOPY

Electron-dense deposits are invariably present in the mesangial and perimesangial areas. Subendothelial and, rarely, sparse subepithelial electron-dense deposits can be observed (Fig. 7-8C).

DIFFERENTIAL DIAGNOSIS

IgA nephropathy can mimic a large variety of diseases morphologically, from lupus nephritis class II, to FSGS, to MPGN, and IF studies are necessary to discriminate between these disorders and IgA nephropathy.

PROGNOSIS AND TREATMENT

IgA nephropathy is a slowly progressive disease, in particular those forms with significant proliferation. Negative prognostic factors are high blood pressure, severe proteinuria, and high serum creatinine. On the other hand, the prognosis for HSP, particularly in children, is more favorable. In approximately 50% of patients, IgA nephropathy recurs in the transplanted kidney.

MEMBRANOPROLIFERATIVE GLOMERULONEPHRITIS

The MPGN pattern can be seen in a variety of diseases, from idiopathic and secondary MPGN to cryoglobulinemia, hepatitis C, lupus nephritis, and postinfectious GN. Idiopathic MPGN is divided into types I, II, and III.

EPIDEMIOLOGY

Idiopathic MPGN is more common in children, whereas secondary forms, discussed later, are more common in adults.

CLINICAL FEATURES

Mixed nephrotic and nephritic syndrome is the common presentation; hypocomplementemia is almost always present. Patients with type I MPGN may also have positive serology for nephritic factor. In adult patients, secondary forms are more common, especially those associated with hepatitis C infection.

MEMBRANOPROLIFERATIVE GLOMERULONEPHRITIS—FACT SHEET

Definition
▶ Immune-complex mediated GN, idiopathic or secondary to other diseases
▶ Characterized by alteration of the GBM, proliferation of glomerular cells, and inflammation
▶ Localization of immune complexes in the mesangium and capillary walls

Incidence
▶ 5% of idiopathic nephrotic syndrome in children, although the most common presentation is nephritic syndrome
▶ More common in underdeveloped countries

Gender, Race, and Age Distribution
▶ More frequent in older children and young adults
▶ Secondary forms are more frequent in adults

Clinical Features
▶ Nephritic syndrome or nephrotic syndrome or a combination of the two
▶ Low serum complement levels

Prognosis and Treatment
▶ Persistent progressive disease
▶ 50% of the patients progress to end-stage renal disease
▶ High recurrence in transplanted kidneys

PATHOLOGIC FEATURES

MICROSCOPIC FINDINGS

The MPGN pattern is characterized by mesangial expansion and mesangial cell proliferation; endocapillary proliferation composed of swollen endothelial cells and sometimes inflammatory cells, leading to obliteration of the capillary lumina; and extensive double contour formation. Double contours are formed by interposition of mesangial cell cytoplasm and deposits between two layers of the capillary basement membrane. The outer layer represents the original GBM, and the inner layer is newly formed by the endothelium, resulting in a "tram track" appearance. Double contours are best seen on silver stain, where both layers of the GBM are silver positive and the deposits and mesangial cell cytoplasm are silver negative (Fig. 7-9). Extracapillary proliferation (i.e., crescents) may be present. Types II and III are generally less proliferative forms than type I MPGN. In particular, type II (dense deposit disease) is characterized by thickening of the capillary walls, which stain strongly with PAS and trichrome but are negative on silver stain (Fig. 7-10A).

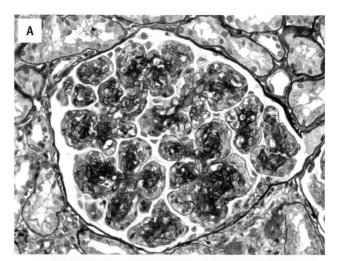

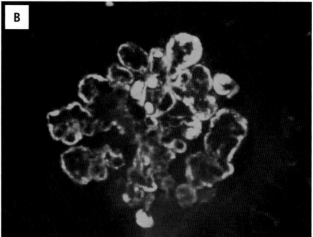

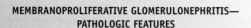

MEMBRANOPROLIFERATIVE GLOMERULONEPHRITIS— PATHOLOGIC FEATURES

Microscopic Findings

▶ Mesangial cell proliferation
▶ Endocapillary proliferation, including endothelial cells and inflammatory cells, with obliteration of the capillary lumina
▶ Double contours of the glomerular capillary basement membrane
▶ Subendothelial deposits
▶ Occasional extracapillary proliferation (crescents)

Immunofluorescence

▶ IgG and C3, occasionally IgM, in mesangium (granular) and subendothelium (semilinear deposits)

Ultrastructural Features

▶ Mesangial and subendothelial deposits; occasional subepithelial deposits are also present
▶ Mesangial cell proliferation
▶ Endothelial cell proliferation
▶ Double contours
▶ Podocyte foot process effacement

Differential Diagnosis

▶ Proliferative IgA NP
▶ Lupus nephritis class IV
▶ Postinfectious GN
▶ Dense deposit disease

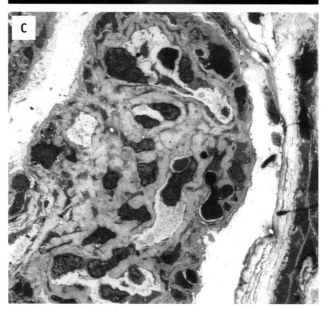

FIGURE 7-9

Membranoproliferative glomerulonephritis. **A,** Silver staining shows large hypercellular glomeruli with numerous double contours. The capillary lumina are obliterated by endocapillary proliferation (40×). **B,** Immunofluorescence reveals deposition of C3 in the capillary walls with a semilinear pattern indicating subendothelial location. **C,** Electron microscopy shows double contours formed by interposition of mesangial cell cytoplasm, with partial obliteration of the capillary lumen. Mesangial expansion and proliferation are also present.

ANCILLARY STUDIES

IMMUNOFLUORESCENCE

IF studies show large glomerular capillary wall (pseudolinear pattern) deposits with more granular mesangial deposits positive for IgG, IgM, and C3. In type II MPGN, the deposits are pseudolinear to linear along the capillary walls (ribbon-like) (Fig. 7-10B).

ELECTRON MICROSCOPY

Glomerular capillaries are obliterated by the presence of double contours, endocapillary proliferation, and mesangial expansion. Electron-dense deposits are pres-

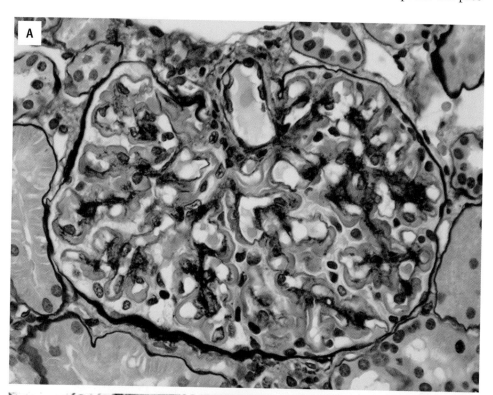

FIGURE 7-10

Dense deposit disease. **A,** Light micrograph of a glomerulus with a ribbon-like thickening of the capillary walls and mild proliferation. The glomerular basement membrane (GBM) is partially silver negative due to the presence of deposits. **B,** On electron microscopy, electron-dense bands replace the extracellular matrix of the GBM. The electron-dense areas correspond to the pink areas noted on silver staining.

ent in the subendothelium, mesangium, and occasionally subepithelium (sparse) (Fig. 7-9C). Type II MPGN is characterized by ribbon-like electron-dense deposits substituting for the GBM (Fig. 7-10B).

DIFFERENTIAL DIAGNOSIS

MPGN can mimic a variety of diseases, and clinical information needs to be integrated with IF and EM findings. The most difficult discrimination is between idiopathic MPGN and postinfectious GN. A positive antistreptolysin-O (ASO) titer and the presence of typical "humps" (in postinfectious GN) should help to discriminate between the two. Lupus nephritis can also manifest with an MPGN pattern, but in this case the clinical history or positive laboratory tests for lupus, positive IF for all immunoglobulins and complement and the presence of tubuloreticular inclusions in endothelial cells guide the diagnosis. In cryoglobulinemia, the presence of monoclonal (type I) organized deposits should help in making the diagnosis. IgA nephropathy with MPGN pattern stains positive for IgA and C3 rather than IgG and C3. Other possible diseases resembling MPGN are LCDD, diabetes, and transplant glomerulopathy. No immunoglobulins or complements are detected by IF in these cases (Table 17-13).

PROGNOSIS AND TREATMENT

MPGN is a progressive disease with a high recurrence in transplanted kidneys.

POSTINFECTIOUS GLOMERULONEPHRITIS

EPIDEMIOLOGY

The acute form of postinfectious (poststreptococcal) GN is less frequent in the United States but still common in underdeveloped countries. Poststreptococcal GN is more common in children, whereas other forms of postinfectious GN—secondary to endocarditis, deep visceral abscess, or infected atrioventricular shunts—are more frequently seen in adults.

CLINICAL FEATURES

The classic presentation is nephritic syndrome. Children develop renal symptoms 2 to 3 weeks after an upper

---

POSTINFECTIOUS GLOMERULONEPHRITIS—FACT SHEET

Definition
▶ Immune complex deposition disease that occurs after exposure to infection, usually by group A β-hemolytic streptococcus (type 12, 4, and 1)

Incidence
▶ Not so frequent in developed countries but still high incidence in underdeveloped countries
▶ Higher incidence in overcrowded environments with poor hygiene (skin infections)

Gender, Race, and Age Distribution
▶ Poststreptococcal GN is common in children, 6-10 years of age
▶ Other forms of postinfectious GN are more common in adults, any age

Clinical Features
▶ Nephritic syndrome after an upper respiratory tract infection, accompanied by high antistreptolysin O titer and low serum complement levels (most commonly in children)
▶ Nephritic syndrome and low serum complement levels in adult patients with bacterial infection

Prognosis and Treatment
▶ 90% of the cases resolve in a few weeks
▶ Adults have a less favorable prognosis: only 60% of the patients recover

---

respiratory tract infection, usually one caused by β-hemolytic *Streptococcus*. Hypocomplementemia and positive serology for ASO are also common findings.

PATHOLOGIC FEATURES

MICROSCOPIC FINDINGS

Glomeruli are enlarged and hypercellular, with obliteration of the capillary lumina due to endocapillary (endothelial cell) proliferation and exudation (especially neutrophils). Mesangial expansion and proliferation and double contours are also noted. In the most aggressive cases, extracapillary proliferation (crescents) is observed. The tubular interstitial compartment may also be affected, and erythrocytes and neutrophils can be seen in tubular lumina. Interstitial inflammation is also frequently noted.

ANCILLARY STUDIES

IMMUNOFLUORESCENCE

The disease is caused by deposition of circulating immune complexes formed by antibodies to strepto-

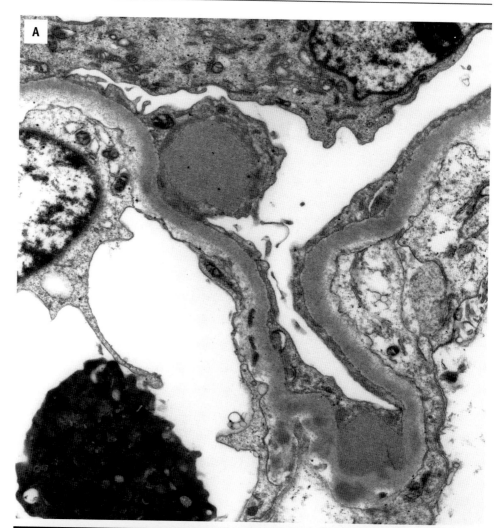

FIGURE 7-11

A, The diagnostic feature of post-infectious glomerulonephritis is the presence of large, sparse, subepithelial electron-dense deposits (humps). **B,** Post infectious GN. C3 staining showing sparse granular staining in mesangium and capillary walls (starry sky).

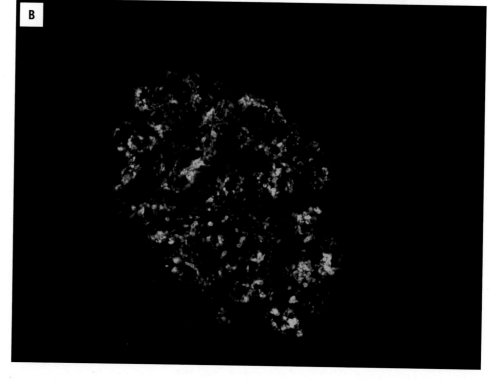

POSTINFECTIOUS GLOMERULONEPHRITIS—PATHOLOGIC FEATURES

Microscopic Findings

▶ Mesangial cell proliferation
▶ Endocapillary proliferation including endothelial cells and neutrophils with obliteration of the capillary lumina
▶ Occasional double contours
▶ Fuchsinophilic capillary wall deposits ("gum drops")
▶ Occasional extracapillary proliferation (crescents)

Immunofluorescence

▶ IgG and C3 with starry sky pattern
▶ In late stages, C3 only

Ultrastructural Features

▶ Humps—large, infrequent subepithelial deposits
▶ Small mesangial and subendothelial deposits

Differential Diagnosis

▶ Proliferative IgA NP
▶ Lupus nephritis class IV
▶ MPGN

---

coccal antigens and complement. IgG and C3 staining, or sometimes C3 alone, is seen, with a granular "lumpy-bumpy" appearance. Deposits are in the capillary walls as well as in the mesangial areas ("starry sky" pattern).

ELECTRON MICROSCOPY

The most characteristic finding is the presence of large, usually sparse subepithelial deposits ("humps"); subendothelial and mesangial electron-dense deposits are also common (Fig. 7-11).

DIFFERENTIAL DIAGNOSIS

For information on the differential diagnosis, see the section on MPGN and Table 7-13.

PROGNOSIS AND TREATMENT

The prognosis is good in children, but in adults it is more variable.

LUPUS NEPHRITIS

SLE is an autoimmune disease. Lupus nephritis, the most common complication, includes a wide range

of glomerular damage. According the World Health Organization classification, six classes of glomerular disease can be identified. They include morphologic patterns that vary from normal, to mesangial proliferative disease, to segmental or global endocapillary proliferation, MGN, and sclerosing lesions. Recently, a revised classification has been proposed.

EPIDEMIOLOGY

Lupus is mainly a disease of young women (male/female ratio, 1:13) and is more common in African American and Asian women.

CLINICAL FEATURES

Patients present with a variety of clinical symptoms. In mesangial proliferative forms, hematuria is the classic presentation, whereas in forms with endocapillary proliferation, nephritic syndrome is more common and is sometimes accompanied by severe proteinuria. Patients with class V (membranous) lupus nephritis usually present with NS.

LUPUS NEPHRITIS—FACT SHEET

Definition

▶ Autoimmune disease characterized by dysregulation and hyperreactivity of B cells, with wide range of morphologic patterns

Incidence

▶ Lupus nephritis is the most common complication of SLE

Gender, Race, and Age Distribution

▶ Female predominance (M/F ratio, 1:13)
▶ Adolescents and young adults
▶ AA and Asian

Clinical Features

▶ The clinical presentation varies according to the class of lupus nephritis
▶ Hematuria, nephritic syndrome, nephrotic syndrome, or a combination of the two
▶ ARF occurs in cases with severe active disease

Prognosis and Treatment

▶ Active disease needs aggressive immunosuppression
▶ High chronicity index is a poor prognostic feature

PATHOLOGIC FEATURES

MICROSCOPIC FINDINGS

Lupus nephritis may manifest with a variety of morphologic patterns:

Class I: normal glomeruli on LM but evidence of deposits on IF and EM

Class II: mesangial expansion and proliferation on LM, accompanied by mesangial deposits on IF and EM

Class III: focal proliferative GN, with segmental or global endocapillary proliferation involving fewer than 50% of the glomeruli, which may be accompanied by extracapillary proliferation

Class IV: diffuse proliferative GN, with endocapillary proliferation, segmental or global, involving 50% or more of the glomeruli, possibly accompanied by extracapillary proliferation and inflammation of the glomerular tuft. Class IV lupus nephritis can resemble MPGN. Large subendothelial deposits (wire loops) or intracapillary deposits (hyaline thrombi) can also be seen. As in idiopathic MPGN, extensive double contours are present (Fig. 7-12A-D).

Class V: diffuse thickening of the GBMs with subendothelial deposits (see MGN), sometimes with mesangial expansion and deposits. MGN pattern may occur in class III or IV. Lesions may be very active or more chronic.

Activity and chronicity indices should be always calculated for proliferative forms. Active lesions are those with crescents, necrosis, large wire loops, endocapillary proliferation, exudation, and interstitial inflammation. For the chronicity index, the amount of glomerular sclerosis, interstitial fibrosis, tubular atrophy, and chronic vascular damage is calculated.

LUPUS NEPHRITIS—PATHOLOGIC FEATURES

Microscopic Findings

▶ Class I: normal histology
▶ Class II: mesangial proliferation
▶ Class III: focal proliferative GN (<50% of glomeruli)
▶ Class IV: diffuse proliferative GN (>50% of glomeruli)
▶ Class V: membranous pattern
▶ Class VI: advanced sclerosing glomerulopathy
▶ *Activity index (0-24):* endocapillary proliferation (0-3+), glomerular inflammation (0-3+), wire loops (0-3+), interstitial inflammation (0-3+), fibrinoid necrosis (0-3+ × 2), cellular crescents (0-3+ × 2)
▶ *Chronicity index (0-12):* glomerular sclerosis (0-3+), fibrous crescents (0-3+), interstitial fibrosis (0-3+), and tubular atrophy (0-3+)

Immunofluorescence

▶ All immunoglobulins and fractions of complement are positive (full house)
▶ Class I and II: mesangial deposits
▶ Class III and IV: mesangial and capillary wall deposits (wire loops)
▶ Class V: granular deposits in the capillary walls
▶ Class VI: sparse, weak granular deposits or negative IF

Ultrastructural Features

▶ Mesangial deposits are always present. According to the class of lupus nephritis, subepithelial and subendothelial deposits can be seen. In class III and IV, the subendothelial deposits are prominent and the subepithelial rare. In class V, numerous granular electron-dense deposits are present between the GBM and podocytes

Differential Diagnosis

▶ Class II: IgA NP
▶ Class III and IV: all forms of MPGN
▶ Class V: all other forms of membranous glomerulopathy
▶ Class VI: FSGS

ANCILLARY STUDIES

IMMUNOFLUORESCENCE

Deposits generally stain for all immunoglobulins and fractions of complement (C3, C4, and C1q are the most frequently tested). The pattern of positive staining varies according to the class of lupus nephritis. In class I and II, positive staining is restricted to the mesangium. Class III and IV show pseudolinear staining in the capillary walls (wire loops) and mesangial staining (Fig. 7-12E). In class V, the staining is mostly granular in the capillary walls. Sclerosing lupus nephritis may have only traces to no staining at all.

ELECTRON MICROSCOPY

Electron-dense deposits are present in the mesangial areas (class I and II), or in the mesangium and subendothelium with occasional subepithelial deposits (class III and IV). Class V shows numerous subepithelial deposits, with or without associated mesangial and subendothelial deposits. In sclerosing lupus nephritis, remodeling of the GBM and mesangial sclerosis may be the only findings. Deposits may be organized in a curvilinear parallel arranged pattern and resemble fingerprints (Fig. 7-12F). Podocyte injury with foot process effacement is a constant finding, especially in class III, IV, and V. A typical finding in lupus nephritis is the presence of tubuloreticular inclusions in endothelial cells.

DIFFERENTIAL DIAGNOSIS

Lupus nephritis can mimic a variety of diseases. Class II can mimic IgA nephropathy; class III and IV may mimic any form of proliferative glomerular disease, idiopathic or secondary. Class V is obviously very similar to

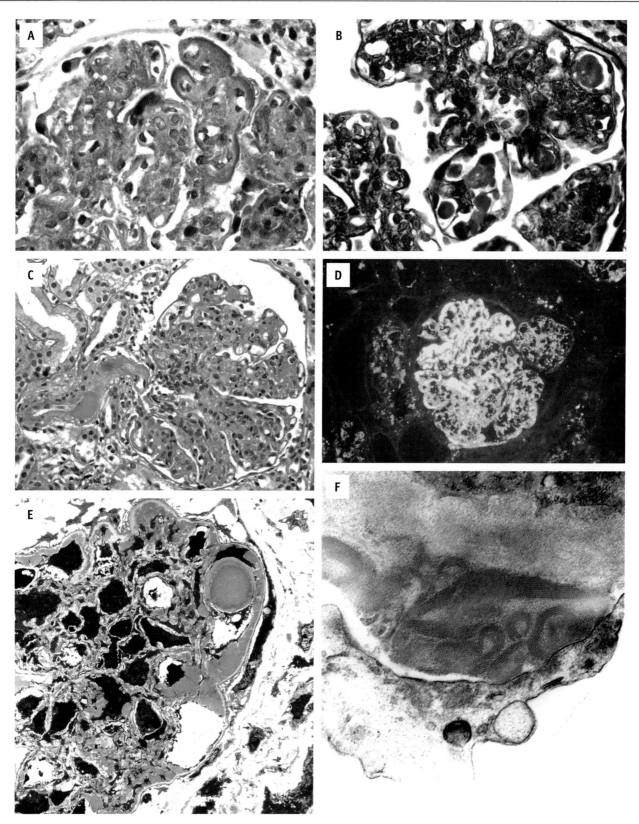

FIGURE 7-12

Lupus nephritis class IV. **A,** This trichrome stain shows large subendothelial deposits *(red)* forming "wire loops") (60×). **B,** Occasionally, endocapillary deposits (hyaline thrombi) are also observed. It is important to discriminate between hyaline thrombi, which are formed by intracapillary precipitation of immune complexes, and thrombi formed by fibrin. Extensive double contours and endocapillary proliferation are also present (silver stain; 60×). **C,** Large deposits can also be seen also in vascular walls (hematoxylin and eosin stain; 40×). **D,** On immunofluorescence, all immunoglobulins and fractions of complement are generally positive. In this image, staining for immunoglobulin M shows pseudolinear staining in the capillary walls, corresponding to the large subendothelial deposits seen in A (wire loops). **E,** The large subendothelial and endocapillary deposits are also seen on electron microscopy. Again, double contours are present. **F,** Occasionally, deposits have an organized substructure in microtubules (fingerprints).

idiopathic or other secondary forms of MGN. Clinical information together with a positive IF result for all immunoglobulins and complement fraction should guide the diagnosis. The presence of tubuloreticular inclusions and positive staining for C1q are strongly suggestive of lupus nephritis.

PROGNOSIS AND TREATMENT

The prognosis varies according to the class and activity or chronicity of the disease. Class II lupus nephritis generally progresses very slowly, whereas class III and IV have a more aggressive course. In approximately one fourth of the cases, transformation from one class to another can occur. Lesions with high activity, including fibrinoid necrosis of glomeruli and vessels and crescents, need aggressive treatment. Lesions with high chronicity index also have a poor prognosis.

GLOMERULOPATHIES WITH ORGANIZED DEPOSITS

Fibrils or microtubules can be observed in a variety of diseases (see Table 7-13) including
- Amyloidosis
- Fibrillary glomerulopathy
- Immunotactoid glomerulopathy
- Cryoglobulinemia
- Lupus nephritis
- Diabetic nephropathy
- Fibronectin glomerulopathy

Fibrils do not have a lumen, do not have periodicity, are randomly arranged, and may be derived from amyloid proteins, immunoglobulins, or extracellular matrix proteins (collagen).

Microtubules have a lumen, are generally oriented in parallel bundles, and are composed of immunoglobulins.

AMYLOIDOSIS

The two most common forms of amyloidosis occur in patients with a plasma cell dyscrasia or long-standing history of chronic inflammation. Familial forms of amyloidosis are rare.

EPIDEMIOLOGY

Among patients with primary amyloidosis, approximately 10% to 20% have myeloma, and the remaining ones have monoclonal spikes in urine or serum only.

Patients with secondary amyloidosis have a history of chronic inflammatory disease such as osteomyelitis, rheumatoid arthritis, tuberculosis, or cancer. This form is the result of increased serum amyloid A (SAA) levels, caused by protracted tissue destruction and inflammation and reduced capacity of liver enzymes to degrade it.

CLINICAL FEATURES

The most common clinical presentation is nephrotic-range proteinuria or NS with or without renal failure.

PATHOLOGIC FEATURES

MICROSCOPIC FINDINGS

Glomeruli, tubules, interstitium, and vessels may be involved by amyloidosis. Amyloid appears as a smudgy accumulation of acellular material, which may involve mesangial areas or capillary walls. It is pale on H&E and PAS staining and is silver negative (Fig. 7-13A). Occasionally, projections of epimembranous spicules may be seen protruding from the capillary walls into the urinary space. Congo red staining is always positive with classic birefringence; this is the most specific stain for amyloidosis (Fig. 7-13B). Crystal violet is also commonly used and stains amyloid in purple. IF for thioflavin T is a very sensitive technique. It is possible to discriminate between primary AL and AA by pretreatment of the sections with potassium permanganate before staining with Congo red. AA amyloid will be Congo red negative, whereas AL amyloid will maintain the classic birefringence. Immunostaining for κ light chain, λ light chain, AA, or other components in familial forms of amyloidosis confirms the diagnosis and further characterizes the disease (Fig. 7-13C,D).

ANCILLARY STUDIES

IMMUNOFLUORESCENCE

The κ light chain, or more frequently λ light chain, is positive in primary AL, whereas staining for AA is positive in secondary forms. Staining for AA amyloid can be performed by IF or by immunohistochemistry (Fig. 7-13C,D). IF can also be performed for TTR in suspected familial amyloidosis or elderly.

ELECTRON MICROSCOPY

The characteristic feature is the presence of subendothelial, mesangial, and subepithelial fibrils, 8 to 11 nm, randomly arranged. They may form pseudospikes where they protrude throughout the basement membranes into the urinary space (Fig. 7-13E).

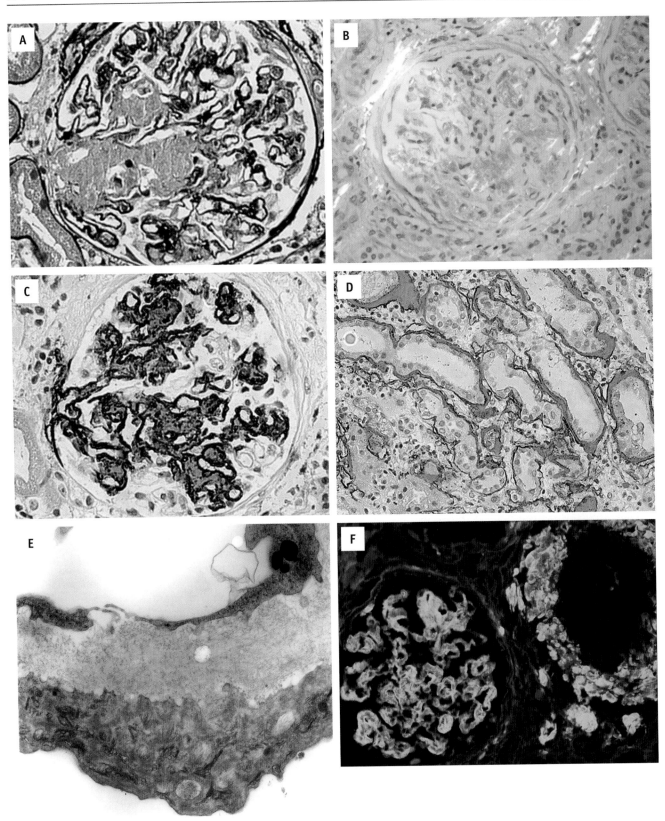

FIGURE 7-13

Amyloidosis. **A,** Amorphous deposition of silver-negative material in the mesangial areas (silver stain, 40×). **B,** Amyloid is Congo red positive and shows typical apple-green birefringence under polarized light (40×). **C,** Secondary amyloidosis stains positive with antibodies against AA in the glomeruli (40×). **D,** Secondary amyloidosis stains positive with antibodies against AA in the tubular basement membranes (40×). **E,** Amyloid fibrils are nonbranching and randomly organized. They are found in the mesangial areas and in the glomerular basement membrane. They measure approximately 9 to 11 nm. **F,** AL amyloidosis, lambda type. On immunofluorescence lambda is positive in the glomerular mesangium and GBM. An interlobular artery also shows extensive deposition of amyloid positive for lambda light chain only.

DIFFERENTIAL DIAGNOSIS

Any lesion with hypocellular expansion of the mesangium may be in the differential diagnosis with amyloidosis (Table 7-13). Nodular sclerosis or hyalinosis can also resemble amyloidosis. Congo red-positive staining is the first step toward the diagnosis of amyloidosis, compared with all the other diseases with organized deposits. Amyloid fibrils are randomly arranged and measure 9 to 11 nm, compared with 12 to 30 nm (usually about 20 nm) in fibrillary glomerulopathy. Moreover, whereas AL amyloid contains only one of the light chains, fibrillary glomerulopathy is always positive for IgG and both light chains. In immunotactoid glomerulopathy, deposits are composed of bundles of microtubules (and not fibrils) with a parallel arrangement, which measure 10 to 90 nm (usually > 30 nm) and are composed of immunoglobulin (IgG), C3, and one or sometimes both of the light chains. Cryoglobulinemia is characterized in most of the cases by curved microtubules, monoclonal, measuring 25 to 35 nm. In diabetic glomerular sclerosis, collagen fibers are negative on IF and argyrophilic on silver staining and measure 5 to 20 nm.

PROGNOSIS AND TREATMENT

The prognosis is generally poor. End-stage renal disease is the major cause of morbidity and mortality in primary forms. Patients with primary amyloidosis have a worse prognosis compared to those with AA amyloidosis. AL forms are treated with chemotherapy.

FIBRILLARY GLOMERULOPATHY

EPIDEMIOLOGY

Fibrillary glomerulopathy is a rare disease, but it is more common in Caucasian Americans than in African Americans. The reported incidence is between 0.8% and 1.5% in native biopsies from adult patients. The peak of occurrence is between 50 and 60 years of age.

CLINICAL FEATURES

The disease is characterized by nephrotic-range proteinuria, often accompanied by hematuria, hypertension, and renal insufficiency.

FIBRILLARY GLOMERULOPATHY—FACT SHEET

Definition
► Deposition of fibrils in mesangium and subepithelium

Incidence
► 0.8-1.5% of native biopsies from adult population

Gender, Race, and Age Distribution
► M = F
► Caucasian
► 50-60 years old

Clinical Features
► Proteinuria, hematuria, HTN and/or renal failure

Prognosis and Treatment
► 50% of patients progress to renal failure in 2-4 years

PATHOLOGIC FEATURES

MICROSCOPIC FINDINGS

Fibrillary glomerulopathy may manifest with a variety of morphologic patterns, but the most frequent is mesangial expansion and thickening of the capillary walls caused by deposition of fibrils. Intracapillary and extracapillary proliferation can also occur. The deposits are generally silver negative. Occasionally, extracapil-

---

FIBRILLARY GLOMERULOPATHY—PATHOLOGIC FEATURES

Light Microscopy
► Thickening of the GBM
► Mesangial expansion with mild hypercellularity
► Silver negative deposition of amorphous material in mesangium and GBM
► Congo red and crytal violet negative

Immunofluorescence
► Granular positive staining for IgG, C3, and both kappa and lambda light chains in the capillary walls and mesangium

Ultrastructural Features
► Non-branching randomly arranged fibrils (12–30 nm) in mesangium and GBM

Differential Diagnosis
► Immunotactoid glomerulopathy
► LCDD
► Amyloidosis
► Lupus nephritis
► Cryoglobulinemia
► Nodular diabetic glomerulosclerosis

lary proliferation can be present. The tubulointerstitial compartment is not significantly affected. Congo red staining is always negative.

ANCILLARY STUDIES

IMMUNOFLUORESCENCE

Characteristic of fibrillary glomerulopathy is smudgy staining for IgG (IgG_4 isotype) in the capillary walls. C3 is present, as well as κ and λ light chains. Thioflavin T is negative.

ELECTRON MICROSCOPY

Diagnosis cannot be made without EM studies. Fibrils are found in the mesangium and capillary walls; they are randomly arranged as in amyloidosis but are generally thicker, in the range of 20 nm (12-30 nm) (Fig. 7-14A).

DIFFERENTIAL DIAGNOSIS

For information on the differential diagnosis, see the section on amyloidosis and Table 7-13.

PROGNOSIS AND TREATMENT

Patients are usually treated with corticosteroids and cytotoxic drugs, but the disease has a slowly progressive course to renal failure within 2 to 4 years. There is high recurrence of the disease in renal transplants (>50%), but usually with a more benign course.

IMMUNOTACTOID GLOMERULOPATHY

EPIDEMIOLOGY

Immunotactoid glomerulopathy is a rare disease, accounting for only 0.08% of all native kidney biopsies. The peak occurrence is at 60 years of age.

CLINICAL FEATURES

The clinical presentation is similar to that of fibrillary glomerulopathy, but patients with the immunotactoid

---

IMMUNOTACTOID GLOMERULOPATHY—FACT SHEET
Definition
▶ Deposition of microtubules in mesangium and subepithelium
▶ Immunotactoid is frequently associated with a lymphoproliferative disorder
Incidence
▶ 0.8-1.5% of native biopsies from adult population
Gender, Race, and Age Distribution
▶ M = F
▶ Caucasian
▶ 50-60 years old
Clinical Features
▶ Proteinuria, hematuria, HTN and/or renal failure
Prognosis and Therapy
▶ 50% of patients progress to renal failure in 2-4 years
▶ If a lymphoproliferative disorder is present, therapy should target the underlying disease. Resolution of the lymphoproliferative disease may result in improvement of the renal function

form tend to have an underlying monoclonal gammopathy or lymphoproliferative disease.

PATHOLOGIC FEATURES

MICROSCOPIC FINDINGS

Mesangial expansion, occasionally with mild mesangial proliferation and thickening of the capillary walls, is the most common feature. The increased thickness of the capillary wall can be subtle or evident, with large subendothelial deposits that are silver negative. Endocapillary and extracapillary proliferation can also be noted (Fig. 7-14B).

ANCILLARY STUDIES

IMMUNOFLUORESCENCE

The IF pattern can be purely mesangial or mixed with a capillary wall component, granular to pseudolinear. IgG is the most common positive immunoglobulin, together with κ and/or λ light chain (20% of the

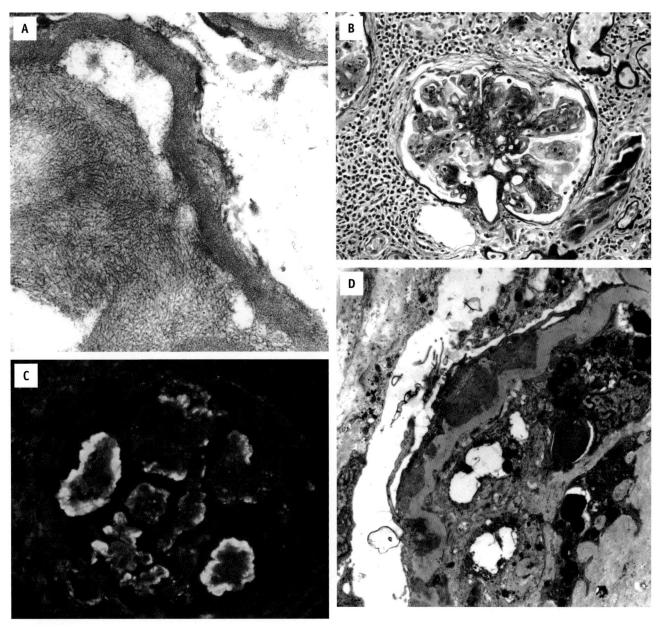

FIGURE 7-14

Fibrillary glomerulopathy. **A,** Fibrillary glomerulopathy is composed of nonbranching, randomly arranged fibrils (20-30 nm in diameter) in the mesangial areas and glomerular basement membrane. **B,** Silver staining shows a diffuse and global proliferative pattern. The capillary walls are markedly thickened and irregular in texture and contour (40×). **C,** Immunofluorescence shows deposits in the capillary walls, with a granular to semilinear pattern (C3). **D,** In immunotactoid glomerulopathy deposits are located in the subendothelium, mesangium, and subepithelium and are composed of parallel-arranged microtubules measuring approximately 30 to 50 nm in diameter.

cases). In approximately 50% of the cases, C3 is also positive (Fig. 7-14C).

ELECTRON MICROSCOPY

The disease is characterized by glomerular extra-cellular deposits of nonbranching, parallel microtubules in bundles. The mesangium is almost always involved, but the deposits can be seen in the subepithelium, resembling MGN, or in the subendothelial space.

Microtubules vary in diameter from 10 to 90 nm, but are usually larger than 30 nm (Fig. 7-14D).

DIFFERENTIAL DIAGNOSIS

For the differential diagnosis, see the section on amyloidosis and Table 7-13.

IMMUNOTACTOID GLOMERULOPATHY—PATHOLOGIC FEATURES

Light Microscopy
▶ Thickening of the GBM
▶ Mesangial expansion with mild hypercellularity
▶ Silver negative deposition of amorphous material in mesangium and GBM
▶ Congo red and crytal violet negative

Immunofluorescence
▶ Granular positive staining for IgG, C3, either kappa or lambda light chains in the capillary walls and mesangium

Ultrastructural Features
▶ Non-branching parallel arranged microtubules in subepithelium, mesangium and subendothelium (10–90 nm) in the GBM and mesangium

Differential Diagnosis
▶ Fibrillary glomerulopathy
▶ LCDD
▶ Amyloidosis
▶ Lupus nephritis
▶ Cryoglobulinemia
▶ Nodular diabetic glomerulosclerosis

PROGNOSIS AND TREATMENT

Approximately 50% of patients present with renal insufficiency and progress to renal failure within 2 to 4 years. Treatment of the lymphoproliferative disorder may result in improvement of renal function.

CRYOGLOBULINEMIA

There is more than one form of cryoglobulinemia: type I, made of isolated monoclonal immunoglobulin; type II, mixed essential cryoglobulinemia with a monoclonal component (with antibody activity toward polyclonal IgG); and type III, in which both components are polyclonal. Types II and III represent circulating immune complexes capable of being deposited in the kidney. Type I cryoglobulinemia is associated with hematologic malignancy. Type II cryoglobulinemia is generally composed of an IgG-IgM complex, where IgM is the monoclonal component to IgG (polyclonal). Type III cryoglobulinemia is secondary to connective tissue disease or infectious disease.

EPIDEMIOLOGY

Cryoglobulinemia is a rare disease that occurs primarily in adults.

CLINICAL FEATURES

The classic presentation is nephritic syndrome, occasionally associated with symptoms of systemic vasculitis.

PATHOLOGIC FEATURES

MICROSCOPIC FINDINGS

MPGN is the classic morphologic pattern. Cryoglobulins can precipitate into the glomerular capillaries, forming "hyaline thrombi" ("pseudothrombi").

ANCILLARY STUDIES

IMMUNOFLUORESCENCE

Pseudolinear deposits of C3, IgG, and IgM in type II cryoglobulinemia and monoclonal IgM in type I cryoglobulinemia are seen. Frequently, hyaline pseudothrombi stain for immunoglobulin.

ELECTRON MICROSCOPY

Subendothelial, intraluminal, and mesangial electron-dense deposits have a characteristic microtubular appearance. Microtubules measure from 25 to 35 nm. Microtubules may not be evident, but in the presence of a clinical history of cryoglobulinemia and MPGN, the ultrastructural evidence of the microtubules is not necessary for the diagnosis.

DIFFERENTIAL DIAGNOSIS

Cryoglobulinemia type I may resemble immunotactoid glomerulopathy or LCDD. In immunotactoid glomerulopathy, the microtubules are generally larger and are arranged in parallel bundles. In LCDD, there are no heavy chains and only one light chain type. Moreover, the glomeruli are in general lobulated but not as hypercellular. Cryoglobulinemia type II must be differentiated from idiopathic MPGN or other secondary MPGNs such as lupus. The clinical history and the IF findings are usually discriminatory. Hyaline pseudothrombi differ from true thrombi because they do not contain fibrin but rather immunoglobulin (Table 7-13).

PROGNOSIS AND TREATMENT

Only one third of the patients recover. In general, surviving patients have persistent renal abnormalities and often develop chronic renal failure.

LIGHT-CHAIN DEPOSITION DISEASE

Patients with multiple myeloma may develop primary amyloidosis, LCDD, or myeloma cast nephropathy. LCDD is caused by deposition of light chains in the GBM and TBM. Whereas amyloidosis is most frequently composed of λ light chains, LCDD more often contains κ light chain. In some cases, both heavy and light chains are deposited.

EPIDEMIOLOGY

LCDD is the second most common renal disease associated with plasma cell dyscrasia. Adults and elderly individuals are most frequently affected. Men are more frequently affected than women (male/female ratio, 4:1).

CLINICAL FEATURES

Microscopic hematuria and nephrotic-range proteinuria, with or without NS, is the most common presentation. Monoclonal spikes in urine and serum are usually present.

PATHOLOGIC FEATURES

MICROSCOPIC FINDINGS

Lobulation of the glomerular tuft is the characteristic lesion. Nodules tend to be hypocellular and resemble diabetic nodular sclerosis. The TBMs are often affected and reveal a typical glassy thickening. Interstitial inflammatory infiltrate is also present and rarely has malignant plasma cells (Fig. 7-15A).

ANCILLARY STUDIES

IMMUNOFLUORESCENCE

Linear staining of the glomerular and TBMs is present for one light-chain type (most frequently κ). Mesangial staining is also present (Fig. 7-15B,C).

ELECTRON MICROSCOPY

Electron-dense, finely granular deposits are present in the inner (subendothelial) side of the GBM and the outer side of the TBM (Fig. 7-15D,E).

DIFFERENTIAL DIAGNOSIS

The major differential diagnosis is with diabetic nephropathy; in the latter entity, the mesangial nodules

---

LIGHT-CHAIN DEPOSITION DISEASE—FACT SHEET

Definition
▶ Monoclonal deposition of light chains, associated with lymphoid malignancy

Incidence
▶ Rare
▶ Second most common renal disease associated with plasma cell dyscrasia

Gender, Race, and Age Distribution
▶ Male predominance (M/F ratio, 4:1)
▶ Adults and elderly

Clinical Features
▶ Renal insufficiency, hematuria, and proteinuria

Prognosis and Treatment
▶ Poor

LIGHT-CHAIN DEPOSITION DISEASE—PATHOLOGIC FEATURES

Light Microscopy
▶ Very mild thickening of the GBM
▶ Acellular mesangial nodules, silver negative
▶ Thickening of the tubular basement membranes
▶ Congo red and crystal violet negative

Immunofluorescence
▶ Linear staining in glomerular and tubular basement membranes and mesangial nodules for either kappa or lambda light chains

Ultrastructural Features
▶ Finely granular electron densities in the subendothelium along the glomerular basement membranes and in the tubular basement membranes

Differential Diagnosis
▶ Fibrillary glomerulopathy
▶ Immunotactoid glomerulopathy
▶ Amyloidosis
▶ Lupus nephritis
▶ Cryoglobulinemia
▶ Nodular diabetic glomerulosclerosis

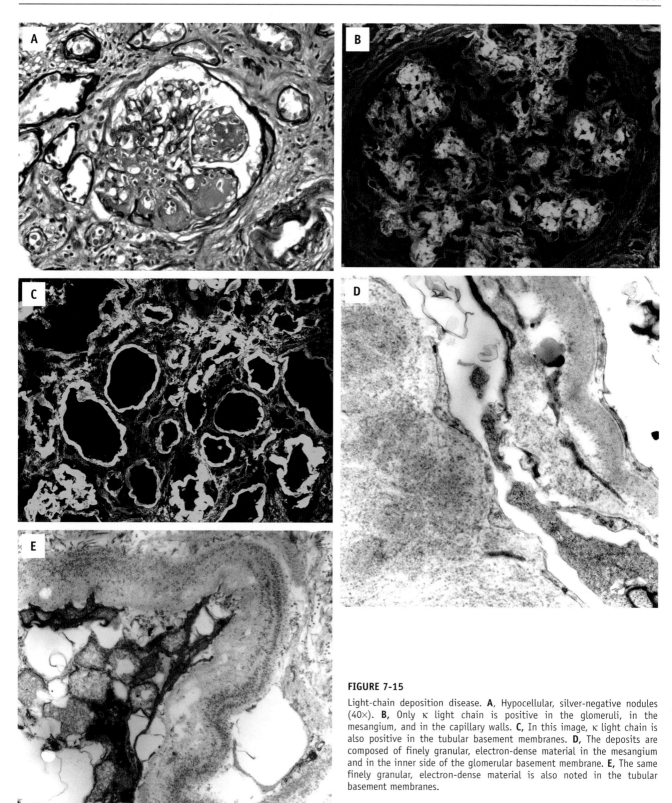

FIGURE 7-15

Light-chain deposition disease. **A,** Hypocellular, silver-negative nodules (40×). **B,** Only κ light chain is positive in the glomeruli, in the mesangium, and in the capillary walls. **C,** In this image, κ light chain is also positive in the tubular basement membranes. **D,** The deposits are composed of finely granular, electron-dense material in the mesangium and in the inner side of the glomerular basement membrane. **E,** The same finely granular, electron-dense material is also noted in the tubular basement membranes.

are composed of collagen and are argyrophilic, and IF is generally negative. Moreover, in diabetic nephropathy, lesions are accompanied by abundant hyalinosis. LCDD must be differentiated from AL amyloidosis. LCDD is Congo red negative and is usually IF positive for κ rather than λ light chain. Moreover, in LCDD the deposits are subendothelial and granular, whereas in amyloidosis they are composed of randomly arranged fibrils. Other diseases such as cryoglobulinemia or immunotactoid glomerulopathy may resemble LCDD morphologically, but they generally contain heavy chains and organized deposits (see earlier discussion and Table 7-13).

PROGNOSIS AND TREATMENT

Most patients progress to renal failure.

GLOMERULONEPHRITIS CHARACTERIZED BY EXTRACAPILLARY PROLIFERATION

CRESCENTIC AND NECROTIZING PAUCI-IMMUNE GLOMERULONEPHRITIS

This group of systemic disorders is characterized by positive antineutrophil cytoplasmic autoantibodies (ANCA) in the serum and crescentic necrotizing GN with or without necrotizing arteritis. Four disorders are included in this group: Wegener's granulomatosis, microscopic polyangiitis, renal limited vasculitis, and Churg-Strauss syndrome. See Table 7-14 for differential diagnosis.

EPIDEMIOLOGY

Studies of European populations indicate an annual incidence of 10 to 20 per year per million population, with a prevalence of 150 to 200 per million. ANCA-associated GN may arise at any age, with a peak at 65 to 75 years. Drugs such as propylthiouracil, penicillamine, and hydralazine may be associated with ANCA-associated disease.

CLINICAL FEATURES

Patients present with rapidly progressive renal failure and nephritic syndrome. The disease is systemic in Wegener's granulomatosis and microscopic polyangiitis and limited to the kidney in renal limited vasculitis.

CRESCENTIC NECROTIZING GLOMERULONEPHRITIS, PAUCI-IMMUNE TYPE—FACT SHEET

Definition
▶ Aggressive disease, neutrophil mediated disease associated with small vessel vasculitis

Incidence
▶ More frequent than in the past

Gender, Race, and Age Distribution
▶ Elderly

Clinical Features
▶ ANCA+
▶ ARF
▶ Pulmonary hemorrhage
▶ ¾ of patients have systemic vasculitis
▶ Rapidly progressive

Morphologic Features
▶ Crescents and fibrinoid necrosis

Immunofluorescence
▶ Pauci immune (rare deposits) or negative

Prognosis and Therapy
▶ Immunosuppression
▶ 25% of patients have renal failure in 5 years

ANCA are detectable in 90% of the patients. ANCA can be directed against myeloperoxidase; in such cases, when patient's serum is incubated with neutrophils, there is a perinuclear positive staining (p-ANCA) on indirect IF. ANCA can also be directed against proteinase 3, and in this case the staining is cytoplasmic (c-ANCA). c-ANCA is generally observed in Wegener's granulomatosis, whereas p-ANCA is more frequent in patients with microscopic polyangiitis or renal limited vasculitis. In a small percentage of ANCA-positive patients, anti-GBM antibodies can also be detected in the serum.

PATHOLOGIC FEATURES

MICROSCOPIC FINDINGS

The classic morphologic features are glomerular fibrinoid necrosis with crescent formation. Crescents have cellular, fibrocellular, and fibrous phases. Cellular crescents are composed of parietal epithelium, inflammatory cells, and podocytes in a fibrin matrix. Fibrin is indicative of rupture of the glomerular capillaries, and breaks in the GBM may be identified on silver stains. Crescents can be associated with rupture of Bowman's

Table 7-14

Differential Diagnosis of Crescentic Glomerulonephritis

IMMUNE-COMPLEX RELATED DISEASES

Includes lupus, MPGN, postinfectious GN, IgA nephropathy

Crescents often a poor prognostic indicator

Diagnosis requires demonstration of immune-complex deposits by IF and/or EM

PAUCI-IMMUNE GLOMERULONEPHRITIS

90% of cases ANCA-positive

Few or no deposits by IF and EM

P-ANCA (anti-myeloperoxidase) positive
Microscopic polyangiitis (MPA); arteritis seen on only about 10% of biopsies

"Idiopathic" crescentic GN; limited to the kidney

Wegener's granulomatosis (more often C-ANCA positive, but not always)

C-ANCA (anti-proteinase-3) positive
Wegener's granulomatosis

Microscopic polyangiitis (more often P-ANCA positive)

"Idiopathic" crescentic GN (more often P-ANCA positive)

Churg-Strauss syndrome

ANTI-GBM DISEASE

Autoantibodies to portion of type IV collagen a3 chain ("Goodpasture antigen")

Diagnosis requires linear IgG in glomerular capillaries by IF

Confirmed by ELISA using patient serum vs Goodpasture antigen; no deposits by EM

Antibody can cross-react with pulmonary alveolar BM ("Goodpasture syndrome")

20-30% of patients are also ANCA-positive. Least common of the three classes of crescentic GN

ANCA, antineutrophil cytoplasmic autoantibodies; BM, basement membrane; c-ANCA, cytoplasmic ANCA; ELISA, enzyme-linked immunoassay; EM, electron microscopy; GBM, glomerular basement membrane; GN, glomerulonephritis; IF, immunofluorescence; IgA, immunoglobulin A; MPGN, membranoproliferative glomerulonephritis; p-ANCA, perinuclear ANCA.

CRESCENTIC NECROTIZING GLOMERULONEPHRITIS, PAUCI-IMMUNE TYPE—PATHOLOGIC FEATURES

Light Microscopy
▶ Cellular crescents in acute phase or fibrocellular and fibrous crescents in chronic phases
▶ Fibrinoid necrosis of the glomerular tuft
▶ No intracapillary proliferation
▶ Rupture of the Bowman's capsule and GBM
▶ Severe acute tubulointerstitial disease with inflammation and numerous red blood cells in tubular lumina
▶ Negative or sparse granular staining positive for complement or Ig

Immunofluorescence
▶ Negative or sparse granular staining positive for complement or Ig

Ultrastructural Features
▶ Fibrin, rupture of the GBM
▶ Epithelial and inflammatory cells in the Bowman's space
▶ Variable amount of food process effacement

Differential Diagnosis
▶ Anti-GBM disease
▶ Any proliferative glomerulonephritis (lupus, MPGN, post-infectious, IgA nephropathy)

granulomatosis (Fig. 7-16B). Arteries may have dyssynchronous lesions with necrotizing and sclerosing vascular lesions in the same tissue specimens. There may be medullary capillaritis with leukocytoclasis.

ANCILLARY STUDIES

IMMUNOFLUORESCENCE

Glomeruli have focal granular staining for immunoglobulin and complement. Fibrin is identified in areas of glomerular necrosis and in cellular crescents. Affected arteries have fibrin/fibrinogen, IgM, and C3 deposition without IgG or IgA.

ELECTRON MICROSCOPY

EM findings are nonspecific and reflect the LM and IF results. Sparse mesangial or capillary wall electron-dense deposits may be present. The relative paucity of detectable immune complexes (by IF and EM) permits the designation "pauci-immune" GN. Fibrin is often seen in glomeruli and vessels. Breaks and ruptures of the GBM may be present, especially where there is fibrin extravasation into the urinary space. Podocytes show a variable degree of foot process effacement. The urinary space may be obliterated by epithelial cells, inflammatory cells, and fibrin, with collagen and fibroblasts in the more advanced forms.

capsule. Over weeks, there is progressive loss of cellularity with fibrosis of Bowman's space. The glomerular lesions are usually accompanied by acute tubulointerstitial inflammation, edema, and acute tubular epithelial injury. Interstitial infiltrates are composed of MNCs, plasma cells, and occasionally eosinophils and neutrophils. RBCs, fibrin, and RBC casts can be seen in tubular lumina. Necrotizing arteritis with mural fibrinoid necrosis and leukocytes are identified in arcuate and interlobular arteries (Fig. 7-16A). Perivascular (or interstitial) granulomas may be observed in Wegener's

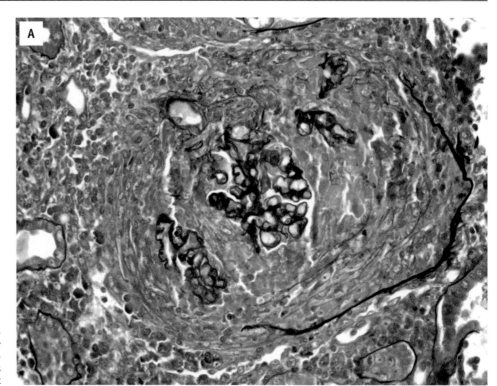

FIGURE 7-16

Crescentic necrotizing glomerulo-nephritis. **A,** Circumferential cellular crescent. Bowman's capsule is ruptured. Fibrin and inflammatory cells are also present in the crescent (silver stain, 40×). **B,** Necrosis can be seen in association with crescents or alone as in this glomerulus with segmental fibrinoid necrosis *(red)* (trichrome stain, 40×).

Continued

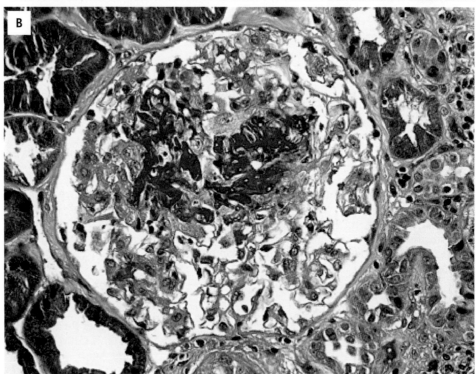

DIFFERENTIAL DIAGNOSIS

The major differential diagnosis is anti-GBM disease. In the absence of serologic studies, IF is the most useful tool to discriminate between the two. Anti-GBM disease has linear staining for IgG by IF along the GBM. Pauci-immune necrotizing GN must also be distinguished from immune-complex mediated GN with crescents and necrosis. Typically, the latter have endocapillary proliferation and abundant immune-complex deposits detectable by IF and EM (Table 7-14).

Renal morphologic findings in ANCA-associated GN are indistinguishable in renal limited vasculitis,

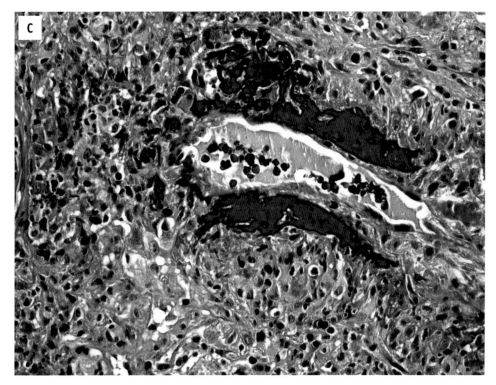

FIGURE 7-16, CONT'D

C, Vasculitis. Transmural vasculitis with fibrinoid necrosis of the arterial wall (in red) (trichrome staining, 40×).

microscopic polyangiitis, and Wegener's granulomatosis. Abundant tubulointerstitial eosinophils raise the possibility of Churg-Strauss syndrome, but clinical correlation is required to confirm this diagnosis. Arteriolitis is uncommon, and fibrinoid necrosis of these vessels raises the possibility of TMA. Acute TMA has prominent thrombi and lacks crescents. Larger arteries have intimal proliferative or mucoid lesions in TMA, in contrast to the fibrinoid change with leukocytoclasis observed in ANCA-associated GN. Classic polyarteritis nodosa has fibrinoid necrosis of arcuate size (or larger) arteries with cortical infarction, without crescents or ANCA.

PROGNOSIS AND TREATMENT

Standard therapy consists of steroids and cyclophosphamide, and remission rates greater than 90% have been reported. Relapse rates of 30-50% are described after cessation of immunosuppression. Mortality rates of 7% at 6 months, 16% at 1 year, and 24% at 5 years are reported despite therapy. End-stage kidney disease develops in 20% to 25% of survivors. Pathologic features predictive of remission or renal survival include acute and focal necrotizing lesions with higher proportions of unaffected glomeruli. Advanced renal scarring with severe glomerular sclerosis, interstitial fibrosis, and tubular atrophy predicts poor renal outcome.

ANTI-GLOMERULAR BASEMENT MEMBRANE DISEASE

EPIDEMIOLOGY

Anti-GBM disease is a rare entity, accounting for fewer than 0.5% of renal biopsies. The disease is very rare in children and more common in Caucasian Americans.

CLINICAL FEATURES

As in other forms of crescentic necrotizing GN, patients with anti-GBM disease present with ARF. When associated with pulmonary hemorrhage, this disease is designated Goodpasture syndrome. Patients have anti-GBM antibodies in the serum that are detectable by enzyme-linked immunoassay (ELISA).

PATHOLOGIC FEATURES

MICROSCOPIC FINDINGS

Glomerular fibrinoid necrosis with crescent formation is commonly seen. As in other forms of crescentic

ANTI-GLOMERULAR BASEMENT MEMBRANE DISEASE—FACT SHEET

Definition
▶ Aggressive disease mediated by antibodies against the non-collagenous domain of collagen type IV

Incidence
▶ Rare

Gender, Race, and Age Distribution
▶ Adults

Clinical Features
▶ Anti GBM +
▶ ARF
▶ Pulmonary hemorrhage
▶ Rapidly progressive

Morphologic Features
▶ Crescents and fibrinoid necrosis

Immunofluorescence
▶ Linear staining for IgG in the GBM

Prognosis and Therapy
▶ Immunosuppression and plasmapheresis

necrotizing GN, crescents may have cellular, fibrocellular, and fibrous phases. Cellular crescents, composed of parietal epithelium, inflammatory cells, and podocytes, indicate high activity of the disease. Rupture of the GBM and/or Bowman's capsule can also be seen. Over weeks, there is progressive loss of cellularity with fibrosis of Bowman's space. The glomerular lesions are usually accompanied by acute tubulointerstitial inflammation, edema, and acute tubular epithelial injury. Interstitial inflammation of MNCs, plasma cells, and occasionally eosinophils and neutrophils is also common. RBCs, fibrin, and RBC casts can be seen in tubular lumina.

ANCILLARY STUDIES

IMMUNOFLUORESCENCE

The diagnostic feature is linear staining along the GBM for IgG by direct IF on frozen tissue (Fig. 7-17). In general, IF on paraffin tissue is not reliable for the detection of anti-GBM antibodies.

ELECTRON MICROSCOPY

Again, the morphologic glomerular damage is indistinguishable from that of other forms of crescentic necrotizing GN.

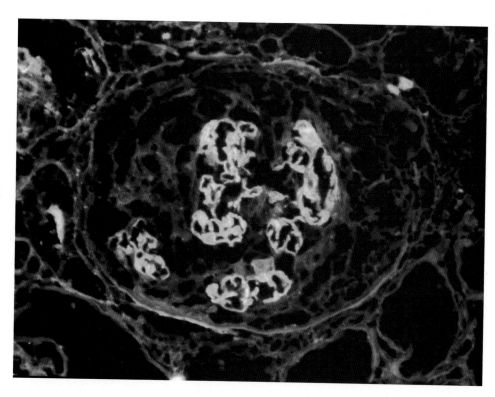

FIGURE 7-17

Anti GBM disease. Linear staining for immunoglobulin G is diagnostic of anti-glomerular basement membrane disease.

DIFFERENTIAL DIAGNOSIS

For information on the differential diagnosis, see the earlier section on ANCA-associated necrotizing and crescentic GN and Table 7-14.

PROGNOSIS AND TREATMENT

The treatment of choice is plasmapheresis and immunosuppression. Despite therapy, patients may require dialysis and transplantation. The recurrence rate in transplanted kidneys is low; these patients tend to have linear staining for IgG in the GBM but only rarely develop necrotizing crescentic GN.

GLOMERULAR DISEASES ASSOCIATED WITH INTRINSIC STRUCTURAL ABNORMALITY OF THE GLOMERULAR BASEMENT MEMBRANES

Alport disease and thin basement membrane disease are characterized by alteration in composition and structure of the basement membranes due to defects in the genes encoding for collagen type IV (COL4).

Alport disease includes the following entities:
1. X-linked disease with mutations of the COL4A5 gene (80% of cases)—nephropathy with end-stage renal disease by age 30 years in 50% of male patients and by 40 years in 12% of female patients
2. X-linked disease with mutations of the COL4A5-A6 gene (rare)
3. Autosomal recessive form with mutations of the COL4A3-A4 genes (10% of cases)— end-stage renal disease by age 35 years in males and females. (Males and females are equally affected by severe disease; disease often appears in families after consanguineous marriage.)
4. Autosomal dominant mutations of the COL4A3-A4 gene (rare)
5. Sporadic cases: up to 10% of the cases are due to de novo mutations, with or without hearing loss.

Patients with thin basement membrane diseases may be heterozygous for mutations of COL4A3-A4; however, cases not linked to this locus have been reported. These mutations are also associated with autosomal recessive Alport syndrome: heterozygotes may present with benign hematuria, the mutation appearing to have a dominant mode of transmission, or with a full Alport syndrome. It is not clear why some heterozygous mutations lead to autosomal dominant Alport syndrome and others to benign familial hematuria.

ALPORT DISEASE

CLINICAL FEATURES

The classic full form of Alport syndrome is characterized by proteinuria, hematuria, progressive renal failure, high-tone sensorineural hearing loss, and ocular abnormalities (anterior lenticonus and perimacular flecks).

PATHOLOGIC FEATURES

MICROSCOPIC FINDINGS

The most common feature at biopsy is FSGS. In addition, on silver staining, irregularities of thickness and texture of the GBM may be present. A variable amount of interstitial fibrosis, foam cells, and nonspecific inflammation accompanies glomerular sclerosis. Erythrocytes are often noted in the tubular lumina.

ANCILLARY STUDIES

IMMUNOFLUORESCENCE

Standard IF studies for immunoglobulin and complement are negative. If Alport disease is suspected,

ALPORT'S DISEASE—FACT SHEET

Definition

▶ Hereditar disease in 90% of the cases, 10% are sporadic. Defect of the α chains of collagen type IV

Incidence

▶ Rare: 0.5% population in US

Gender, Race, and Age Distribution

▶ Male predominance (80% of the cases are X linked)

Clinical Features

▶ Hematuria and proteinuria, occasionally within nephrotic range

Morphologic Features

▶ FSGS and irregular thickness of the GBM

Immunofluorescence

▶ Abnormal Alport panel: negative staining for α3 or α3 and α5 in GBM
▶ Women may have a mosaic pattern

Ultrastructural Features

▶ Thick and thin GBM. Electron lucent areas alternating with electron dense curvilinear areas (basketweave)

Prognosis and Therapy

▶ Renal failure by the age of 30. Patients may develop anti GBM disease after renal transplant

ALPORT DISEASE—PATHOLOGIC FEATURES

Light Microscopy

▶ Abnormal GBM with thinning alternating to thickening of the GBM
▶ Focal segmental glomerulosclerosis
▶ Interstitial foam cells
▶ Interstitial fibrosis and tubular atrophy

Immunofluorescence

▶ X-linked form: negative staining for collagen type IV alpha 3 and 5 chains in GBM. Alpha 5 chain is also negative in Bowman's capsule and tubular basement membranes
▶ Autosomal recessive or dominant form: negative staining for collagen type IV alpha 3 and 5 chains in GBM. Alpha 5 chain is positive in Bowman's capsule and tubular basement membranes
▶ Negative IF for complement and Ig

Ultrastructural Features

▶ Thinning the GBM in early phases
▶ Thinning and thickening of the GBM
▶ Occasional brakes in the GBM
▶ "Basket wave" appearance
▶ Foot process effacement

Differential Diagnosis

▶ Focal segmental glomerulosclerosis
▶ Thin basement membranes
▶ Remodeling of the GBM secondary to glomerulonephritis

staining for collagen type IV α1, α3, and α5 chains should be performed. Normal adult kidney has α1 the mesangium and TBMs and α3 and α5 in the GBMs and, focally, TBMs. The Bowman's capsule contains α5 and α6 chains. In Alport disease, due to a mutation in the α5 chain, no staining for α3 or α5 is detected in both GBM and Bowman's capsule, whereas in forms caused by a mutation of α3 chain, the GBM are negative for α3 and α5 but the Bowman's capsule maintains a positive staining for α5 (Fig. 7-18A,B). Heterozygous women may have a mosaic pattern.

ELECTRON MICROSCOPY

Ultrastructural analysis shows areas of thickening alternating with areas of thinning of the GBM, with splitting and lamination of the lamina densa ("basket-weave" appearance). Podocytes may have foot process effacement (Fig. 7-18C).

DIFFERENTIAL DIAGNOSIS

The major differential diagnosis on LM is with FSGS. Family history of renal failure and EM and IF findings

are helpful. In early stages, no specific alterations of the texture of the GBM may have developed, and the GBM may simply appear thinner than usual; in these cases, IF may be the only diagnostic tool to discriminate between thin basement membrane disease and Alport disease.

PROGNOSIS AND TREATMENT

Patients undergo renal failure by the age of 30 years. Renal transplantation may be associated with development of antibodies to collagen type IV α3 or α5 chains, because these are neoantigens in these patients. Therefore, there is a potential to develop anti-GBM antibodies, although these are rarely of clinical consequence.

THIN BASEMENT MEMBRANE DISEASE

CLINICAL FEATURES

Patients with persistent asymptomatic hematuria may have thin basement membrane disease. This disease

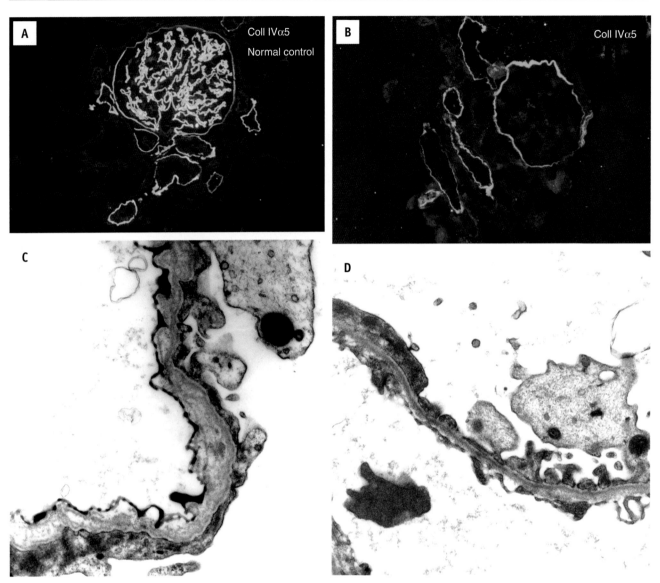

FIGURE 7-18
Hereditary nephritis. **A,** Staining for collagen type IV α5 chain in normal control. The glomerular basement membrane (GBM) and Bowman's capsule show a linear positive staining. **B,** In patients with mutations in the α3 chain of collagen type IV, staining for α3 and α5 is negative in the GBM, but staining for α5 is still positive in the Bowman's capsule. **C,** In patients with Alport disease, the GBM is irregular in thickness, texture, and contour. Electron dense curvilinear areas alternate with electron lucent areas (basketweave pattern). **D,** Patients with benign hematuria have diffuse thinning of the GBM, which in this case measures approximately 100 nm.

may occur in families, or it may be sporadic. Children and adults are equally affected.

PATHOLOGIC FEATURES

MICROSCOPIC FINDINGS

Occasional RBCs in tubular lumina can be observed. The GBMs may have weak argyrophilia because they are thin.

ANCILLARY STUDIES

IMMUNOFLUORESCENCE

IF studies are negative for immunoglobulin and complement. The Alport panel shows normal staining for collagen type IV α chains.

ELECTRON MICROSCOPY

EM shows diffuse thinning of the GBM. Because GBM thickness is variable and normal thickness varies

THIN BASEMENT MEMBRANES DISEASE—FACT SHEET

Definition
► Hereditary disease in 90% of the cases, 10% are sporadic. Defect of the α chains of collagen type IV

Incidence
► 3-8% of population in US

Gender, Race, and Age Distribution
► Female predominance

Clinical Features
► Hematuria

Morphologic Features
► Normal histology

Immunofluorescence
► Normal Alport panel

Ultrastructural Features
► GBM is <250 nm in thickness
► (normal 300-350 nm)

Prognosis and Therapy
► Good, almost never progress

from laboratory to laboratory, normal kidney values for adults and children should be determined in each laboratory. In general, normal thickness in adults varies between 300 and 480 nm. The GBM is thicker in males than in females by approximately 50 nm. In children up to 10 years of age, normal thickness is about 150 nm. It has been suggested that a cutoff value of normal minus 2 standard deviations may be consistent with thin basement membrane disease (Fig. 7-18D).

THIN BASEMENT MEMBRANES DISEASE—PATHOLOGIC FEATURES

Light Microscopy
► Normal parenchyma
► Occasionally, diffuse thinning of the GBM can be appreciated with silver staining
► Tubular basement membranes can be thin too

Immunofluorescence
► Normal Alport panel
► Negative IF for complement and Ig

Ultrastructural Features
► Thinning the GBM

Differential Diagnosis
► Alport disease early phase

DIFFERENTIAL DIAGNOSIS

The major differential diagnosis is with Alport disease. In general, in Alport disease there is alteration of the texture of the GBM, with both thickening and thinning; in some cases, these changes are very focal and undetectable. Immunostaining for collagen type IV α chain may discriminate between these disorders.

PROGNOSIS AND TREATMENT

The prognosis is generally benign; however, there is a mildly increased risk of progressive glomerular sclerosis, hypertension, and decline of renal function with advancing age.

TUBULOINTERSTITIAL DISEASES

The category of tubulointerstitial diseases is one with diverse causes but few histologic patterns. Tubules can undergo acute injury, as in ATN or with inflammation of the tubules (tubulitis), or they can become atrophic in response to chronic disease. The interstitium can become expanded by three conditions which often overlap: edema, inflammation, and fibrosis. The pattern of tubular injury, the amount and characteristics of the inflammatory infiltrates, and the degrees of tubular atrophy and interstitial fibrosis are key features used to distinguish the underlying pathogenesis. Despite these clues, the inciting event can be difficult to differentiate in many cases. Entities that are included in this category include ATN and acute and chronic pyelonephritis, which are discussed in a separate chapter.

MYELOMA CAST NEPHROPATHY

Myeloma cast nephropathy (also known as Bence Jones cast nephropathy, or simply cast nephropathy) is an injury to the renal tubules caused by the toxic effects of light chains excreted in the urine in high amounts in individuals with multiple myeloma.

CLINICAL FEATURES

The clinical features vary among individuals but may include renal failure, proteinuria, defects in tubular transport, hypercalcemia, and other signs and symptoms associated with multiple myeloma. Renal failure occurs in more than half of individuals with multiple myeloma and is most often caused by cast nephropathy.

ARF can be precipitated in myeloma patients after administration of contrast dyes or in association with dehydration or infection. Proteinuria can be massive and is often in nephrotic range. Light chains are not detected on routine urinalysis testing, and other tests should be done in elderly patients with evidence of NS, notably serum and urine electrophoresis and immunofixation. The proteinuria is selective; rarely is albumin a significant portion. The light chain is more often κ than λ.

PATHOLOGIC FEATURES

MICROSCOPIC FINDINGS

The classic finding is tubular cast material that has fractures, angulated shapes, and giant cells engulfing the cast material (Fig. 7-19). Other associated features include epithelial cell injury similar to that seen in ATN and a mild to moderate interstitial inflammation. Sometimes, neutrophils are prominent and can be found within the tubule lumina associated with the cast material. The cast material usually stains strongly eosinophilic with H&E and can be polychromatic with a trichrome stain. Occasionally, Congo red staining is positive by standard LM, but it lacks birefringence on polarization. In rare cases, amyloid fibrils can be found within the cast material. Some of the casts can have a layered appearance with a central pale region. Staining of the cast material with antibodies sometimes shows restriction to the specific light chain found in the patient's urine, but in many cases this finding is not specific and the cast material stains with antibodies for both light chains, as well as immunoglobulins, albumin, and fibrinogen.

Over time, tubular atrophy and interstitial fibrosis occur in response to the inflammation.

DIFFERENTIAL DIAGNOSIS

Other conditions that injure the tubule can cause Tamm-Horsfall protein to leak from the tubule lumen into the interstitium, and its presence can induce an inflammatory response which at times will include giant cells. Special stains for basement membrane aid in distinguishing leakage into the interstitium from true cast nephropathy. Hyaline casts of Tamm-Horsfall protein are found in many biopsy specimens and should not be confused with those of cast nephropathy. Cast nephropathy should always be kept in the differential diagnosis of a biopsy specimen containing an interstitial

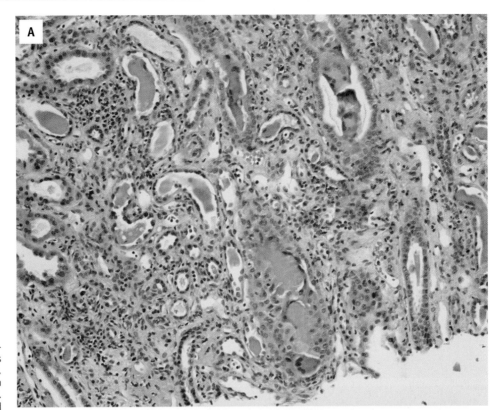

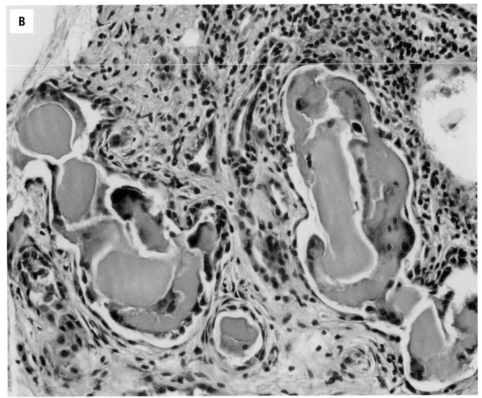

FIGURE 7-19

Myeloma cast nephropathy. **A,** Low-power micrograph demonstrates eosinophilic dense tubular casts, tubular epithelial cell injury, and an interstitial inflammatory infiltrate. Some of the cast material has elicited a cellular reaction within the tubule lumen (hematoxylin and eosin stain [H&E], 10×). **B,** Higher-power view shows irregularly shaped cast material surrounded by a cellular reaction with features of giant cells (H&E, 20×). *Continued*

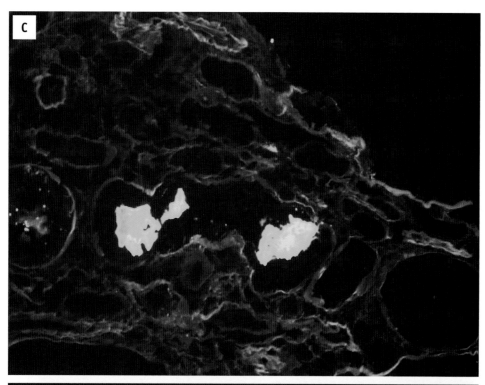

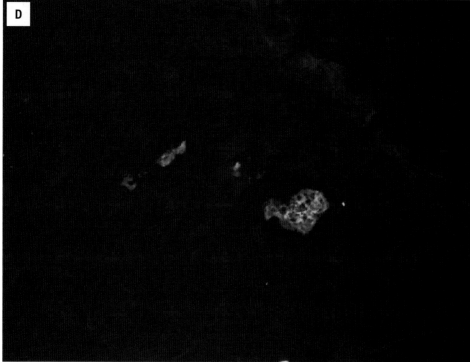

FIGURE 7-19, CONT'D
C, Myeloma cast nephropathy. Kappa light chain is positive in intratubular casts on immunofluorescence (20×). **D,** Myeloma cast nephropathy. Lambda light chain is negative in the same intratubular casts on immunofluorescence (20×).

nephritis in the appropriate clinical setting, even if diagnostic casts are not seen, because they can be focal. Multiple sections can uncover the diagnostic features. Tubular injury can be a prominent feature and is similar to that found with ATN, but in ATN there is no intratubular giant cell reaction.

PROGNOSIS AND TREATMENT

Mortality from multiple myeloma is frequently caused by infection, although renal failure can be a contributing cause. Treatment of the myeloma with reduction

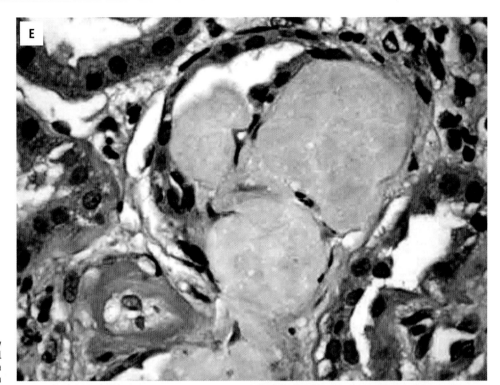

FIGURE 7-19, CONT'D

E, Tamm Horsfoll casts. Differently from myeloma casts, Tamm Horsfoll casts are pale on H&E and have a mucoid appearance. On occasion cellular reaction may also be present making the differential diagnosis difficult (H&E 40×). **F,** Tamm Horsfoll casts may leak outside the tubules (silver 40×).

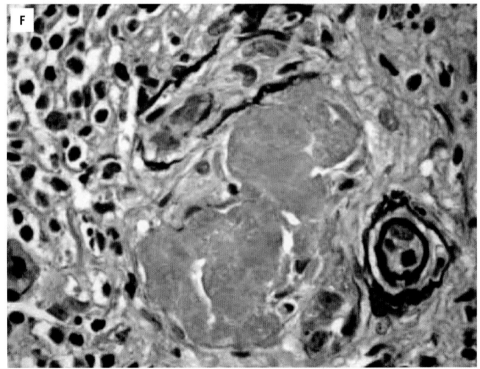

of light chain production improves renal function if significant scarring has not taken place. Dialysis can be used for renal replacement therapy. Transplantation is rarely undertaken. Avoiding situations that promote cast formation (e.g., dehydration, contrast dyes, NSAIDs, infection) reduces the likelihood of renal failure due to cast nephropathy.

SARCOIDOSIS

Sarcoidosis in the kidney is, as in other tissues, a diagnosis of exclusion. In many instances of renal sarcoid, there is nonspecific tubulointerstitial nephritis with a mixture of infiltrating cells. Typically, there is a granulomatous-type inflammation (Fig. 7-20). This is distinguished from tuberculosis by the lack of caseation in sarcoid. Calcium deposition may be present but is a nonspecific finding. In a suspected case of sarcoid, special histologic stains to rule out other causes must be employed. If no other infectious process can be identified and medication-induced granulomatous inflammation can be ruled out as well, a diagnosis of changes consistent with renal sarcoidosis can be rendered. No specific test is available to give a definitive diagnosis of sarcoidosis. The renal findings should be correlated with serologic testing, including calcium and angiotensin-converting enzyme levels (both of which are elevated in sarcoidosis), as well as other tests such as chest radiograph showing typical infiltrates. In the United States, the incidence of sarcoidosis is approximately 1 in 10,000, and African Americans tend to be affected more often than Caucasian Americans.

MEDICATION-ASSOCIATED (ALLERGIC OR HYPERSENSITIVITY) INTERSTITIAL NEPHRITIS

A host of medications are known to induce acute tubulointerstitial nephritis. The most common offending agents, probably because of their high frequency of use, are antibiotics, NSAIDs, and diuretics. The histologic features vary slightly, depending on the circumstances, but are typically of two types: a diffuse mononuclear inflammatory infiltrate, often con- taining eosinophils, or a noncaseating granulomatous inflammation.

CLINICAL FEATURES

The signs and symptoms of AIN are nonspecific and can include the classic triad of fever, joint pain, and rash, but often one or more of these features are absent. Patients may present with common features of ARF, with nausea, vomiting, and malaise. They may have flank pain. As in other causes of ARF, urine output may be reduced. Laboratory tests of renal function indicate reduced clearance, and urinalysis often shows low levels of hematuria and proteinuria. Eosinophils in the urine can be a clue to AIN, but often they are absent.

PATHOLOGIC FEATURES

MICROSCOPIC FINDINGS

In AIN, the interstitium is infiltrated by inflammatory cells, predominantly mononuclear; however, in many cases a striking number of eosinophils can be identified. The presence of eosinophils is not diagnostic for medication-associated interstitial nephritis, because they can be seen in other forms of acute interstitial nephritis. When they are seen, they are often accompanied by peripheral eosinophilia. Neutrophils are

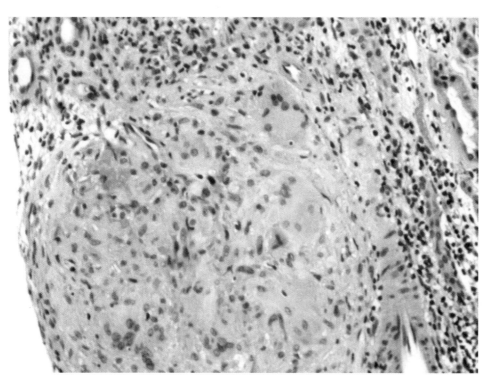

FIGURE 7-20

Sarcoidosis. Granulomatous inflammation in a case of renal sarcoid. Giant cells are present within the granuloma, and lymphocytes can be identified around the periphery (H&E 20×).

ALLERGIC INTERSTITIAL NEPHRITIS—FACT SHEET

Definition

▶ Acute inflammation of the interstitium secondary to allergic or immunologic reaction to a medication or toxic agent

Incidence

▶ Commonly caused by antibiotics and NSAIDs, but can occur with any drug
▶ Risk is increased in the elderly and in those taking multiple medications
▶ Accounts for approximately 15% of ARF

Morbidity and Mortality

▶ Renal function usually returns to normal in 4-6 weeks after elimination of drug
▶ In severe cases, chronic insufficiency or renal failure can occur

Clinical Features

▶ ARF
▶ Oliguria or anuria
▶ Nausea and vomiting
▶ Flank pain

Laboratory Findings

▶ Increased creatinine and blood urea nitrogen
▶ Urine may contain white cells, including eosinophils, and occasionally RBCs

Prognosis and Treatment

▶ Good prognosis for full renal recovery in most patients
▶ Poor renal outcome in chronic cases
▶ Patients may require dialysis during recovery
▶ Corticosteroids may be used in unrelenting cases

ALLERGIC INTERSTITIAL NEPHRITIS—PATHOLOGIC FEATURES

Microscopic Findings

▶ Often intense interstitial inflammation with mononuclear cells and eosinophils
▶ Interstitial edema
▶ Certain drugs may produce a granulomatous inflammation
▶ Chronic cases show less inflammation, more tubular atrophy and interstitial fibrosis

Differential Diagnosis

▶ Both acute pyelonephritis and ATN can have interstitial inflammation and tubule cell injury, the preponderance of neutrophils is more characteristic of acute pyelonephritis, whereas lymphocytes and eosinophils are more likely with AIN
▶ Sloughing of necrotic epithelial cells into the tubule lumens is not a prominent feature of AIN

uncommon in AIN. Some medications have a tendency to cause a granulomatous reaction. In these cases, eosinophils may not be a prominent feature. In most cases of AIN, there is an associated interstitial edema. Tubulitis can also be found (Fig. 7-21). Chronic forms have sparse mononuclear infiltrates with tubular atrophy and interstitial fibrosis.

DIFFERENTIAL DIAGNOSIS

AIN may need to be distinguished from acute pyelonephritis or ATN. In most cases of ATN, there is less of an interstitial infiltrate compared with AIN, whereas in AIN the interstitial component is more prominent and tubular injury is present to a lesser degree than in ATN. The presence of neutrophils and particularly neutrophil casts should readily distinguish acute pyelonephritis from AIN. In many cases of long-standing AIN, the clinician may be interested in knowing the degree of active inflammation compared to the level of chronicity,

and the diagnosis of chronic tubulointerstitial nephritis may be in the differential diagnosis. The degree of inflammation and presence of edema versus fibrosis in the interstitium are useful indicators to determine reversibility of the condition and recovery of function.

PROGNOSIS AND TREATMENT

Recovery from AIN is promising if the medication or toxic agent is discontinued before the development of significant scarring. Recovery of renal function can occasionally take 4 to 6 weeks, and temporary renal replacement therapy may be required. In some cases, steroid therapy is instituted in resistant cases.

VASCULAR DISEASES OF THE KIDNEY

A range of renal vascular diseases, including nephrosclerosis, renal arterial stenosis, embolic diseases, and renal arterial aneurysm and dissection, are discussed in a separate chapter. This section briefly reviews thrombotic microangiopathy (TMA) and renal vasculitis.

THROMBOTIC MICROANGIOPATHY

TMA is a collective term for a group of systemic disorders with renal involvement characterized by glomerular, arteriolar, and arterial endothelial injury and thrombosis. TMA in the native kidney may be associated with infection (Shiga or Shiga-like toxin-associated hemolytic-uremic syndrome [HUS], CMV, hepatitis C, HIV), an inherited condition (complement

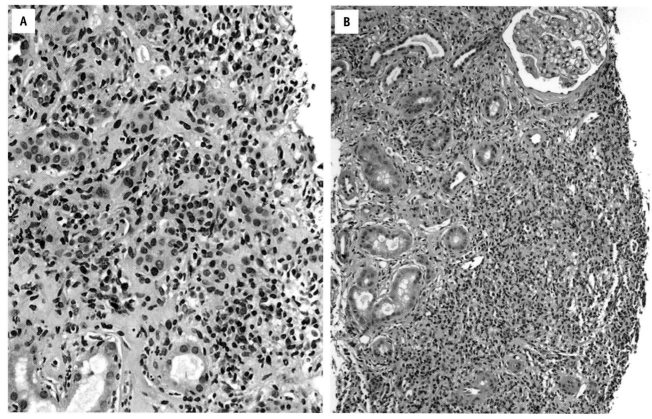

FIGURE 7-21

Acute interstitial nephritis. **A,** An intense interstitial inflammation consisting mainly of mononuclear cells, with scattered eosinophils. Foci of tubulitis are present. A limited number of neutrophils can be seen (H&E 40×). **B,** A case of drug-induced granulomatous interstitial inflammation (H&E, 20×).

factor H deficiency and others), malignant hypertension, systemic sclerosis, pharmacologic agents (oral contraceptives, mitomycin, calcineurin inhibitors), radiation nephropathy, bone marrow transplantation, pregnancy (eclampsia, preeclampsia, postpartum), or malignancy (prostate, stomach, breast, pancreas), or it may be idiopathic (HUS, thrombotic thrombocytopenic purpura, antiphospholipid [APL] syndrome nephropathy).

CLINICAL FEATURES

The disorders associated with TMA are diverse but are characterized by renal failure, microangiopathic (nonimmune) hemolytic anemia, thrombocytopenia, and elevated serum lactate dehydrogenase. Sporadic HUS is most frequently associated with diarrheal infection by toxin-producing *Escherichia coli*. HUS with classic history and clinical findings typically affects children, and biopsy is rarely ordered. Atypical features such as microscopic hematuria and proteinuria (rarely nephrotic) with subacute or chronic renal failure lead to kidney biopsy.

PATHOLOGIC FEATURES

MICROSCOPIC FINDINGS

Glomeruli, arteries, and arterioles are the principal foci of injury, with secondary parenchymal ischemia. The earliest acute glomerular lesions include endothelial swelling, capillary thrombi, GBM duplication (Fig. 7-22), and mesangiolysis, characterized by an edematous mesangium with erythrocytolysis, appearing as mesangial RBC fragments. Glomeruli with global lesions appear shrunken and solidified. Chronic glomerular lesions have widespread glomerular capillary basement membrane duplication (chronic microangiopathy) with an expanded sclerotic mesangium or ischemic wrinkling of the GBM. Thrombi are inconspicuous in chronic glomerular lesions.

Arterioles have two principal lesions in the acute phase of TMA: thrombosis with mural fibrinoid change and obliterative arteriolopathy. These arteriolopathic lesions are identical to those of malignant hypertension. Small arteries have marked myxoid intimal thickening and endothelial swelling. ATN with scant interstitial infiltrates and edema or parenchymal coagulation necrosis may be evident. Chronic arteriolopathy is

THROMBOTIC MICROANGIOPATHY—FACT SHEET

Definition

▶ A group of disorders characterized by glomerular, arteriolar, and arterial endothelial injury with luminal narrowing and thrombosis; it can be secondary to the following:
▶ Infection—Shiga(-like) toxin-associated HUS, CMV, HIV
▶ Inherited condition—factor H deficiency, others
▶ Malignant hypertension
▶ Scleroderma/systemic sclerosis
▶ Pharmacologic agents—oral contraceptive, mitomycin, calcineurin inhibitors
▶ Cancer chemotherapy, irradiation, bone marrow transplantation
▶ Pregnancy—(pre)eclampsia, postpartum renal failure
▶ Malignancy—prostate, stomach, breast, pancreas
▶ Idiopathic—atypical HUS, thrombotic thrombocytopenic purpura (TTP), antiphospholipid syndrome nephropathy

Incidence

▶ TTP ~ 4/million in United States
▶ HUS predominantly a disease of children

Clinical Features

▶ (Acute) renal failure
▶ Nonimmune hemolytic anemia
▶ Schistocytes
▶ Thrombocytopenia

Prognosis and Treatment

▶ Treat underlying disorder
▶ Children, 66% recovery
▶ Adults, <30% recovery

THROMBOTIC MICROANGIOPATHY—PATHOLOGIC FEATURES

Microscopic Findings

▶ Glomerular endothelial swelling, thrombi, mesangiolysis, GBM duplication, solidification
▶ Arteriolar thrombi, fibrinoid change, obliterative arteriolopathy, arterial mucoid intimal thickening
▶ Acute ischemic tubular necrosis, cortical necrosis

Immunofluorescence

▶ Fibrin in glomeruli, arterioles; IgM, C3 in arteriolar walls

Ultrastructural Features

▶ Glomerular endothelial swelling and detachment from GBM, duplication of GBM, mesangial swelling
▶ Arteriolar fibrin/platelet thrombi, smooth muscle necrosis and apoptosis

Differential Diagnosis

▶ TMA from all causes is morphologically similar
▶ MPGN types 1 and 2
▶ Proliferative lupus nephritis
▶ Cryoglobulinemic glomerulonephritis
▶ Sickle cell nephropathy

characterized by transmural hyaline and intimal fibrosis (arteriolosclerosis) with luminal narrowing. None of these pathologic features is disease specific.

ANCILLARY STUDIES

IMMUNOFLUORESCENCE

Fibrin/fibrinogen deposits in lumina and walls of glomerular capillaries, mesangium, and arterioles are identified by IF. Arterioles and glomerular capillaries may also have IgM and C3 in acute fibrinoid and chronic hyalinizing lesions. Staining of glomerular capillaries for immunoglobulins and complement is scant or nil.

ELECTRON MICROSCOPY

Acute arteriolar and glomerular lesions have endothelial swelling and detachment with subendothelial lucency containing wispy, weakly electron-dense material. Chronic lesions have GBM duplication. Medial smooth muscle cells are separated in an edematous matrix containing platelets and their microparticles, fibrin tactoids, and cell debris. Immune complex-type electron-dense deposits are absent.

DIFFERENTIAL DIAGNOSIS

Acute TMA often cannot be further classified into specific causes on the basis of renal biopsy pathologic features, and diagnosis requires clinical correlation. Predominance of arteriolopathic lesions with glomerular ischemia may suggest malignant hypertension but this is not a pathognomonic finding. The acute glomerular findings should be distinguished from immune complex GN, including membranoproliferative, cryoglobulinemic, and lupus GN, and, in addition, sickle cell glomerulopathy. Rarely, TMA may coexist with immune complex GN, including postinfectious, lupus (with or without APL syndrome), and IgA nephropathy. Acute arteriolopathic changes should be distinguished from cryoglobulinemic arteriolopathy (with or without hepatitis C infection), macroglobulinemia, and crystalglobulinemia associated with monoclonal gammopathies and B-cell neoplasia. Severe chronic hyalinizing arteriolopathy may be difficult to distinguish from diabetic and hypertensive arteriolopathy or amyloid deposition. Severe arterial luminal stenosis with concentric duplication of the internal elastica is suggestive of systemic sclerosis in the appropriate clinical context.

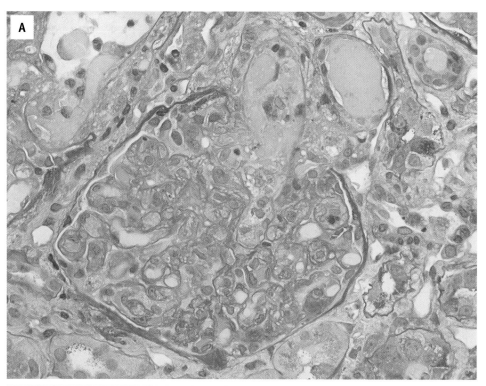

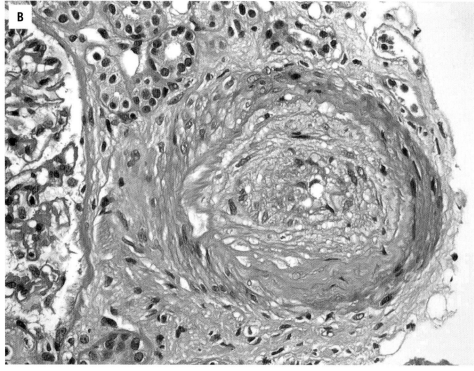

FIGURE 7-22

Thrombotic microangiopathy. **A,** Glomerular hilar and capillary thrombi with segmental capillary wall basement membrane duplication (periodic acid-Schiff stain, 400×). **B,** Scleroderma. The arterial wall is markedly thickened with sub-occlusion of the arterial lumen.

PROGNOSIS AND TREATMENT

Features predictive of poor renal outcome in acute TMA include the extent of cortical necrosis and the severity of glomerular and arteriolar lesions. Cortical necrosis is most frequently observed in infants, and its extent determines the prognosis. Diffuse cortical necrosis predicts irreversible renal dysfunction. Diffuse glomerulopathy with or without arteriolopathy is most frequently seen in young children with TMA, and outcome is related to the extent of glomerular involvement. Predominant involvement of arterioles and arteries is observed in older children, adolescents, and adults and predicts a worse prognosis than TMA with predominant glomerular involvement in these age groups. In general, biopsy specimens with acute changes, given the caveats described, indicate a greater chance of reversibility than do those with predominantly chronic changes, and it is important to convey the relative proportion and significance of these findings in pathology reports of TMA. About 66 % of childhood disease leads to complete recovery; in adults, this diminishes to less than 30 %. Treatment administered depends on the underlying cause. Plasmapheresis or plasma exchange, with dialysis, steroids, intravenous immunoglobulins, antiplatelet agents, and antihypertensives, are among the battery of agents used in treatment of this group of disorders.

Thrombotic Microangiopathy in Specific Circumstances

ANTIPHOSPHOLIPID SYNDROME NEPHROPATHY

Nephropathy may arise in primary or lupus-associated secondary forms of APL syndrome and is characterized by vaso-occlusive renal disease in patients with APL antibodies, anticardiolipin antibodies, or lupus anticoagulant.

EPIDEMIOLOGY

Renal involvement occurs in 25 % of patients with primary APL syndrome. One third of lupus patients have vascular lesions consistent with APL nephropathy.

CLINICAL FEATURES

These patients typically have hypertension, renal insufficiency, subnephrotic-range proteinuria, and hematuria.

PATHOLOGIC FEATURES

MICROSCOPIC FINDINGS

Acute lesions include arteriolar and glomerular TMA and arterial thrombi. Chronic lesions include myointimal hyperplasia and intimal fibrosis of arteries and arterioles, recanalizing thrombi in arteries and arterioles (fibrocellular cushion-like intimal projections), arteriolar hyalinization, and intimal fibrous occlusions. Glomeruli may show double contours with or without thrombi, ischemic collapse, or FSGS. The most charac-

teristic finding is fibrous cortical atrophy, consisting of subcapsular ischemic glomerular collapse, glomerular microcysts, tubular atrophy, and interstitial fibrosis in wedge-shaped scars.

ANCILLARY STUDIES

IMMUNOFLUORESCENCE

Fibrin/fibrinogen, IgM, and C3 are detected in affected arteries and arterioles. Glomeruli lack significant immunoglobulin and complement deposits in primary APL syndrome nephropathy.

ELECTRON MICROSCOPY

For EM findings, see the earlier discussion of TMA and malignant hypertension.

SYSTEMIC SCLEROSIS

The kidney is affected when there is acute oliguric renal failure with malignant hypertension arising in the course of systemic sclerosis (scleroderma renal crisis).

EPIDEMIOLOGY

Scleroderma renal crisis arises in 20 % of patients with systemic sclerosis.

PATHOLOGIC FEATURES

MICROSCOPIC FINDINGS

The acute phase shows severe mucoid intimal thickening of arteries and arterioles, with luminal stenosis. Thrombosis, intimal fibrin, and erythrocytolysis may be observed. Periadventitial fibrosis may also be evident. Glomeruli show ischemic collapse. Chronic arteriopathy produces severe arterial luminal stenosis with marked concentric duplication of the internal elastica (Fig. 7-22B).

ANCILLARY STUDIES

IMMUNOFLUORESCENCE

Fibrin/fibrinogen, IgM, and C3 are detected in affected arteries and arterioles by IF.

ELECTRON MICROSCOPY

For EM findings, see the earlier discussion of TMA and malignant hypertension.

RENAL VASCULITIS

Renal vasculitis is a collective term for a heterogenous group of disorders characterized by inflammation of arteries, arterioles, and venules with or without GN. The lesions may be immune complex-mediated, or they may have no detectable immune complex deposits.

Disorders include the following: (1) ANCA-associated vasculitides (Wegener's granulomatosis, microscopic polyangiitis, renal limited vasculitis, Churg-Strauss syndrome)—see earlier discussion of glomerular disease with extracapillary proliferation and Table 7-14; (2) immune complex-mediated vasculitis (postinfectious [rare], SLE, HSP, cryoglobulinemia)—see respective sections on glomerular disease; and (3) classic polyarteritis nodosa, a disorder rarely encountered in the renal biopsy.

LUPUS-ASSOCIATED VASCULAR LESIONS

Arterial and arteriolar lesions are observed in the context of SLE.

EPIDEMIOLOGY

Lupus-associated vascular lesions are observed in 25% to 30% of biopsies for lupus nephritis.

PATHOLOGIC FEATURES

Pathologic findings of renal biopsies in lupus-associated disease may include the following:
1. Immune complex deposition without arteriopathy—minimal wall thickening; intimal IgG, C3, and C1q by IF
2. Immune complex deposition with arteriopathy (lupus vasculopathy)—intimal and medial eosinophilic fibrinoid/hyaline material without significant inflammation or necrosis; fibrin/fibrinogen, IgG, C3, and C1q by IF
3. Necrotizing lupus vasculitis—fibrinoid necrosis and leukocytoclasis; fibrin/fibrinogen, IgG, C3, and C1q by IF

4. Arteriosclerosis and arteriolosclerosis—nonspecific, common
5. Thrombotic microangiopathy—morphologically identical to TMA as described earlier; fibrin/fibrinogen with no IgG by IF; may be associated with APL antibodies or mixed connective tissue disease (scleroderma overlap).

For additional features of lupus nephritis, see the earlier section on GN.

PROGNOSIS AND TREATMENT

Five- and 10-year renal survival rates are reduced in patients with lupus nephritis and vascular lesions, compared to patients lacking these lesions (74% versus 90% at 5 years, and 58% versus 86% at 10 years).

RENAL TRANSPLANT PATHOLOGY

This section describes commonly encountered disorders of renal allografts selected from the pathologic classification presented in Table 7-15. International standardized criteria for rejection, as specified by the Banff system, are used throughout.

Immunologic Rejection

HYPERACUTE REJECTION

Preformed antidonor antibodies against blood group or major histocompatibility antigens bind to graft endothelium and cause severe endothelial injury and activation, with intravascular platelet-fibrin thrombi, extravasation of erythrocytes, and irreversible graft necrosis.

EPIDEMIOLOGY

Hyperacute rejection is rare in current practice.

CLINICAL FEATURE

The transplant surgeon sees the graft become mottled and later hemorrhagic soon after revascularization, often accompanied by cessation of urinary output.

Table 7-15
Diagnostic Classification of Renal Allograft Lesions

IMMUNOLOGICALLY MEDIATED REJECTION

Primarily T cell-mediated
Acute cellular rejection
    Tubulointerstitial: type 1*
    Vascular (endarteritis): type 2*
    Glomerular: transplant glomerulitis

Primarily antibody-mediated
Hyperacute rejection

Acute humoral rejection (C4d positive)
    Acute tubular necrosis-like
    Capillaritis (glomerular, peritubular)
    Arterial transmural inflammation and/or fibrinoid necrosis
      (necrotizing arteritis): type 3*

Thrombotic microangiopathy

Chronic rejection
Chronic arteriopathy (chronic endarteritis)

Chronic allograft glomerulopathy

GRAFT INJURY DUE TO CAUSES OTHER THAN REJECTION

Acute ischemic tubular necrosis
Perfusion injury
Calcineurin inhibitor toxicity
    Functional
    Tubular
    Vascular

Thrombosis of major vessels
    Renal vein thrombosis
    Renal artery thrombosis

Urinary obstruction
Graft infection
    Viral: polyomavirus, cytomegalovirus, adenovirus
    Bacterial: acute pyelonephritis
    Post-transplantation lymphoproliferative disorder: Epstein-
      Barr virus (EBV)

Drug-induced interstitial nephritis
Recurrent glomerular disease
De novo glomerular disease
Chronic allograft nephropathy

---

*Types as defined by Banff 1997 criteria. (Racusen LC, Solez K, Colvin RB, et al: The Banff 97 working classification of renal allograft pathology. Kidney Int 1999;55:713.)

PATHOLOGIC FEATURES

Grossly, there is massive enlargement, with subcapsular petechial hemorrhages and focal yellow white necrotic areas.

MICROSCOPIC FINDINGS

Diffuse glomerular and peritubular capillary (PTC) thrombosis with interstitial hemorrhages, ischemic ATN, and infarction. Capillary neutrophils and platelets are abundant.

ANCILLARY STUDIES

IMMUNOFLUORESCENCE

Focal IgG, IgM, and C3 may be detectable in the PTCs by direct IF. C4d may be detectable in PTCs.

ELECTRON MICROSCOPY

Diffuse capillary endothelial swelling and detachment from the basement membrane, platelet-fibrin thrombi, neutrophils, macrophages, and capillary rupture are observed on EM.

PROGNOSIS AND TREATMENT

Once the process is established, graft loss is inevitable. There is no effective therapy. Prevention and preoperative cross-matching are key.

ACUTE REJECTION

DEFINITION

Acute allograft inflammation and injury mediated by a donor-specific immune reaction. Cellular effectors include T and B lymphocytes, and humoral effectors include donor-specific antibodies (DSA), complement activation, and recruitment of innate effectors such as macrophages, neutrophils, and platelets.

Types of acute rejection and their frequencies are humoral (10%), cellular (30% to 60%), and mixed humoral and cellular (30% to 60%).

EPIDEMIOLOGY

Cadaveric allografts have higher rates of acute rejection than living related allografts. The frequency among first recipients of cadaveric grafts is approximately 10% to 20%.

CLINICAL FEATURES

Patients typically are asymptomatic. Acute rejection is recognized by acute deterioration of graft function with elevation of the serum creatinine. If there is a history of cessation or reduction of immunosuppression (noncompliance), the clinical suspicion is acute rejection. Acute rejection may arise days to years after transplantation.

PATHOLOGIC FEATURES—ACUTE HUMORAL REJECTION

MICROSCOPIC FINDINGS

Pure acute humoral rejection (i.e., with little evidence of cellular rejection) has (1) neutrophilic peritubular capillaritis, (2) acute glomerulitis, (3) capillary thrombosis, (4) interstitial hemorrhage, (5) ATN, (6) necrotizing arteritis, and (7) PTC C4d by immunohistochemistry. More than two neutrophils, in two or more PTCs, typically with endothelial swelling or detachment and capillary luminal dilation, indicate neutrophilic capillaritis (Fig. 7-23A). Acute transplant glomerulitis has endocapillary inflammation with MNCs, neutrophils, swollen endothelium, and segmental double contours (Fig. 7-23B). Interstitial hemorrhage and intracapillary platelet margination are frequently observed. ATN, with epithelial simplification, focal epithelial necrosis, and detachment with cast formation may be the only morphologic feature observed. Rarely, acute humoral rejection has predominantly glomerular TMA.

ACUTE RENAL ALLOGRAFT REJECTION—FACT SHEET

Definition
▶ Immunologic graft injury from recipient immune reaction to donor antigens expressed in the graft

Incidence
▶ 10-20% of cadaveric grafts in current practice

Clinical Features
▶ Asymptomatic acute elevation of serum creatinine arising from days to years after transplantation

Prognosis and Treatment
▶ Acute cellular rejection—intravenous corticosteroids, anti-T cell antibodies
▶ Acute humoral rejection—plasmapheresis, intravenous immunoglobulin, anti-B cell antibodies
▶ Graft survival 1 year after diagnosis: 90-95% with acute cellular rejection, 60% with acute cellular and humoral rejection

---

ACUTE RENAL ALLOGRAFT REJECTION—PATHOLOGIC FEATURES

Microscopic Findings
▶ Subtypes
▶ 30-60% cellular
▶ 30-60% mixed cellular and humoral
▶ 10% humoral
▶ *Acute cellular rejection:* interstitial mononuclear inflammation, edema, tubulitis, intimal arteritis (acute endarteritis) ± acute transplant glomerulitis
▶ *Acute humoral rejection:* acute capillaritis, glomerular + PTC, ATN, TMA (rare), necrotizing arteritis

Immunofluorescence
▶ Indirect IF reveals diffuse PTC C4d in acute humoral rejection
▶ Direct IF reveals little immunoglobulin or other complement components in vasculature

Ultrastructural Features
▶ Useful to distinguish recurrent glomerular disease from transplant glomerulitis

Differential diagnosis
▶ Polyoma virus nephropathy
▶ EBV (PTLD)
▶ Acute pyelonephritis, septicemia, reperfusion injury
▶ Drug-induced interstitial nephritis
▶ Recurrent glomerulonephritis
▶ Recurrent vasculitis (rarely)

ANCILLARY STUDIES—ACUTE HUMORAL REJECTION

IMMUNOFLUORESCENCE

Indirect IF studies on frozen sections or immunohistochemistry on paraffin sections for the C4d component of the classic complement pathway reveals linear staining of PTC walls. Diffuse PTC C4d (Fig. 7-23C) may be detectable with or without typical histology. PTC C4d is the hallmark of humoral rejection. Immunoglobulins and complement are typically undetectable in the vasculature. Necrotizing arteritis may have fibrin/fibrinogen, IgM, and C3 in affected artery walls. Acute transplant glomerulitis typically has no or minor amounts of IgG, IgM, and C3; however, C4d is prominent in capillary walls and in the mesangium.

Serologic evidence of DSA may be detectable by flow cytometry or by lymphocytotoxicity assays, typically with anti-major histocompatibility complex (MHC) class I or class II specificity. The Banff criteria for renal allograft rejection, as updated in 2003, specify that DSA must be demonstrated to establish the diagnosis of humoral rejection. In the absence of demonstrable DSA, biopsy findings are suspicious for acute humoral rejection but not diagnostic.

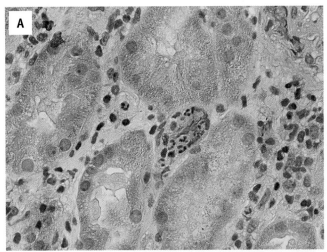

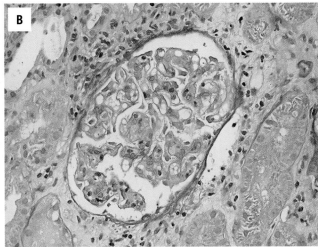

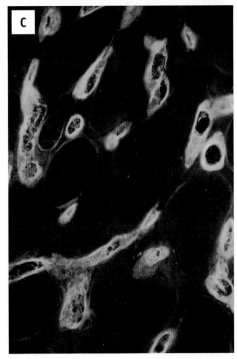

FIGURE 7-23

Acute humoral rejection. **A,** Congested peritubular capillary with marginating neutrophils and focal interstitial mononuclear infiltrate without tubulitis (hematoxylin and eosin stain, H&E, 60×). **B,** Glomerulus with endocapillary hypercellularity attributable to mononuclear inflammatory cells in lower half of tuft (periodic acid-Schiff stain [PAS], 40×). **C,** Indirect immunofluorescence reveals diffuse capillary C4d (40×).

ELECTRON MICROSCOPY

EM is used to exclude immune complex-mediated GN in cases of acute transplant glomerulitis. Capillaritis has endothelial swelling with fenestral loss, detachment from the basement membrane, and luminal macrophages, platelets, and neutrophils.

PATHOLOGIC FEATURES—ACUTE CELLULAR REJECTION

MICROSCOPIC FINDINGS

Diagnosis of acute rejection depends on identification of specific tubulointerstitial inflammation and/or arterial inflammation. Between 25% and 35% of biopsy specimens showing acute rejection have both tubulo-interstitial and arterial inflammation. An interstitial mononuclear infiltrate composed of lymphocytes, macrophages, and occasional granulocytes with edema is typical. Lymphoid cells are polymorphous, with cells in varying stages of activation. Interstitial clusters or sheets of mature plasma cells may be numerous, especially in acute rejection of later onset. Plasma cells in acute rejection are polyclonal and are associated with interstitial hemorrhage, eosinophils, and frequently PTC C4d, suggesting mixed humoral and cellular rejection. Neutrophils are uncommon. Tubules have intraepithelial or subepithelial mononuclear inflammation in tubulitis, best identified on PAS-stained sections inside the confines of the TBM (Fig. 7-24A). Tubular epithelial injury, with epithelial flattening and mitoses, in foci with or without inflammation, is frequent. Intimal arteritis or acute endarteritis is pathognomonic of acute cellular rejection. Focal lesions are usual

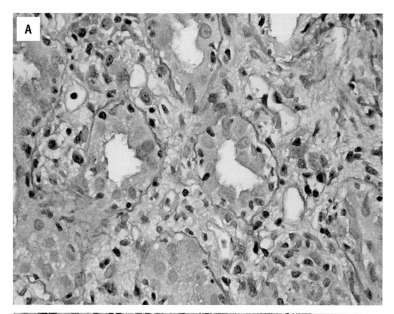

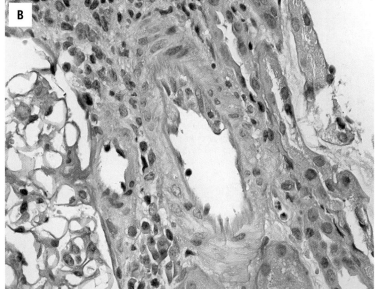

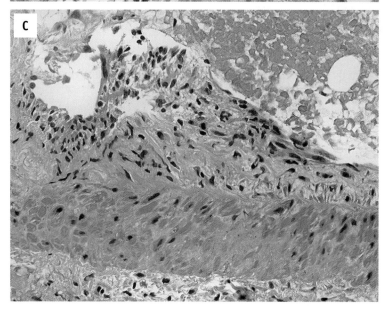

FIGURE 7-24

Acute rejection. **A,** Tubulitis with mononuclear inflammatory cells lying between the epithelium and the basement membrane with interstitial mononuclear cells PAS, 40×). **B,** Small artery with subendothelial mononuclear inflammation (intimal arteritis or endothelialitis (PAS, 40×). **C,** Intimal arteritis superimposed on an artery with intimal fibrosis (donor arteriosclerosis) (H&E, 40×).

and may be identified as subendothelial infiltration of MNCs (T cells and macrophages) resulting in loss of endothelial adhesion to the basement membrane with subendothelial widening (Fig. 7-24B). Acute endarteritis may involve arteries with preexisting arteriosclerosis (Fig. 7-24C). If the inflammation extends through the media or adventitia (i.e., transmural arteritis), there may be medial fibrinoid necrosis, a lesion with important implications for the severity of acute rejection. Arteriolar intimal arteritis may also be observed and typically accompanies arteritis in larger arteries. Approximately 10% of biopsy specimens showing acute rejection also have acute transplant glomerulitis. This lesion is characterized by endocapillary hypercellularity with margination and aggregation of mononuclear inflammatory cells (T cells and macrophages) and endothelial swelling (Fig. 7-23B).

ANCILLARY STUDIES—ACUTE CELLULAR REJECTION

IMMUNOFLUORESCENCE

Immunoglobulins and complement components are undetectable in the vasculature in acute cellular rejection.

PATHOLOGIC FEATURES—MIXED ACUTE CELLULAR AND HUMORAL REJECTION

Overlapping histologic features of acute humoral and acute cellular rejection are observed, with diffuse PTC C4d and DSA by serology.

Diffuse PTC C4d is observed in 30% to 60% of biopsy specimens with acute cellular rejection and provides evidence of humoral in addition to cellular injury of the allograft.

DIAGNOSIS OF ACUTE REJECTION USING THE BANFF 97 CLASSIFICATION SYSTEM

For acute cellular rejection, the extent of cortical interstitial mononuclear inflammation, composed principally of lymphocytes and macrophages, is subjectively scored in nonscarred renal cortex as follows: none = i0, 10% to 25% = i1, 26% to 50% = i2, and 50% or greater = i3. Tubulitis is scored by the severity of tubular mononuclear inflammation in tubular cross-sections or per 10 tubular epithelial cells, when evaluating oblique or longitudinal tubular profiles, as follows: none = t0, 1 to 4 MNCs per tubular cross-section = t1, 5 to 10 MNCs = t2, and more than 10 MNCs = t3; tubular rupture with t2 is also scored as t3. Scoring is performed on sections stained with PAS (or methenamine silver). Scoring of the severity of intimal arteritis is determined by the luminal cross-sectional area, internal to the elastic lamina, that is occluded by intimal inflammatory infiltrates. The lesions are scored as follows: none = v0, less than 25% luminal occlusion = v1, more than 25% luminal occlusion = v2, transmural inflammation and/or fibrinoid necrosis = v3. Synthesis of the findings for arteries and the tubulo-interstitial compartments allows classification of intragraft mononuclear inflammatory ("cellular") infiltrates into borderline infiltrates or acute rejection type 1, 2, or 3 as shown in Table 7-16.

Table 7-16

Classification of Allograft Mononuclear Inflammation and Acute (Cellular) Rejection by the Banff 97 System

Classification	Interstitial inflammation (i) (% cortex)*	Tubulitis (t) (MNCs/TCS)†	Intimal Arteritis (v)
Nonspecific infiltrates	1 to 10 (i0)	1 to >10	None
Borderline infiltrates	10 to 25 (i1)	<5 or ≥5	None
	≥25 (i2, i3)	<5	None
Acute cellular rejection			
Type 1A	≥25	5-10 (t2)	None
Type 1B	≥25	>10 (t3)	None
Type 2A	0 to >25	1 to >10	Mild (<25% occlusion)
Type 2B	0 to >25	1 to >10	Moderate/severe (>25% occlusion)
Type 3	0 to >25	1 to >10	Transmural

*Percentage of cortical interstitium with inflammatory mononuclear infiltrate.
†Number of mononuclear cells per tubular cross-section.

DIFFERENTIAL DIAGNOSIS

Neutrophils, congestion, hemorrhage: Intracapillary neutrophils and platelets may be seen as a nonspecific response to tissue coagulative necrosis from any cause. In renal vein thrombosis, there may be capillary congestion, interstitial hemorrhage and edema, and capillary neutrophils; however, PTCs are C4d negative and necrosis is prominent. Neutrophilic capillaritis may also be seen in septicemia and ischemia-reperfusion injury; however, PTC C4d staining is absent. Prominent neutrophilic tubulitis suggests acute pyelonephritis.

Tubulointerstitial mononuclear inflammation: Inflammatory infiltrates resembling acute cellular rejection may be seen in post-transplantation lymphoproliferative disease (PTLD) and polyomavirus BK-type infection. CMV and adenovirus may also produce tubulointerstitial inflammation. Capillary endothelium and podocytes may have inclusions in CMV infection. Adenovirus infection typically has distinctive smudged nuclear inclusions in tubules. The diagnosis is confirmed by immunohistochemistry for viral antigens or by in situ hybridization for viral DNA. Acute rejection may coexist with or follow polyomavirus infection and may follow CMV infection.

Arteritis, endarteritis: Intimal or transmural arteritis is virtually pathognomonic of acute rejection. Recurrent ANCA-type vasculitis may mimic type 2 or 3 acute rejection; however, crescentic GN is identifiable in this situation. Neutrophils and/or erythrocytes (hematomedia) permeating artery walls may be evident in reperfusion injury in the absence of fibrinoid necrosis.

Acute transplant glomerulitis/glomerulopathy: These lesions ought to be distinguished from MPGN type 1. Immunofluorescence and EM studies reveal immune complex-type deposits in MPGN type 1. Microangiopathy of calcineurin inhibitor toxicity has GBM duplication, mesangiolysis, and thrombi, with little endocapillary inflammation.

PROGNOSIS AND TREATMENT

Acute humoral rejection is reversible if appropriately treated, by plasmapheresis or intravenous immunoglobulin. Acute cellular rejection tends to be responsive to intravenous steroid therapy in Banff type 1, and steroid resistant in Banff types 2, 3 and acute humoral rejection; however, this depends on the time of onset of acute rejection, because late rejection is generally less steroid responsive. Follow-up biopsies after treatment reveal reduction of interstitial inflammation with slower reduction of tubulitis. Graft survival at 1 year after diagnosis in early acute rejection is approximately 90% to 95%; for later acute rejection (> 6 months), it is 65% to 70%. Survival decreases with diffuse PTC C4d (i.e., mixed cellular and humoral rejection), to 60% (early) and 35% (late).

BORDERLINE INFILTRATES

Borderline infiltrates may represent the crescendo or decrescendo phases of type 1 acute rejection. If identified early in the post-transplantation period (< 3 months), these features should be considered suspicious for acute rejection, especially if there is no other explanation for acute graft dysfunction. Borderline infiltrates in biopsy specimens after treatment with antirejection therapy are probably regressive lesions and in a minority of instances may progress to recurrence of acute rejection.

CHRONIC REJECTION

DEFINITION

Chronic rejection is prolonged alloimmune injury to graft tissue that is characterized by chronic glomerulopathy, inflammatory intimal fibrosis (chronic endarteritis), and PTC basement membrane duplication as specific vascular markers. Chronic vascular injury may be accompanied by ischemic or inflammatory tubular atrophy and interstitial fibrosis.

EPIDEMIOLOGY

About 40% of graft biopsy specimens obtained for chronic dysfunction have chronic rejection. The lesion accounts for approximately 25% of graft losses.

CHRONIC RENAL ALLOGRAFT REJECTION—FACT SHEET

Definition
▶ Prolonged alloimmune graft injury characterized by chronic glomerulopathy, chronic endarteritis, and peritubular capillary basement membrane duplication

Incidence
▶ 40% of biopsies for chronic dysfunction
▶ 25% of late graft losses

Clinical Features
▶ Asymptomatic slow elevation of serum creatinine over months to years.
▶ Proteinuria typically subnephrotic

Prognosis and Treatment
▶ Increased oral immunosuppression
▶ Graft loss 1 year after diagnosis in ~50%

PATHOLOGIC FEATURES

MICROSCOPIC FINDINGS

Chronic transplant glomerulopathy is characterized by diffuse, often segmental GBM duplication on PAS-stained sections (Fig. 7-25A) and variable mesangial sclerosis with segmental adhesion of the glomerular tufts to Bowman's capsule. Global and segmental glomerular sclerosis and hyalinosis may be prominent. PTCs have basement membrane thickening and multi-layering. Arteries have intimal fibrous thickening with small amounts of infiltrating T cells and foamy macrophages, features diagnostic of chronic endarteritis (Fig. 7-25B). Interstitial inflammation and fibrosis with tubular atrophy are variable.

ANCILLARY STUDIES

IMMUNOFLUORESCENCE

IF reveals little IgG, IgM, or C3 in glomeruli. PTC, glomerular capillary, and mesangial C4d deposition is frequent in biopsy specimens with chronic transplant

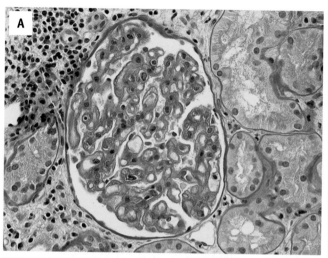

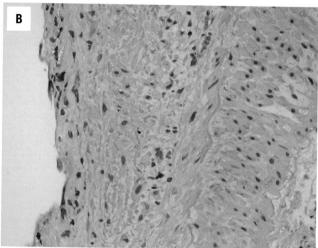

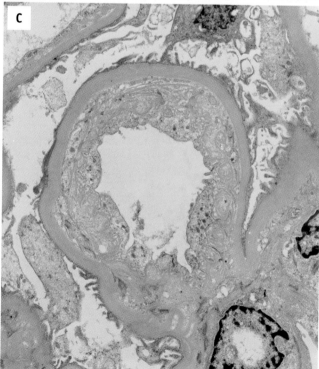

FIGURE 7-25

Chronic allograft nephropathy. **A,** Glomerulus with global capillary basement membrane duplication, mesangial thickening, and mild hypercellularity typical of chronic transplant glomerulopathy PAS, 40×). **B,** Chronic allograft arteriopathy (endarteritis) with intimal thickening, myointimal cells, mononuclear inflammation, and foam cells *(upper left)* (H&E, 40×). **C,** Chronic allograft glomerulopathy with endothelial swelling and sub-endothelial new basement membrane formation in the absence of electron-dense deposits (electron micrograph, 5200×).

Graft Injury Due to Causes Other Than Rejection

CALCINEURIN INHIBITOR TOXICITY

Calcineurin inhibitor therapy includes tacrolimus or cyclosporine, used as immunosuppressives in combination with prednisone and other agents. Toxicity is defined as graft dysfunction attributable to direct injury to the graft tissues. This can be difficult to prove in practice. Tacrolimus and cyclosporine each have functional and morphologic toxic effects. Toxic effects can be considered under three headings:

1. Functional toxicity: reversible dysfunction attributable to vasoconstriction
2. Acute and chronic tubular toxicity: a consequence of functional vasoconstriction with additional direct toxic sublethal injury of tubular epithelium
3. Acute and chronic vascular toxicity: direct endothelial and smooth muscle injury principally affecting arterioles and glomeruli

Tubular and vascular toxicity may coexist.

glomerulopathy. Diffuse PTC C4d correlates with the presence of circulating DSA in chronic rejection.

ELECTRON MICROSCOPY

Glomerular capillaries have swollen endothelium, fenestral loss, detachment from the basement membrane, and formation of new subendothelial strands of basement membrane (Fig. 7-25C). Cellular interposition may be evident; however, electron-dense deposits of the immune complex type are absent. Mesangial sclerosis is prominent. Podocyte foot processes are effaced. PTCs have swollen endothelium and multiple periendothelial layers of new basement membrane.

CLINICAL FEATURES

Toxic effects may arise at any time in the posttransplantation period. Typically, there is acute or chronic elevation of the serum creatinine as the only clinical manifestation. Knowledge of trough blood levels of calcineurin inhibitor may be of help in biopsy interpretation; however, the severity of tissue injury and

DIFFERENTIAL DIAGNOSIS

Chronic transplant glomerulopathy must be distinguished from recurrent or de novo MPGN type 1, notably in patients with hepatitis C infection. Immune complex deposits are detectable by IF and EM in MPGN type 1. Chronic hypertension may be associated with arterial intimal fibrosis (arteriosclerosis); however, inflammatory cells are absent.

PROGNOSIS AND TREATMENT

Treatment of chronic rejection may require increased oral immunosuppression. Graft loss rates of 50% at 1 year and 75% at 3 years after diagnosis are described.

blood levels of calcineurin inhibitor are not strongly correlated.

PATHOLOGIC FEATURES

MICROSCOPIC FINDINGS

Functional Toxicity

Functional toxicity by definition has no morphologic tissue changes.

Acute Tubular Toxicity

Acute tubular toxicity is characterized by focal or diffuse epithelial isometric vacuolization imparting a foam cell appearance (Fig. 7-26A); it may affect tubules with ATN. Straight portions of the proximal tubules and small clusters of profiles representing convoluted segments may be affected. Epithelial megamitochondria are rare and appear as large eosinophilic granules. Confirmation requires EM examination. Tubular calcium phosphate or hydroxyapatite (von Kossa positive) may be seen. Glomeruli are typically normal. Arterioles may have minor nonspecific changes, including smooth muscle vacuolization.

CALCINEURIN INHIBITOR TOXICITY—PATHOLOGIC FEATURES

Microscopic Findings
▶ *Acute tubular toxicity:* isometric vacuolization of tubular epithelial cell cytoplasm, acute tubular injury, megamitochondria, tubular calcium phosphate/hydroxyapatite
▶ *Acute vascular toxicity:* afferent arterioles predominantly affected with mural myxoid swelling, smooth muscle vacuolization and necrosis, myxoid intimal swelling of arteries, TMA (arteriolar and glomerular)
▶ Subacute/chronic toxicity: peripheral nodular hyaline arteriolosclerosis, tubular atrophy, striped interstitial fibrosis

Immunofluorescence
▶ Fibrin in affected vessel walls and lumens
▶ Arteriolar mural IgM and C3 (nonspecific trapping)

Ultrastructural Features
▶ Tubular megamitochondria
▶ Nodular medial (peripheral) hyaline arteriolosclerosis

Differential Diagnosis
▶ *TMA:* recurrent HUS, malignant hypertension, acute humoral rejection, hepatitis C infection with antiphospholipid antibodies
▶ *Acute tubular toxicity:* osmolar nephrosis
▶ *Hyaline arteriolosclerosis:* hypertension, diabetes

Chronic Tubular Toxicity

Chronic tubular toxicity has tubular atrophy with interstitial fibrosis and shrinkage of the parenchyma often observed as condensation of glomeruli. This may have bands of interstitial fibrosis beside areas of nonatrophic tubules, imparting a striped appearance. Typically, glomeruli exhibit ischemic collapse.

Acute Vascular Toxicity

Acute vascular calcineurin inhibitor toxicity affects the preglomerular arterioles.

In acute arteriolopathy, there is loss of definition of smooth muscle cells, accumulation of clear/myxoid basophilic matrix (Fig. 7-26B), increased medial PAS-positive matrix, and loss of smooth muscle cell nuclei. Medial apoptotic bodies and necrotic cells may be observed.

In thrombotic microangiopathy, arterioles have luminal thrombi, endothelial detachment or necrosis, intimal and medial fibrinoid exudates, and medial swelling with concentric smooth muscle separation. Obliterative arteriopathy has marked mural interstitial swelling, thickening, intramural erythrocyte fragmentation, myointimal proliferation, and severe luminal stenosis without luminal thrombosis. Thrombotic and obliterative arteriolopathic lesions tend to be focal in calcineurin inhibitor toxicity. Glomerular capillary platelet-fibrin thrombi, endothelial swelling, capillary obliteration, and mesangiolysis affect a minority of glomeruli. Ischemic glomerulopathy and wrinkling and collapse of glomerular capillaries may be prominent.

Chronic Vascular Toxicity

Chronic vascular calcineurin inhibitor-associated toxicity has distinctive nodular hyaline arteriolosclerosis, beginning as hyaline replacement of smooth muscle in the outer media, which imparts a "beaded necklace" appearance (Fig. 7-26C), progressing with time to involve the entire media and intima. Arteriolosclerosis with chronic ischemia may explain the striped pattern of fibrosis. Glomeruli have ischemic collapse.

ANCILLARY STUDIES

IMMUNOFLUORESCENCE

Direct IF reveals fibrin/fibrinogen, IgM, and C3 in glomeruli and arterioles in acute TMA. Platelets are detectable by immunohistochemistry for CD61 or CD62.

ELECTRON MICROSCOPY

EM is rarely used for diagnosis. Tubular microcalcifications and megamitochondria with vascular erythrocytolysis, intimal and medial platelets, mesangiolysis, and glomerular capillary endothelial detachment can all be observed ultrastructurally. Nodular hyalinization can

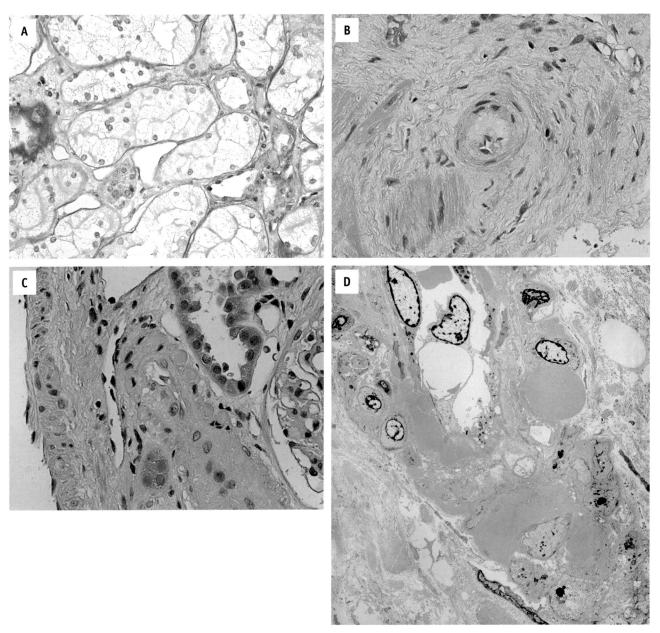

FIGURE 7-26

A, Tubular isometric vacuolization affecting proximal tubular segments in acute tubular toxicity. This appearance is indistinguishable from osmolar nephrosis (PAS, 40×). **B,** Acute arteriolopathy with myxoid intimal and medial thickening (H&E, 40×). **C,** Longitudinal section of an arteriole with intimal thickening and nodular hyalinization of periadventitial myocytes from a patient receiving tacrolimus after transplantation of small intestine. The findings illustrate acute and chronic vascular calcineurin inhibitor toxicity (H&E, 40×). **D,** Arteriolar intimal hyaline and medial hyaline replacing smooth muscle cells from the same kidney as in **C** (electron micrograph, 1650×).

be observed as electron-dense material replacing smooth muscle (Fig. 7-26D).

DIFFERENTIAL DIAGNOSIS

ISOMETRIC VACUOLIZATION

Acute tubular calcineurin inhibitor toxicity with isometric vacuolization must be distinguished from osmotic nephrosis associated with the use of hyper-

osmolar agents such as preparations of intravenous immunoglobulin or radiocontrast agents. Vacuolization is widespread in osmotic nephrosis and tends to be focal in calcineurin inhibitor toxicity.

HYALINE ARTERIOLOSCLEROSIS

Hyaline arteriolosclerosis of diabetic nephropathy and hypertension is initially intimal, progresses to involve the media, and is not typically nodular. Advanced transmural hyaline arteriolosclerosis may present a difficult dilemma.

THROMBOTIC MICROANGIOPATHY

APL antibodies with or without hepatitis C infection may be associated with allograft TMA. Recurrent HUS is morphologically identical to calcineurin inhibitor-associated TMA but tends to be diffuse and severe and has much higher graft loss rates. Perfusion nephropathy should be considered if there is TMA in the first few days after transplantation in a patient with a history of perfusion-preservation and poor early graft function. Acute humoral rejection with TMA typically has diffuse PTC C4d and circulating DSA.

PROGNOSIS AND TREATMENT

Reduction of dosage or temporary or permanent cessation of calcineurin inhibitor therapy is the basis of treatment. Graft loss from acute calcineurin inhibitor toxicity is rare, and even TMA is reversible. Late allograft failure (8-10 years) may be associated with prominent arteriolar hyalinosis.

POLYOMAVIRUS NEPHROPATHY

Renal allograft tubular invasion by polyomavirus, with or without tubulointerstitial inflammation and fibrosis, is in most instances attributable to BK virus and uncommonly to JC virus.

EPIDEMIOLOGY

Polyomavirus nephropathy occurs in 5% to 8% of renal allografts.

CLINICAL FEATURES

There is asymptomatic acute or chronic renal allograft dysfunction. Patient presents from 6 weeks to more than 5 years after transplantation, with a median time of 9 months.

PATHOLOGIC FEATURES

MICROSCOPIC FINDINGS

Polyoma virus-infected cells exhibit a spectrum of nuclear changes in the same biopsy specimen, including (1) slight enlargement with clumping of chromatin; (2)

> **POLYOMAVIRUS NEPHROPATHY—FACT SHEET**
>
> **Definition**
> ▶ Direct infection of renal tubular epithelium by polyomavirus, mainly BK type
>
> **Incidence**
> ▶ 5-8% of allografts
>
> **Clinical Features**
> ▶ Asymptomatic acute and chronic graft dysfunction
> ▶ Plasma and urinary polyomavirus DNA
>
> **Prognosis and Treatment**
> ▶ No specific antiviral therapy
> ▶ Reduction of immunosuppression
> ▶ 45-65% graft loss

marked enlargement with two or more macronucleoli, nuclear pallor, and vesicular chromatin; (3) basophilic or amphophilic intranuclear inclusions with clear outlines; and (4) deeply basophilic ground-glass nuclei (Fig. 7-27A). Infected cells have cytoplasmic PAS-positive granules, loss of adhesion to the TBM, and cellular casts of necrotic epithelium with nuclear inclusions. Initially, medullary collecting ducts are involved. Cortical infection initially involves collecting ducts and distal tubules and later proximal tubules and Bowman's capsule. Tubulointerstitial inflammation consists of predominantly lymphocytes and macrophages and plasma cells, with lesser amounts of eosinophils, neutrophils, or

---

> **POLYOMAVIRUS NEPHROPATHY—PATHOLOGIC FEATURES**
>
> **Microscopic Findings**
> ▶ Tubular epithelial nuclear enlargement with inclusions: circumscribed basophilic, amphophilic, ground-glass coarse macronucleoli
> ▶ Cytoplasmic granularity and loss of cellular adhesion
> ▶ Tubulointerstitial inflammation with lymphocytes, macrophages, neutrophils
> ▶ Tubular atrophy with marked thickening of the basement membranes
>
> **Immunohistologic Findings**
> ▶ SV40-T antigen detectable in tubular epithelial nuclei
>
> **Ultrastructural Features**
> ▶ Nuclear 40-45 nm particles in paracrystalline arrays
>
> **Differential Diagnosis**
> ▶ Adenovirus, herpes simplex virus, CMV
> ▶ Acute rejection

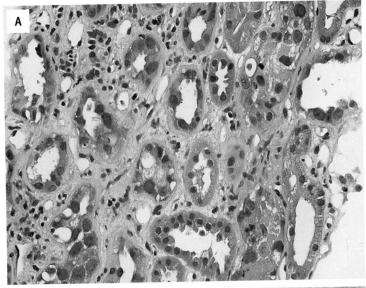

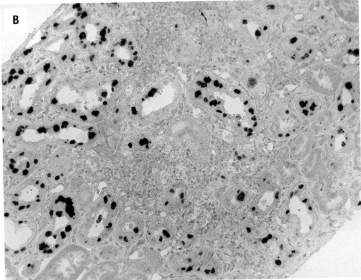

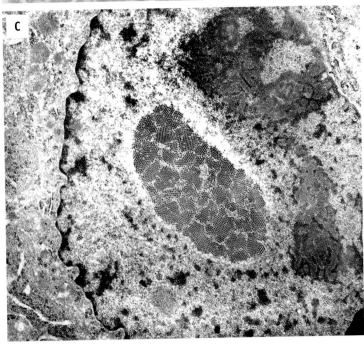

FIGURE 7-27

Polyomavirus nephropathy. **A,** Tubular segments with enlarged hyperchromatic nuclei containing circumscribed basophilic inclusions and large coarse nucleoli, with epithelial necrosis and dyshesion *(upper* and *lower right)*. There is interstitial edema and mononuclear inflammatory cell infiltrate (H&E, 40×). **B,** Polyomavirus large T antigen expression in epithelial nuclei (immunoalkaline phosphatase, naphthol red, 20×). **C,** Intranuclear paracrystalline arrays of polyomavirus (electron micrograph, 15,500×).

granulomas. Tubulitis affects tubules with and without viral cytopathic changes. Tubular atrophy with inflammation, marked TBM thickening, epithelial cell loss, and tubular shrinkage is seen with interstitial fibrosis. Lymphoid nodules containing T and B cells may be observed.

ANCILLARY STUDIES

IMMUNOHISTOLOGY

Polyomavirus large T antigen (SV40-T antigen) is detectable in tubular nuclei (Fig. 7-27B). Lymphoid nodules have predominantly B cells (CD20 positive) with lesser amounts of T cells (CD3 positive).

ELECTRON MICROSCOPY

EM detects nuclear or cytoplasmic virions of 40 to 45 nm, typically in clusters or paracrystalline arrays (Fig. 7-27C).

DIFFERENTIAL DIAGNOSIS

CMV nephropathy is characterized by glomerular and PTC endothelial, visceral epithelial, and (rarely) tubular karyomegaly with eosinophilic inclusions surrounded by a halo and a thickened nuclear envelope. Infected cells have basophilic cytoplasm with granular inclusions. Adenovirus infection is characterized by prominent epithelial necrosis and deeply basophilic smudged nuclear inclusions in viable and necrotic tubular cells. Peritubular granulomas may be evident. Herpes simplex infection is rare and is associated with epithelial necrosis and slate grey intranuclear inclusions. CMV and herpes simplex virus can be detected immunohistochemically with the use of monoclonal antibodies. Adenovirus is detected by in situ hybridization using virus-specific DNA probes. Evidence of concomitant acute rejection and polyomavirus infection includes diffuse tubulointerstitial inflammation with very focal polyomavirus infection, intimal arteritis, and PTC C4d.

PROGNOSIS AND TREATMENT

Currently, there is no specific antiviral therapy for polyomavirus infection. Reduced immunosuppression may allow viral clearance from graft tissue, with increased risk of development of acute rejection. Interstitial fibrosis with tubular atrophy develops within months after onset of tubular infection and is irreversible. Graft loss rates range from 45% to 65%.

POST-TRANSPLANTATION LYMPHOPROLIFERATIVE DISEASE

PTLD is a multicentric disease characterized by predominantly B cell proliferation that ranges from a benign, reversible condition to progressive, malignant disease. These disorders are EBV driven in most instances.

EPIDEMIOLOGY

Between 1% and 5% of allograft recipients develop PTLD. Lesions most frequently arise within 2 years after transplantation. An EBV-negative recipient of a kidney from an EBV-positive donor (also a CMV-negative recipient with a CMV-positive donor) is at increased risk, as are all recipients in childhood. These tend to be multisystem diseases that may or may not involve the allograft.

PATHOLOGIC FEATURES

MICROSCOPIC FINDINGS

Renal allograft biopsy specimens may exhibit plasmacytic hyperplasia, polymorphous B-cell hyperplasia and lymphoma, and monomorphous non-Hodgkin's lymphomas (NHL) (immunoblastic, plasmacytoid immunoblastic, and plasmacytoma-like NHL). T cell and NK cell NHLs are very rare. Infiltrates have a high content of blastic lymphoid cells (Fig. 7-28A) in clusters or

---

POST-TRANSPLANTATION LYMPHOPROLIFERATIVE DISEASE—FACT SHEET

Definition
▶ Lymphoproliferative disease with a spectrum of features from mononucleosis-like disease to benign reversible lymphoid proliferations to non-Hodgkin's lymphoma

Incidence
▶ 1-5% of allograft recipients

Clinical Features
▶ Fever, lymphadenopathy, organomegaly
▶ Incidental discovery in biopsy for acute graft dysfunction
▶ 30-40% have involvement of transplanted organ

Prognosis and Treatment
▶ Reduced immunosuppression
▶ High mortality

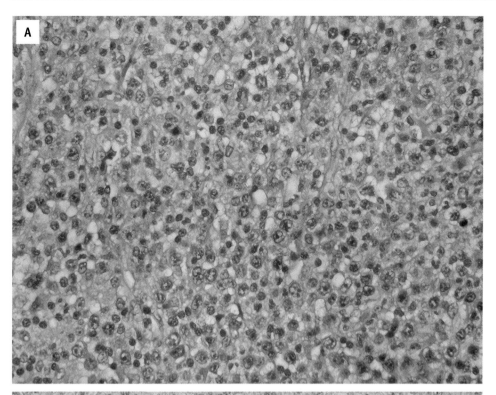

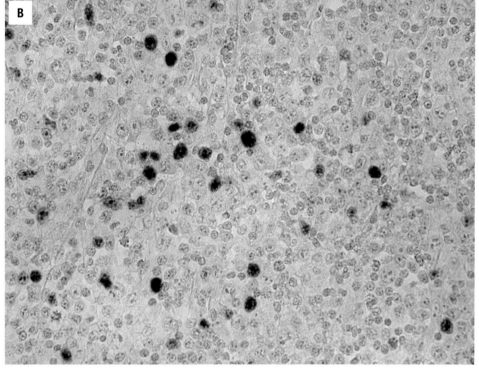

FIGURE 7-28

A, Dense infiltrate of lymphoid blasts with plasmacytoid differentiation and scattered eosinophils from a lymph node with polymorphous B-cell hyperplasia (H&E, 40×). **B,** Epstein-Barr virus–encoded RNA detected by in situ hybridization (EBER-RNA-2 probe with nitroblue tetrazolium, fast red counterstain, 40×).

nodules that expand the interstitium. Nodules lack tingible body macrophages and dendritic cells (CD21 negative) in lymphomatous infiltrates. Serpiginous necrosis and extrarenal invasion may be evident. Tubulitis is not prominent. Endarteritis is absent. Glomeruli are unremarkable.

ANCILLARY STUDIES

IMMUNOHISTOLOGY AND IN SITU HYBRIDIZATION

Early lesions (< 2 years) have EBV-encoded RNA (EBER) expression by in situ hybridization and are

POST-TRANSPLANTATION LYMPHOPROLIFERATIVE DISEASE—PATHOLOGIC FEATURES

Microscopic Findings
▶ B cell types: plasmacytic hyperplasia, polymorphous B-cell hyperplasia, monomorphous B-cell lymphoma
▶ T cell and NK cell lymphomas: very rare
▶ Expansile nodules with atypical lymphoid blasts ± necrosis
▶ Immunohistology, in situ hybridization, gene rearrangements
▶ Lymphoid markers: CD20+ in B cell types
▶ κ:λ light chains by immunoperoxidase or in situ RNA hybridization
▶ EBV encoded RNA: typically in PTLD arising <2 years after transplantation (PTLD arising >2 years after transplantation tends to be EBV negative)
▶ Immunoglobulin heavy chain or T-cell receptor rearrangements

Ultrastructural Features
▶ No diagnostic role

Differential diagnosis
▶ Acute rejection Banff 97 type 1
▶ Polyomavirus nephropathy

composed predominantly of B cells (CD20 positive). Diagnosis of PTLD may be established by in situ hybridization for EBER, revealing nuclear expression of EBER in many infiltrating cells (Fig. 7-28B). PTLD arising later than 2 years after transplantation may be EBV negative and rarely involves the renal allograft. In situ hybridization for light-chain messenger RNA, immunohistochemistry for light chains, and molecular studies for immunoglobulin heavy chain or (rarely) T-cell receptor gene rearrangements help establish the clonality of the infiltrates.

DIFFERENTIAL DIAGNOSIS

Acute rejection type 1 may have focal lymphoid nodules containing T and B cells. Acute rejection with abundant plasma cells has clusters of interstitial mature cells and prominent lymphocytic tubulitis. Plasma cells are polytypic, and PTC C4d may be present. Polyomavirus nephropathy may have numerous lymphoid nodules composed of T and B cells.

PROGNOSIS AND TREATMENT

Reduction of immunosuppression (immune reconstitution) and antiviral agents are used for polyclonal EBV-positive PTLD. Radiation and chemotherapy are used for monomorphic lymphoma. Mortality rates as high as 60% to 80% have been reported in lymphomas.

RECURRENT AND DE NOVO GLOMERULAR DISEASE

Recurrent disease refers to graft dysfunction caused by recurrence of the renal disease responsible for end-stage failure of the native kidney. De novo disease refers to glomerular disease, arising after renal transplantation, in recipients with end-stage failure of the native kidney attributable to a different disease.

EPIDEMIOLOGY

Between 1% and 5% of allograft failures are attributable to recurrent disease. Isografts have higher recurrence rates. The frequencies of recurrent diseases are given in Table 7-17. By comparison, between 3% and 5% of allograft recipients develop de novo disease, the most common of which are summarized in Table 7-18. Hepatitis C virus infection is a risk factor for de novo MPGN type 1.

PATHOLOGIC FEATURES

Glomerular diseases included in these categories are classifiable using criteria for GN of the native kidney.

DIFFERENTIAL DIAGNOSIS

MPGN type 1 must be distinguished from acute or chronic transplant glomerulopathy.

PROGNOSIS AND TREATMENT

Graft loss rates are given in Tables 7-17 and 7-18.

CHRONIC ALLOGRAFT NEPHROPATHY

Chronic allograft nephropathy is a nonspecific term for renal allograft interstitial fibrosis and tubular atrophy of indeterminate cause (Table 7-19). The term is used only if there is no evidence of chronic rejection, chronic calcineurin inhibitor toxicity, hypertensive vascular disease, chronic infection, urinary obstruction, recurrent or de novo glomerular disease; it is a diagnosis of exclusion. About 35% of biopsies with late graft dysfunction have these nonspecific findings. Grading of the

Table 7-17
Recurrent Glomerular Disease in Renal Allografts

Disease	% Recurrence	Time of Recurrence	% Graft Loss*
Diabetic nephropathy	50	3-5 years	~50
Immunoglobulin A nephropathy	45-50	Months to years	7
Primary FSGS	25-30	7.5 months	10
Hemolytic-uremic syndrome	25-30	<1 month	67
MPGN type 1	25-70	2 months to 7.5 years	10
ANCA-associated necrotizing GN	10-25	30 months	13
Membranous glomerulopathy	20-25	Weeks to months	10
Amyloid glomerulopathy	12	1-3 years	0
Fibrillary glomerulopathy	43	Years	22
MPGN type 2 (dense deposit disease)	90	Weeks	15

ANCA, antineutrophil cytoplasmic autoantibodies; FSGS, focal segmental glomerulosclerosis; GN, glomerulonephritis; MPGN, membranoproliferative glomerulonephritis.
*Estimated graft loss attributable to recurrent disease.

Table 7-18
De Novo Glomerular Disease in Renal Allografts

Disease	Frequency (%)	Time of Onset	% Graft Loss*
MGN	0.5-9	1-54 months	38-52
FSGS	8	1-53 months	40-100
MPGN type 1 (hepatitis C related)	3.3	3 months to 10 years	>60

FSGS, focal segmental glomerulosclerosis; MGN, membranous glomerulopathy; MPGN, membranoproliferative glomerulonephritis.
*Estimated graft loss attributable to de novo disease.

Table 7-19
Causes of Chronic Allograft Nephropathy

Chronic rejection

Chronic calcineurin inhibitor toxicity

Hypertensive nephrosclerosis

Urinary obstruction with or without reflux

Infection (polyomavirus, bacterial, other)

Recurrent or de novo glomerular disease

Chronic allograft nephropathy, not otherwise specified, nonspecific

extent of interstitial fibrosis and tubular atrophy as mild (< 25% of cortex), moderate (26% to 50%), or severe (> 50%) may provide important prognostic information.

SUGGESTED READING

Podocytopathies

Barisoni L, Kriz W, Mundel P, D'Agati V: The dysregulated podocyte phenotype: A novel concept in the pathogenesis of collapsing idiopathic focal segmental glomerulosclerosis and HIV-associated nephropathy. J Am Soc Nephrol 1999;10:51–61.

Glassock RJ: Secondary minimal change disease. Nephrol Dial Transplant 2003;18(Suppl 6):vi52–58.

Glassock RJ, Adler S, Cohen AH: Promary glomerular diseases. In Brenner

B (ed): The Kidney, 5th ed. Philadelphia, WB Saunders, 1996, pp 1435–1444.

Howie AJ: Pathology of minimal change nephropathy and segmental sclerosing glomerular disorders [review]. Nephrol Dial Transplant 2003;18(Suppl 6):vi33–38.

Laurinavicius A, Rennke HG: Collapsing glomerulopathy: A new pattern of renal injury [review]. Semin Diagn Pathol 2002;19:106–115.

Olson J, Schwartz M: Heptinstall's Pathology of the Kidney, 5th ed. Philadelphia, Lippincott-Raven, 1998, pp 187–258.

Pollak MR: The genetic basis of FSGS and steroid-resistant nephrosis [review]. Semin Nephrol 2003;23:141–146.

Valeri A, Barisoni L, Appel GB, et al: Idiopathic collapsing focal segmental glomerulosclerosis: A clinicopathologic study. Kidney Int 1996;50:1734–1746.

Membranous Glomerulopathy

Glassock RJ: Diagnosis and natural course of membranous nephropathy [review]. Semin Nephrol 2003;23:324–332.

Markowitz G: Membranous glomerulopathy: Emphasis on secondary forms and disease variants [review]. Adv Anat Pathol 2001;8:119–125.

Schwartz M: Heptinstall's Pathology of the Kidney, 5th ed. Phildelphia, Lippincot-Raven, 1998, pp 259–308.

Immunoglobulin A Nephropathy

D'Amico G: Natural history of idiopathic IgA nephropathy: Role of clinical and histological prognostic factors [review]. Am J Kidney Dis 2000;36:227–237.

Ferrario F, Rastaldi MP: Histopathological atlas of renal diseases: IgA nephropathy. J Nephrol 2004;17:351–353.

Haas M: Histologic subclassification of IgA nephropathy: A clinicopathologic study of 244 cases. Am J Kidney Dis 1997;29:829–842.

Hall YN, Fuentes EF, Chertow GM, Olson JL: Race/ethnicity and disease severity in IgA nephropathy. BMC Nephrol 2004;5:10.

Membranoproliferative Glomerulonephritis

Silva F: Heptinstall's Pathology of the Kidney, 5th ed. Philadelphia, Lippincot-Raven, 1998, pp 309–368.

Postinfectious Glomerulonephritis

Silva F: Heptinstall's Pathology of the Kidney, 5th ed. Philadelphia, Lippincot-Raven, 1998, pp 389–454.

Lupus Nephritis

Austin HA, Balow JE: Natural history and treatment of lupus nephritis [review]. Semin Nephrol 1999;19:2–11.

Lewis EJ, Schwartz MM: Pathology of lupus nephritis. Lupus 2005;14:31–38.

Mittal B, Rennke H, Singh AK: The role of kidney biopsy in the management of lupus nephritis. Curr Opin Nephrol Hypertens 2005;14:1–8.

Tahir H, Isenberg DA: Novel therapies in lupus nephritis. Lupus 2005;14:77–82.

Weening JJ, D'Agati VD, Schwartz MM, et al: The classification of glomerulonephritis in systemic lupus erythematosus revisited. J Am Soc Nephrol 2004;15:241–250. Erratum in J Am Soc Nephrol 2004;15:835–836.

Glomerulonephritis with Organized Deposits

Beddhu S, Bastacky S, Johnson JP: The clinical and morphologic spectrum of renal cryoglobulinemia. Medicine (Baltimore) 2002;81:398–409.

Bridoux F, Hugue V, Coldefy O, et al: Fibrillary glomerulonephritis and immunotactoid (microtubular) glomerulopathy are associated with distinct immunologic features. Kidney Int 2002;62:1764–1775.

Gertz MA, Lacy MQ, Dispenzieri A: Immunoglobulin light chain amyloidosis and the kidney. Kidney Int 2002;61:1–9.

Iskandar SS, Herrera GA: Glomerulopathies with organized deposits. Semin Diagn Pathol 2002;19:116–132.

Markowitz GS: Dysproteinemia and the kidney. Adv Anat Pathol 2004;11:49–63.

Meyers CM, Seeff LB, Stehman-Breen CO, Hoofnagle JH:Hepatitis C and renal disease: An update. Am J Kidney Dis 2003;42:631–657.

Olson J: Heptinstall's Pathology of the Kidney, 5th ed. Philadelphia, Lippincot-Raven, 1998, pp 1247–1286.

Pozzi C, Locatelli F: Kidney and liver involvement in monoclonal light chain disorders. Semin Nephrol 2002;22:319–330.

Light-Chain Deposition Disease

Markowitz GS: Dysproteinemia and the kidney. Adv Anat Pathol 2004;11:49–63.

Pozzi C, D'Amico M, Fogazzi GB, et al: Light chain deposition disease with renal involvement: Clinical characteristics and prognostic factors. Am J Kidney Dis 2003;42:1154–1163.

Glomerular Disease Characterized by Extracapillary Proliferation

Booth AD, Pusey CD, Jayne DR: Renal vasculitis: An update in 2004. Nephrol Dial Transplant 2004;19:1964–1968.

Falk RJ, Jennette JC: Thoughts about the classification of small vessel vasculitis. J Nephrol 2004;17(Suppl 8):S3–S9.

Jennette JC: Heptinstall's Pathology of the Kidney, 5th ed. Philadelphia, Lippincot-Raven, 1998, pp. 625–656.

Kalluri L: Goodpasture syndrome. Kidney Int 1999;55:1120–1122.

Kluth DC, Rees AJ: Anti-glomerular basement membrane disease. J Am Soc Nephrol 1999;10:2446–2453.

Langford CA, Balow JE: New insights into the immunopathogenesis and treatment of small vessel vasculitis of the kidney. Curr Opin Nephrol Hypertens 2003;12:267–272.

Glomerular Diseases Associated with Intrinsic Structural Abnormality of the Glomerular Basement Membranes

Kashtan CE: Alport syndrome and thin glomerular basement membrane disease. J Am Soc Nephrol 1998;9:1736–1750.

Kashtan CE: Familial hematuria due to type IV collagen mutations: Alport syndrome and thin basement membrane nephropathy. Curr Opin Pediatr 2004;16:177–181.

Mazzucco G, De Marchi M, Monga G: Renal biopsy interpretation in Alport syndrome. Semin Diagn Pathol 2002;19:133–145.

Monnens LA: Thin glomerular basement membrane disease. Kidney Int 2001;60:799–800.

Noel LH: Renal pathology and ultrastructural findings in Alport's syndrome. Ren Fail 2000;22:751–758.

Pescucci C, Longo I, Bruttini M, et al: Type-IV collagen related diseases. J Nephrol 2003;16:314–316.

Savige J, Rana K, Tonna S, et al: Thin basement membrane nephropathy. Kidney Int 2003;64:1169–1178.

Medication-Induced (Allergic or Hypersensitivity) Interstitial Nephritis

Baker RJ, Pusey CD: The changing profile of acute tubulointerstitial nephritis. Nephrol Dial Transplant 2004;19:8–11.

Buysen JG, Houthoff HJ, Krediet RT, Arisz L: Acute interstitial nephritis: A clinical and morphological study in 27 patients. Nephrol Dial Transplant 1990;5:94–99.

Kodner CM, Kudrimoti A: Diagnosis and management of acute interstitial nephritis. Am Family Physician 2003;67:2527–2534.

Schwarz A, Krause PH, Kunzendorf U, et al: The outcome of acute interstitial nephritis: Risk factors for the transition from acute to chronic interstitial nephritis. Clin Nephrol 2000;54:179–190.

Silva FG: Chemical-induced nephropathy: A review of the renal tubulointerstitial lesions in humans. Toxicol Pathol 2004;32(Suppl 2):71–84.

Thrombotic Microangiopathy

Moake JL: Thrombotic microangiopathies. N Engl J Med 2002;347:589–600.

Nochy D, Daugas E, Droz D, et al: The intrarenal vascular lesions associated with primary antiphospholipid syndrome. J Am Soc Nephrol 1999;10:507–518.

Wolf G: Not known from ADAM(TS-13): Novel insights into the pathophysiology of thrombotic microangiopathies. Nephrol Dial Transplant 2004;19:1687–1693.

Renal Vasculitis

Bajema I, Haagen EC, Hermans J, et al: Kidney biopsy as a predictor for renal outcome in ANCA-associated necrotizing glomerulonephritis. Kidney Int 1999;56:1751–1758.

Jeanette JC, Falk RJ: Small vessel vasculitis. N Engl J Med 1997;337:1512–1523.

Savige J, Davies D, Falk RJ, Jennette JC: Antineutrophil cytoplasmic autoantibodies and associated disease: A review of clinical and laboratory features. Kidney Int 2000;57:846–862.

Lupus-Associated Vascular Lesions

D'Agati VD: Renal disease in systemic lupus erythematosus, mixed connective tissue disease, Sjogrens syndrome and rheumatoid arthritis. In Jenette JC, Olson JL, Schwartz MM, Silva FG (eds): Heptinstall's Pathology of the Kidney, 5th ed. Philadelphia, Lippincot-Raven, 1998, pp 541–624.

Renal Transplant Pathology

Colvin RB: Chronic allograft nephropathy. N Engl J Med 2003;349:2288–2290.

Michaels PJ, Fishbein MC, Colvin RB: Humoral rejection of human organ transplants. Springer Semin Immunopathol 2003;25:119.

Nickeleit V, Mihatsch MJ: Kidney transplants, antibodies, and rejection: Is C4d a magic marker? Nephrol Dial Transplant 2003;18:2232.

Poduval RD, Kadambi PV, Josephson MA, et al: Implications of immunohistochemical detection of C4d along peritubular capillaries in late acute renal allograft rejection. Transplantation 2005;79:228–235.

Racusen LC, Colvin RB, Solez K, et al: Antibody mediated rejection criteria: An addition to the Banff 97 classification of renal allograft rejection. Am J Transplant 2003;3:708–714.

Racusen LC, Solez K, Colvin RB, et al: The Banff 97 working classification of renal allograft pathology. Kidney Int 1999;55:713.

Regele H, Bohmig GA, Habicht A, et al: Capillary deposition of complement split product C4d in renal allografts is associated with basement membrane injury in peritubular and glomerular capillaries: A contribution of humoral immunity to chronic rejection. J Am Soc Nephrol 2002;13:2371–2380.

Calcineurin Inhibitor Toxicity

Mihatsch MJ, Antonovych T, Bohman SO, et al: Cyclosporin A nephropathy: Standardization of evaluation of kidney biopsies. Clin Nephrol 1994;41:23–32.

Mihatsch MJ, Kyo M, Morozumi K, et al: The side-effects of ciclosporine-A and tacrolimus. Clin Nephrol 1998;49:356–363.

Nankivell BJ, Borrows RJ, Fung CLS, et al: Calcineurin inhibitor nephrotoxicity: Longitudinal assessment by protocol histology. Transplantation 2004;78:557–565.

Trimarchi HM, Truong LD, Brennan S, et al: FK506-associated thrombotic microangiopathy Transplantation 1999;67:539–544.

Zarifian A, Meleg-Smith S, O'Donovan R, et al: Cyclosporine-associated thrombotic microangiopathy in renal allografts. Kidney Int 1999;55:2457–2466.

Polyomavirus Nephropathy

Drachenberg C, Papadimitriou JC, Hirsch HH, et al: Histological patterns of polyoma virus nephropathy: Correlation with graft outcome and viral load. Am J Transplant 2004;4:2082–2092.

Nickeleit V, Steiger J, Mihatsch MJ: BK virus infection after kidney transplantation. Graft 2002;5:S46–S57.

Randhawa PS, Finkelstein S, Scantlebury V, et al: Human polyoma virus-associated interstitial nephritis in the allograft kidney. Transplantation 1999;67:103–109.

Post-Transplantation Lymphoproliferative Disease

Knowles DM, Cesarman E, Chadburn A, et al: Correlative morphologic and genetic analysis demonstrates three distinct categories of posttransplantation lymphoproliferative disroders. Blood 1995;85:552–565.

Nelson BP, Nalesnik MA, Bahler DW, et al: Epstein-Barr virus-negative post-transplant lymphoproliferative disorders. Am J Surg Pathol 2000;24:375–385.

Randhawa PS, Magnone M, Jordan M, et al: Renal allograft involvement by Epstein-Barr virus associated post-transplant lymphoproliferative disease. Am J Surg Pathol 1996;20:563–571.

Recurrent and De Novo Glomerular Disease

Baid S, Cosimi AB, Tolkoff-Rubin N, et al: Renal disease associated with hepatitis C infection after kidney and liver transplantation. Transplantation 2000;70:255–261.

Hariharan S, Adams MB, Brennan DC, et al: Recurrent and de novo glomerular disease after renal transplantation. Transplantation 1999;68:635–641.

Kotanko P, Pusey CD, Levy JB: Recurrent glomerulonephritis following renal transplantation Transplantation 1997;63:1045–1052.

8 Diseases of the Penis, Urethra, and Scrotum

Rajal B. Shah • Mahul B. Amin

DISEASES OF THE PENIS

ANATOMY AND HISTOLOGY

The penis is composed of three parts: the body (shaft), which makes up the central portion; the glans, coronal sulcus, and foreskin (prepuce), which comprise the anterior end; and the root portion, which constitutes the posterior end. The glans is a conical extension of the urethral corpus spongiosum, with a central vertical cleft, the meatus. The urethra opens at the meatus. The meatus is attached to the foreskin by a ventral triangular portion of the mucosa, referred to as frenulum. The corona is a slightly elevated, circular ridge surrounding the glans and represents the base of the cone. The coronal sulcus, which is behind or below the corona, separates the glans from the foreskin (Fig. 8-1).

GLANS PENIS

The glans is composed of the following layers: stratified nonkeratinizing mucosa, lamina propria, corpus spongiosum, tunica albuginea, and corpora cavernosa. Most epithelial neoplasms of the penis originate from the glans mucosa. The lamina propria is a loose connective tissue layer, 1 to 3 mm thick, which separates the mucosa from the corpus spongiosum. The corpus spongiosum is the main component of the glans and is composed of specialized erectile tissues, with numerous anastomosing venous sinuses of varying caliber having multiple peripheral nerves between them (Fig. 8-2). The glans corpus spongiosum is about 8 to 10 mm thick. The transition from the lamina propria frequently is not sharp and sometimes is difficult to determine. However, this distinction has important staging implications (Table 8-1). The tunica albuginea is a very dense, fibrous and elastic membrane that separates the spongiosum from underlying cavernosa and constitutes an important barrier to the spread of cancer.

FORESKIN

The foreskin is a double membrane that encases the glans. Microscopically, it has five histologic layers: (1) innermost mucosal epithelium, similar to the glans; (2) 2- to 3-mm thick lamina propria; (3) 6- to 10-mm thick dartos muscle, composed of a double layer of smooth muscle fibers situated within the loose connective tissue; (4) dermis; and (5) epidermis, which is the outermost, thin, wrinkled, squamous epithelium containing scant adnexal structures.

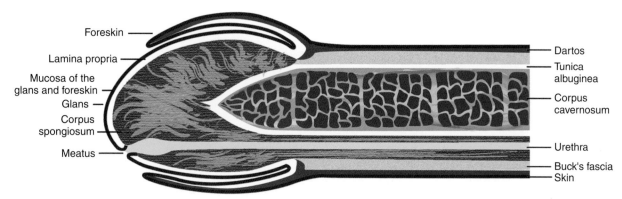

FIGURE 8-1

Diagrammatic representation of the anatomy of the penis: cut section view. (Modified from Young RH, Srigley JR, Amin MB, et al: Tumors of the Prostate Gland, Seminal Vesicles, Male Urethra, and Penis. AFIP Atlas of Tumor Pathology. Washington, DC, Armed Forces Institute of Pathology, 2000, p 404, Figure 10-4.)

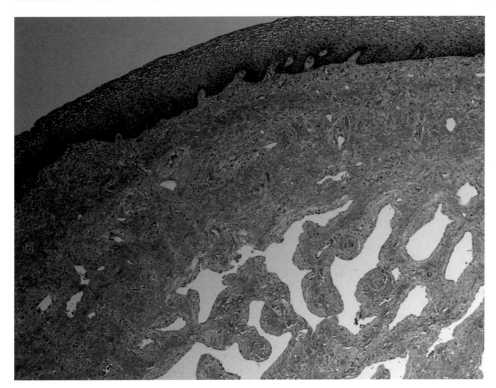

FIGURE 8-2
Low-power view of section of the glans penis, demonstrating three histologic levels: nonkeratinizing squamous epithelium, lamina propria, and corpora spongiosum with richly vascular erectile tissue. Note that the separation between the lamina propria and the corpora is abrupt.

Table 8-1
TNM Classification of Carcinomas of the Penis

TNM CLASSIFICATION

T—Primary tumor

TX	Primary tumor cannot be assessed
T0	No evidence of primary tumor
Tis	Carcinoma in situ
Ta	Noninvasive verrucous carcinoma
T1	Tumor invades subepithelial connective tissue
T2	Tumor invades corpus spongiosum or cavernosum
T3	Tumor invades urethra or prostate
T4	Tumor invades other adjacent structures

N—Regional lymph nodes

NX	Regional lymph nodes cannot be assessed
N0	No regional lymph node metastasis
N1	Metastasis in a single superficial inguinal lymph node
N2	Metastasis in multiple or bilateral superficial inguinal lymph nodes
N3	Metastasis in deep inguinal or pelvic lymph node or nodes, unilateral or bilateral

M—Distant metastasis

MX	Distant metastasis cannot be assessed
M0	No distant metastasis
M1	Distant metastasis

STAGE GROUPING

Stage	T	N	M
Stage 0	Tis	N0	M0
	Ta	N0	M0
Stage I	T1	N0	M0
Stage II	T1	N1	M0
	T2	N0,N1	M0
Stage III	T1,T2	N2	M0
	T3	N0,N1,N2	M0
Stage IV	T4	Any N	M0
	Any T	N3	M0
	Any T	Any N	M1

Adapted from Greene FL, Page DL, Fleming ID, Fritz A, et al. (eds): AJCC Cancer Staging Manual, 6th ed. New York, Springer; 2002, pp 303–308.

BODY

Microscopically, the body of the penis shows the following layers: (1) outer epidermis layer similar to foreskin; (2) dermis; (3) dartos muscle; (4) adipose tissue; (5) Buck's fascia, with numerous vessels and nerves; (6) tunica albuginea; and (7) erectile tissue of the corpora cavernosa and spongiosum, the latter encasing the urethra. Both the corpora cavernosa and the corpus spongiosum are covered by the tunica albuginea and encased in Buck's fascia (Fig. 8-3).

MALIGNANT NEOPLASMS

The incidence of penile malignancy varies throughout the world, with the highest incidence in developing countries, especially parts of Africa such as Uganda; parts of South America such as Brazil and Paraguay; Mexico; Jamaica; and Haiti, where it represents 10% to 12% of all malignancies. In western countries, the incidence of penile cancer is, in general, quite low accounting for fewer than 0.5% of all male neoplasms. Age-adjusted incidence rates in the western world are in the range of 0.3 to 1.0 cases per 100,000 population. This geographic difference in incidence indicates that environmental factors play an important role. More than 95% of malignant neoplasms are carcinomas, and

squamous cell carcinomas are by far the most common type of penile carcinoma (Table 8-2).

SQUAMOUS CELL CARCINOMA, USUAL TYPE

ETIOLOGIC FACTORS AND ASSOCIATION WITH HUMAN PAPILLOMAVIRUS INFECTION

Environmental factors play a much more important role than genetic factors in the pathogenesis of penile carcinoma. Epidemiologic studies have identified several risk ractors, including phimosis, particularly when

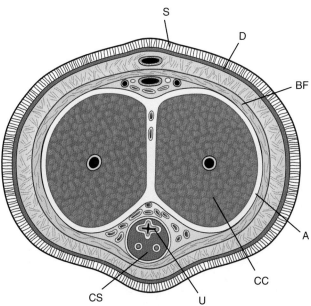

FIGURE 8-3

Diagrammatic representation of the cross-sectional anatomy of the body (shaft) of the penis. The dartos (D) is closely attached to the skin (S). Buck's fascia (BF) covers the inferior part of the urethra (U). The corpus spongiosum (CS) and the urethra are located in the groove between the corpora cavernosa (CC) and Buck's fascia. The tunica albuginea (A) encases the corpora cavernosa. (From Young RH, Srigley JR, Amin MB, et al: Tumors of the Prostate Gland, Seminal Vesicles, Male Urethra, and Penis. AFIP Atlas of Tumor Pathology. Washington, DC, Armed Forces Institute of Pathology, 2000, p 407, Figure 10-8.)

Table 8-2
WHO Histologic Classification of Tumors of the Penis

MALIGNANT EPITHELIAL TUMORS OF THE PENIS

Squamous cell carcinoma

Basaloid carcinoma

Warty (condylomatous) carcinoma

Verrucous carcinoma

Papillary carcinoma, NOS

Sarcomatous carcinoma

Mixed carcinomas

Adenosquamous carcinoma

Paget disease

Merkel cell carcinoma

Small cell carcinoma of neuroendocrine type

Sebaceous carcinoma

Clear cell carcinoma

Basal cell carcinoma

PRECURSOR LESIONS

Intraepithelial neoplasia grade III

Bowen disease

Erythroplasia of Queyrat

MELANOCYTIC TUMORS

Melanocytic nevi

Melanoma

MESENCHYMAL TUMORS

HEMATOPOIETIC TUMORS

SECONDARY TUMORS

NOS, not otherwise specified.
Adapted from Eble JN, Sauter G, Epstein JI, Sesterhenn IA: WHO Classification: Tumours of the Urinary System and Male Genital Organs. Lyon, France, IARC Press, 2004, p 280.

associated with long foreskin; chronic inflammatory conditions, especially balanitis xerotica obliterans (lichen sclerosus et atrophicus); smoking; ultraviolet irradiation; and human papillomavirus (HPV) infection. In a recent case-control study, circumcision neonatally, but not after neonatal period, was associated with a threefold decreased risk of penile cancer, although 20% of the patients with penile cancer had been circumcised neonatally.

There is growing awareness of the role of HPV infection in the pathogenesis of penile carcinoma. HPV is believed to play a role in penile cancer through progression of HPV-associated penile intraepithelial lesions, which are consistently positive for HPV DNA. However, HPV infection is present in only about one third of penile squamous cell carcinomas, with HPV type 16 being the most frequent type. HPV DNA is preferentially found in subtypes of squamous carcinomas with basaloid and/or warty features, and it is only weakly correlated with conventional keratinizing squamous cell carcinoma. The cumulative evidence on risk factors for penile cancer suggests prevention of phimosis, treatment of chronic inflammatory conditions, limiting treatment with psoralens and ultraviolet A irradiation (PUVA), smoking cessation, and prophylactic prevention of HPV infection as preventive measures that could be considered.

CLINICAL FEATURES

Patients usually present with an exophytic, ulcerative or fungated mass, or occasionally with a flat, erythematous and granular lesion (Fig. 8-4). In patients with long phimotic foreskin, a submucosal mass may delay the clinical presentation, with metastasis as a presenting sign. Mean age at presentation is 60 years. Most penile squamous carcinomas originate in the squamous epithelium lining in one of three penile compartments: mucosa of glans (75% to 80%), mucosa of the foreskin (15%), and coronal sulcus (5%), with 2% being multicentric. Only a few arise in the skin of the foreskin and shaft. Adjacent precancerous lesions (see later discussion) often can be seen as a marble-white thickening ("leukoplakia") or a moist, erythematous lesion (Fig. 8-4).

PATHOLOGIC FEATURES

GROSS FINDINGS

Growth Patterns of Penile Squamous Carcinoma

The gross characteristics depend on the overall growth pattern, which strongly correlates with prognosis. Three main growth patterns are recognized (Fig. 8-5).
1. *Superficial spreading* (up to 40% of cases): a flat, white, plaque-like or granular, firm tumor growing

---

SQUAMOUS CELL CARCINOMA, USUAL TYPE, PENIS—FACT SHEET

Definition
► A malignant epithelial neoplasm with usual squamous, nonpapillary differentiation

Incidence and Location
► The most common malignant neoplasm and the most common type of all penile carcinomas
► Accounts for 70% of all squamous carcinomas
► Most originate from mucosa of glans (80%), mucosa of the foreskin (15%), or coronal sulcus (5%)
► Only few arise in the skin of foreskin and shaft

Morbidity and Mortality
► Depends on histologic grade, depth of invasion, and status of metastasis
► Mortality in patients with superficially spreading carcinoma is 10%, compared with 67% for patients with vertical growth pattern

Gender, Race, and Age Distribution
► Males, with mean age at presentation of 60 years
► Incidence varies worldwide, with the highest incidence in Uganda and in South America, where it accounts for 10-12% of malignancies
► In Western countries, it accounts for 0.5% of all male neoplasms, in the range of 0.3 to 1.0 case per 100,000 population

Clinical Features
► Patients present with an exophytic or ulcerative mass, or occasionally with a flat, erythematous and granular lesion

Prognosis and Treatment
► Depends on pathologic stage, grade, and vascular invasion. The threshold for penile metastasis is 4 to 6 mm invasion in the corpus spongiosum. Surgery is the preferred treatment option.

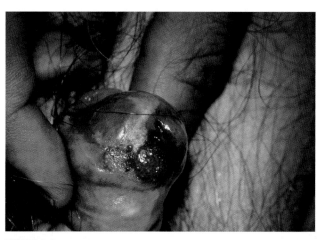

FIGURE 8-4
Squamous carcinoma, usual type. A nodular red/tan tumor involves the glans. Surrounding mucosa is flat, moist, and erythematous and demonstrates histologic changes of intraepithelial neoplasia. (Courtesy of Cheryl Lee, University of Michigan, Ann Arbor, MI.)

Superficial spreading

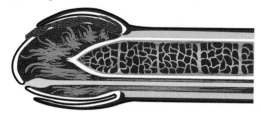

Vertical growth

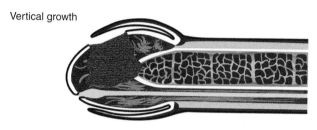

Verruciform growth

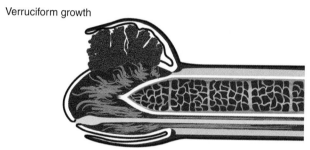

FIGURE 8-5

Diagrammatic representation of the growth patterns of squamous carcinoma of the penis.

SQUAMOUS CELL CARCINOMA, USUAL TYPE, PENIS— PATHOLOGIC FEATURES

Gross Findings

▶ Depends on the growth pattern

▶ Ranges from an exophytic and cauliflower-like appearance to a flat or slightly elevated and/or deeply ulcerated lesion

Microscopic Findings

▶ Majority of squamous carcinomas are similar to their counterparts in other organs and exhibit usual, nonpapillary differentiation and range of differentiation from good to moderate to poor

▶ Characteristic features include keratinizing nests of squamous cells with variable atypia surrounded by reactive fibrous stroma

▶ Superficially invasive tumors tend to be well differentiated, and deep tumors tend to be poorly differentiated

▶ Adjacent squamous epithelium may show changes of penile intraepithelial neoplasia with koilocytic atypia

Immunohistochemical Features

▶ Cytokeratins are positive

Pathologic Differential Diagnosis

▶ Pseudoepitheliomatous hyperplasia for superficial well-differentiated tumor

▶ Urothelial carcinoma

▶ Malignant melanoma

---

horizontally that usually shows a prominent intra-epithelial component and invasion, chiefly superficial, of the anatomic layers of the penis. Frequently, more than one epithelial compartment (glans, sulcus, or foreskin) is involved.

2. *Vertical growth pattern* (up to 30% of cases): large, ulcerated or fungating, white-gray or hemorrhagic mass that spreads down deeply, is often of high grade, and has a high rate of inguinal lymph node metastasis.

3. *Verruciform growth pattern* (up to 18% to 20% of cases): composed of several histologic subtypes of well-differentiated papillary neoplasms, as discussed later, with a low incidence of metastasis. The glans is the most commonly involved site, but the foreskin or coronal sulcus may be involved. Grossly, these are large, granular, white to gray, exophytic, cauliflower-like neoplasms.

Mixtures of the above growth patterns can occur in about 10% to 15% of carcinomas.

MICROSCOPIC FINDINGS

Histologic Subtypes

Histologically, the majority of squamous carcinomas of the penis (about 70%) are similar to their counter-parts in other organs, demonstrating usual nonpapillary-type growth and ranging from good, to moderate, to poor differentiation. The remaining 30% have a predominant histologic appearance that is different. These types include basaloid carcinoma; the spectrum of verruciform carcinomas (warty [condylomatous] carcinoma, verrucous carcinoma, and papillary carcinoma, not otherwise specified [NOS]); and the very rare pseudo-hyperplastic carcinoma. Clinical and histologic features of subtypes of squamous carcinoma are discussed in detail in the following section.

Characteristic histologic features of the usual well to moderately differentiated squamous carcinomas include keratinizing nests of squamous cells with variable cytologic atypia, surrounded by reactive fibrous stroma (Fig. 8-6). Very well differentiated carcinomas and solid nonkeratinizing poorly differentiated carcinomas are unusual. Invasion can be seen as individual cells, cords, or large cohesive sheets present in the lamina propria or corpus spongiosum (see Fig. 8-6). Superficially invasive tumors tend to be well differentiated, and deep tumors tend to be poorly differentiated. The adjacent squamous epithelium frequently shows changes that are known to be associated with squamous carcinoma, ranging from hyperplasia to penile intraepithelial neoplasia (PeIN) and well-developed balanitis xerotica obliterans.

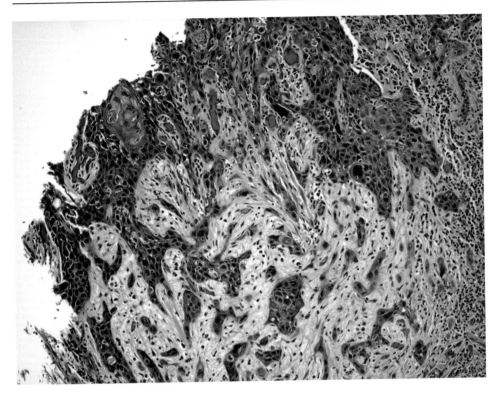

FIGURE 8-6

Low-power view of invasive, well to moderately differentiated squamous carcinoma. Invasive nests demonstrate cytologic atypia, paradoxical maturation, and pronounced stromal desmoplasia.

ANCILLARY STUDIES

IMMUNOHISTOCHEMISTRY

Immunohistochemistry is rarely needed in the diagnosis of conventional squamous carcinoma. Poorly differentiated squamous carcinomas are positive for cytokeratins, at least focally. The presence of HPV DNA can be tested by in situ hybridization studies; it is preferentially found in tumors with higher grade and more aggressive basaloid morphology.

DIFFERENTIAL DIAGNOSIS

Superficially invasive, well-differentiated squamous carcinoma should be distinguished from pseudoepitheliomatous hyperplasia. In the latter, the acanthotic epithelium has long, slender, often angulated rete ridges which, when cut tangentially, appear as "infiltrating" nests in the stroma (Fig. 8-7). The presence of nests detached from overlying epithelium, demonstrating disorderly maturation; paradoxical differentiation characterized by keratinization; more eosinophilia; and nuclear atypia, favor the diagnosis of carcinoma over hyperplasia (Fig. 8-6). Desmoplasia may be seen in both conditions, but it is more pronounced and more frequent in carcinomas. The presence of nests deep in the dartos or corpora favors the diagnosis of carcinoma. Cubilla and colleagues recently described 10 cases of very well-differentiated nonverruciform squamous

carcinoma of the penis that demonstrated "pseudo-hyperplastic" features, posing diagnostic difficulty with pseudoepitheliomatous hyperplasia, particularly in superficial biopsies. Emphasis on the similar diagnostic features discussed should be helpful. The presence of adjacent PeIN or balanitis xerotica obliterans may also aid the diagnosis.

Urothelial cell carcinoma may sometimes be in the differential diagnosis. The presence of typical foci of squamous cell differentiation, continuity with PeIN, and lack of urothelial carcinoma in situ (CIS) are helpful features. Poorly differentiated squamous carcinoma may be confused with amelanotic melanoma. The presence of focal individual cell with cytoplasmic keratinization supports the diagnosis of squamous carcinoma. Malignant melanomas are usually located on the shaft and usually are biphasic tumors with epithelioid and spindle cell morphology. Immunohistochemical stains for S-100, HMB-45, melan A, and cytokeratins are useful in difficult cases.

PROGNOSIS AND TREATMENT

The prognosis of squamous carcinoma largely depends on the stage of disease as determined by both local invasion and involvement of inguinal nodes (see Table 8-1). Pathologic parameters related to the prognosis of penile carcinomas are site of the primary tumor, histologic type, grade, depth of invasion, and vascular invasion. Of these, histologic grade, depth of invasion,

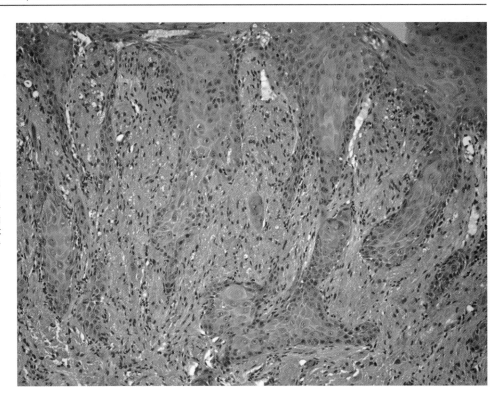

FIGURE 8-7

Pseudoepitheliomatous hyperplasia. Low-power view of glans mucosa demonstrates downward proliferation of squamous nests with focal keratinization. However, the proliferating nests are superficial, mature without cytologic atypia, and lack the desmoplastic response.

and vascular invasion have been most strongly correlated with final outcome. Tumors limited to the foreskin carry a better prognosis because of the frequent superficial invasive nature of the tumor. In one large series, inguinal lymph node metastasis was found in 82%, 42%, and 33% of tumors with vertical growth, superficial spreading, and multicentricity, respectively. Verrucous tumors without conventional or destructive invasion did not demonstrate metastasis. In another large series, Banon Perez and associates demonstrated that patients with pT1 tumor and good cell differentiation showed no metastatic adenopathy on long follow-up. Overall mortality for patients with superficially spreading carcinomas is 10%, compared with 67% for patients with vertical growth pattern. Therefore, the depth of invasion is important to evaluate on all penile resection specimens. Measurement of depth of invasion should be performed from the basement membrane of adjacent squamous epithelium to the deepest point of invasion. For large exophytic (verrucous) tumors, depth should be measured from the nonkeratinizing surface of the tumor to the deepest point of invasion. The threshold for penile metastasis is about 4- to 6-mm invasion into the corpus spongiosum.

Cubilla and colleagues proposed a prognostic index system on a scale of 1 to 6, combining numerical values for histologic grade (scoring 1 to 3) and anatomic level of invasion (scoring 1 for lamina propria, 2 for corpus spongiosum, and 3 for corpora cavernosa invasion for glans tumors and 1 for lamina propria, 2 for dartos, and 3 for skin for foreskin tumors). Indices totalling 1 to 3 are associated with no mortality, whereas the high indices of 5 and 6 are associated with a high metastatic rate and high mortality. Molecular markers have also

been studied as prognostic factors. P53 appears to be an independent risk factor for nodal metastasis, progression of disease, and survival. Recently, tissue-associated eosinophilia has also been suggested to predict improved survival in patients with penile cancer.

Penile carcinomas demonstrate a fairly predictable dissemination pattern: initially to superficial lymph nodes, then to deep groin and pelvic nodes, and finally to retroperitoneal nodes. The first metastatic site is usually a superficial inguinal lymph node located in the groin upper inner quadrant (sentinel node). This pattern of metastasis is present in about 70% of cases. Skip pattern of metastasis is rare. Systemic bloodborne metastasis occurs late and usually to liver, heart, lungs, and bone.

Surgery is the preferred treatment option. Partial penile resection is the treatment of choice for superficially invasive primary lesions. Deeply invasive tumors require total penectomy with inguinal node dissection. Radiotherapy provides no demonstrable benefit. Patient follow-up is fundamental to detect recurrence or metastatic adenopathy.

Several recent works have identified many variants of squamous cell carcinoma with unique clinical and prognostic implications.

Squamous Carcinoma Variants with Verruciform Growth Pattern

There are two principal forms of verruciform tumors: noncondylomatous verruciform tumors, which comprise verrucous carcinoma and the closely related papillary carcinoma, NOS type, and condylomatous verruciform tumors, which comprise condyloma and warty carcinoma.

VERRUCOUS CARCINOMA

Verrucous carcinomas are slow-growing tumors that locally invade in a pushing manner but usually do not metastasize and are not related to HPV infection.

The true frequency of verrucous carcinoma is difficult to assess, but the reported incidence ranges from 3% to 13% of all penile cancers and up to 20% of all the verruciform tumors. The frequency is probably much lower than reported in the literature, because many of the giant condylomas, warty carcinomas, and papillary squamous cell carcinomas, NOS type, have been misinterpreted as verrucous carcinomas.

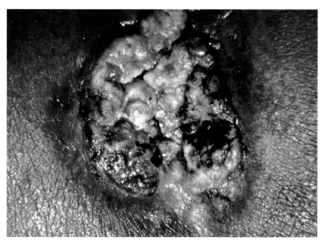

FIGURE 8-8
In verrucous carcinoma, a large, cauliflower-like, gray-white mass involves the skin. (Courtesy of Lori Lowe, University of Michigan, Ann Arbor, MI.)

CLINICAL FEATURES

Patients usually present with a large (average, 3 cm) cauliflower-like mass (Fig. 8-8) of relatively long duration (average, 56 months). Most of them involve the glans and coronal sulcus, with frequent involvement of preputial skin.

PATHOLOGIC FEATURES

GROSS FINDINGS

Grossly, verrucous carcinomas are often large, gray-white, cauliflower-like, frequently ulcerated masses that on sectioning reveal burrowing through the normal tissues.

MICROSCOPIC FINDINGS

Microscopically, verrucous carcinoma is a very well-differentiated squamous carcinoma demonstrating an exophytic papillary growth pattern, acanthosis, and hyperkeratosis. The papillae usually do not contain

---

VERRUCOUS CARCINOMA—FACT SHEET

Definition
▶ Variant of squamous carcinoma with verruciform growth pattern
▶ No association with HPV infection

Incidence and Location
▶ Rarest (3%) of all penile cancers
▶ Most start on coronal sulcus and spread to glans and preputial skin

Morbidity and Mortality
▶ Slow-growing tumor, potentially curable if adequately excised

Gender, Race, and Age Distribution
▶ Similar to that of squamous carcinoma, usual type

Clinical Features
▶ Patients present with a slow-growing, large, cauliflower-like mass of long duration

Prognosis and Treatment
▶ Excellent prognosis for pure tumor
▶ Wide excision or partial penectomy is usually sufficient treatment

---

VERRUCOUS CARCINOMA—PATHOLOGIC FEATURES

Gross Findings
▶ Cauliflower-like, frequently ulcerated, gray-white mass that burrows deeply into normal tissues

Microscopic Findings
▶ Very well-differentiated squamous cell carcinoma with prominent papillomatosis, acanthosis, and hyperkeratosis
▶ The papillae do not contain fibrovascular cores and show broad-based regular bulbous infiltration into soft tissues
▶ Minimal cytologic atypia
▶ No koilocytic changes

Differential Diagnosis
▶ Verrucous hyperplasia
▶ Giant condyloma
▶ Papillary carcinoma, NOS type
▶ Warty carcinoma

any fibrovascular cores. Cross-sections of the tip of the papilla show a central keratin plug, with neoplastic cells at the periphery. Characteristically, the tumor shows a pattern of broad-based bulbous infiltration into underlying stroma (Fig. 8-9A). Deeper infiltration into corpora cavernosa is unusual. Cytologic atypia is minimal, and mitosis is rare and usually confined to the deeper portion of the tumor. A dense inflammatory cell infiltrate may be present at the interface between tumor and stroma and occasionally may obscure it. Koilocytic

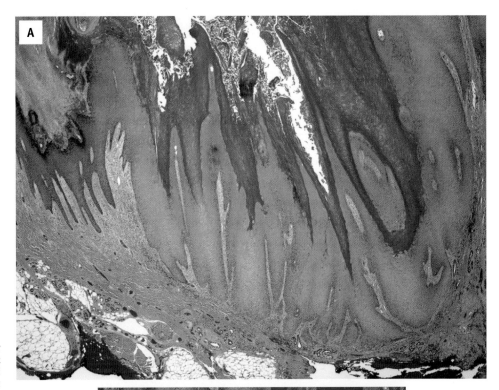

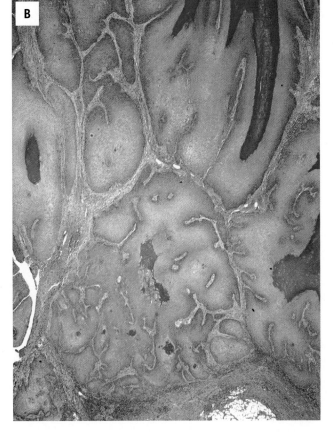

FIGURE 8-9

Verrucous carcinoma. **A,** Low-power view of the mass shows prominent papillomatosis, hyperkeratosis, and acanthosis. The interface between the tumor and stroma is relatively sharp, with a broad, bulbous pattern of infiltration. **B,** High-power view of same tumor shows very well-differentiated squamous epithelium without evidence of human papilloma virus (HPV)-related cytologic atypia. (Courtesy of Doug Fullen, University of Michigan, Ann Arbor, MI.)

change is absent or minimal (see Fig. 8-9B). Extensive sampling of the tumor is essential, because up to 5% of verrucous carcinomas demonstrate foci of conventional squamous carcinoma (hybrid tumor).

DIFFERENTIAL DIAGNOSIS

Verrucous carcinomas should be distinguished from other verruciform neoplasms. The morphologic features that are helpful in separating them are summarized in the Table 8-3 and illustrated in Figure 8-10. Verrucous carcinomas lack the HPV-related cellular changes characteristically seen in giant condylomas and warty carcinomas. Papillary carcinoma, NOS type exhibits more cytologic atypia than verrucous carcinoma and has an irregular invasive front. In a superficial biopsy, the distinction of verrucous carcinoma from squamous cell hyperplasia, or of papillary from verrucous type, may be impossible. Wide excision is necessary in such situations to assess the tumor and stroma interaction.

PROGNOSIS AND TREATMENT

Pure verrucous carcinomas demonstrate an aggressive behavior locally, but not biologically, and do not metastasize. However, one third of verrucous carcinomas recur, usually because of insufficient surgery or multicentricity. Verrucous carcinomas containing a component of conventional squamous carcinoma (hybrid tumor) may metastasize. The preferred treatment is surgery. Wide surgical excision, usually requiring partial penectomy, is the treatment of choice. Anaplastic transformation of penile verrucous carcinoma has also been reported after radiotherapy.

WARTY CARCINOMA

Warty carcinomas are unusual, low- to intermediate-grade, verruciform tumors with many morphologic similarities to condylomas because of their prominent HPV-related changes. They account for 6% to 10% of all penile carcinomas and 20% to 35% of all verruciform neoplasms.

CLINICAL FEATURES

These are relatively slow-growing lesions that are frequently present for several years before pathologic diagnosis. Average age at presentation is 61 years. The most common site is the glans, but multiple sites can be involved. Inguinal lymphadenopathy is infrequent.

Table 8-3
Comparison of Verruciform Neoplasms

Feature	Giant Condyloma	Warty Carcinoma	Verrucous Carcinoma	Papillary Carcinoma
Papillae	Arborizing, non-undulating, rounded	Long and undulating, condylomatous, complex	Straight with keratin cysts	Variable, complex
Fibrovascular cores	Prominent	Prominent	Rare	Present
Invasive borders	None	Irregular and jagged	Regular, broad, and pushing	Irregular and jagged
Differentiation	Well differentiated	Well to moderately differentiated	Well differentiated	Well to moderately differentiated
Koilocytotic atypia	Present at surface	Prominent and diffuse	Absent	Absent or very focal
HPV association	Types 6 and 11	Type 16	Usually absent	Absent
Metastasis	No	Yes	No	Yes

Adapted from Young RH, Srigley JR, Amin MB, et al: Tumors of the Prostate Gland, Seminal Vesicles, Male Urethra, and Penis. AFIP Atlas of Tumor Pathology. Washington, DC, Armed Forces Institute of Pathology, 2000, p 424, Table 10-3.

FIGURE 8-10

Diagrammatic comparison of the histo-logic differences among tumors with verruciform growth pattern. **A,** Verrucous carcinoma: regular papillae with broad bulbous base and prominent hyperker-atosis *(red)*. Keratinized cysts are promi-nent (seen at the base). **B,** Papillary carcinoma, NOS type: papillae are more irregular than in **A,** and many have fibrovascular cores. Infiltration is seen at the base, and koilocytosis is absent. **C,** Giant condyloma: arborescent hyper-keratotic papillae with broad bases and koilocytosis (indicated by white dots) at the surface. **D,** Warty (condylomatous) carcinoma: papillae are more irregular than in **C,** koilocytosis is diffuse, and the interface between tumor and stroma is irregular. (From Young RH, Srigley JR, Amin MB, et al: Tumors of the Prostate Gland, Seminal Vesicles, Male Urethra, and Penis. AFIP Atlas of Tumor Patho-logy. Washington, DC, Armed Forces Institute of Pathology, 2000, p 424, Figure 10-31.)

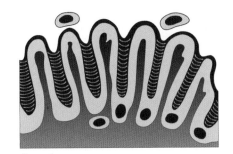

A

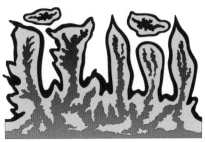

B

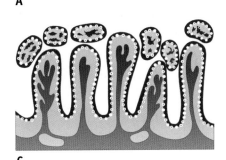

C

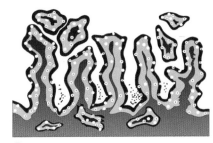

D

WARTY CARCINOMA—FACT SHEET

Definition
▶ Variant of squamous carcinoma with verruciform growth pattern and strong association with HPV infection

Incidence and Location
▶ Accounts for 6% of all penile carcinomas and 20-30% of verruciform tumors
▶ Most common location is glans

Morbidity and Mortality
▶ Very low
▶ Inguinal metastasis is infrequent
▶ 5-year survival rate is 100%

Gender, Race, and Age Distribution
▶ Similar to squamous carcinoma, usual type

Clinical Features
▶ Patient presents with slow-growing lesions that have been present for several years
▶ Lesions are large, firm, and papillary

Prognosis and Treatment
▶ Excellent prognosis for pure tumor
▶ Partial penectomy is usually sufficient treatment

WARTY CARCINOMA—PATHOLOGIC FEATURES

Gross Findings
▶ A cauliflower-like, firm, white-gray granular mass measuring up to 7 to 8 cm (average, 4 cm)
▶ The cut surface demonstrates deep invasion into lamina propria and corpus spongiosum, but the cavernosa are rarely involved

Microscopic Findings
▶ Hyperparakeratotic, arborizing, papillomatous growth with central fibrovascular cores
▶ Prominent koilocytic atypia
▶ Base of the tumor shows irregular, deep infiltration into soft tissues

Differential Diagnosis
▶ Verrucous carcinoma
▶ Papillary carcinoma, NOS type
▶ Giant condyloma

PATHOLOGIC FEATURES

GROSS FINDINGS

As with other verruciform tumors, patients with warty carcinoma present with a big, cauliflower-like,

firm, white, granular mass. The cut surface shows both prominent exophytic and endophytic growth pattern. The interface between tumor and underlying tissues is often well demarcated, although they typically show a jagged or serrated appearance at the base. There is usually gross involvement of the lamina propria and corpus spongiosum, but the corpora cavernosa is infrequently involved.

MICROSCOPIC FINDINGS

Microscopically, warty carcinoma shows hyperpara-keratotic, arborizing, papillomatous growth. The papil-

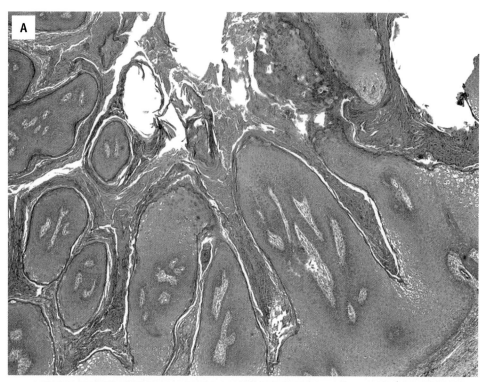

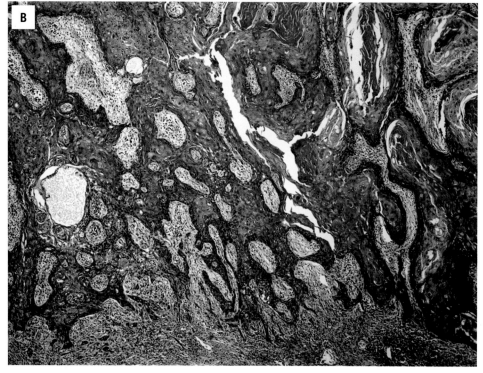

FIGURE 8-11

Warty carcinoma. **A,** Low-power view demonstrates undulating, complex, hyperkeratotic papillary growth with prominent koilocytic atypia. (Courtesy of Anuradha Radhakrishnan, Emory University Hospital, Atlanta, GA.) **B,** High-power view shows an irregular interface between tumor and underlying stroma.

lae are long, with a complex undulating appearance, and have a central fibrovascular core; the tips are variably rounded or tapered. Koilocytic atypia in the neoplastic cells is conspicuous and is the definitional feature. Intraepithelial abscesses may be prominent, especially in the basal areas. Tumors may infiltrate deeply, and the interface of tumor with stroma is usually irregular (Fig. 8-11).

DIFFERENTIAL DIAGNOSIS

Warty carcinomas should be distinguished from other verruciform neoplasms, which are summarized in Table 8-3 and Figure 8-10. Giant condyloma may be histologically similar to warty carcinoma, but the pleomorphism is less marked and, most importantly, the base of the tumor is broad, with "pushing" margins rather than the irregular, infiltrative appearance seen with warty carcinomas. Verrucous and papillary carcinomas do not show HPV-related changes.

PROGNOSIS AND TREATMENT

Some warty carcinomas have metastasized to regional lymph nodes, usually associated with deeply invasive tumors. In one reported large series, 2 of 11 warty carcinomas demonstrated metastasis to the inguinal nodes.

PAPILLARY CARCINOMA, NOT OTHERWISE SPECIFIED

CLINICAL FEATURES

Papillary carcinoma, NOS type is the most common of all the verruciform cancers, accounting for approximately 15% of penile cancers. The average age at presentation is 60 years. The most common sites of involvement are the glans and foreskin. Patients often present with a large, cauliflower-like mass.

PAPILLARY CARCINOMA, NOS TYPE, PENIS—FACT SHEET

Definition
▶ Variant of squamous carcinoma with verruciform growth pattern
▶ No association with HPV infection

Incidence and Location
▶ The most common of all verruciform tumors, accounting for approximately 15% of all penile carcinomas
▶ The most common site of involvement is glans and foreskin

Morbidity and Mortality
▶ Very low
▶ The reported 5-year survival rate is approximately 90%

Gender, Race, and Age Distribution
▶ Similar to squamous carcinoma, usual type

Clinical Features
▶ Patient presents with slow-growing, bulky, cauliflower-like mass

Prognosis and Treatment
▶ Excellent
▶ Deep invasion can occur, but inguinal metastasis rare
▶ Wide excision or partial penectomy is treatment of choice

PATHOLOGIC FEATURES

GROSS FINDINGS

The gross features are similar to those of verrucous carcinoma; however, on sectioning, the tumors typically show jagged or irregular borders with deeper invasion into dartos muscle, corpora spongiosum, and, rarely, cavernosa.

MICROSCOPIC FINDINGS

Histologically, well to moderately differentiated, hyperkeratotic lesions with irregular, complex papillae, with or without fibrovascular cores, are typical. Cytologic atypia is usually obvious, differentiating these tumors from verrucous carcinoma. The key feature is the absence of HPV-associated cytologic changes, which, if present, would put the tumor in the category of a warty carcinoma. The base of the lesion is characteristically jagged, with irregular nests infiltrating into deeper soft tissues. Irregular wide areas of keratinization, referred to as "keratin lakes," are frequently present between adjacent papillae and sometimes reach to the tip (Fig. 8-12).

DIFFERENTIAL DIAGNOSIS

Papillary carcinomas should be distinguished from other verruciform neoplasms, which are summarized in the Table 8-3 and Figure 8-10. Warty carcinomas and giant condylomas have distinctive HPV-related cellular changes in the majority of the cells. Verrucous carcinomas demonstrate neither cytologic atypia nor irregular stromal infiltration. Papillary carcinoma also should be distinguished from typical squamous cell

---

PAPILLARY CARCINOMA, NOS TYPE, PENIS—PATHOLOGIC FEATURES

Gross Findings
▶ Large, cauliflower-like or papillary mass
▶ On cut sections, tumor demonstrates invasion into lamina propria or corpus spongiosum; infiltration into cavernosa is uncommon

Microscopic Findings
▶ Well to moderately differentiated, hyperkeratotic lesion with irregular, complex papillae with or without fibrovascular cores are typical
▶ Obvious cytologic atypia, with base of lesion demonstrating characteristic jagged, irregular infiltration into soft tissues
▶ Koilocytotic cytologic atypia absent

Differential Diagnosis
▶ Giant condyloma
▶ Verrucous carcinoma
▶ Warty carcinoma
▶ Squamous carcinoma, usual type

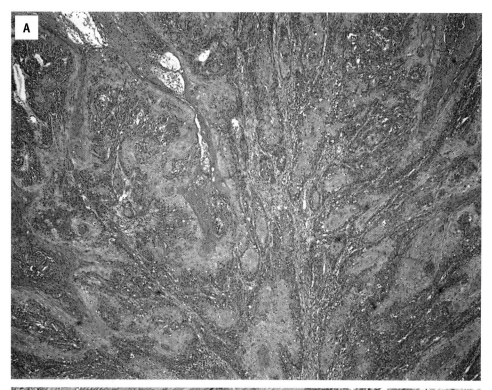

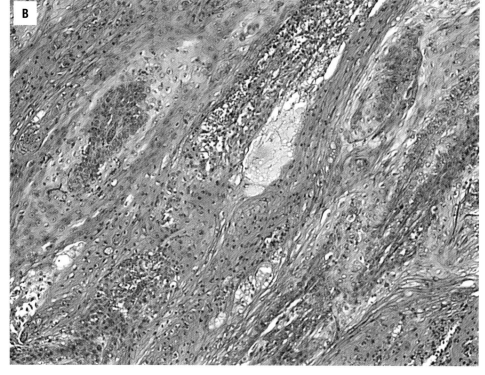

FIGURE 8-12
Papillary carcinoma, NOS type. **A,** Tumor demonstrates irregular papillary growth pattern with prominent fibrovascular cores. The interface between tumor and stroma is jagged. (Courtesy of Anuradha Radhakrishnan, Emory University Hospital, Atlanta, GA.) **B,** Note prominent wide areas of keratinization between papillae and the absence of koilocytic changes at higher magnification.

carcinoma, in which papillary features and a high degree of differentiation are not prominent.

survival rate is approximately 90%. Surgery is the treatment of choice.

PROGNOSIS AND TREATMENT

Despite the fact that deep invasion can occur, regional lymph node metastasis is usually rare. The 5-year

CARCINOMA CUNICULATUM

Barreto JE et al recently reported a series of variant penile squamous cell carcinomas with verruciform growth pattern, characterized by its peculiar deeply penetrating and burrowing sinous pattern of growth. Microscopically, the lesions corresponded to well-differentiated carcinomas with bulbous front of invasion. These neoplasms were similar to the plantar epithelioma cunniculatum originally described by Ayrd in 1954. Unlike most subtypes of penile SCCs and despite the deep invasion, none of the tumors showed groin or systemic dissemination at the time of diagnosis.

BASALOID CARCINOMA

Basaloid carcinoma is an HPV-related, aggressive variant of squamous carcinoma that accounts for 5 % to 10 % of penile cancers.

CLINICAL FEATURES

Most commonly, basaloid carcinoma arises in the glans in the perimeatal region. The median age at presentation is 52 years. Patients present with a flat, ulcerated, firm, and deeply infiltrative mass. More than half of the patients present with enlarged inguinal lymph nodes due to metastatic disease.

BASALOID CARCINOMA OF THE PENIS—FACT SHEET

Definition
► An aggressive variant of squamous carcinoma of the penis with basaloid features

Incidence and Location
► Accounts for 5-10% of penile cancers
► Most commonly involves glans

Morbidity and Mortality
► One of the aggressive variants of squamous carcinomas
► In one series, >50% patients died of disease in 3 years

Gender, Race, and Age Distribution
► Mean age of 55 years, other characteristics similar to squamous carcinoma, usual type

Clinical Features
► Patient presents with large, ulcerated mass in the glans
► Presentation with inguinal lymphadenopathy is common

Prognosis and Treatment
► Two-thirds of patients present with positive inguinal lymph nodes
► Prognosis is poor
► May need total penectomy with inguinal lymph node dissection and/or adjuvant chemotherapy

---

BASALOID CARCINOMA OF THE PENIS—PATHOLOGIC FEATURES

Gross Findings
► Flat, ulcerated, firm, gray-white mass
► Cut sections demonstrate deep infiltration into underlying soft tissues

Microscopic Findings
► Nests of monotonous small basaloid tumor cells with scant cytoplasm, oval to round, hyperchromatic nuclei, and inconspicuous nucleoli
► Brisk mitotic rate
► Abrupt keratinization with central comedo-type necrosis is common

Immunohistochemical Features
► Cytokeratins positive

Differential Diagnosis
► Squamous cell carcinoma, usual type and urothelial carcinoma
► Basal cell carcinoma
► Malignant melanoma
► Small cell neuroendocrine carcinoma and metastatic carcinoma

---

PATHOLOGIC FEATURES

GROSS FINDINGS

Tumors grossly are gray-white, firm, and ulcerated. Cut surfaces demonstrate a vertical growth pattern with deep infiltration into underlying soft tissues.

MICROSCOPIC FINDINGS

Microscopically, basaloid carcinoma is composed of packed nests of basaloid tumor cells, often associated with comedo-type necrosis. The cells are small, with scant cytoplasm and oval to round, hyperchromatic nuclei and inconspicuous nucleoli. The mitotic rate is usually brisk. Palisading at the periphery of the nests and abrupt central keratinization are occasionally seen (Fig. 8-13). These tumors tend to infiltrate deeply into corpora cavernosa. A striking "starry sky" appearance may be noted due to the high amount of apoptotic cells. Perineural and angiolymphatic invasion are frequent. Atypical basal cell hyperplasia and basaloid CIS are frequently associated lesions. Basaloid carcinoma may coexist with conventional squamous cell carcinoma or, infrequently, with warty carcinoma.

ANCILLARY STUDIES

In situ hybridization studies demonstrate that the majority are positive for high-risk HPV-16 and -18. Basaloid carcinomas are positive for cytokeratins.

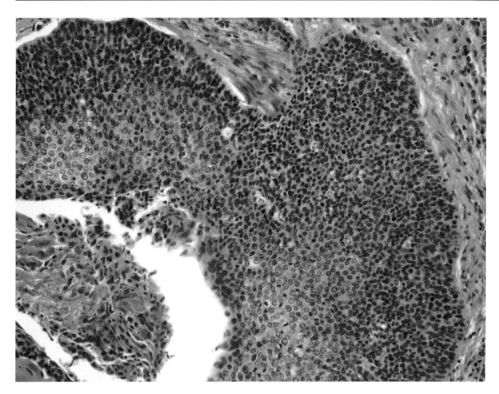

FIGURE 8-13

Basaloid carcinoma. High-power view demonstrates nodule of tumor cells with relatively monotonous hyperchromatic basaloid cells. In the center, tumor shows focal comedotype necrosis and abrupt keratinization. There is high number of apoptotic tumor cells.

DIFFERENTIAL DIAGNOSIS

Basaloid carcinoma differs from the usual poorly differentiated squamous cell carcinoma by having smaller, more regular cells with a high nuclear/cytoplasmic ratio, compared with the large, more pleomorphic cells with appreciable eosinophilic cytoplasm of the latter (Fig. 8-13). Keratinization in basaloid carcinoma is usually abrupt and focal, within the center of solid nests, and does not have the irregular distribution that is typical of a squamous carcinoma. Basaloid carcinomas are more malignant in appearance than basal cell carcinomas, and the latter characteristically occur in the skin of the shaft, in contrast to the typical glans location of the basaloid carcinoma. The peripheral palisading is either absent or not conspicuous in basaloid carcinoma compared with basal cell carcinoma. Basal cell carcinomas lack the comedo-type necrosis and high number of apoptotic tumor cells. Urothelial carcinomas occasionally may present with relatively small cells and commonly have nesting similar to basaloid carcinomas; however, conventional urothelial differentiation is usually apparent in other areas. Urothelial carcinomas also have frequent squamous and glandular differential, and the epicenter of mass is around the urethra, which has urothelial CIS changes.

Other differential diagnoses include small cell neuroendocrine carcinoma and metastatic carcinoma. Small cell carcinomas are also highly proliferating and mitotically active tumors; however, the presence of spindling and crushing, nuclear molding, and the characteristic nuclear chromatin pattern distinguishes them from basaloid carcinoma.

PROGNOSIS AND TREATMENT

In comparison to the usual squamous carcinomas, basaloid carcinomas tend to have higher histologic grade, a deeper invasion of the penile anatomic layers, and higher mortality. It is one of the aggressive variants of squamous carcinoma, with a high rate of inguinal lymph node metastasis and a mortality rate of 59% at 5 years.

PSEUDOHYPERPLASTIC CARCINOMA

This is a rare, nonverruciform, very well-differentiated squamous cell carcinoma variant that exhibits pseudohyperplastic features (Fig. 8-14). Cubilla and colleagues recently reported 10 such cases of penile carcinomas with pseudohyperplastic features. Pseudoepitheliomatous hyperplasia was the principal differential diagnosis, particularly in the superficial biopsy specimens. Well-developed lichen sclerosus was seen in all cases, suggesting a precancerous role.

SARCOMATOID (SPINDLE-CELL) CARCINOMA

Squamous carcinoma with sarcomatoid differentiation may arise as dedifferentiation of the primary tumor, de novo, or after the radiation therapy.

cell component. The spindle cell component may predominate. Areas resembling fibrosarcoma, malignant fibrous histiocytoma, or leiomyosarcoma can be seen. Differentiation into bone or cartilage can also be seen. Careful examination may reveal the focal presence of typical epithelial differentiation of carcinoma or the presence of penile intraepithelial lesions. Necrosis is often prominent.

ANCILLARY STUDIES

IMMUNOHISTOCHEMISTRY

Sarcomatoid carcinomas usually demonstrate positivity for cytokeratins, and p63, at least focally. Broad-spectrum cytokeratins, including high-molecular-weight cytokeratin, should be included in the panel. S-100, HMB-45, and melan A markers are negative.

ULTRASTRUCTURAL FEATURES

Poorly developed desmosomes and cytoplasmic filaments and the absence of specific ultrastructural features for sarcoma or melanoma aid the diagnosis.

DIFFERENTIAL DIAGNOSIS

The usual differential diagnosis is from sarcoma or malignant melanoma. Tumors demonstrating focal presence of squamous CIS or differentiated carcinoma favor the diagnosis of sarcomatoid carcinoma. Diagnosis can be made in the absence of typical squamous carcinoma if there is a history of pure squamous carcinoma at that site that was not treated with radiation. Pure spindle cell tumors without such history may pose a diagnostic problem, and additional immunohistochemical stains and electron microscopy may be useful to rule out sarcoma and melanoma. Sometimes, squamous carcinomas have pseudoangiomatoid areas, which may raise possibility of angiosarcoma.

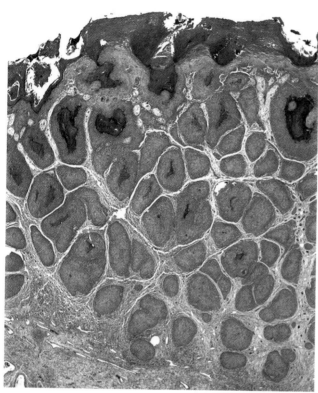

FIGURE 8-14

Pseudohyperplastic carcinoma. Low-power view demonstrates nests of well-differentiated carcinoma proliferating downward, involving the lamina propria. Surface nests show keratinization. Surface changes mimic pseudoepitheliomatous hyperplasia. (Courtesy of Anuradha Radhakrishnan, Emory University Hospital, Atlanta, GA.)

CLINICAL FEATURES

Patients present with a large, ulcerated or exophytic mass that usually is situated on the glans but may occur on the mucosal side of the foreskin. It accounts for approximately 1% to 3% of penile carcinomas. The average patient age is 60 years.

PATHOLOGIC FEATURES

GROSS FINDINGS

Sarcomatoid carcinomas are frequently large (5 to 7 cm), irregular, gray-white tumors with exophytic and prominent endophytic components. On cut surface, the tumor deeply infiltrates into the corpus spongiosum and cavernosa.

MICROSCOPIC FINDINGS

Histologically, sarcomatoid carcinoma is a biphasic tumor composed of a malignant spindle and epithelial

PROGNOSIS AND TREATMENT

Sarcomatoid carcinomas are associated with a high rate of regional lymph node metastasis and carry a bad prognosis. Recurrence is common, with mortality rate of 60%.

ADENOSQUAMOUS CARCINOMA

Squamous cell carcinoma with glandular differentiation usually arises from the surface epithelium. Embryologically misplaced glands of the perimeatal region of the glans or metaplastic mucinous glands have been postulated as a possible source for the origin of these tumors. Grossly, the tumor is similar to conventional squamous carcinoma involving the glans. Microscopically, the squamous component predominates over the glandular component. In one series of three cases reported, two demonstrated a prominent "warty" component of squamous carcinoma and a third demonstrated the usual squamous differentiation. The glandular component stains positive for carcinoembryonic antigen (CEA). Tumors similar to mucoepidermoid carcinoma have also been reported.

If squamous carcinoma secondarily involves the periurethral glands, it may mimic adenosquamous carcinoma. However, in such cases the glands appear morphologically benign.

MIXED CARCINOMAS

About one fourth of penile carcinomas demonstrate some mixture of various histologic types. The most common mixed pattern of neoplasia is the focal presence of moderate- to high-grade squamous carcinoma with typical verrucous carcinoma, referred to as hybrid verrucous carcinoma. Such tumors demonstrate metastatic potential, and the prognosis usually depends on the worst growth pattern. The presence of a basaloid carcinoma component in an otherwise typical squamous carcinoma also portends a higher incidence of groin metastasis. Other recognized combinations include a mixture of warty and basaloid carcinoma, combinations of adenocarcinoma and basaloid carcinoma (adenobasaloid), and a mixture of squamous and neuroendocrine carcinoma.

OTHER RARE PRIMARY PENILE CARCINOMAS

Other rare pure primary penile carcinomas reported include clear cell carcinoma, Merkel cell carcinoma, small cell neuroendocrine carcinoma, and sebaceous carcinoma.

Liegl and Reuager recently reported five cases of **clear cell carcinoma** of the penis distinct from the usual penile squamous cell carcinomas. Histologically, the tumors were composed of large clear cells with intracytoplasmic periodic acid-Schiff (PAS)-positive material and demonstrated propensity for extensive lymphatic and blood vessel invasion. Tumor cells characteristically stained for Muc-1, epithelial membrane antigen (EMA), and CEA. All carcinomas were positive for HPV-16 DNA, though HPV-related cytologic changes were rarely seen. All patients presented with inguinal lymph node metastasis, and the prognosis was uniformly poor despite adjuvant chemotherapy and radiation therapy.

Other Malignant Neoplasms of the Penis

EXTRAMAMMARY PAGET DISEASE OF THE PENIS

The detailed discussion of anogenital Paget disease is presented in the section of scrotum pathology.

MALIGNANT MELANOMA

Malignant melanomas of the penis are rare, with slightly more than 100 cases reported in the literature. They affect white men between the ages of 50 and 70 years. Risk factors include exposure to ultraviolet radiation, history of melanoma, and preexisting nevi. Most of the melanomas (60% to 80%) arise from the glans penis, fewer than 10% affect the prepuce, and the remainder arise from the skin of the shaft. Grossly, they can manifest as an ulcer, papule, or nodule that is blue, brown, or red. Reported histologic subtypes include nodular, superficial spreading, and mucosal lentiginous. Prognosis is poor, and management is similar to that for melanomas of other regions.

BASAL CELL CARCINOMA

Basal cell carcinoma affecting the penis is a rare, indolent neoplasm similar to basal cell carcinomas arising from other sun-exposed sites. They may be unicentric or multicentric, and they usually occur on the shaft of the penis. They are superficially invasive, with limited metastatic potential. It is important not to confuse basal cell carcinoma with basaloid squamous cell carcinoma, because the prognosis is very different. Basaloid carcinomas are aggressive tumors that affect the glans and are characterized by more pronounced cytologic atypia, mitoses, comedo-type necrosis, and less conspicuous palisading of the peripheral cells. Wide local surgical excision is the treatment of choice for basal cell carcinoma.

RARE MESENCHYMAL TUMORS

Mesenchymal tumors are very uncommon in the penis, although many subtypes have been reported in the literature. The most frequently encountered benign mesenchymal tumors of the penis are vascular related. The most common malignant ones also include vascular tumors as well as leiomyosarcoma. All of these tumors conform to definitions provided at other body sites and are not discussed further here.

SECONDARY TUMORS

Metastasis to the penis is rare. The corpus cavernosum is the most common site of metastasis, followed by penile skin, spongiosum, and glans. Metastatic disease should be suspected in patients who develop priapism and have a known history of cancer.

Prostate and bladder are the most common primary sites, with kidney and colon least frequent. A multinodular growth pattern is characteristic.

PRECANCEROUS SQUAMOUS LESIONS

Precursor lesions of penile carcinoma comprise a heterogeneous spectrum of epithelial alterations affecting the squamous epithelium of penile anatomic compartments. One of the major areas of confusion in the nomenclature of penile lesions is the terminology used for premalignant epithelial proliferations.

Various designations such as squamous intraepithelial lesion, low grade (LGSIL) and high grade (HGSIL); mild, moderate, and severe dysplasia, with or without HPV changes; PeIN I, II, and III; and CIS have been used with similar significance. SILs of low and high grade, or PeIN, is the recommended terminology. In our routine practice, we prefer the use of former terminology. Erythroplasia of Queyrat and Bowen disease are both synonymous with HGSIL/PeIN III or squamous CIS, the former term usually used for lesions of the glans and foreskin mucosa, and the latter for lesions of the body. Other probable precursor lesions are squamous hyperplasia and bowenoid papulosis. Bowenoid papulosis shares similar histologic features with Bowen disease but has a different clinical presentation and clinical significance and will be discussed separately.

HPV DNA is consistently positive in the majority (70% to 100%) of PeIN cases and is believed to play a role in progression to penile carcinoma. However, HPV DNA is not so strongly correlated with the usual invasive squamous carcinomas. A possible explanation is that HPV-negative invasive carcinoma does not arise from HPV-positive, but from unrecognized HPV-negative precursor lesions. The "high risk" HPVs—most commonly types 16 and 18—are predominantly associated with subclinical lesions.

PRECANCEROUS SQUAMOUS LESIONS, PENIS—FACT SHEET

Definition

▶ A spectrum of atypical intraepithelial squamous lesions with various designations such as squamous intraepithelial lesion (SIL), low grade (LGSIL) and high grade (HGSIL); mild, moderate, and severe dysplasia; penile intraepithelial neoplasia (PeIN) I, II, and III; carcinoma in situ; Bowen disease; and erythroplasia of Queyrat
▶ The terms erythroplasia of Queyrat and Bowen disease are synonymous with HGSIL or PeIN III; SIL or PeIN is the preferred term

Incidence and Location

▶ Seen in sexually active men where HPV infection is at epidemic proportions
▶ Most commonly involves the glans, prepuce, and shaft of penis

Gender, Race, and Age Distribution

▶ Males in fourth to sixth decade
▶ The lesions occur, on average, at a later age than in cases of bowenoid papulosis

Clinical Features

▶ Patients present with moist erythematous or scaly plaques, as discrete or diffuse lesions with irregular borders
▶ May be multiple
▶ Also may manifest as white patches of "leukoplakia"
▶ Frequently seen in association with squamous carcinoma

Prognosis and Treatment

▶ Up to 10% progress to carcinoma
▶ Patients with pernicious HPV infection or with an immunocompromised state are at higher risk
▶ Wide excision of the lesion is the preferred treatment
▶ Topical chemotherapy is also frequently used

PRECANCEROUS SQUAMOUS LESIONS, PENIS— PATHOLOGIC FEATURES

Gross Findings

▶ Irregular or discrete, moist and erythematous or scaly plaques

Microscopic Findings

▶ Graded according to proportion of atypical cells occupying the epithelial thickness and degree of cytologic atypia
▶ The surface is often hyperkeratotic
▶ The nuclei are enlarged, pleomorphic, and hyperchromatic, with irregular nuclear membranes
▶ Koilocytotic atypia frequently prominent

Immunohistochemical Features

▶ 70-100% of lesions are positive for HPV DNA

Differential Diagnosis

▶ Bowenoid papulosis
▶ Urothelial carcinoma in situ

SQUAMOUS INTRAEPITHELIAL LESIONS/PENILE INTRAEPITHELIAL NEOPLASIA

CLINICAL FEATURES

Patients with HGSIL are typically in the middle to later years of life, with a peak frequency in the sixth decade. These lesions occur, on average, at a later age than cases of bowenoid papulosis. They may be solitary but more frequently are associated with adjacent invasive squamous cell carcinoma (see Fig. 8-4). The lesions typically manifest as irregular, moist, and erythematous areas or scaly plaques (Fig. 8-15). LGSILs may not be clinically apparent, or they may manifest as white patches of "leukoplakia."

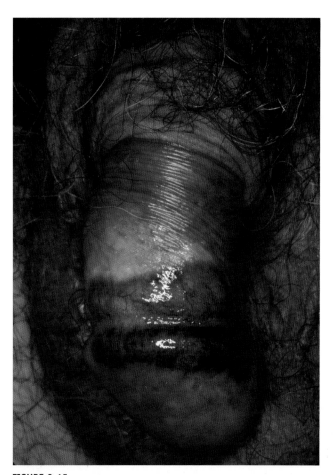

FIGURE 8-15

Bowen disease. An irregular, moist, erythematous, flat lesion involves part of the shaft and glans penis. (Courtesy of Lori Lowe, University of Michigan, Ann Arbor, MI.)

PATHOLOGIC FEATURES

GROSS FINDINGS

Grossly, the lesions appear as an irregular, moist, erythematous to scaly plaque.

MICROSCOPIC FINDINGS

PeIN is graded in proportion to the epithelial thickness occupied by the transformed basaloid cells and the degree of cytologic atypia. The cells vary in size and shape, and the nuclei are pleomorphic and hyperchromatic, with loss of polarity. Mitosis is frequent. In LGSILs, atypia is confined to the lower one third or there is only minimal patchy cytologic atypia; in HGSILs, atypical cells affect at least the lower two thirds of the epithelium or there is a moderate degree of cytologic atypia. Full-thickness atypia is also referred to as "Bowen atypia" or squamous CIS (Fig. 8-16). SILs may be further classified based on architecture as squamous or simplex type (most frequent) or as warty (condylomatous) and basaloid type.

DIFFERENTIAL DIAGNOSIS

Various skin conditions may produce penile lesions that are difficult to distinguish from SILs, particularly from the clinical spectrum of erythroplasia of Queyrat and Bowen disease. Zoon's balanitis closely mimics erythroplasia of Queyrat. However, on microscopic examination the interpretation should be straightforward. The distinction of SILs from bowenoid papulosis may be impossible on purely histologic grounds, but clinical differences are usually suggestive and are summarized in Table 8-4. Squamous carcinoma in situ lesions also must be distinguished from urothelial CIS, which may secondarily involve the glans mucosa.

PROGNOSIS AND TREATMENT

If untreated, 5% to 10% of HGSILs progress to invasive squamous cell carcinoma. Longitudinal studies demonstrate that patients who cannot clear high-risk HPV infections within a year are at higher risk for the malignant transformation. It is clinically impossible to determine which individual will develop pernicious HPV infection and progress to invasive cancer. Therefore, in patients older than 40 years of age, as well as immunosuppressed individuals at earlier ages, lesions should always be approached as premalignant and treated surgically. Topical chemotherapy 5-flurouracil is also frequently used. Treatment failure may be related to indistinct margin or involvement of lesion down in the hair follicles and unrecognized foci of invasive tumor.

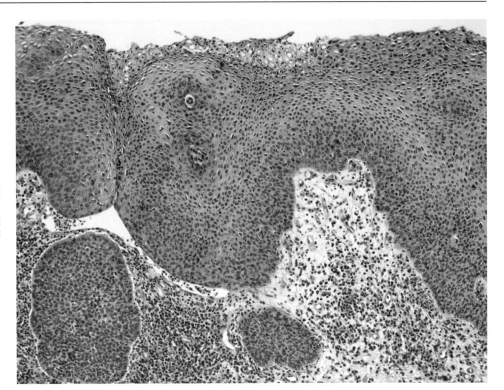

FIGURE 8-16

In this high-grade squamous intra-epithelial lesion (PeIN III), the squamous epithelium demonstrates hyperkeratosis, parakeratosis, acanthosis, and full-thickness cytologic atypia. Note that the koilocytic atypia is prominent.

Table 8-4

Comparison between Penile Intraepithelial Neoplasia III (Bowen's Disease and Erythroplasia of Queyrat) and Bowenoid Papulosis

Feature	Penile Intraepithelial Neoplasia III (Includes BD and EQ)	Bowenoid Papulosis
Site	Glans, prepuce (EQ); shaft (BD)	Shaft
Age	4th-6th decade	3rd-4th decades
Lesion	Scaly (BD); erythematous plaque (EQ)	Papules
Maturation	−	+
Sweat gland involvement	−	+
Pilosebaceous involvement	±	−
Precancerous potential	5-10%	−
Spontaneous regression	−	+
HPV	+	+

BD, Bowen disease; EQ, erythroplasia of Queyrat; HPV, human papillomavirus.
Modified from Young RH, Srigley JR, Amin MB, et al: Tumors of the Prostate Gland, Seminal Vesicles, Male Urethra, and Penis. AFIP Atlas of Tumor Pathology. Washington, DC, Armed Forces Institute of Pathology, 2000, p 412, Table 10-2.

BOWENOID PAPULOSIS

CLINICAL FEATURES

Bowenoid papulosis is an HPV-related condition that affects young men; the median age at presentation is 30 years. Clinically, patients typically present with multiple red papules, resembling persistent warts, affecting the shaft of the penis, or occasionally the glans or foreskin. Some evidence suggests a viral origin on the basis of infection with high-risk oncogenic genotypes of HPV-16/18 and an association with cervical carcinoma.

PATHOLOGIC FEATURES

GROSS FINDINGS

Lesions grossly appear as solitary or multiple, small, red papules.

MICROSCOPIC FINDINGS

The histologic features are indistinguishable from those of HGSIL/Bowen disease lesions. However, there is, in general, a more spotty distribution of atypical cells and greater maturation of keratinocytes than seen in Bowen disease (Fig. 8-17).

BOWENOID PAPULOSIS—FACT SHEET

Definition
▶ HPV-related lesions in young, sexually active men that display histologic features of penile intraepithelial neoplasia III (Bowen disease)

Incidence and Location
▶ Most common location is shaft of penis, but occasionally on the glans or foreskin

Gender, Race, and Age Distribution
▶ Seen in young, sexually active people 16 to 35 years of age (mean, 28 years)
▶ Typically encountered in younger men than those with PeIN

Clinical Features
▶ Patient presents with multiple or sometimes single red papules, most commonly affecting the shaft of the penis

Prognosis and Treatment
▶ Predominantly transient, self-limited, and benign condition
▶ Spontaneous regression is common
▶ Because of association with high-risk HPV-16 and HPV-18, close surveillance is necessary

---

DIFFERENTIAL DIAGNOSIS

Diagnosis of bowenoid papulosis is made purely on a clinicopathologic basis. Young patients presenting with

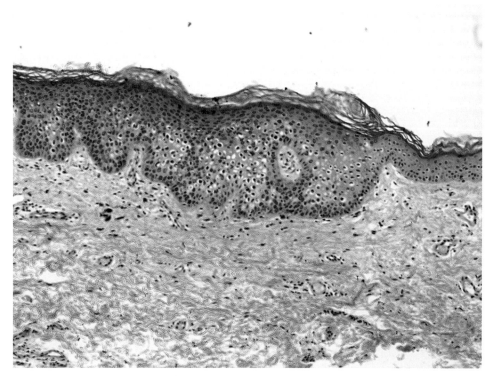

FIGURE 8-17

In bowenoid papulosis, squamous epithelium demonstrates cytologic atypia, similar to that seen in squamous intraepithelial lesions; however, it is spotty in distribution and demonstrates surface maturation. (Courtesy of Doug Fullen, University of Michigan, Ann Arbor, MI.)

BOWENOID PAPULOSIS—PATHOLOGIC FEATURES

Gross Findings
▶ Small red nodules or papules

Microscopic Findings
▶ Histologic features are essentially similar to usual HGSIL
▶ In general, a more spotty distribution of atypical cells and greater maturation of keratinocytes than in HGSIL

Immunohistochemical Features
▶ Oncogenic HPV DNA, most commonly type 16, but also type 18 and/or 33-35 has been reported

Differential Diagnosis
▶ Bowen disease (HGSIL/PeIN III)

---

multiple lesions and spotty cytologic atypia are typical for bowenoid papulosis.

PROGNOSIS AND TREATMENT

Malignant transformation in bowenoid papulosis is rare, and many lesions spontaneously regress. Recent reports suggest good response to immunomodulatory treatment. In view of the oncogenic potential of high-risk HPV infections (types 16 and 18), regardless of the treatment used, all patients with bowenoid papulosis and their sexual partners must be included in long-term follow-up and regularly examined for the malignant transformation.

BALANITIS XEROTICA OBLITERANS (LICHEN SCLEROSUS ET ATROPHICUS)

CLINICAL FEATURES

Balanitis xerotica obliterans is an unusual chronic mucocutaneous inflammatory condition of the penis that usually affects the foreskin or glans penis lamina and is identical to vulvar lichen sclerosus et atrophicus. It usually manifests with phimosis, with severe narrowing of the preputial orifice or the urethral meatus. The mucosa demonstrates irregular, gray-white, atrophic-appearing patches (Fig. 8-18). Most cases are seen in the third to fifth decades of life, although they may occur at the extremes of age. Frequently, it coexists with penile carcinoma. The etiology of this condition is unknown at present.

BALANITIS XEROTICA OBLITERANS—FACT SHEET

Definition
▶ Lesion is similar to the lichen sclerosus et atrophicus of the vulva, characterized by diffuse atrophy of epithelium and condensation of connective tissues

Incidence and Location
▶ Relatively common condition, associated with phimosis or with carcinomas
▶ In one series the lesion was present in 37% of cases associated with carcinomas
▶ Commonly affects glans and prepuce, in the perimeatal region

Gender, Race, and Age Distribution
▶ Male patients
▶ Analogous lesion in female is lichen sclerosus et atrophicus
▶ Usually affects elderly men

Clinical Features
▶ Patients typically present with phimosis with severe narrowing of preputial orifice or meatus
▶ Mucosa appears gray-white, irregular, and atrophic
▶ It may coexist with carcinoma

Prognosis and Treatment
▶ Has been proposed as a possible risk factor for carcinoma
▶ Early diagnosis and treatment are important to avoid urologic complications
▶ Treatment varies from topical corticosteroids and laser in early cases, to meatoplasty and urethroplasty in severe cases

---

PATHOLOGIC FEATURES

GROSS FINDINGS

Grossly, the mucosa appears to have gray-white, irregular, atrophic areas.

MICROSCOPIC FINDINGS

Microscopically, overlying epithelium demonstrates hyperkeratosis and atrophy with loss of rete ridges. Hyperplastic variant may also be present. The characteristic finding is the early edema and chronic inflammation, and later hyalinization with a band of dense eosinophilic fibrosis in the lamina propria (Fig. 8-19).

DIFFERENTIAL DIAGNOSIS

The microscopic features of well-developed balanitis xerotica obliterans are straightforward. Nonspecific dermatitis, lichen planus, may get confused with it if the band of eosinophilic fibrosis is not well developed. Amyloid deposition also may rarely be confused with balanitis xerotica obliterans, when it demonstrates prominent eosinophilic fibrosis.

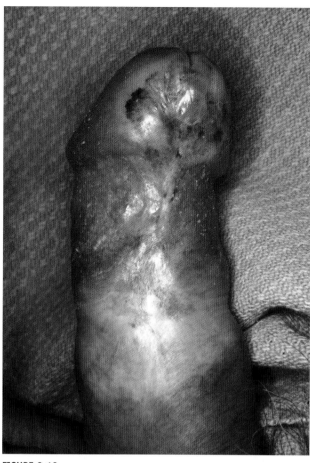

FIGURE 8-18

In balanitis xerotica obliterans, a gray-white, irregular, atrophic-appearing lesion involves the perimeal area of the glans penis. (Courtesy of Lori Lowe, University of Michigan, Ann Arbor, MI.)

BALANITIS XEROTICA OBLITERANS—PATHOLOGIC FEATURES

Gross Findings

▶ White-gray, flat, irregular geographic atrophic areas involving the foreskin or glans, especially perimeal region

Microscopic Findings

▶ Atrophy of squamous epithelium with hyperkeratosis
▶ The rete ridges are flat
▶ In early lesions, lamina propria demonstrates edema and chronic inflammation; in later cases, there is a characteristic band of eosinophilic fibrosis, frequently with vacuolar interface dermatitis.
▶ The lesion is superficial, 3 to 4 mm in depth

Differential Diagnosis

▶ Nonspecific dermatitis
▶ Lichen planus
▶ Amyloidosis deposition
▶ Fibrosis

PROGNOSIS AND TREATMENT

Early diagnosis and treatment is important in preventing the urologic complications of the disease (e.g., urethral stricture). Treatment depends on the anatomic location of the lesion and its severity. The treatment varies from topical corticosteroids and laser ablation in early cases to meatoplasty and urethroplasty in severe cases.

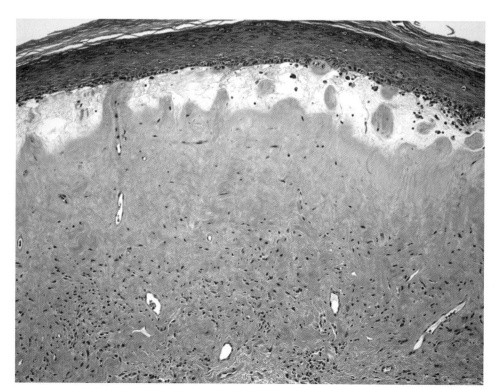

FIGURE 8-19

In balanitis xerotica obliterans, the lamina propria is edematous, with a characteristic eosinophilic band of hyalinization. The overlying epithelium demonstrates hyperkeratosis, atrophy, and loss of rete ridges.

Balanitis xerotica obliterans has been suggested as one of the etiologic factors for squamous carcinoma of the penis, because of its frequent association with it.

SQUAMOUS HYPERPLASIA

Squamous hyperplasia is an epithelial abnormality that is frequently associated with squamous cell carcinomas, particularly those demonstrating verruciform growth pattern. It is commonly present in the mucosa of the glans, coronal sulcus, and foreskin, adjacent to, distant from, or in continuity with the carcinoma. Microscopically, squamous hyperplasia is characterized by acanthosis, hyperkeratosis, and normal maturation of the epithelium. Cytologic atypia is absent. The overall growth pattern can be flat or papillary.

TUMOR-LIKE LESIONS

CONDYLOMA

Condyloma accounts for the most common tumor-like condition of the penis and is caused by HPV infections.

CLINICAL FEATURES

Condylomas are seen in sexually active young men, among whom HPV infections are at epidemic proportions. Most cases are sexually transmitted, as underlined by the higher incidence of condyloma among men whose partners have HPV-related cervical lesions. The incidence of condyloma is reported to be about 5% among adults aged 20 to 40 years. If it is seen in a child, sexual abuse should be strongly suspected.

Condylomas manifest as either flat or cauliflower-like lesions that are usually located on the corona of the glans, fossa navicularis, or meatus, but involvement of scrotal or perineal skin may also be seen.

PATHOLOGIC FEATURES

GROSS FINDINGS

Lesions grossly have a papillary or cauliflower-like appearance and range from multiple, small warts (1 to 2 mm) to large growths 5 to 10 cm in diameter in rare instances.

CONDYLOMA, PENIS—FACT SHEET

Definition
▶ Most common tumor-like condition of penis, caused by HPV infection

Incidence and Location
▶ About 5% of sexually active adults of 20 to 40 years
▶ Rare in children; if present, sexual abuse should be suspected.
▶ Most common locations include corona of glans, fossa navicularis, meatus, and shaft
▶ Scrotal or perineal skin may be involved

Gender, Race, and Age Distribution
▶ Common in sexually active men 20 to 40 years of age, among whom HPV infections are epidemic
▶ Giant condyloma affects slightly older patients than typical condyloma acuminata

Clinical Features
▶ Patient may present with multiple papillary, warty lesions or small, flat lesions that may be clinically inapparent

Prognosis and Treatment
▶ After initial infections, reactivation is common
▶ May be associated with squamous cell carcinoma but is not considered precancerous
▶ Cryotherapy common treatment

MICROSCOPIC FINDINGS

Microscopic features include prominent papillary growth with hyperkeratosis. Fibrovascular cores are prominent, with surface koilocytosis and benign histology (Fig. 8-20). Condylomas may also manifest with

---

CONDYLOMA, PENIS—PATHOLOGIC FEATURES

Gross Findings
▶ Papillary, warty, cauliflower-like lesions
▶ Also can be small, flat lesions

Microscopic Findings
▶ Varying degree of papillomatosis, acanthosis, parakeratosis, and hyperkeratosis, with prominent to inconspicuous koilocytic atypia and cytoplasmic vacuolization, raisinoid nuclei, and binucleation
▶ True condyloma, including giant variant, should not have irregular, infiltrative appearance

Immunohistochemical Features
▶ Most are positive for HPV-6 and HPV-11 by in situ hybridization

Differential Diagnosis
▶ Warty carcinoma
▶ Papillary carcinoma, NOS type
▶ Verrucous carcinoma
▶ Squamous papilloma

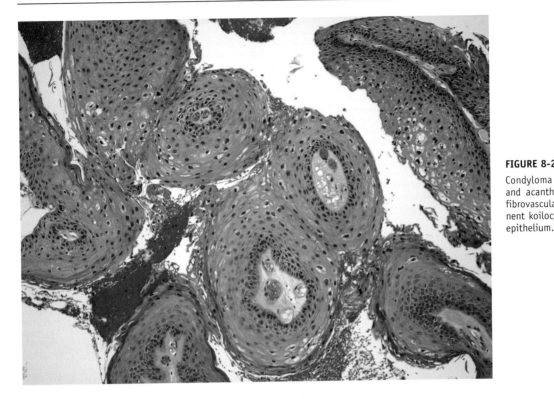

FIGURE 8-20
Condyloma shows papillomatosis and acanthosis with well-developed fibrovascular cores. Note the prominent koilocytic atypia of the surface epithelium.

a flat growth pattern. The base of the lesion is well demarcated from the underlying stroma.

ANCILLARY STUDIES

HPV DNA types 6 and 11 are the most commonly associated types.

DIFFERENTIAL DIAGNOSIS

In cases with not well-developed koilocytic atypia, squamous papilloma may enter the differential diagnosis. In difficult cases, confirmation with HPV DNA by in situ hybridization or immunohistochemistry may be helpful.

PROGNOSIS AND TREATMENT

Recurrence of the genital warts is very common. They are typically treated with cryotherapy and topical immunomodulatory agents.

GIANT CONDYLOMA ACUMINATUM

Giant condyloma is a benign, very rare verruciform, arborescent, papillomatous growth of the penis, which is also referred to as Buschke-Lowenstein tumor. The literature is confusing about these tumors, because many have been called verrucous carcinoma. They occur in patients slightly older than those with common condyloma and younger than those with warty carcinoma, the other two HPV-related lesions of the penis. Clinically, they manifest with large (5 to 10 cm), cauliflower-like tumors. Microscopic features are identical to the common type of condyloma but demonstrate more cellular histology with slight atypia. The growth is also more exuberant, and the base of the lesion shows a bulbous expansion into underlying tissues.

The major differential diagnosis is with warty carcinoma, a closely related tumor, which is malignant histologically, with the borders between tumor and stroma being preferentially jagged. In the literature, giant condylomas and verrucous carcinomas have often been considered the same tumors due to their large size. However, verrucous carcinomas do not show evidence of koilocytic atypia and papillae with prominent fibrovascular cores. The differential diagnostic features are summarized in Table 8-3 and Figure 8-10.

PEYRONIE'S DISEASE

The cause of Peyronie's disease is still largely unknown, even though it has been recognized since the 17th century. Some authors suggest that it is related to fibromatosis, based on its association, in approximately 10% of patients, with other types of fibromatosis such as Dupuytren's contracture or palmar or plantar fibromatosis. Others postulate that this disease is caused by an inflammatory/fibrosing reaction secondary to urethritis. Other contributing factors include repeated mechanical trauma, hypertension, diabetes, and immune reactions.

CLINICAL FEATURES

The disease typically affects middle-aged or older men and is rare among those under 40 years of age. The lesion is often palpated as a firm plaque or nodule on the dorsal surface of the erect penile shaft. The inelasticity of the fibrous tissue leads to plaques that cause penile curvature and pain during erection.

PATHOLOGIC FEATURES

GROSS FINDINGS

In resection specimens, grossly there is proliferation of vaguely circumscribed, firm, fibrous tissue between the corpora cavernosa and the tunica albuginea.

MICROSCOPIC FINDINGS

Histologically, fibrosis is the main finding (Fig. 8-21). Depending on the stage of development of the lesion, slight variations can be seen. An inflammatory cell component is usually present in the early-stage lesions. Hyalinization with areas of bone and cartilage formation is usually seen in advanced lesions.

DIFFERENTIAL DIAGNOSIS

Nonspecific inflammation and fibrosis may mimic Peyronie's disease. Microscopically, the diagnosis is usually straightforward in the right clinical context.

PROGNOSIS AND TREATMENT

The clinical course of Peyronie's disease is variable. The lesion resolves spontaneously in one third of patients. Radiotherapy, steroid injections, anti-inflammatory metalloproteins, or surgical resection with graft placement can alleviate the symptoms.

PEYRONIE'S DISEASE—FACT SHEET

Definition
▶ An unusual variant of superficial fibromatosis affecting mainly the tunica albuginea

Incidence and Location
▶ Uncommon condition
▶ Affects the shaft of the penis

Gender, Race, and Age Distribution
▶ The disease typically affects middle-aged or older men and is rare among those younger than 40 years of age

Clinical Features
▶ Patients usually complain of painful erection with bending of penis
▶ A firm, plaque-like area is detected on the dorsal aspect of the erect penis, creating confusion sometimes with neoplasm

Prognosis and Treatment
▶ Clinical course is variable
▶ The lesion resolves spontaneously in one third of patients
▶ Radiotherapy, steroid injections, or surgical resection can alleviate the symptoms

---

PEYRONIE'S DISEASE—PATHOLOGIC FEATURES

Gross Findings
▶ Characterized by gray-white, firm, fibrous tissue between the corpora cavernosa and tunica albuginea

Microscopic Findings
▶ Appearance similar to that of fibromatosis at other sites, although it tends to be less cellular and more sclerotic
▶ A perivascular lymphoid infiltrate is seen in early stage of disease
▶ Rarely, calcification or ossification is seen in advanced lesions

Differential Diagnosis
▶ Pathologic features are usually straightforward
▶ Injection of pharmacologic agents may simulate the clinical and microscopic presentation of Peyronie's disease

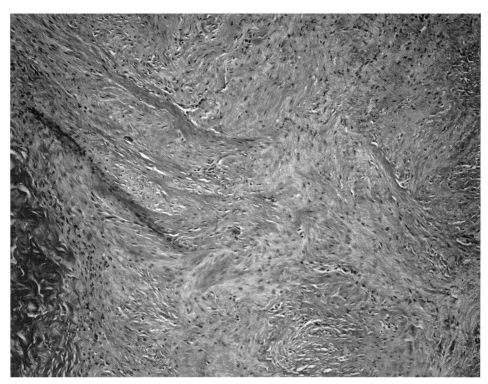

FIGURE 8-21
High-power view demonstrates typical microscopic features of Peyronie's disease. There is proliferation of spindle cells in the sclerotic and collagenized stroma. (Courtesy of David Lucas, University of Michigan, Ann Arbor, MI.)

VERRUCIFORM XANTHOMA

Verruciform xanthoma is a rare benign lesion that occurs primarily in the oral mucosa but infrequently also arises in the skin at several sites, more notably at the anogenital skin. Only a few lesions occurring in the penis and scrotum have been reported. The cause of this lesion remains elusive. Because of peculiar occurrence of this lesion in the oral cavity and genital skin, the possible role of infection by a transmittable virus such as HPV has been considered; however, researchers have not been able to document HPV by DNA in situ hybridization or more sensitive techniques, including polymerase chain reaction and RNA whole-genome probe to HPV.

CLINICAL FEATURES

The lesions are solitary, slow-growing nodules that range from 0.2 to 2 cm in diameter, mimicking a wart or cyst of hidradenitis suppurativa.

PATHOLOGIC FEATURES

GROSS FINDINGS

Grossly, lesions are small, tan/yellow, and polypoid.

VERRUCIFORM XANTHOMA—FACT SHEET

Definition
► Rare, tumor-like condition affecting anogenital skin, of uncertain cause, with propensity to involve the oral mucosa

Incidence and Location
► Rare condition in anogenital area
► Most common locations within anogenital skin include scrotal skin and penis

Morbidity and Mortality
► Benign condition

Clinical Features
► Lesions are 0.2- to 2-cm, slow-growing papules, that clinically may simulate warts or cysts of hidradenitis suppurativa

MICROSCOPIC FINDINGS

On microscopic examination, the surface is verrucoid, papillary, or crater-shaped. The epidermis displays acanthosis, papillomatosis, and hyperkeratosis; the granular layer is absent. Parakeratosis is prominent between the papillomatous epidermis, and it is associated with a variably intense but prominent neutrophilic infiltrate at the junction of the parakeratotic layer and stratum spinosum. The epidermis lacks koilocytotic atypia. In addition to the verrucoid appearance, the hallmark of this lesion is the presence of plump, round, foamy histiocytes, which fill the papillary dermis, between and at the tips of the papillae. A band-like, lymphoplasmacytic infiltrate may be present at the base of the lesion (Fig. 8-22).

DIFFERENTIAL DIAGNOSIS

The differential diagnosis includes verrucous lesions of the genital skin, particularly condyloma acuminatum and verrucous carcinoma. Condyloma and verrucous carcinoma lack the characteristic plump, foamy histiocytes. Verruciform xanthoma lacks the koilocytic atypia and does not have an invasive front. Fungal infections rarely can mimic verruciform xanthoma; therefore, fungal stains may be worthwhile, especially if the lesion is accompanied by neutrophilic infiltrate within the parakeratotic layer of the epidermis.

PROGNOSIS AND TREATMENT

Prognosis is excellent, and the treatment of choice is simple excision of the lesions.

VERRUCIFORM XANTHOMA—PATHOLOGIC FEATURES

Gross Findings

▶ Papules or nodules ranging from 0.2 to 2 cm

Microscopic Findings

▶ The epidermis has a verrucoid, papillary, or crater-shaped appearance
▶ The epidermis displays acanthosis, papillomatosis, and hyperkeratosis
▶ Granular layer absent
▶ Parakeratosis prominent between the papillomatous epidermis, and associated with a variably intense neutrophilic infiltrate
▶ The hallmark of the lesion is the presence of foamy histiocytes, which fill the papillary dermis, between and at the tips of papillae

Immunohistochemistry

▶ Rarely needed.
▶ Foamy macrophages are positive for histiocytic marker CD68

Differential Diagnosis

▶ Verrucous lesions: condyloma, verrucous carcinoma

FIGURE 8-22

Low-power view of a verrucoid lesion demonstrating papillary epithelial hyperplasia, hyperkeratosis and para-keratosis, and a collection of characteristic stromal histiocytes with foamy cytoplasm between elongated rete ridges. (Courtesy of Doug Fullen, University of Michigan, Ann Arbor, MI.)

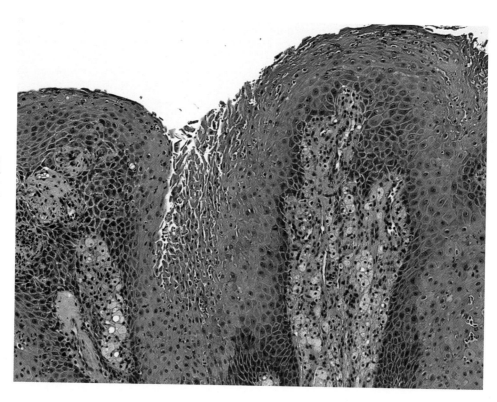

HIRSUTOID PAPILLOMA (PEARLY PENILE PAPULES)

Hirsutoid papillomas are common penile lesions without clinical significance and are present in approximately 20% to 30% of normal men. They most likely represent embryologic remnants of a copulative organ that is well developed in other mammals.

CLINICAL FEATURES

The characteristic lesions are yellow-white papules (1 to 3 mm in diameter), usually located on the corona, or rarely on the frenulum of the penis. The individual lesions are dome-like, resembling hair follicles, and are usually arranged in a row.

PATHOLOGIC FEATURES

Histologically, they show epithelial thickening associated with a central fibrovascular core (angiofibroma).

PROGNOSIS AND TREATMENT

They are not associated with any infectious agents, particularly HPV infection, have no potential for malignant transformation, and require no treatment. Psychological and cosmetic concerns often prompt patients to seek therapeutic removal of these lesions. Use of carbon dioxide laser has proven to be the most effective cosmetic treatment.

SCLEROSING LIPOGRANULOMA

A detailed clinicopathologic spectrum of sclerosing lipogranuloma is presented in the section on scrotum pathology.

DISEASES OF THE URETHRA

ANATOMY AND HISTOLOGY

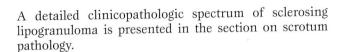

The dissimilarity in the spectrum of epithelial neoplasms between the female and the male urethra may be chiefly attributable to the distinct differences in anatomy and histology of the urethra in the two sexes (Tables 8-5 and 8-6). Both are discussed separately here.

FEMALE URETHRA

The female urethra is a conduit 2.5 to 4 cm long that is located between the urinary bladder proximally and the vulva distally. Frequently, for pathologic and prognostic considerations, the female urethra is subdivided roughly on the basis of histology into the proximal one third (posterior), which is lined by urothelium, and the distal two thirds (anterior), which is lined by stratified squamous epithelium. Patches of pseudostratified or stratified columnar epithelium may interrupt the squamous epithelium. Paraurethral glands in females (Skene glands) are believed to be homologs of prostatic tissue, as judged by their expression of prostate-specific antigen (PSA). The lamina propria is composed of loose fibroconnective tissue with many elastic fibers and

---

Table 8-5
Anatomic and Histologic Correlation of Urethral Carcinomas in Women

Region	Histology	Type of Carcinoma	Frequency (%)
Anterior (distal two-thirds of urethra)	Stratified squamous epithelium	Squamous carcinoma	70
Posterior (proximal third of urethra)	Urothelium Pseudostratified columnar epithelium	Urothelial Adenocarcinoma	20 10

Table 8-6
Anatomic and Histologic Correlation of Urethral Carcinomas in Men

Region	Histology	Type of Carcinoma (%)	Frequency (%)
Penile urethra	Stratified nonkeratinizing squamous epithelium Urothelium	Squamous (90) Urothelial (10)	34
Bulbomembranous urethra	Stratified/pseudostratified columnar epithelium	Squamous (82) Urothelial (8) Adenocarcinoma (8) Undifferentiated (2)	59
Prostatic urethra	Urothelium	Urothelial (86) Squamous (14)	7

Modified from Young RH, Srigley JR, Amin MB, et al: Tumors of the Prostate Gland, Seminal Vesicles, Male Urethra, and Penis. AFIP Atlas of Tumor Pathology. Washington, DC, Armed Forces Institute of Pathology, 2000, p 367, Figure 8-1.

prominent venous channels. Muscularis propria has two layers in which smooth muscle is oriented concentrically.

MALE URETHRA

The male urethra is also subdivided into an anterior (distal) portion, consisting of the bulbous and penile segments, and a posterior (proximal) portion, comprising the prostatic and membranous segments. Tumors involving the bulbous and membranous urethra have similar features and are considered clinically together as bulbomembranous. The prostatic urethra is 3 to 4 cm long, originates at the bladder neck, and merges with the membranous urethra and the urogenital diaphragm. Paraurethral prostatic glands open along the urethra proximal to the verumontanum. The 2- to 2.5-cm membranous urethra is completely engulfed by muscle fibers as it traverses the urogenital diaphragm. The secretory ducts of Cowper's (bulbourethral) glands, a pair of tubuloalveolar glands, lie in the skeletal muscle of the urogenital diaphragm and enter in the posterior aspect of the bulbous urethra. The bulbous urethra is 3 to 4 cm long and merges with the penile urethra, which lies in the corpus spongiosum. The prostatic urethra is lined by urothelium, similar to the urinary bladder. The bulbomembranous and proximal portion of penile urethra is lined by stratified or pseudostratified columnar epithelium, whereas the distal penile urethra, including the fossa navicularis, is lined by stratified nonkeratinizing squamous epithelium. Occasional goblet cells may be dispersed throughout the penile urethra. The lamina propria is composed of loose connective tissue contain-ing occasional smooth muscle bundles. The membranous urethra is surrounded by striated muscle, whereas the penile urethra is enveloped by Buck's fascia containing the corpus spongiosum.

MALIGNANT NEOPLASMS

EPITHELIAL NEOPLASMS

Primary carcinomas of the urethra comprise less than 1% of all urothelial neoplasms. Although the spectrum of tumors occurring in the urethra is almost identical to that of bladder lesions (Table 8-7), urethral lesions also differ in several important respects. Epithelial tumors of the urethra are distinctly rare but are almost exclusively carcinomas; they are three to four times more common in women; a greater percentage are high-grade invasive tumors; a greater percentage are squamous cell carcinomas; there is a greater likelihood of high stage at the time of diagnosis; and they usually demonstrate poor prognosis. Urethral carcinomas occurring in men are strikingly different from those in women in clinical and pathologic features.

The cause of urethral carcinomas is not entirely clear, but there is a growing appreciation for the role of HPV infection in certain types. Squamous cell carcinoma of the urethra is associated with HPV infection in both female and male patients. High-risk HPV-16 or -18 is detected in up to 60% of urethral carcinomas in women. There is no convincing evidence for an association of urothelial carcinoma or adenocarcinoma with HPV.

Table 8-7

Histologic Classification of Carcinomas of the Urethra

1. Primary tumors
   A. Carcinomas
      1. Squamous cell carcinoma
      2. Urothelial (transitional cell) carcinoma
      3. Carcinoma in situ
         a. Primary
         b. Secondary
      4. Adenocarcinoma
         a. Clear cell carcinoma
         b. Non-clear cell carcinoma
            (1) Enteric
            (2) Colloid (mucinous) carcinoma
            (3) Signet-ring cell carcinoma
            (4) Adenocarcinoma, not otherwise specified (NOS)
            (5) Adenoid cystic carcinoma
      5. Others
         a. Undifferentiated carcinoma
         b. Adenosquamous carcinoma
         c. Mixed "cloacogenic" carcinoma
2. Secondary tumors

EPITHELIAL NEOPLASMS OF THE URETHRA—FACT SHEET

Definition

▶ A spectrum similar to urinary bladder, but almost all are exclusively carcinomas, with predilection for females

Incidence and Location

▶ Rare as pure urethral tumor
▶ Comprise about 1% of all urothelial neoplasms
▶ Tumors involving the distal urethra and meatus are most common
▶ Proximal urethral tumors are less common

Morbidity and Mortality

▶ Tumors involving the anterior urethra (distal urethra and meatus) do better than posterior urethral tumors (proximal one third of urethra); overall 5-year survival rate is 51% for anterior and 6-20% for posterior tumors

Gender, Race, and Age Distribution

▶ M/F ratio, 1:4
▶ Mean age, 60 years

Clinical Features

▶ Patients are typically postmenopausal women or men in their sixth or seventh decade
▶ Common presentations include vaginal or urethral bleeding, dysuria, urinary frequency or incontinence, urinary tract infection, and perineal mass or obstruction
▶ Urethral carcinomas may clinically mimic "caruncle"

Prognosis and Treatment

▶ The prognosis is relatively poor
▶ Tumors involving "anterior" urethra do better than "posterior" urethra tumors
▶ Usually need radical surgery
▶ Adjuvant chemotherapy and radiotherapy for advanced tumors

CLINICAL FEATURES

Urethral carcinomas typically occur in the postmenopausal female or male in sixth to seventh decade (male/female ratio, 1:4), with a mean age of 60 years. Sex has an effect on the frequency of different histologic types of carcinoma, with most adenocarcinomas occurring in women. The most common presentation includes vaginal or urethral bleeding, dysuria, urinary frequency and incontinence, urinary tract infection, and perineal mass or obstruction. Patients with an anterior urethral mass (distal urethra) usually present with a palpable mass. In men, painful erection, priapism, penile erosions, and sexual impotence are also frequently associated with anterior tumors.

Urethral carcinoma clinically may be confused with urethral caruncle or polyp. Therefore, caruncles should be removed early for pathologic examination.

PATHOLOGIC FEATURES

GROSS FINDINGS

Tumors involving the distal urethra and meatus are most common; they appear as exophytic, nodular, infiltrative or papillary lesions with frequent ulcerations. Tumors involving the proximal urethra that are urothelial in differentiation exhibit the gross diversity of bladder neoplasia: papillary or nodular, flat or ulcerative. Adenocarcinomas are often large infiltrative or expansile neoplasms with a variable surface exophytic component and are mucinous, gelatinous, or cystic in consistency.

MICROSCOPIC FINDINGS

The pathology of the carcinoma usually depends on the location of the tumor along the urethral tract (see Tables 8-5 and 8-6). The tumors of the distal urethra/ meatus are squamous cell carcinomas (70%), and tumors of the proximal urethra are urothelial carcinoma (20%) or adenocarcinoma (10%). In men, the majority of carcinomas arise in bulbomembranous urethra (59%) or penile urethra (34%) and are usually squamous carcinomas; the remaining lesions arise in the prostatic urethra (7%) are mostly urothelial carcinomas.

Squamous cell carcinomas: Squamous carcinomas are the most common urethral carcinomas in both male and female patients. They range from well-differentiated types, including rare verrucous carcinoma, to moderately differentiated and poorly differentiated lesions. Most squamous carcinomas are moderately differentiated and deeply infiltrative at the time of presentation.

EPITHELIAL NEOPLASMS OF THE URETHRA—PATHOLOGIC FEATURES

Gross Findings

▶ Tumors involving the distal urethra and meatus grossly appear as exophytic nodular, infiltrative, or papillary lesions with frequent ulcerations

▶ Tumors involving the proximal urethra are usually urothelial and exhibit macroscopic diversity of papillary or nodular, flat or ulcerative lesions

Microscopic Findings

▶ Majority are squamous carcinomas (70%), followed by urothelial carcinomas (20%) and adenocarcinomas (10%), although other types may occur rarely

▶ The histologic subtype varies with the location

▶ Distal urethral tumors are usually squamous carcinoma in both sexes, whereas proximal tumors tend to be urothelial carcinomas or adenocarcinomas

▶ Most adenocarcinomas occur in women

Immunohistochemistry

▶ Enteric type adenocarcinoma positive for CDX2, CK20, negative for CK7 and β-catenin

Differential Diagnosis

▶ Prostate type adenocarcinoma with ductal features in men

▶ Nephrogenic adenoma if clear cell adenocarcinoma is in the differential diagnosis

▶ Clear cell adenocarcinoma versus adenocarcinoma, NOS type

▶ Melanoma for poorly differentiated carcinomas

Urothelial (transitional cell) carcinomas: The second most common urethral carcinomas, urothelial carcinomas, may exhibit the same diversity of presentation as they do in urinary bladder, which includes noninvasive, papillary tumors (papilloma, neoplasm of low malignant potential, low grade and high grade carcinoma, flat CIS, and invasive carcinoma). Most are carcinomas that secondarily involve the urethra after bladder cancer or as part of multifocal urinary tract tumors. Invasive carcinomas are usually high-grade, with or without a papillary component, and are characterized by a desmoplastic and/or inflammatory response. Tumors may exhibit variable squamous and/or glandular differentiation. Rarely, urothelial carcinoma can have an uncommon morphology, including nested, microcystic, micropapillary, clear cell, and plasmacytoid differentiation. Small cell and sarcomatoid differentiation is extremely uncommon. Tumors involving the paraurethral glands or prostatic ducts may mimic invasive disease. Prostatic duct involvement should be distinguished from that involving the prostatic stroma, because the latter indicates a much worse prognosis.

Adenocarcinoma: Adenocarcinoma involving the urethra can be broadly divided into clear cell adenocarcinoma (40%) and non-clear cell adenocarcinoma (60%). The non-clear cell adenocarcinomas can demonstrate myriad growth patterns, including enteric, mucinous, and signet-ring cell types; adenocarcinoma, NOS; and adenoid cystic carcinoma. Adenocarcinomas are thought to arise from the paraurethral glands or through a metaplastic process of the surface epithelium.

Clear cell adenocarcinoma is of special interest because of its unique propensity to involve the urethra and its exclusive occurrence in women. These tumors usually arise in paraurethral glands or urethral diverticulum. The microscopic features are distinctive. Tumor is composed of sheets of tubules and papillae lined by uniform ovoid cells with clear to eosinophilic cytoplasm and well-defined cytoplasmic borders. Cells lining the tubules often have a "hobnail" appearance. Pleomorphism is frequently noted, with areas of necrosis. Mitoses are readily found. Tumor usually infiltrates deep into the soft tissues (Fig. 8-23).

ANCILLARY STUDIES

Enteric-type adenocarcinomas are usually negative for CK7 and β-catenin and positive for CK20 and CDX2. Clear cell adenocarcinomas are positive for CEA, CA-125, and CK7 and usually negative for PSA, prostate-specific acid phosphatase (PSAP), and CK20.

DIFFERENTIAL DIAGNOSIS

The differential diagnosis of most primary urethral tumors follows the guidelines established for bladder

---

CLEAR CELL ADENOCARCINOMA—FACT SHEET

Definition

▶ Subtype of adenocarcinoma with distinctive histologic features and propensity to involve exclusively the urethra of female patients

Incidence and Location

▶ Relatively rare tumor

▶ Most frequent in women, in whom they may arise in paraurethral glands or diverticulum

Gender, Race, and Age Distribution

▶ Age range, 22 to 83 years (mean, 57 years)

▶ Almost all female patients

Clinical Features

▶ Gross hematuria, dysuria, suprapubic pain, and discharge are the usual presenting features

Prognosis and Treatment

▶ Mixed prognosis

▶ It is not uniformly unfavorable as initially proposed

▶ Metastasis is reported in up to 15% of patients, with death from disease reported in 25-30%

▶ Most patients require radical surgery

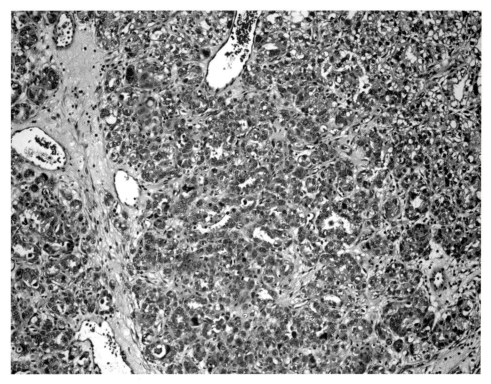

FIGURE 8-23

In clear cell adenocarcinoma, there is a crowded proliferation of small tubules and glands with granular to focally clear cytoplasm. The growth pattern resembles nephrogenic adenoma, but there is an obvious cytologic pleomorphism.

neoplasms and usually does not present significant diagnostic problems.

In male patients, prostatic adenocarcinoma, particularly with ductal differentiation, may manifest as a intraurethral mass and therefore should always be included in the differential diagnosis of urethral adenocarcinoma and papillary urothelial carcinoma. Centrally occurring ductal carcinomas have an epicenter in the urethral region and display an exuberant papillary/ tubular growth, characterized by papillary fronds lined by tumor cells ranging from single-layer to stratified tall columnar epithelium (Fig. 8-24). Prostatic ductal carcinomas are positive for PSA and PSAP, a diagnostically useful profile. Primary urethral adenocarcinomas with villoglandular growth pattern and papillary urothelial carcinoma are negative for PSA and PSAP. In our recent experience, a panel of PSA, high-molecular weight cytokeratin (clone 34BE12), and/or p63 antibodies was optimal to differentiate poorly differentiated prostate adenocarcinoma from urothelial carcinoma. Enteric-type primary adenocarcinoma closely mimics metastatic colon cancer both morphologically and immunophenotypically. Recently, β-catenin has been reported to be of help in separating these tumors. Adenocarcinomas also should be distinguished from the common adenosquamous carcinomas and urothelial carcinoma demonstrating glandular differentiation. Clear cell adenocarcinoma must be differentiated from other types of adenocarcinoma, nephrogenic adenoma, urothelial carcinoma with clear cell features, and metastatic carcinoma, in particular from renal cell carcinoma and prostate adenocarcinoma in men. The histologic pattern of small tubules, papillae, and sheets, frequently lined

by hobnail-type cells without significant intraluminal mucin, distinguishes them from other adenocarcinomas. Nephrogenic adenoma is histologically similar to clear cell adenocarcinoma, but the presence of necrosis, cellular anaplasia, and infiltration into deeper portions separates the latter from nephrogenic adenoma. The presence of thick, hyalinized basement membrane-type material favors the diagnosis of nephrogenic adenoma.

CLEAR CELL ADENOCARCINOMA—PATHOLOGIC FEATURES

Gross Findings
► Polypoid mass

Microscopic Findings
► Sheets of tubules and papillae lined by uniform cells with clear to eosinophilic cytoplasm
► Hobnailing common
► Cytologic atypia, mitoses, and necrosis frequent

Immunohistochemical Features
► Cytokeratin, CA-125, and CEA are positive; PSA and PSAP are negative

Differential Diagnosis
► Nephrogenic adenoma
► Prostate adenocarcinoma in male patient
► Adenocarcinoma, NOS type
► Metastatic renal cell carcinoma

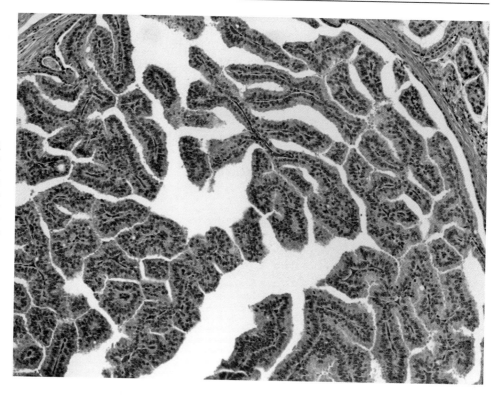

FIGURE 8-24

Prostate adenocarcinoma with ductal features. Polypoid mass with an epicenter at prostatic urethra demonstrates papillae, lined by tumor cells ranging from a single layer to pseudostratified columnar epithelium. This growth pattern may be confused with papillary urothelial carcinoma or adenocarcinoma, NOS type.

Clear cell adenocarcinomas are extremely unusual in men and are usually negative for PSA and PSAP and positive for CEA. Rare immunostaining of clear cell adenocarcinoma for PSA and PSAP has been reported, although recent studies have consistently demonstrated negativity for these antigens. The distinction from metastatic renal carcinoma especially may be difficult on histologic grounds alone. Clinical and radiographic studies may aid in selected cases.

PROGNOSIS AND TREATMENT

There is a separate TNM staging system for tumors of the urethra (Table 8-8), as well as the system proposed by Grabstald. The prognosis of urethral carcinomas is relatively poor except when disease is diagnosed in the early stages and treated aggressively. Grabstald described the tumors as being either "anterior" (limited to the meatus or distal third of the urethra) or "posterior and/or entire" (i.e., tumor involving the entire urethra or the proximal two thirds of the urethra). Tumors restricted to the anterior urethra are more amenable to localized surgery with more favorable outcome than are tumors of the posterior or entire urethra, which require radical surgery and have a poor prognosis. The overall 5-year survival rate for anterior urethral tumors is 51%, compared with 6% for posterior tumors in female patients.

As with female urethral carcinomas, the prognosis for anterior tumors occurring in men is considerably better than for posterior tumors. The difference in prognosis is related to earlier diagnosis and greater amenability to penile amputation. The 5-year survival rate for anterior tumors is approximately 50%, versus 20% for the posterior tumors. Tumors of the anterior urethra typically metastasize to inguinal and external iliac lymph nodes, whereas posterior tumors spread to internal iliac and hypogastric lymph nodes.

In localized, noninvasive carcinoma of the distal (anterior) urethra, partial urethrectomy may be adequate. In advanced cases, after local excision and lymphadenectomy, adjuvant chemotherapy seems to be beneficial. The proximal urethral tumors are best treated by the combined treatment modality of surgery and radiotherapy/chemotherapy.

UROTHELIAL CARCINOMA IN SITU

CIS rarely occurs as a primary urethral neoplasm, but it has been documented in about 10% of urethras after cystoprostatectomy for bladder cancer, when the urethra was left in situ.

CLINICAL FEATURES

Patients present with hematuria, dysuria, or urinary frequency. However, some patients are detected through regular cytology screening after surgery, and not because of symptoms.

Table 8-8

Staging of Urethra Neoplasms: American Joint Committee on Cancer

T, M, or N Stage	Description
TX	Primary tumor cannot be assessed
T0	No tumor
Ta	Noninvasive tumor (papillary, polypoid, verrucous)
Tis	Carcinoma in situ
T1	Invasion of subepithelial connective tissue
T2	Invasion of: Corpus spongiosum Periurethral muscle Prostate gland
T3	Invasion of: Corpus cavernosum Extraprostatic tissue Anterior vagina Bladder neck
T4	Invasion of other adjacent organs
NX	Regional lymph nodes cannot be assessed
N0	No regional lymph node metastases
N1	One nodal metastasis, ≤2.0 cm
N2	Multiple nodal metastases or one metastasis, >2.0 cm
MX	Distant metastases cannot be assessed
M0	No distant metastases
M1	Distant metastases

Adapted from Greene FL, Page DL, Fleming ID, Fritz A, et al. (eds): AJCC Cancer Staging Manual, 6th ed. New York, Springer; 2002, pp 341–346.

PATHOLOGIC FEATURES

GROSS FINDINGS

CIS usually appears as a flat, erythematous, velvety lesion.

MICROSCOPIC FINDINGS

Histologically, CIS may manifest with several growth patterns, similar to what is seen in the urinary bladder. Most often, large pleomorphic cells with a high nuclear/cytoplasmic ratio, thick homogeneous eosinophilic cytoplasm, irregular nuclear membranes, and lumpy chromatin are arranged over discrete or full-thickness areas of the urothelium. Full-thickness atypia is not necessary for the diagnosis, and, similarly, CIS cells may not always demonstrate high nuclear/cytoplasmic ratio.

UROTHELIAL CARCINOMA IN SITU, URETHRA—FACT SHEET

Definition
▶ Urothelial CIS involving the urethra

Incidence and Location
▶ Rare as primary urethral neoplasm, but can be seen in 10% of cases with bladder cancer or as part of multifocal urinary tract neoplasms
▶ May involve any part of the urethra

Morbidity and Mortality
▶ Involvement of urethra by CIS in patients with bladder cancer significantly increases the chances of disease relapse

Gender, Race, and Age Distribution
▶ Equal distribution for both sexes, similar to bladder cancer

Clinical Features
▶ Gross hematuria or as a part of palpable mass
▶ Sometimes asymptomatic and detected through regular cytology screening after radical cystectomy

Prognosis and Treatment
▶ Prognosis is worse for bladder cancer patients having CIS in the urethra and prostatic ducts, with high chances of disease relapse
▶ May necessitate radical surgery including total urethrectomy

CIS demonstrating pagetoid (Fig. 8-25) and denuding growth patterns are important to recognize, because they often remain underdiagnosed.

DIFFERENTIAL DIAGNOSIS

In patients with CIS of the urethra, an important diagnostic pitfall is the involvement of urethral glands or prostatic glands, mimicking invasion (Fig. 8-26). Therefore, diagnosis of invasion should be made using strict criteria, as for urinary bladder carcinomas. Reactive or therapy-induced atypia may also mimic CIS. The diagnosis of CIS should be made using strict cytologic features. In some difficult cases, immunohistochemical stains for CK20, p53, and CD44 may provide an objective support for urothelial CIS.

PROGNOSIS AND TREATMENT

Involvement of urethra by CIS is an adverse risk factor in the management of urothelial carcinoma and may necessitate urethrectomy in resistant cases. CIS of the prostatic urethra, particularly involving the margin of resection, is associated with an increased risk of disease

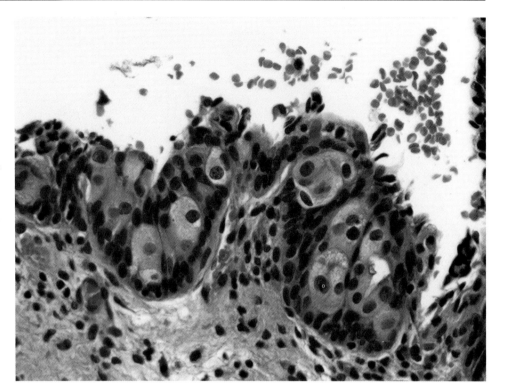

FIGURE 8-25

Urothelial carcinoma in situ (CIS) of the urethra. Large atypical cells with abundant vacuolated cytoplasm are present scattered within the urothelium. This pagetoid growth pattern is important to recognize to avoid underdiagnosis of CIS.

UROTHELIAL CARCINOMA IN SITU—PATHOLOGIC FEATURES

Gross Findings

▶ Red velvety lesions

Microscopic Findings

▶ Similar to spectrum seen in the urinary bladder
▶ Denuding and pagetoid forms of CIS are important morphologic variations to recognize
▶ Involvement of peraurethral glands and prostate glands may mimic invasion

Immunohistochemical Features

▶ In selected cases CK20, p53, and/or CD44 markers may be a useful panel to differentiate urothelial CIS from reactive/therapy-induced atypia

Differential Diagnosis

▶ Reactive/therapy-induced atypia

---

recurrence and may be an indication for total urethrectomy. If the entire urethra is not removed at the time of radical surgery, pathologic evaluation of the resected portion is essential to assess CIS in the urethra, prostatic ducts, or the grossly uninvolved bladder mucosa.

Because of its clinical significance, patients treated with cystectomy or cystoprostatectomy need to undergo lengthy follow-up for recurrence. The best current method for monitoring the penile urethra after cystoprostatectomy is urethral wash cytopathology. The

tumor cells in urethral washings may appear poorly preserved, but they can be distinguished by their eccentric nuclei, high nuclear/cytoplasmic ratio, pleomorphism, and granular chromatin (Fig. 8-27). The presence of neoplastic cells in specimens obtained at periodic intervals from asymptomatic patients signals the presence of disease. Considering the major surgery that may be provoked by a positive urethral wash interpretation, a conservative approach to pathologic diagnosis is warranted.

MALIGNANT MELANOMA

The urethra is the most common site of primary melanoma in the genitourinary tract. Melanomas are more common in women than in men. In men, the distal urethra is the most common site. Clinically, patients present with a polypoid or ulcerated mass that may mimic urethral caruncles. The pathology does not differ from melanoma at other sites of the body, except that significant proportions of the tumors are amelanotic and tend to be spindled. More than half are amelanotic and hence potentially serious mimics of carcinoma (Fig. 8-28). The presence of mixed epithelioid and spindle morphology or high-grade pleomorphic nuclei and the absence of CIS may raise the suspicion for malignant melanoma. Pagetoid growth also occurs on the surface. Immunohistochemical stains for S-100, melan A, HMB-45, and the cytokeratin profile establish the diagnosis in difficult cases. Most urethral melanomas

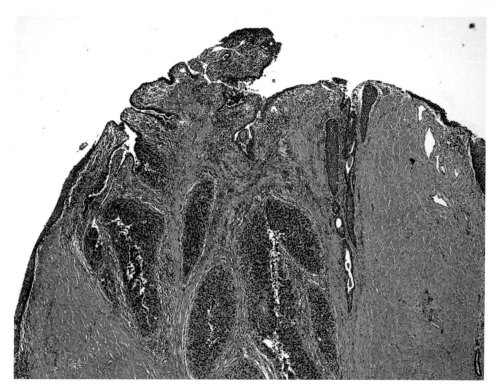

FIGURE 8-26

Urothelial carcinoma in situ (CIS) with spread to urethral glands. CIS of the urethra with spread of the tumor cells into the periurethral glands. This growth pattern should not be misinterpreted as invasion.

FIGURE 8-27

Urothelial carcinoma in situ. Urothelial cells demonstrate a high nuclear/cytoplasmic ratio, eccentric nuclei, hyperchromatism, and irregular nuclear membranes. (Courtesy of Robert Pu, University of Michigan, Ann Arbor, MI.)

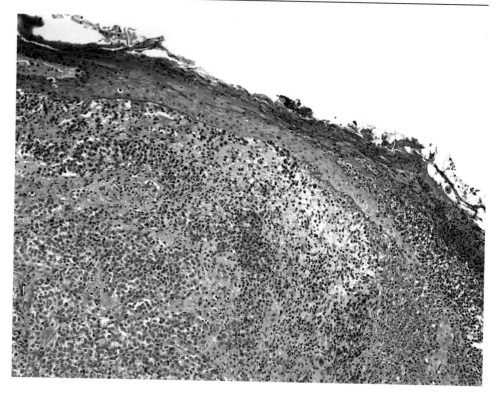

FIGURE 8-28

Malignant melanoma of the urethra. Low-power view demonstrates an ulcerated mucosa with proliferation of nests of epithelioid tumor cells without pigment. This feature may be confused with carcinoma. (Courtesy of Anuradha Radhakrishman, Emory University Hospital, Atlanta, GA.)

are localized at the time of diagnosis, although the prognosis is usually poor, with few patients surviving longer than 5 years after diagnosis.

BENIGN TUMORS

UROTHELIAL PAPILLOMAS

Both typical and inverted types of urothelial papillomas can occur in the urethra, and they account for a subset of urethral "polyps." The typical urothelial papilloma is small and solitary, with delicate, finger-like papillae lined by cytologically and architecturally normal urothelium with normal maturation, intact superficial umbrella cells, and no mitotic figures. They are usually seen in patients younger than 50 years of age. The diagnosis should be based strictly on these criteria. These are benign tumors with rare recurrence.

VILLOUS ADENOMA

Villous adenomas arising in the urethra are rare and usually represent a form of recurrence of villous adenoma occurring in the urinary bladder or ureter. A single example of this lesion occurring in the pure form has been reported in the male urethra. The lesions appear similar to the typical colonic lesion (Fig. 8-29). Coexisting in situ or infiltrating adenocarcinoma can be seen, and therefore the diagnosis should be made cautiously and only after the lesion has been entirely resected and examined. Pure villous adenoma without associated invasive carcinoma or CIS portends a favorable prognosis. Villous adenoma of the urethra associated with tubulovillous adenoma and adenocarcinoma of the rectum has also been reported.

Tumor-Like Conditions

URETHRAL CARUNCLE

The term "caruncle" is by convention restricted to a relatively common distal urethral polypoid lesion of women that microscopically exhibits inflammation of the lamina propria.

CLINICAL FEATURES

Patients are usually postmenopausal women who complain of dysuria and spotting. Clinically, caruncles appear as polypoid lesions at the meatus. Rarely, an essentially similar lesion may be seen in the distal male urethra.

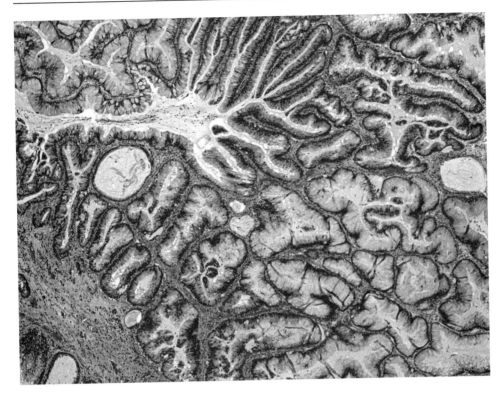

FIGURE 8-29
Villous adenoma. Polypoid lesion demonstrates tubules and papillae lined by dysplastic cells containing tall columnar epithelium with abundant mucin, histologic features similar to those seen in colon.

PATHOLOGIC FEATURES

GROSS FINDINGS

Grossly, urethral caruncles are nodular or pedunculated lesions.

MICROSCOPIC FINDINGS

Microscopically, caruncles are composed of a nodular proliferation of polymorphous inflammatory infiltrate within the lamina propria, rich in lymphocytes and small blood vessels, mimicking granulation tissue (Fig. 8-30). Epithelial hyperplasia and metaplasia may occur.

DIFFERENTIAL DIAGNOSIS

The clinical background and bland cytologic features of the lesional cells should facilitate the correct interpretation in most cases. Frequently, urethral carcinoma or metastatic carcinoma may mimic caruncle. Histologic examination in these cases correctly establishes the diagnosis.

If the epithelial hyperplasia is exuberant and finger-like, it can be confused with carcinoma. In such cases,

---

URETHRAL CARUNCLE—FACT SHEET

Definition
▶ A relatively common distal urethral polypoid lesion of women that microscopically exhibits inflammation of lamina propria

Incidence and Location
▶ Common lesion
▶ Distal urethra (meatus)

Morbidity and Mortality
▶ Benign condition

Gender, Race, and Age Distribution
▶ Almost exclusively affects women of postmenopausal age

Clinical Features
▶ Postmenopausal women who complain of dysuria and spotting
▶ Manifests as a polypoid mass at the urethral opening
▶ Urethral carcinoma or metastatic carcinoma may clinically mimic urethral caruncle

Prognosis and Treatment
▶ Excellent
▶ Surgical excision treatment of choice

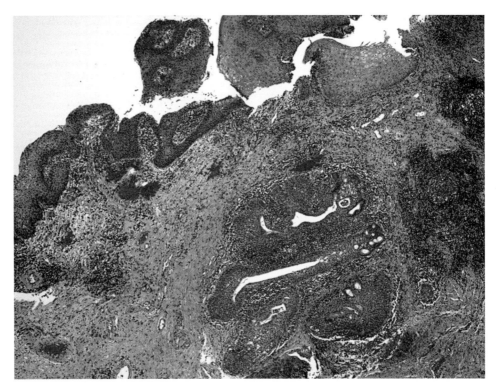

FIGURE 8-30

Caruncle. Low-power view demonstrates polypoid lesion lined by stratified squamous epithelium with collection of chronic inflammation within lamina propria.

URETHRAL CARUNCLE—PATHOLOGIC FEATURES

Gross Findings
▶ Nodular or pedunculated lesions of urethra

Microscopic Findings
▶ Dense polymorphous infiltrate in the lamina propria, rich in lymphocytes and small blood vessels, mimicking granulation tissue
▶ Epithelial hyperplasia and metaplasia may occur
▶ Infrequently, stromal cells may show prominent atypia

Immunohistochemical Features
▶ Rarely needed

Differential Diagnosis
▶ Carcinoma
▶ Sarcoma in cases with prominent stromal atypia

---

islands of epithelium may seem to be deep in the lamina propria. However, the nests maintain their cytologic organization and lack significant cellular atypia. Infrequently, stromal cells of caruncle may show prominent atypia and be confused for sarcoma or lymphoma. The atypical cells represent a variant of the atypical mesenchymal cell seen relatively commonly in the lower female genital tract. Awareness of this phenomenon, its microscopic nature, and the lack of significant mitotic activity should help avoid the erroneous diagnosis of malignant tumor.

NEPHROGENIC ADENOMA

Nephrogenic adenoma is a metaplastic process of the urothelium that may occur anywhere along the urinary system. Recently, it has been postulated that nephrogenic adenoma in renal transplant patients originate from the renal tubular epithelium. They are commonly associated with a history of genitourinary trauma, surgical resection, calculi, or renal transplantation.

CLINICAL FEATURES

Approximately 10% of nephrogenic adenomas occur in the urethra. In men, they commonly involve the bulbous or, more often, the prostatic urethra. In women, they are more frequently associated with urethral diverticulum. Hematuria is a common presentation.

PATHOLOGIC FEATURES

GROSS FINDINGS

Nephrogenic adenomas are small, papillary, polypoid, or sessile lesions, and approximately 18% are multiple.

NEPHROGENIC ADENOMA, URETHRA—FACT SHEET

Definition
▶ Metaplasia of the urothelium, similar to that seen in bladder

Incidence and Location
▶ Approximately 10% of nephrogenic adenomas occur in the urethra
▶ In men, it commonly involves either the bulbous or prostatic urethra
▶ In women, it is frequently associated with urethral diverticulum

Morbidity and Mortality
▶ Benign condition

Gender, Race, and Age Distribution
▶ Seen in both sexes, common in elder population

Clinical Features
▶ Patients may present with hematuria, usually with a history of transurethral resection, trauma, stones, or transplantation

Prognosis and Treatment
▶ Benign metaplastic condition
▶ No known or proven association with cancer

MICROSCOPIC FINDINGS

Microscopic examination shows proliferation of single or combinations of tubules, and papillae lined by cuboidal nonstratified cells that have scant clear to eosinophilic cytoplasm. Focal atypia may be seen but is degenerative in nature. Mitoses are absent or rare. Tubules are frequently surrounded by PAS-positive, thick, hyalinized basement membrane. Background inflammation is common. The process is usually superficial and limited to the lamina propria (Fig. 8-31).

ANCILLARY STUDIES

IMMUNOHISTOCHEMISTRY

Nephrogenic adenomas are negative for PSA and PSAP, and significant proportions are positive for α-methylacyl-coenzyme A racemase (AMACR). Recently, PAX2, a renal transcription factor marker, has been reported to be positive in both transplant related and not-related nephrogenic adenomas.

DIFFERENTIAL DIAGNOSIS

The major differential diagnoses include clear cell adenocarcinoma, particularly in female patients. Clear cell adenocarcinoma tends to show frank cytologic atypia, with frequent necrosis. Invasion of the deeper soft tissue is common. The presence of thick hyalinized basement membrane material favors nephrogenic adenoma. In men, prostate adenocarcinoma is a major diagnostic problem. A significant proportion of nephrogenic adenomas involving the prostatic urethra are posi-

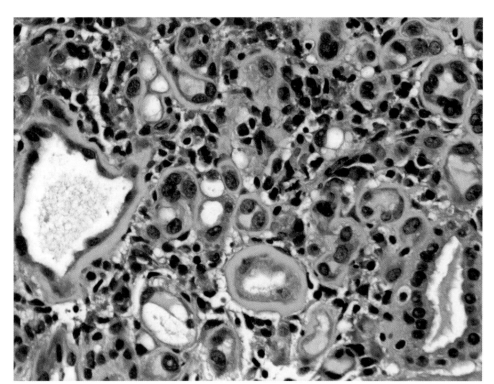

FIGURE 8-31

Nephrogenic adenoma. High-power view demonstrates proliferation of characteristic small- to medium-sized tubules with thick hyalinized basement membrane surrounding them. Cells lining the tubules are cuboidal and lack cytologic atypia.

NEPHROGENIC ADENOMA, URETHRA—PATHOLOGIC FEATURES

Gross Findings

▶ Small, 2- to 4-mm, polypoid mucosal lesions

Microscopic Findings

▶ Spectrum of papillary, tubular, and cystic growth patterns
▶ Tubules and papillae lined by cuboidal cells with clear or eosinophilic cytoplasm and small, discrete nuclei
▶ Process limited within mucosa
▶ The tubules surrounded by a thickened and hyalinized basement membrane
▶ Background inflammation is common

Immunohistochemical Features

▶ PSA and PSAP negative, CEA negative, P504S (monoclonal antibody to AMACR) marker used for prostate carcinoma positive in significant proportion of cases and PAX2, a renal transcription factor marker also has been reported to be positive in majority of cases

Differential Diagnosis

▶ Prostate adenocarcinoma
▶ Clear cell adenocarcinoma
▶ Adenocarcinoma, NOS type
▶ Papillary urothelial carcinoma

---

tive for α-methylacyl-coenzyme A racemase (AMACR), a biomarker increasingly used in the workup of prostate cancer diagnosis. Nephrogenic adenomas are negative for PSA and PSAP; these tests, along with the morphology, would be the best approach to resolve the diagnosis in such situations.

Nephrogenic adenoma with a predominant papillary component may also be confused with low-grade papillary urothelial neoplasm. The presence of non-stratified cuboidal lining epithelium would favor the diagnosis of nephrogenic adenoma over the urothelial neoplasm.

PROGNOSIS AND TREATMENT

Nephrogenic adenomas are not typically considered to be a precursor lesion. Recently, one study has demonstrated molecular evidence for progression of nephrogenic adenoma to clear cell adenocarcinoma.

POLYPOID URETHRITIS

Polypoid urethritis is similar to papillary-polypoid cystitis. The urethral variant is more common. Papillae have abundant edematous stroma without well-developed fibrovascular cores. Background inflammation is com-

mon. The common differential diagnosis is papillary urothelial neoplasm.

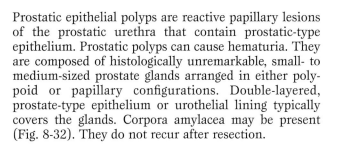

PROSTATIC EPITHELIAL POLYP

Prostatic epithelial polyps are reactive papillary lesions of the prostatic urethra that contain prostatic-type epithelium. Prostatic polyps can cause hematuria. They are composed of histologically unremarkable, small- to medium-sized prostate glands arranged in either polypoid or papillary configurations. Double-layered, prostate-type epithelium or urothelial lining typically covers the glands. Corpora amylacea may be present (Fig. 8-32). They do not recur after resection.

CONDYLOMA

The urethra is usually involved by direct extension from lesions arising at adjacent sites, but primary urethral condyloma can occur. Evidence of HPV infection is demonstrated in almost all cases. HPV types 6 and 11 are the most common types identified. Condylomas of the urethra are especially common in men in whom they may account for 30% of tumor-like lesions. Most patients are sexually active, ages 20 to 40 years. Multiplicity and reactivation of infection are common. The pathologic features of condyloma do not differ from those occurring in common other genital sites. They may manifest as papillary or flat lesions.

DISEASES OF THE SCROTUM

Malignant Epithelial Tumors

SQUAMOUS CELL CARCINOMA

The incidence of squamous cell carcinoma, the most common malignant tumor of the scrotum, has dramatically decreased over the past half-century. Now, these tumors are extraordinarily infrequent; recent large series from tertiary care centers in the United States, including Memorial Sloan-Kettering Cancer Center, Mayo Clinic, and Johns Hopkins Hospital, all averaged only 1 patient every 2 to 3 years. This tumor is of great historical interest, however, because it was the first cancer to be directly linked to exposure to occupational carcinogens. Numerous industrial and occupational carcinogens have been linked to development of this tumor; for example, it was a common occurrence among chimney workers. Excluding cases with occupational exposure to carcinogens, social class is an important

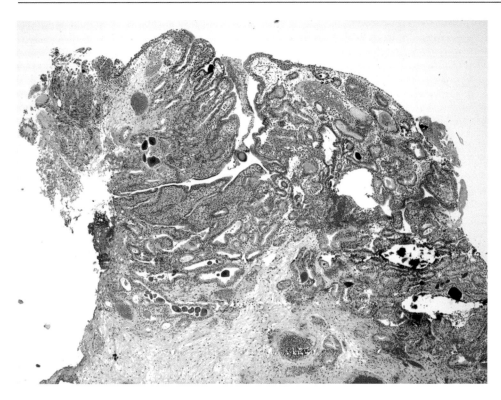

FIGURE 8-32
Prostatic epithelial polyp. Polypoid lesion containing crowded collection of small- and medium-sized prostatic-type glands. Surface is lined by the urothelium, and glands contain brown to orange corpora amylacea secretions.

predisposing factor. Disease is very infrequent in blacks. More recently, PUVA treatments have been shown to be associated with male genital malignancies. The risk to genitalia (penis and scrotum) for development of squamous cell carcinoma is 5 to 15 times greater than for other parts of the body at similar dosage levels of exposure. This risk is dose dependent. Another risk factor is HPV infection; of 14 cases of scrotal cancer with long-term follow-up from the Mayo Clinic files, 45% had documented HPV infection. Currently, most cases reported in the United States are not associated with any occupational exposure. Lowe reviewed in detail the epidemiologic and etiologic factors of scrotal cancer.

CLINICAL FEATURES

Squamous cell carcinoma is usually a solitary lesion affecting men in their 50s (range, 51 to 60 years) in major reported series. In patients with occupational exposure, the left side and anterolateral aspect of the scrotum are more commonly involved; this proclivity for side is not significant when cases with occupational exposure are excluded.

The lesion presents as slow-growing nodules, "warts," or pimples that persist for several months before ulcerating. At the time of the presentation, most are ulcerated, with rolled edges and an indurated base. Advanced lesions show invasion of the testis or penis.

Approximately 50% of the patients have palpable ipsilateral inguinal lymphadenopathy at presentation.

PATHOLOGIC FEATURES

GROSS FINDINGS

Grossly, the tumors range from nodules to an ulcerated mass with heaped-up edges and an indurated base.

MICROSCOPIC FINDINGS

The tumor is usually well to moderately differentiated, keratinizing, and identical to conventional cutaneous squamous cell carcinoma. Rare variants such as verrucous carcinoma have been reported. The epidermis adjacent to the ulcerated neoplasm may show dysplastic changes and is frequently acanthotic with hyperkeratosis. Squamous cell CIS (Bowen disease) accounted for 6 of 14 cases in one series; HPV infection was identified in 4 of these cases. The tumor may be heavily pigmented.

DIFFERENTIAL DIAGNOSIS

The clinical differential diagnosis is wide and comprises a variety of lesions, including epidermoid cysts, nevus,

SQUAMOUS CELL CARCINOMA, SCROTUM—FACT SHEET

Definition

▶ Most common malignant neoplasm of the scrotum; incidence has dramatically decreased over the past half-century due to elimination of exposures to occupational hazards

Incidence and Location

▶ Now extraordinarily infrequent in Western world
▶ One patient every 2 to 3 years reported from large cancer centers
▶ May involve left side and anterolateral aspect of the scrotum in patients with a history of occupational hazards; no such association without history

Morbidity and Mortality

▶ Data regarding survival are limited, but overall outcome is poor for invasive cancers
▶ Reported survival rates vary from 56-67% at 2 years and from 22-52% at 5 years

Gender, Race, and Age Distribution

▶ Men in their 50s (range, 51-60 years)
▶ Rare in black men

Clinical Features

▶ Patient presents with slow-growing nodules or pimples, resembling "warts," which persist for several months before ulcerating
▶ At presentation, most are ulcerated with rolled edges
▶ Advanced lesions may show invasion of penis or testis
▶ Fifty percent of patients present with palpable ipsilateral inguinal lymphadenopathy

Prognosis and Treatment

▶ Overall prognosis is poor for invasive cancers and is based on the extent of local disease and metastasis. Patients may require total scrotectomy.

SQUAMOUS CELL CARCINOMA, SCROTUM—PATHOLOGIC FEATURES

Gross Findings

▶ Nodule or ulcerated mass with rolled edges and indurated base
▶ Sectioning may demonstrate invasion of penis and testis in advanced lesions

Microscopic Findings

▶ The tumor is usually well to moderately differentiated, keratinizing, and identical to conventional cutaneous squamous cell carcinoma
▶ Rare variants include verrucous carcinoma
▶ Adjacent epidermis may show dysplastic or in situ changes
▶ HPV-related koilocytic changes may be seen

Differential Diagnosis

▶ Clinically may mimic many conditions, including epidermoid cysts, Paget disease, basal cell carcinoma, malignant melanoma, and sarcoma
▶ Usually easily distinguishable on pathologic examination

Table 8-9

Staging System for Scrotal Carcinoma

Stage	Description
A1	Disease localized to the scrotum
A2	Locally extensive tumor invading adjacent structures such as testis, spermatic cord, penis, pubic bone, and perineum
B	Metastatic disease involving inguinal lymph nodes only
C	Metastatic disease involving pelvic lymph nodes without evidence of distant spread
D	Metastasis beyond the pelvic lymph nodes, to involve distant organs

From Lowe FC: Squamous cell carcinoma of the scrotum.
J Urol 1983;130:423–427.

tuberculosis, and other malignant tumors such as basal cell carcinoma, malignant melanoma, Paget disease, and sarcoma. These entities are easily distinguishable on microscopic examination.

PROGNOSIS AND TREATMENT

The significance of histologic grade is uncertain because very few cases have been analyzed. The most commonly used staging system is Lowe's modification of the system proposed by Ray and Whitmore. It is based on the extent of local disease and the level of metastasis (Table 8-9). Data regarding survival are limited, but overall outcome is poor for invasive carcinoma. The survival rates in reported series vary from 67% to 56% at 2 years and 22% to 52% at 5 years. Surgery is the preferred treatment.

EXTRAMAMMARY PAGET DISEASE OF PENIS AND SCROTUM

CLINICAL FEATURES

Clinically, patients present with red, thick plaques with scaling or oozing (Fig. 8-33). The lesion may be clinically misdiagnosed as eczema or dermatitis, delaying therapy.

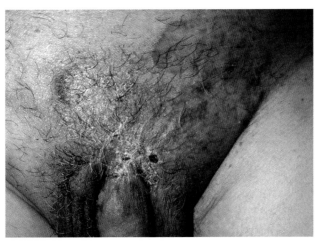

FIGURE 8-33

Extramammary Paget disease of scrotum. An irregular eczematous, scaly, erythematous lesion involves the scrotum and a portion of the penis, extending to other parts of the genital skin. (Courtesy of Lori Lowe, University of Michigan, Ann Arbor, MI.)

As in mammary Paget disease, the lesion in the scrotum and genital area may be a consequence of epidermotropic spread from an underlying colorectal, urogenital, or cutaneous adnexal malignancy. Many patients have synchronous or metachronous visceral malignancy. However, an underlying malignancy is not identified in many cases, and some view it as an epidermotropic spread from an underlying apocrine adnexal adenocarcinoma.

PATHOLOGIC FEATURES

GROSS FINDINGS

The lesion appears as an erythematous or eczematous scaly lesion.

MICROSCOPIC FINDINGS

There is an intraepithelial proliferation of large atypical cells with an abundant pale, granular, vacuolated cytoplasm. Nuclei are vesicular with prominent nucleoli. Tumor cells are scattered throughout the dermis or are seen as small clusters (Fig. 8-34). Invasion into the dermis may result in metastasis to groin or widespread dissemination.

ANCILLARY STUDIES

HISTOCHEMISTRY

Intracytoplasmic mucin is demonstrated in most cases.

EXTRAMAMMARY PAGET DISEASE—FACT SHEET

Definition
▶ Form of an intraepidermal adenocarcinoma similar to mammary Paget disease and frequently a consequence of epidermotropic spread from an underlying malignancy

Incidence and Location
▶ This is a rare lesion, usually affecting inguinal and scrotal regions, with frequent spread to penis
▶ Pure penile lesions are rare

Morbidity and Mortality
▶ The outcome depends on the extent of local disease and underlying evolution of associated malignancy

Clinical Features
▶ Presents with geographic areas of erythematous, scaly lesions in anogenital skin
▶ Clinically mimics eczema or dermatitis, which may delay appropriate therapy

Prognosis and Treatment
▶ The treatment of Paget disease of scrotum is wide surgical excision of involved skin
▶ Combination of irradiation and topical chemotherapy may also be effective

---

EXTRAMAMMARY PAGET DISEASE—PATHOLOGIC FEATURES

Gross Findings
▶ The lesion appears as an erythematous or eczematous scaly lesion

Microscopic Findings
▶ Characterized by atypical large cells with abundant vacuolated cytoplasm, scattered within the epidermis
▶ Underlying invasive carcinoma may be present

Histochemistry
▶ Mucin stains positive

Immunohistochemical Features
▶ CEA, EMA, and MUC 5AC are positive
▶ S-100, HMB-45, and melan A are negative

Differential Diagnosis
▶ Superficial spreading malignant melanoma, Bowen's disease, pagetoid spread of urothelial carcinoma or prostate carcinoma

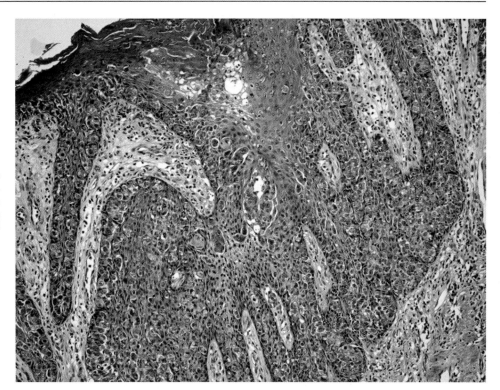

FIGURE 8-34
Extramammary Paget disease of scrotum. Low-power view demonstrates intraepidermal proliferation of large atypical cells with abundant vacuolated cytoplasm scattered throughout the epidermis.

IMMUNOHISTOCHEMISTRY

Paget tumor cells are positive for cytokeratin (low molecular weight), CEA, EMA, and mucin MUC 5AC and are negative for S-100 and PSA.

DIFFERENTIAL DIAGNOSIS

Primary extramammary Paget disease should be distinguished from pagetoid spread of urothelial carcinoma. Other cancers that may demonstrate pagetoid spread include prostate carcinoma. Proper clinical background is important to the workup of the case. Rarely, Bowen disease can have a pagetoid growth pattern, although typical full-thickness cytologic atypia is present focally in most cases. Superficial spreading malignant melanoma may mimic Paget disease. Immunohistochemical stains may aid in the differential diagnosis in difficult cases.

PROGNOSIS AND TREATMENT

Treatment consists of wide surgical excision of involved scrotal skin, with negative surgical margins, to avoid recurrence. Topical treatment with 5-fluorouracil also has been used. Invasion into the dermis may result in metastasis to groin or widespread dissemination. The outcome depends on the extent of local disease and the evolution of associated malignancy.

BASAL CELL CARCINOMA

Basal cell carcinoma is a rare scrotal tumor. It is usually an indolent tumor, similar to its nongenital cutaneous counterpart. However, metastases have been documented in some. Wide local excision with negative margins probably constitutes adequate therapy, and there appears to be no rationale for inguinal lymph node dissection. Radiation therapy has been administered in up to 15 % of cases, usually in combination with surgery. The patients with reported metastatic disease received additional chemotherapy.

MESENCHYMAL NEOPLASMS

A wide range of tumors in this category have been reported, but all are rare. Leiomyosarcoma and liposarcoma are the most common sarcomas reported in this category. The descriptions of these tumors follow the guidelines established for other body sites and are not discussed further here due to their rarity.

Non-neoplastic Lesions

SCLEROSING LIPOGRANULOMA

Lipogranulomas are also known as paraffinomas or Tancho's nodules. They involve the penile or scrotal skin. The cause of this lesion has generated considerable interest, and it appears that multiple causes result in a similar histology. Oertel and Johnson reported 23 cases from the Armed Forces Institute of Pathology, 14 of them in the scrotum; their findings and those of others suggested that the lesions were secondary to injections or topical applications of oil-based substances such as paraffin, silicone, oil, or wax, either for cosmetic purposes (enlargement of genitals) or for therapeutic use. Although most penile lipogranulomas are secondary to injections of oils, additionally they may be caused by trauma or by cold weather.

CLINICAL FEATURES

Most lesions are seen in men younger than 40 years of age, who complain of a localized plaque or mass that

SCLEROSING LIPOGRANULOMA—FACT SHEET

Definition
► Uncommon tumor-like condition affecting scrotal or penile skin
► Also referred to as paraffinoma and Tancho's nodules

Incidence and Location
► Rare condition
► Largest series from AFIP demonstrates >50% occurring in scrotal skin, remainder in penis

Morbidity and Mortality
► Benign condition

Gender, Race, and Age Distribution
► Most lesions are seen in men younger than 40 years of age

Clinical Features
► Patients complain of a localized plaque or mass, which may be tender and indurated and is usually a few centimeters in diameter but may be massive
► History of injections or topical applications of oil-based substances such as paraffin, silicone, oil, or wax for cosmetic reasons (enlargement of genitals) or therapeutic purpose may be elicited

Prognosis and Treatment
► Benign course.
► Excision mandatory to exclude a neoplasm

SCLEROSING LIPOGRANULOMA—PATHOLOGIC FEATURES

Gross Findings
► Gross specimens are usually fragmented, with ill-defined margins
► The tissue is firm, yellow to grayish-white, and solid with a trabecular and cystic appearance

Microscopic Findings
► Lesions consist of lipid vacuoles of varying sizes, embedded in densely sclerotic stroma
► Marked variation in the size of the vacuoles is a very useful feature
► Foreign body-type granulomatous reaction may be present

Immunohistochemical Features
► Frozen tissue may demonstrate positivity for Oil Red O stain
► Osmium tetroxide fails to blacken the lipid, characteristic of paraffin hydrocarbons

Differential Diagnosis
► Sclerosing liposarcoma
► Signet-ring cell carcinoma
► Adenomatoid tumor

may be tender and indurated and is usually a few centimeters in diameter but can become massive and replace the scrotal wall. Biopsy and/or excision is mandatory to exclude a neoplasm, especially in the absence of a clinical history of injection.

PATHOLOGIC FEATURES

GROSS FINDINGS

The gross specimens are usually fragmented, because the lesion is removed in pieces due to the location and its ill-defined margins. The tissue is firm, yellow to grayish-white, and solid with a trabecular and cystic appearance.

MICROSCOPIC FINDINGS

Microscopically, the lesions consist of lipid vacuoles of varying sizes embedded in a variably sclerotic stroma. Marked variation in the size of the vacuoles is a useful feature. They are devoid of a cellular lining, although multinucleated giant cells may line a few. The inflammatory response is also variable, with nodular or interspersed aggregates of inflammatory cells. A histiocytic or foreign-body granulomatous infiltrate with or without eosinophils is usually present (Fig. 8-35). The diagnosis is not difficult in most cases and may be confirmed by lipid stains. Sections from frozen tissue show positivity for Oil Red O, and osmium tetroxide fails to blacken the lipid, which is characteristic of paraffin hydrocarbons.

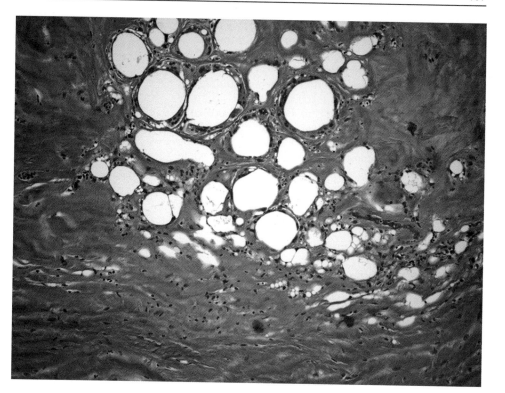

FIGURE 8-35

Sclerosing lipogranuloma. There is a collection of multiple, variably sized vacuoles within the dense sclerotic stroma. There is a focal foreign body-type granulomatous response. (Courtesy of Lakshmi Priya Kunju, University of Michigan, Ann Arbor, MI.)

DIFFERENTIAL DIAGNOSIS

The histologic differential diagnosis may include signet-ring carcinoma, sclerosing liposarcoma, and adenomatoid tumor, but distinction is usually straightforward. Sclerosing lipogranulomas demonstrate the fatty nature of the vacuoles, compared to the mucin material in the signet-ring carcinomas. The presence of multinucleated giant cells associated with vacuoles is helpful to separate them from sclerosing liposarcoma.

"IDIOPATHIC" SCROTAL CALCINOSIS AND EPIDERMOID CYSTS

Scrotal calcinosis is an uncommon disorder characterized by the progressive development of calcific nodules in the scrotal skin which, if untreated, may result in dramatic distortion and destruction of the scrotum. The cause of this lesion has been debated. Calcinosis may be dystrophic, metastatic, or idiopathic. In most patients, a lack of clinical history such as hyperparathyroidism, advanced renal failure, systemic sarcoidosis fails to support metastatic calcification as a mechanism of causation. Dystrophic calcification is currently the favored

SCROTAL CALCINOSIS—FACT SHEET

Definition

▶ Uncommon disorder characterized by the progressive development of calcific nodules in the scrotal skin. Dystrophic calcification is now a favored etiology

Incidence and Location

▶ Rare condition, affects scrotal skin

Morbidity and Mortality

▶ Benign but can be destructive condition

Gender, Race, and Age Distribution

▶ Males
▶ Ninety percent of the lesions occur before 40 years of age

Clinical Features

▶ Patients present with multiple, nontender, gray-white, firm nodules, which may be associated with discharge of chalky-white material

Prognosis and Treatment

▶ Most cases are managed effectively by local excision of scrotal skin
▶ Pronounced cases with destruction of scrotum may require total scrotectomy

mechanism. Dare and Axelsen showed small cysts lined by stratified squamous epithelium in three of four cases in their series of typical scrotal calcinosis. It is, therefore, plausible that idiopathic scrotal calcinosis represents an end-stage phenomenon in which numerous "old" epidermal cysts have lost their walls over time. Dare and Axelsen concluded that, because the evidence strongly suggests a dystrophic rather than an idiopathic origin for this disease, the term idiopathic should be dropped from the nomenclature. It is unclear why some cysts show a predilection for calcification and others do not.

CLINICAL FEATURES

The lesions first appear in childhood or early adulthood (90% before 40 years of age), and they may be solitary or multiple with a tendency to slowly enlarge. The lesions vary in size from a few millimeters to lesions that assume a nodular, bosselated configuration. The lesions are nontender and usually asymptomatic, but they may be associated with a discharge of chalky-white material from ulcerated lesions, or they may be pruritic.

PATHOLOGIC FEATURES

GROSS FINDINGS

The gross features of scrotal calcinosis are highly characteristic. They demonstrate multiple gray-white, firm nodules involving the skin; on sectioning, chalky white material is frequently demonstrated (Fig. 8-36).

MICROSCOPIC FINDINGS

Histologically, granules and globules of basophilic calcific material in the dermis characterize the lesions

---

SCROTAL CALCINOSIS—PATHOLOGIC FEATURES

Gross Findings
▶ Multiple, firm, gray-white nodules
▶ Cut surfaces may demonstrate chalky-white granular material

Microscopic Findings
▶ Granules and globules of basophilic calcific material within the dermis, frequently with foreign-body giant cell granulomatous reaction
▶ Sometimes, a recognizable cyst wall lining, representing ruptured epidermoid cyst, is present

Differential Diagnosis
▶ Dystrophic calcifications due to parasites

(Fig. 8-37). A foreign-body giant cell granulomatous reaction may be present, and infrequently a recognizable cyst wall lining is seen. Clinically well-characterized, noncoalescent dermal nodules, which histologically show characteristic features of epidermoid cysts including keratinizing squamous epithelium and keratinaceous material, should be regarded as such.

DIFFERENTIAL DIAGNOSIS

The differential diagnosis includes dystrophic calcification due to parasites.

PROGNOSIS AND TREATMENT

Most cases of scrotal calcinosis are managed effectively by local excision; however, pronounced cases with destruction of scrotum require partial or total scrotectomy.

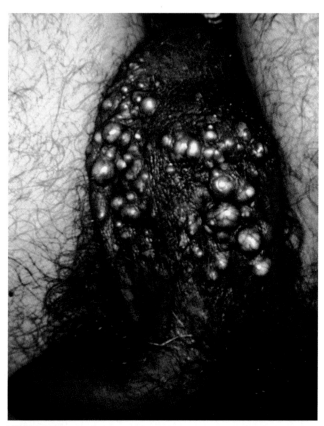

FIGURE 8-36

In scrotal calcinosis, the scrotal skin is replaced by multiple, variable-sized, gray-white nodules. (Courtesy of Lori Lowe, University of Michigan, Ann Arbor, MI.)

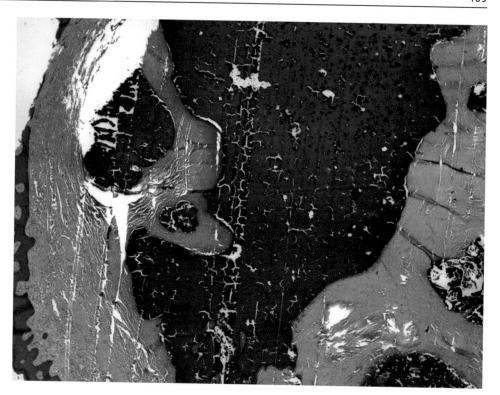

FIGURE 8-37
Low-power view of scrotal calcinosis demonstrates variably sized multiple nodules of basophilic calcified material within the dermis. (Courtesy of Lakshmi Priya Kunju, University of Michigan, Ann Arbor, MI.)

ANGIOKERATOMA

Angiokeratoma is a distinctive vascular lesion of the scrotum, regarded as a variant distinct from diffuse systemic angiokeratoma corporis diffusum, that is associated with Febry's disease, angiokeratoma of Mibelli, solitary papillary angiokeratoma, and plaque-like angiokeratoma circumscriptum. Angiokeratoma of Fordyce is the most common type of angiokeratoma affecting the scrotal skin.

CLINICAL FEATURES

Patients present with 1- to 4-mm, red to blue, soft, compressible lesions that are usually multiple. Some patients present with diffuse redness of the scrotum. The lesions typically affect middle-aged to elderly patients.

PATHOLOGIC FEATURES

GROSS FINDINGS

Angiokeratomas are multiple, soft, and small (1 to 4 mm) red papules.

ANGIOKERATOMA, SCROTUM—FACT SHEET

Definition
▶ A distinctive vascular lesion of the scrotum, regarded as a variant of angiokeratoma distinct from diffuse systemic angiokeratoma

Incidence and Location
▶ Uncommon condition
▶ Angiokeratoma of Fordyce is the most common angiokeratoma affecting the scrotal skin

Morbidity and Mortality
▶ Benign condition

Gender, Race, and Age Distribution
▶ Males
▶ Typically affects middle-aged to elderly patients

Clinical Features
▶ Patients present with 1- to 4-mm, red to blue, soft, compressible lesions that are usually multiple in the presentation
▶ Rarely may manifest as cause of red scrotum

Prognosis and Treatment
▶ Benign course
▶ Conditions that predispose to increased venous pressure have been suggested as a predisposing factor for angiokeratomas and should be sought

---

ANGIOKERATOMA, SCROTUM—PATHOLOGIC FEATURES

Gross Findings

▶ Multiple, soft, and small (1 to 4 mm) red papules

Microscopic Findings

▶ Classic histologic features include marked dilatation of the papillary dermal vasculature with or without thrombi
▶ Acanthosis and elongation of rete ridges, forming a collarette engulfing vascular lacunae
▶ Moderate to marked hyperkeratosis
▶ Parakeratosis
▶ Direct communication between the cystic vascular spaces and underlying dilated veins in the deeper dermis

Differential Diagnosis

▶ Other benign vascular tumors

MICROSCOPIC FINDINGS

Classic histologic features of angiokeratomas include marked dilatation of the papillary dermal vasculature with or without thrombi; acanthosis and elongation of rete ridges forming a collarette partly or circumferentially engulfing vascular lacunae; moderate to marked hyperkeratosis; parakeratosis; and a direct communication between the cystic vascular spaces and underlying dilated veins in the deeper dermis. Dermal fibrosis, chronic inflammation, atrophy of the dartos

muscle, and degeneration of the elastic tissue may also be present (Fig. 8-38).

DIFFERENTIAL DIAGNOSIS

Other potential differential diagnoses include benign vascular tumors. Angiokeratomas have distinctive histologic features, as described here, which should help the pathologist arrive at correct diagnosis.

PROGNOSIS AND TREATMENT

Angiokeratomas are benign lesions. Conditions that predispose to increased venous pressure have been suggested as predisposing factors for angiokeratomas and should be sought.

SCROTAL FAT NECROSIS

Scrotal fat necrosis is frequently bilateral and occurs in obese prepubertal boys, who present with a swollen scrotum that is firm and tender. The lesion may appear as an ill-defined, gray-yellow mass, which histologically shows the typical features of fat necrosis with asso-

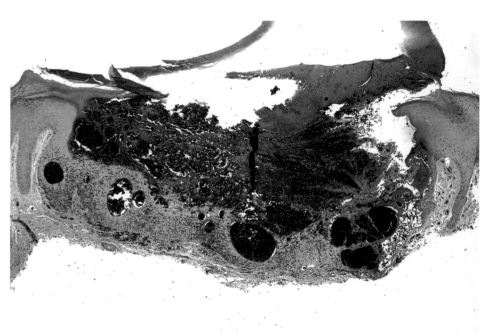

FIGURE 8-38

Angiokeratoma of scrotum. Low-power view shows a cup-shaped lesion with marked vascular dilation filling the papillary dermis. Some vascular spaces contain thrombus. (Courtesy of Doug Fullen, University of Michigan, Ann Arbor, MI.)

ciated inflammation. The cause is unknown, but hypo-thermia, as produced by swimming in very cold water, may play a role.

SUGGESTED READINGS

Diseases of the Penis: Anatomy and Histology

Cubilla AL, Piris A, Pfannl R, et al: Anatomic levels—Important landmarks in penectomy specimens: A detailed anatomic and histologic study based on examination of 44 cases. Am J Surg Pathol 2001;25:1091–1094.

Young RH, Srigley JR, Amin MB, et al: Tumors of the Prostate Gland, Seminal Vesicles, Male Urethra, and Penis. AFIP Atlas of Tumor Pathology, 3rd ed, Fascicle 28. Washington, DC, Armed Forces Institute of Pathology, 2000.Squamous Cell Carcinoma, Usual Type

Squamous cell carcinoma, usual type

Banon Perez VJ, Nicolas Torralba JA, Valdelvira Nadal P, et al: [Squamous carcinoma of the penis]. Arch Esp Urol 2000;53:693–699.

Cubilla AL, Piris A, Pfannl R, et al: Anatomic levels—Important landmarks in penectomy specimens: A detailed anatomic and histologic study based on examination of 44 cases. Am J Surg Pathol 2001;25:1091–1094.

Cubilla AL, Caballero C, Piris A, et al: Prognostic Index (PI): A novel method to predict mortality in squamous carcinoma of the penis. Lab Invest 2000;80:97A.

Cubilla AL, Barreto J, Caballero C, et al: Pathologic features of epidermoid carcinoma of the penis: A prospective study of 66 cases. Am J Surg Pathol 1993;17:753–763.

Cupp MR, Malek RS, Goellner JR, et al: The detection of human papillomavirus deoxyribonucleic acid in intraepithelial, in situ, verrucous and invasive carcinoma of the penis. J Urol 1995;154:1024–1029.

Dillner J, von Krogh G, Horenblas S, Meijer CJ: Etiology of squamous cell carcinoma of the penis. Scand J Urol Nephrol Suppl 2000;(205):189–193.

Eble JN, Sauter G, Epstein JI, Sesterhenn IA: WHO Classification: Tumours of the Urinary System and Male Genital Organs. Lyon, France, IARC Press, 2004.

Ficarra V, Zattoni F, Cunico SC, et al: Lymphatic and vascular embolizations are independent predictive variables of inguinal lymph node involvement in patients with squamous cell carcinoma of penis. (Northeast UroOncological Group) Penile cancer data base date. Cancer 2005;103(12):2507–2516.

Johnson DE, Fuerst DE, Ayala AG: Carcinoma of the penis: Experience with 153 cases. Urology 1973;1:404–408.

Lopes A, Bezerra AL, Pinto CA, et al: P53 as a new prognostic factor for lymph node metastasis in penile carcinoma: Analysis of 82 patients treated with amputation and bilateral lymphadenectomy. J Urol 2002;168:81–86.

Lopes A, Hidalgo GS, Kowalski LP, et al: Prognostic factors in carcinoma of the penis: Multivariate analysis of 145 patients treated with amputation and lymphadenectomy. J Urol 1996;156:1637–1642.

Maiche AG, Pyrhonen S, Karkinen M: Histological grading of squamous cell carcinoma of the penis: A new scoring system. Br J Urol 1991;67:522–526.

Micali G, Innocenzi D, Nasca MR, et al: Squamous cell carcinoma of the penis. J Am Acad Dermatol 1996;35(3 Pt 1):432–451.

Ornellas AA, Seixas AL, Marota A, et al: Surgical treatment of invasive squamous cell carcinoma of the penis: Retrospective analysis of 350 cases. J Urol 1994;151:1244–1249.

Powell J, Robson A, Cranston D, et al: High incidence of lichen sclerosus in patients with squamous cell carcinoma of the penis. Br J Dermatol 2001;145:85–89.

Rubin MA, Kleter B, Zhou M, et al: Detection and typing of human papillomavirus DNA in penile carcinoma: Evidence for multiple independent pathways of penile carcinogenesis. Am J Pathol 2001;159:1211–1218.

Sarin R, Norman AR, Steel GG, Horwich A: Treatment results and prognostic factors in 101 men treated for squamous carcinoma of the penis. Int J Radiat Oncol Biol Phys 1997;38:713–722.

Sarkar FH, Miles BJ, Plieth DH, Crissman JD: Detection of human papillomavirus in squamous neoplasm of the penis. J Urol 1992;147:389–392.

Velazquez EF, Bock A, Soskin A, et al: Preputial variability and preferential association of long phimotic foreskins with penile cancer: An anatomic comparative study of types of foreskin in a general population and cancer patients. Am J Surg Pathol 2003;27:994–998.

Velazquez EF, Cubilla AL: Lichen sclerosus in 68 patients with squamous cell carcinoma of the penis: Frequent atypias and correlation with special carcinoma variants suggests a precancerous role. Am J Surg Pathol 2003;27:1448–1453.

Young RH, Srigley JR, Amin MB, et al: Tumors of the Prostate Gland, Seminal Vesicles, Male Urethra, and Penis. AFIP Atlas of Tumor Pathology, 3rd ed, Fascicle 28. Washington, DC, Armed Forces Institute of Pathology, 2000.Squamous Cell Carcinoma, Usual Type

Verrucous Carcinoma

Banon Perez V, Nicolas Torralba JA, Valdelvira Nadal P, et al: [Penile verrucous carcinoma]. Arch Esp Urol 1999;52:937–940.

Clemente Ramos LM, Maganto Pavon E, Garcia Gonzalez R, et al: [Verrucous carcinoma of the penis. A report of 6 new cases and a review of the diagnostic and therapeutic aspects]. Actas Urol Esp 1997;21:372–376.

Fukunaga M, Yokoi K, Miyazawa Y, et al: Penile verrucous carcinoma with anaplastic transformation following radiotherapy: A case report with human papillomavirus typing and flow cytometric DNA studies. Am J Surg Pathol 1994;18:501–505.

Johnson DE, Lo RK, Srigley J, Ayala AG: Verrucous carcinoma of the penis. J Urol 1985;133:216–218.

Masih AS, Stoler MH, Farrow GM, et al: Penile verrucous carcinoma: A clinicopathologic, human papillomavirus typing and flow cytometric analysis. Mod Pathol 1992;5:48–55.

McKee PH, Lowe D, Haigh RJ: Penile verrucous carcinoma. Histopathology 1983;7:897–906.

Schwartz RA: Buschke-Loewenstein tumor: Verrucous carcinoma of the penis. J Am Acad Dermatol 1990;23(4 Pt 1):723–727.

Seixas AL, Ornellas AA, Marota A, et al: Verrucous carcinoma of the penis: Retrospective analysis of 32 cases. J Urol 1994;152(5 Pt 1):1476–1478; discussion 1478–1479.

Warty Carcinoma

Bezerra AL, Lopes A, Landman G, et al: Clinicopathologic features and human papillomavirus DNA prevalence of warty and squamous cell carcinoma of the penis. Am J Surg Pathol 2001;25:673–678.

Cubilla AL, Velazquez EF, Reuter VE, et al: Warty (condylomatous) squamous cell carcinoma of the penis: A report of 11 cases and proposed classification of "verruciform" penile tumors. Am J Surg Pathol 2000;24:505–512.

Papillary Carcinoma, Not Otherwise Specified

Barreto JE, Velazquez EF, Ayala E, et al: Carcinoma Cuniculatum: A Distinctive Variant of Penile Squamous Cell Carcinoma. Am J Surg Pathol 2007;31:71–75.

Cubilla AL, Reuter V, Velazquez E, et al: Histologic classification of penile carcinoma and its relation to outcome in 61 patients with primary resection. Int J Surg Pathol 2001;9:111–120.

Young RH, Srigley JR, Amin MB, et al: Tumors of the Prostate Gland, Seminal Vesicles, Male Urethra, and Penis. AFIP Atlas of Tumor Pathology, 3rd ed, Fascicle 28. Washington, DC, Armed Forces Institute of Pathology, 2000.

Basaloid Carcinoma

Cubilla AL, Reuter VE, Gregoire L, et al: Basaloid squamous cell carcinoma: A distinctive human papilloma virus-related penile neoplasm. A report of 20 cases. Am J Surg Pathol 1998;22:755–761.

Gregoire L, Cubilla AL, Reuter VE, et al: Preferential association of human papillomavirus with high-grade histologic variants of penile-invasive squamous cell carcinoma. J Natl Cancer Inst 1995;87:1705–1709.

Pseudohyperplastic Carcinoma

Cubilla AL, Velazquez EF, Young RH: Pseudohyperplastic squamous cell carcinoma of the penis associated with lichen sclerosus: An extremely well-differentiated, nonverruciform neoplasm that preferentially affects the foreskin and is frequently misdiagnosed. A report of 10 cases of a distinctive clinicopathologic entity. Am J Surg Pathol 2004;28:895–900.

Sarcomatoid (Spindle-Cell) Carcinoma

Manglani KS, Manaligod JR, Ray B: Spindle cell carcinoma of the glans penis: A light and electron microscopic study. Cancer 1980;46:2266–2272.

Velazuez EF, Melamed J, Barreto JE, et al: Sarcomatoid carcinoma of the penis: a clinicopathologic study of 15 cases. Am J Surg Pathol 2005;29(9):1152–1158

Wood EW, Gardner WA Jr, Brown FM: Spindle cell squamous carcinoma of the penis. J Urol 1972;107:990–991.

Adenosquamous Carcinoma

Cubilla AL, Ayala MT, Barreto JE, et al: Surface adenosquamous carcinoma of the penis: A report of three cases. Am J Surg Pathol 1996;20:156–160.

Froehner M, Schobl R, Wirth MP: Mucoepidermoid penile carcinoma: Clinical, histologic, and immunohistochemical characterization of an uncommon neoplasm. Urology 2000;56:154.

Jamieson NV, Bullock KN, Barker TH: Adenosquamous carcinoma of the penis associated with balanitis xerotica obliterans. Br J Urol 1986;58:730–731.

Layfield LJ, Liu K: Mucoepidermoid carcinoma arising in the glans penis. Arch Pathol Lab Med 2000;124:148–151.

Masera A, Ovcak Z, Volavsek M, Bracko M: Adenosquamous carcinoma of the penis. J Urol 1997;157:2261.

Mixed Carcinomas

Clemente Ramos LM, Garcia Gonzalez R, Burgos Revilla FJ, et al: [Hybrid tumor of the penis: Is this denomination correct?]. Arch Esp Urol 1998;51:821–823.

Cubilla AL, Velazques EF, Barreto J, Ayala G: The penis. In Sternberg SS (ed.): Diagnostic Surgical Pathology, 4th ed. Philadelphia, Lippincott Williams & Wilkins, 2004.

Tamboli P, Tran KP, Ro JY, et al: Mixed basaloid-condylomatous (warty) squamous carcinoma of the penis: A report of 17 cases. Lab Invest 2000;80:115A.

Other Rare Primary Penile Carcinomas

Galanis E, Frytak S, Lloyd RV: Extrapulmonary small cell carcinoma. Cancer 1997;79:1729–1736.

Liegl B, Regauer S: Penile clear cell carcinoma: A report of 5 cases of a distinct entity. Am J Surg Pathol 2004;28:1513–1517.

Oppenheim AR: Sebaceous carcinoma of the penis. Arch Dermatol 1981;117:306–307.

Tomic S, Warner TF, Messing E, Wilding G: Penile Merkel cell carcinoma. Urology 1995;45:1062–1065.

Malignant Melanoma

Banon Perez VJ, Server Pastor G, Valdelvira Nadal P, et al: [Malignant melanoma of the penis]. Arch Esp Urol 2001;54:828–830.

Creagh TA, Murphy DM: Malignant melanoma of the penis. Aust N Z J Surg 1993;63:820–821.

de Bree E, Sanidas E, Tzardi M, et al: Malignant melanoma of the penis. Eur J Surg Oncol 1997;23:277–279.

Fenn NJ, Johnson RC, Sharma AK, et al: Malignant melanoma of the penis. Eur J Surg Oncol 1996;22:548–549.

Basal Cell Carcinoma

Banon Perez VJ, Martinez Barba E, Rigabert Montiel M, et al:[Basal cell carcinoma of the penis]. Arch Esp Urol 2000;53:841–843.

Kim ED, Kroft S, Dalton DP: Basal cell carcinoma of the penis: Case report and review of the literature. J Urol 1994;152(5 Pt 1):1557–1559.

Ladocsi LT, Siebert CF Jr, Rickert RR, Fletcher HS: Basal cell carcinoma of the penis. Cutis 1998;61:25–27.

Peison B, Benisch B, Nicora B: Multicentric basal cell carcinoma of penile skin. Urology 1985;25:322–323.

Rare Mesenchymal Tumors

Al-Rikabi AC, Diab AR, Buckai A, et al: Primary synovial sarcoma of the penis: Case report and literature review. Scand J Urol Nephrol 1999;33:413–415.

Bryant J: Granular cell tumor of penis and scrotum. Urology 1995;45:332–334.

Dehner LP, Smith BH: Soft tissue tumors of the penis: A clinicopathologic study of 46 cases. Cancer 1970;25:1431–1447.

Khanna S: Cavernous haemangioma of the glans penis. Br J Urol 1991;67:332.

Moran CA, Kaneko M: Malignant fibrous histiocytoma of the glans penis. Am J Dermatopathol 1990;12:182–187.

Pow-Sang MR, Orihuela E: Leiomyosarcoma of the penis. J Urol 1994;151:1643–1645.

Sacker AR, Oyama KK, Kessler S: Primary osteosarcoma of the penis. Am J Dermatopathol 1994;16:285–287.

Saw D, Tse CH, Chan J, et al: Clear cell sarcoma of the penis. Hum Pathol 1986;17:423–425.

Webber RJ, Alsaffar N, Bissett D, Langlois NE: Angiosarcoma of the penis. Urology 1998;51:130–131.

Secondary Tumors

Mukamel E, Farrer J, Smith RB, deKernion JB: Metastatic carcinoma to penis: When is total penectomy indicated? Urology 1987;29:15–18.

Perez-Mesa C, Oxenhandler R: Metastatic tumor of the penis. J Surg Oncol 1989;42:11–15.

Precancerous Squamous Lesions

Aynaud O, Bergeron C. [Penile intraepithelial neoplasia]. Prog Urol 2004;14:100–104.

Cubilla AL, Velazquez EF, Young RH: Epithelial lesions associated with invasive penile squamous cell carcinoma: A pathologic study of 288 cases. Int J Surg Pathol 2004;12:351–364.

Cubilla AL, Meijer CJ, Young RH: Morphological features of epithelial abnormalities and precancerous lesions of the penis. Scand J Urol Nephrol Suppl 2000;(205):215–219.

Horenblas S, von Krogh G, Cubilla AL, et al: Squamous cell carcinoma of the penis: Premalignant lesions. Scand J Urol Nephrol Suppl 2000;(205):187–188.

Malek RS, Goellner JR, Smith TF, et al: Human papillomavirus infection and intraepithelial, in situ, and invasive carcinoma of penis. Urology 1993;42:159–170.

Porter WM, Francis N, Hawkins D, et al: Penile intraepithelial neoplasia: Clinical spectrum and treatment of 35 cases. Br J Dermatol 2002;147:1159–1165.

von Krogh G, Horenblas S: Diagnosis and clinical presentation of premalignant lesions of the penis. Scand J Urol Nephrol Suppl 2000;(205):201–214.

Bowenoid Papulosis

Bhojwani A, Biyani CS, Nicol A, Powell CS: Bowenoid papulosis of the penis. Br J Urol 1997;80:508.

Schwartz RA, Janniger CK. Bowenoid papulosis. J Am Acad Dermatol 1991;24(2 Pt 1):261–264.

Snoeck R, Van Laethem Y, De Clercq E, et al: Treatment of a bowenoid papulosis of the penis with local applications of cidofovir in a patient with acquired immunodeficiency syndrome. Arch Intern Med 2001;1611:2382–2384.

Su CK, Shipley WU: Bowenoid papulosis: A benign lesion of the shaft of the penis misdiagnosed as squamous carcinoma. J Urol 1997;157:1361–1362.

Wigbels B, Luger T, Metze D: [Imiquimod: a new treatment possibility in bowenoid papulosis?]. Hautarzt 2001;52:128–131.

Balanitis Xerotica Obliterans (Lichen Sclerosus Atrophicus)

Das S, Tunuguntla HS: Balanitis xerotica obliterans: A review. World J Urol 2000;18:382–387.

Depasquale I, Park AJ, Bracka A: The treatment of balanitis xerotica obliterans. BJU Int 2000;86:459–465.

Finkbeiner AE: Balanitis xerotica obliterans: A form of lichen sclerosus. South Med J 2003;96:7–8.

Giannakopoulos X, Basioukas K, Dimou S, Agnantis N: Squamous cell carcinoma of the penis arising from balanitis xerotica obliterans. Int Urol Nephrol 1996;28:223–227.

Neuhaus IM, Skidmore RA: Balanitis xerotica obliterans and its differential diagnosis. J Am Board Fam Pract 1999;12:473–476.

Pride HB, Miller OF 3rd, Tyler WB: Penile squamous cell carcinoma arising from balanitis xerotica obliterans. J Am Acad Dermatol 1993;29:469–473.

Squamous Hyperplasia

Young RH, Srigley JR, Amin MB, et al: Tumors of the Prostate Gland, Seminal Vesicles, Male Urethra, and Penis. AFIP Atlas of Tumor Pathology, 3rd ed, Fascicle 28. Washington, DC, Armed Forces Institute of Pathology, 2000.

Condyloma and Giant Condyloma Acuminatum

Buffet M, Aynaud O, Piron D, et al: [Buschke-Lowenstein penile tumor]. Prog Urol 2002;12:332–336.

Davies SW: Giant condyloma acuminata: Incidence among cases diagnosed as carcinoma of the penis. J Clin Pathol 1965;18:142–149.

Dawson DF, Duckworth JK, Bernhardt H, Young JM: Giant condyloma and verrucous carcinoma of the genital area. Arch Pathol 1965;79:225–231.

Lal MM, Yadav MS, Dhall JC: Giant condyloma acuminata (Buschke-Loewenstein tumour) of penis (report of two cases). Indian J Dermatol 1975;20:51–55.

Niederauer HH, Weindorf N, Schultz-Ehrenburg U: [A case of giant condyloma acuminatum. On differential diagnosis of giant condylomas from Buschke-Lowenstein tumors and verrucous carcinoma]. Hautarzt 1993;44:795–799.

Peyronie's Diease

Arena F, Peracchia G, di Stefano C, et al: Peyronie's disease: Incision and dorsal vein grafting combined with contralateral plication in straightening the penis. Scand J Urol Nephrol 1999;33:181–185.

Primus G: Orgotein in the treatment of plastic induration of the penis (Peyronie's disease). Int Urol Nephrol 1993;25:169–172.

Wilson SK, Cleves MA, Delk JR 2nd: Long-term followup of treatment for Peyronie's disease: Modeling the penis over an inflatable penile prosthesis. J Urol 2001;165:825–829.

Verruciform Xanthoma

Canillot S, Stamm C, Balme B, Perrot H: [Verruciform xanthoma of the penis]. Ann Dermatol Venereol 1994;121:404–407.

Geiss DF, Del Rosso JQ, Murphy J: Verruciform xanthoma of the glans penis: A benign clinical simulant of genital malignancy. Cutis 1993;51:369–372.

Laguna Urraca G, Concha Lopez A, Tudela Paton MP: [Verruciform xanthoma of the penis]. Actas Urol Esp 1990;14:210–213.

Nakamura S, Kanamori S, Nakayama K, Aoki M: Verruciform xanthoma on the scrotum. J Dermatol 1989;16:397–401.

Torrecilla Ortiz C, Marco Perez LM, Dinares Prat J, Autonell J. [Verruciform xanthoma of the penis]. Actas Urol Esp 1997;21:797–799.

Xia TL, Li GZ, Na YQ, Guo YL: Verruciform xanthoma of the penis: Report of a case. Chin Med J (Engl) 2004;117:150–152.

Hirsutoid Papilloma (Pearly Penile Papules)

Agrawal SK, Bhattacharya SN, Singh N: Pearly penile papules: A review. Int J Dermatol 2004;43:199–201.

Ferenczy A, Richart RM, Wright TC: Pearly penile papules: Absence of human papillomavirus DNA by the polymerase chain reaction. Obstet Gynecol 1991;78:118–122.

Hogewoning CJ, Bleeker MC, van den Brule AJ, et al: Pearly penile papules: Still no reason for uneasiness. J Am Acad Dermatol 2003;49:50–54.

Oates JK: Pearly penile papules. Genitourin Med 1997;73:137–138.

Porter WM, Bunker CB: Treatment of pearly penile papules with cryotherapy. Br J Dermatol 2000;142:847–848.

Sonnex C, Dockerty WG: Pearly penile papules: A common cause of concern. Int J STD AIDS 1999;10:726–727.

Sclerosing Lipogranuloma

Holscher AH, Rahlf G, Zimmermann A: [Sclerosing lipogranuloma of male genitalia (author's transl)]. Urologe A 1979;18:106–108.

Diseases of the Urethra: Anatomy and Histology

Tepper SL, Jagirdar J, Heath D, Geller SA: Homology between the female paraurethral (Skene's) glands and the prostate: Immunohistochemical demonstration. Arch Pathol Lab Med 1984;108:423–425.

Young RH, Srigley JR, Amin MB, et al: Tumors of the Prostate Gland, Seminal Vesicles, Male Urethra, and Penis. AFIP Atlas of Tumor Pathology, 3rd ed, Fascicle 28. Washington, DC, Armed Forces Institute of Pathology, 2000.

Epithelial Neoplasms

Allen R, Nelson RP: Primary urethral malignancy: Review of 22 cases. South Med J 1978;71:547–550.

Amin MB, Young RH: Primary carcinomas of the urethra. Semin Diagn Pathol 1997;14:147–160.

Dinney CP, Johnson DE, Swanson DA, et al: Therapy and prognosis for male anterior urethral carcinoma: An update. Urology 1994;43:506–514.

Dodson MK, Cliby WA, Pettavel PP, et al: Female urethral adenocarcinoma: Evidence for more than one tissue of origin? Gynecol Oncol 1995;59:352–357.

Gonzalez MO, Harrison ML, Boileau MA: Carcinoma in diverticulum of female urethra. Urology 1985;26:328–332.

Grabstald H: Proceedings: Tumors of the urethra in men and women. Cancer 1973;32:1236–1255.

Hakenberg OW, Franke HJ, Froehner M. Wirth MP: The treatment of primary urethral carcinoma—The dilemmas of a rare condition: Experience with partial urethrectomy and adjuvant chemotherapy. Onkologie 2001;24:48–52.

Hopkins SC, Nag SK, Soloway MS: Primary carcinoma of male urethra. Urology 1984;23:128–133.

Johnson DE, O'Connell JR: Primary carcinoma of female urethra. Urology 1983;21:42–45.

Karjn LP, Mehra R, Snyder M and Shah RB: Prostate-specific antigen, high-molecular-weight cytokeratin (clone 34BE12), and/or p63: an optimal immunohistochemical panel to distinguish poorly differentiated prostate adenocarcinoma from urothelial carcinoma. Am J Clinc Pathol; 2006;125:675-681.

Mayer R, Fowler JE Jr, Clayton M: Localized urethral cancer in women. Cancer 1987;60:1548–1551.

Meis JM, Ayala AG, Johnson DE: Adenocarcinoma of the urethra in women: A clinicopathologic study. Cancer 1987;60:1038–1052.

Mostofi FK, Davis CJ Jr, Sesterhenn IA: Carcinoma of the male and female urethra. Urol Clin North Am 1992;19:347–358.

Murphy DP, Pantuck AJ, Amenta PS, et al: Female urethral adenocarcinoma: Immunohistochemical evidence of more than 1 tissue of origin. J Urol 1999;161:1881–1884.

Roberts TW, Melicow MM: Pathology and natural history of urethral tumors in females: Review of 65 cases. Urology 1977;10:583–589.

Wang HL, Lu DW, Yerian LM, et al: Immunohistochemical detection between primary adenocarcinoma of the bladder and secondary colorectal adenocarcinoma. Am J Surg Pathol 2001;25:1380–1387.

Clear Cell Adenocarcinoma

Davis R, Peterson AC, Lance R: Clear cell adenocarcinoma in a female urethral diverticulum. Urology 2003;61:644.

Drew PA, Murphy WM, Civantos F, Speights VO: The histogenesis of clear cell adenocarcinoma of the lower urinary tract: Case series and review of the literature. Hum Pathol 1996;27:248–252.

Ebisuno S, Miyai M, Nagareda T: Clear cell adenocarcinoma of the female urethra showing positive staining with antibodies to prostate-specific antigen and prostatic acid phosphatase. Urology 1995;45:682–685.

Gilcrease MZ, Delgado R, Vuitch F, Albores-Saavedra J: Clear cell adenocarcinoma and nephrogenic adenoma of the urethra and urinary bladder: A histopathologic and immunohistochemical comparison. Hum Pathol 1998;29:1451–1456.

Oliva E, Young RH: Clear cell adenocarcinoma of the urethra: A clinicopathologic analysis of 19 cases. Mod Pathol 1996;9:513–520.

Seballos RM, Rich RR: Clear cell adenocarcinoma arising from a urethral diverticulum. J Urol 1995;153:1914–1915.

Spencer JR, Brodin AG, Ignatoff JM: Clear cell adenocarcinoma of the urethra: Evidence for origin within paraurethral ducts. J Urol 1990;143:122–125.

Young RH, Scully RE: Clear cell adenocarcinoma of the bladder and urethra: A report of three cases and review of the literature. Am J Surg Pathol 1985;9:816–826.

Urothelial Carcinoma In Situ

Begin LR, Deschenes J, Mitmaker B:Pagetoid carcinomatous involvement of the penile urethra in association with high-grade transitional cell carcinoma of the urinary bladder. Arch Pathol Lab Med 1991;115:632–635.

Freeman JA, Esrig D, Stein JP, Skinner DG: Management of the patient with bladder cancer: Urethral recurrence. Urol Clin North Am 1994;21:645–651.

Hardeman SW, Soloway MS: Urethral recurrence following radical cystectomy. J Urol 1990;144:666–669.

Knapik JA, Murphy WM: Urethral wash cytopathology for monitoring patients after cystoprostatectomy with urinary diversion. Cancer 2003;99:352–356.

Kunju LP, Lee C, Montie J, Shah RB: Cytokeratin 20(CK 20) and Ki-67 as markers of urothelial dysplasia. Pathology International 2005;55:248–254.

Lin DW, Herr HW, Dalbagni G: Value of urethral wash cytology in the retained male urethra after radical cystoprostatectomy. J Urol 2003;169:961–963.

Mallofre C, Castillo M, Morente V, Sole M: Immunohistochemical expression of CK20, p53, and Ki-67 as objective markers of urothelial dysplasia. Mod Pathol 2003;16:187–191.

McKenney JK, Desai S, Cohen C, Amin MB: Discriminatory immunohistochemical staining of urothelial carcinoma in situ and non-neoplastic urothelium: An analysis of cytokeratin 20, p53, and CD44 antigens. Am J Surg Pathol 2001;25:1074–1078.

Nixon RG, Chang SS, Lafleur BJ, et al: Carcinoma in situ and tumor multifocality predict the risk of prostatic urethral involvement at radical cystectomy in men with transitional cell carcinoma of the bladder. J Urol 2002;167(2 Pt 1):502–505.

Robert M, Burgel JS, Serre I, et al: [Urethral recurrence after cysto-prostatectomy for bladder tumor]. Prog Urol 1996;6:558–563.

Sarosdy MF: Management of the male urethra after cystectomy for bladder cancer. Urol Clin North Am 1992;19:391–396.

Malignant Melanoma

Blaumeiser B, Tjalma W, Swaegers M, et al: [Primary malignant melanoma of the female urethra]. Zentralbl Gynakol 2000;122:179–182.

DiMarco DS, DiMarco CS, Zincke H, et al: Outcome of surgical treatment for primary malignant melanoma of the female urethra. J Urol 2004;171(2 Pt 1):765–767.

Kim CJ, Pak K, Hamaguchi A, et al: Primary malignant melanoma of the female urethra. Cancer 1993;71:448–451.

Kubo H, Miyawaki I, Kawagoe M, et al: Primary malignant melanoma of the male urethra. Int J Urol 2002;9:268–271.

Oliva E, Quinn TR, Amin MB, et al: Primary malignant melanoma of the urethra: A clinicopathologic analysis of 15 cases. Am J Surg Pathol 2000;24:785–796.

Urothelial Papillomas

McKenney JK, Amin MB, Young RH: Urothelial (transitional cell) papilloma of the urinary bladder: A clinicopathologic study of 26 cases. Mod Pathol 2003;16:623–629.

Villous Adenoma

Algaba F, Matias-Guiu X, Badia F, Sole-Balcells F: Villous adenoma of the prostatic urethra. Eur Urol 1988;14:255–257.

Morgan DR, Dixon MF, Harnden P: Villous adenoma of urethra associated with tubulovillous adenoma and adenocarcinoma of rectum. Histopathology 1998;32:87–89.

Powell I, Cartwright H, Jano F: Villous adenoma and adenocarcinoma of female urethra. Urology 1981;18:612–614.

Raju GC, Roopnarinesingh A, Woo J: Villous adenoma of female urethra. Urology 1987;29:446–447.

Seibel JL, Prasad S, Weiss RE, et al: Villous adenoma of the urinary tract: A lesion frequently associated with malignancy. Hum Pathol 2002;33:236–241.

Urethral Caruncle

Hammadeh MY, Thomas K, Philp T: Urethral caruncle: An unusual presentation of ovarian tumour. Gynecol Obstet Invest 1996;42:279–280.

Karthikeyan K, Kaviarasan PK, Thappa DM: Urethral caruncle in a male: A case report. J Eur Acad Dermatol Venereol 2002;16:72–73.

Khatib RA, Khalil AM, Tawil AN, et al: Non-Hodgkin's lymphoma presenting as a urethral caruncle. Gynecol Oncol 1993;50:389–393.

Lopez JI, Angulo JC, Ibanez T: Primary malignant melanoma mimicking urethral caruncle: Case report. Scand J Urol Nephrol 1993;27:125–126.

Young RH, Oliva E, Garcia JA, et al: Urethral caruncle with atypical stromal cells simulating lymphoma or sarcoma—A distinctive pseudoneoplastic lesion of females: A report of six cases. Am J Surg Pathol 1996;20:1190–1195.

Nephrogenic Adenoma

Gilcrease MZ, Delgado R, Vuitch F, Albores-Saavedra J: Clear cell adenocarcinoma and nephrogenic adenoma of the urethra and urinary bladder: A histopathologic and immunohistochemical comparison. Hum Pathol 1998;29:1451–1456.

Gupta A, Wang HL, Policarpio-Nicolas ML, et al: Expression of alpha-methylacyl-coenzyme A racemase in nephrogenic adenoma. Am J Surg Pathol 2004;28:1224–1229.

Hartmann A, Jumker K, Dietmaier W, et al: Molecular evidence for progression of nephrogenic metaplasia of the urinary bladder to clear cell adenocarcinoma. Hum Pathol 2006;37(1):117–120.

McIntire TL, Soloway MS, Murphy WM: Nephrogenic adenoma. Urology 1987;29:237–241.

Skinnider BF, Oliva E, Young RH, Amin MB. Expression of alpha-methylacyl-CoA racemase (P504S) in nephrogenic adenoma: A significant immunohistochemical pitfall compounding the differential diagnosis with prostatic adenocarcinoma. Am J Surg Pathol 2004;28:701–705.

Tong GX, Melamed J, Mansukhani M, et al: PAX2: a reliable marker for nephrogenic adenoma. Mod Pathol 2006;19(3):356–363.

Young RH, Scully RE: Nephrogenic adenoma: A report of 15 cases, review of the literature, and comparison with clear cell adenocarcinoma of the urinary tract. Am J Surg Pathol 1986;10:268–275.

Polypoid Urethritis

Schinella R, Thurm J, Feiner H: Papillary pseudotumor of the prostatic urethra: Proliferative papillary urethritis. J Urol 1974;111:38–40.

Prostatic Epithelial Polyp

Fan K, Schaefer RF,Venable M:Urethral verumontanal polyp: Evidence of prostatic origin. Urology 1984;24:499–501.

Inoue K, Sakurai H, Hoshino M, et al: [Urethral polyp of prostatic-type epithelium: A report of two cases]. Nippon Hinyokika Gakkai Zasshi 1987;78:2195–2198.

Murphy WM, Grignon DJ, Perlman EJ: Tumors of the Kidney, Bladder, and Related Urinary Structures, Fascicle 1, 4th series. Washington, DC: American Registry of Pathology, 2004.

Sekine H, Mine M, Kaneoya F, et al: Benign polyp with prostatic-type epithelium in the anterior urethra accompanied with urethral stricture. Urol Int 1993;50:114–116.

Condyloma

Murphy WM, Fu YS, Lancaster WD, Jenson AB: Papillomavirus structural antigens in condyloma acuminatum of the male urethra. J Urol 1983;130:84–85.

Young RH: Pseudoneoplastic lesions of the urinary bladder and urethra: A selective review with emphasis on recent information. Semin Diagn Pathol 1997;14:133–146.

Diseases of the Scrotum: Squamous Cell Carcinoma

Andrews PE, Farrow GM, Oesterling JE: Squamous cell carcinoma of the scrotum: Long-term followup of 14 patients. J Urol 1991;146:1299–1304.

Angulo JC, Lopez JI, Flores N: Squamous cell carcinoma of the scrotum in an aluminium worker. Postgrad Med J 1993;69:960–961.

Arias Funez F, Fernandez Fernandez E, Perales Cabanas L, et al: [Epidermoid carcinoma of the scrotum]. Arch Esp Urol 2000;53:937–940.

Buck VR: Cutting oil hazards: Prevention of carcinoma of scrotum. Occup Health (Lond) 1970;22:67–85.

Burmer GC, True LD, Krieger JN: Squamous cell carcinoma of the scrotum associated with human papillomaviruses. J Urol 1993;149:374–377.

Gross DJ, Schosser RH: Squamous cell carcinoma of the scrotum. Cutis 1991;47:402–404.

Grundy D, Jones AC, Powley PH: Carcinoma of the scrotum associated with rubber urinals: Case report. Paraplegia 1993;31:616–617.

Larkin JC Jr, Murdock WT, Phillips S: Carcinoma of the scrotum in a tire recap worker. Arch Dermatol 1964;89:247–249.

Lowe FC: Squamous-cell carcinoma of the scrotum. Urol Clin North Am 1992;19:397–405.

McDonald MW: Carcinoma of scrotum. Urology 1982;19:269–274.

Parys BT, Hutton JL: Fifteen-year experience of carcinoma of the scrotum. Br J Urol 1991;684:414–417.

Redondo Martinez E, Rey Lopez A, Sanchez Lobo V: [Surgical pathology of the scrotum: An analysis of a series of 56 cases]. Arch Esp Urol 1999;52:11–16.

Saracoglu M, Ugras S: Squamous cell carcinoma of the scrotum. Int Urol Nephrol 1994;26:571–572.

Taniguchi S, Furukawa M, Kutsuna H, et al: Squamous cell carcinoma of the scrotum. Dermatology 1996;193:253–254.

Extramammary Paget Disease of Penis and Scrotum

Bewley AP, Bracka A, Staughton RC, Bunker CB: Extramammary Paget's disease of the scrotum: Treatment with topical 5-fluorouracil and plastic surgery. Br J Dermatol 1994;131:445–446.

Helwig EB, Graham JH: Anogenital (extramammary) Paget's disease: A clinicopathological study. Cancer 1963;16:387–403.

Koga F, Gotoh S, Suzuki S: [A case of invasive bladder cancer with Pagetoid skin lesion of the vulva and anogenital Paget's disease]. Nippon Hinyokika Gakkai Zasshi 1997;88:503–506.

Koh KB, Nazarina AR: Paget's disease of the scrotum: Report of a case with underlying carcinoma of the prostate. Br J Dermatol 1995;133:306–307.

Kuan SF, Montag AG, Hart J, et al: Differential expression of mucin genes in mammary and extramammary Paget's disease. Am J Surg Pathol 2001;25:1469–1477.

Kvist E, Osmundsen PE, Sjolin KE: Primary Paget's disease of the penis: Case report. Scand J Urol Nephrol 1992;26:187–190.

Macedo A Jr, Fichtner J, Hohenfellner R: Extramammary Paget's disease of the penis. Eur Urol 1997;31:382–384.

Michimoto O, Buzou S, Nakashima K: Simultaneous prostatic carcinoma and genital Paget's disease associated with subjacent adenocarcinoma. Br J Urol 1979;51:49.

Quinn AM, Sienko A, Basrawala Z, Campbell SC: Extramammary Paget disease of the scrotum with features of Bowen disease. Arch Pathol Lab Med 2004;128:84–86.

Saidi JA, Bose S, Sawczuk IS: Eccrine sweat gland carcinoma of the scrotum with associated extramammary Paget's disease. Urology 1997;50:789–791.

Tomaszewski JE, van Randenborgh H, Paul R, et al: Extramammary Paget's disease of penis and scrotum. J Urol 2002;168:2540–2541.

Yang WJ, Kom DS, Im YJ, et al: Extramammary Paget's disease of penis and scrotum. Urology 2005; 65(5):972–975.

Yoshii N, Kitajima S, Yonezawa S, et al: Expression of mucin core proteins in extramammary Paget's disease. Pathol Int 2002;52:390–399.

Basal Cell Carcinoma

Ho WS, King WW, Chan WY, Li AK: Basal cell carcinoma of the scrotum. Natl Med J India 1995;8:195.

Nahass GT, Blauvelt A, Leonardi CL, Penneys NS: Basal cell carcinoma of the scrotum: Report of three cases and review of the literature. J Am Acad Dermatol 1992;26:574–578.

Redondo Martinez E, Lopez AR, Cruz Benavides F, Camacho Galan R: [Basal cell carcinoma of the scrotum: A rare localization linked to a bad prognosis]. Arch Esp Urol 2000;53:642–644.

Vandeweyer E, Deraemaecker R. Basal cell carcinoma of the scrotum. J Urol 2000;163:914.

Mesenchymal Neoplasms

Bauer JJ, Sesterhenn IA, Costabile RA: Myxoid liposarcoma of the scrotal wall. J Urol 1995;153:1938–1939.

Newman PL, Fletcher CD: Smooth muscle tumours of the external genitalia: Clinicopathological analysis of a series. Histopathology 1991;18:523–529.

Ray B, Huvos AG, Whitmore WF Jr: Unusual malignant tumors of the scrotum: Review of 5 cases. J Urol 1972;108:760–766.

Washecka RM, Sidhu G, Surya B: Leiomyosarcoma of scrotum. Urology 1989;34:144–146.

Sclerosing Lipogranuloma

Holscher AH, Rahlf G, Zimmermann A: [Sclerosing lipogranuloma of male genitalia (author's transl)]. Urologe A 1979;18:106–108.

Kodama K, Yotsuyanagi S, Fuse H, et al: [Sclerosing lipogranuloma of the scrotum: A case report]. Hinyokika Kiyo 1999;45:211–214.

Terada T, Minami S, Onda H, et al: Primary sclerosing lipogranuloma with broad necrosis of the scrotum. Pathol Int 2003;53:121–125.

Watanabe K, Hoshi N, Baba K, et al: Immunohistochemical profile of primary sclerosing lipogranuloma of the scrotum: Report of five cases. Pathol Int 1995;45:854–859.

"Idiopathic" Scrotal Calcinosis and Epidermoid Cysts

Dare AJ, Axelsen RA: Scrotal calcinosis: Origin from dystrophic calcification of eccrine duct milia. J Cutan Pathol 1988;15:142–149.

Dini M, Colafranceschi M: Should scrotal calcinosis still be termed idiopathic? Am J Dermatopathol 1998;20:399–402.

el Fassi MJ, el Ammari JE, Khallouk A, et al: [Scrotal calcinosis]. Prog Urol 2003;13:332–333.

Ozgenel GY, Kahveci R, Filiz G, Ozcan M: Idiopathic scrotal calcinosis. Ann Plast Surg 2002;48:453–454.

Saladi RN, Persaud AN, Phelps RG, Cohen SR: Scrotal calcinosis: Is the cause still unknown? J Am Acad Dermatol 2004;51(2 Suppl):S97–S101.

Swinehart JM, Golitz LE: Scrotal calcinosis: Dystrophic calcification of epidermoid cysts. Arch Dermatol 1982;118:985–988.

Angiokeratoma

Fordyce JA: Angiokeratoma of the scrotum. J Cutan Genitourin Dis 1896;(14):81–87.

Imperial R, Helwig EB. Angiokeratoma of the scrotum (Fordyce type). J Urol 1967;98:379–387.

Jansen T, Bechara FG, Stucker M, Altmeyer P: Angiokeratoma of the scrotum (Fordyce type) associated with angiokeratoma of the oral cavity. Acta Derm Venereol 2002;82:208–210.

Karthikeyan K, Sethuraman G, Thappa DM: Angiokeratoma of the oral cavity and scrotum. J Dermatol 2000;27:131–132.

Miller C, James WD: Angiokeratoma of Fordyce as a cause of red scrotum. Cutis 2002;69:50–51.

Scrotal Fat Necrosis

Hollander JB, Begun FP, Lee RD: Scrotal fat necrosis. J Urol 1985;134:150–151.

Koster LH, Antoon SJ: Fat necrosis in the scrotum. J Urol 1980;123:599–600.

Levine SP: Fat necrosis of the scrotum. J Urol 1980;12:578.

9 Non-neoplastic Diseases of the Testis

Howard S. Levin

Testicular specimens are relative rarities in the surgical pathology laboratory. This chapter describes, illustrates, and compares the most common pathologic entities. Specimens may be obtained from patients who are newborn, prepubertal, or postpubertal. It is therefore important to have knowledge of the embryology and anatomy of the testes and paratesticular structures.

EMBRYOLOGY

The development of the testis depends on fertilization of an X-bearing ovum by a Y-bearing sperm. On the Y chromosome is a gene named sex determining region Y (SRY). Celomic epithelial cells develop at about 5 weeks of gestation, and the mesenchyme along the medial portion of the mesonephros thickens and is known as the genital ridge. Primary sex cords develop in the genital ridges and extend into underlying mesenchyme. Primordial germ cells migrate from the yolk sac and, by week 6, are in the sex cords. Straight tubules, rete testis, and Leydig cells develop from mesenchyme. Sertoli cells develop from sex cords; together with germ cells, they comprise the seminiferous tubules. Mesonephric tubules develop into efferent ducts and connect the rete testis and the epididymis. Localized testosterone production from Leydig cells stimulates the ipsilateral mesonephric duct to form epididymis, vas deferens, and seminal vesicles. Sertoli cells produce anti-müllerian hormone (AMH), which causes regression of the müllerian duct. This is an intricately timed scenario, and abnormalities in timing or in cell or organ precursors lead to abnormalities in structure and function of the testis and the excurrent duct system, and possibly to persistence of müllerian duct structures.

ANATOMY

Each adult testis weighs 12 to 19 g, averages 4.5 × 2.5 × 3 cm in dimension, and is suspended in the scrotum by a spermatic cord. The rete testis at the mediastinum of the testis connects to the head of the epididymis, which is apposed to the testis posteriorly. The epididymis is a convoluted tubular structure, about 5 cm long, that extends to the inferior pole. The tail of the epididymis is attached to the vas deferens, a thick muscular tubular structure that extends superiorly within the spermatic cord and joins the seminal vesicle, becoming the ejaculatory duct within the prostate gland. The lumens of the rete testis, epididymis, vas deferens, and ejaculatory duct are continuous. The testis is covered by a collagenous capsule, the tunica albuginea. Within the substance of the testis are many lobules of tan, convoluted, seminiferous tubules divided into microscopic lobules.

It is important to distinguish between prepubertal and postpubertal testes, in order to understand normal growth and development and whether there is an intact hypothalamic-pituitary-testicular axis. At the time of birth, although Leydig cells have begun to regress, they are still numerous (Fig. 9-1). They usually disappear by age 4 months and reappear at the time of puberty (Fig. 9-2). Seminiferous tubules are small at the time of birth, with small or no lumina. Seminiferous tubules are mostly populated by prepubertal Sertoli cells, with dark round to oval nuclei. A few primordial germ cells are present within each cross-section of tubule. These cells have large nuclei and cleared cytoplasm (Fig. 9-3). Tubules start to enlarge and primary spermatocytes may be recognized by age 8 years. Leydig cells may appear as early as 8 years of age. Sertoli cells acquire more eosinophilic cytoplasm and spermatogenesis may occur by age 11 years (Fig. 9-4). Postpubertal Sertoli cells do not undergo mitosis. Postpubertal seminiferous tubules are larger than prepubertal seminiferous tubules (Fig. 9-5). They have a variable appearance, because the tubules have developed lumina and are in different stages of spermatogenesis.

In adults, all tubules have the least mature cells against the basement membrane and the most mature cells, elongate spermatids, at the luminal border. Along the basement membrane, spermatogonia with enlarged nuclei and clear to dark cytoplasm are present. Sertoli cells are oriented perpendicular to the basement membrane and have round to oval, sometimes indented nuclei with nucleoli. Elongate spermatids may be seen within Sertoli cell cytoplasm. Ultrastructurally, tight junctions form between Sertoli cells, creating basal (outer) and adlumenal (inner) compartments. Primary spermatocytes in three stages are present in cell layers toward the lumen. Primary spermatocytes divide into secondary spermatocytes, which usually are not recognized on light microscopy. These divide into round spermatids, which lose their cytoplasm and develop

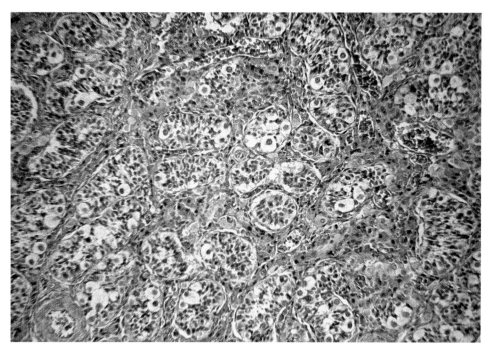

FIGURE 9-1

Aluminal seminiferous tubules contain numerous prepubertal Sertoli cells and primordial germ cells in the testis of a newborn. Between tubules, there are large numbers of eosinophilic Leydig cells.

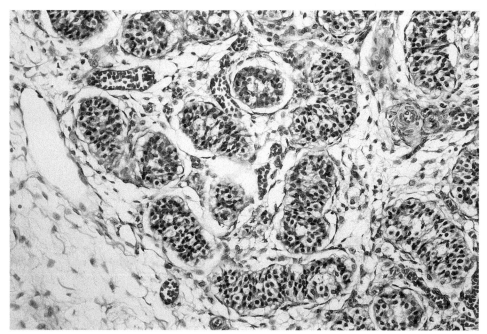

FIGURE 9-2

Small aluminal tubules are present within a loose mesenchyme in the testis of a 4 month old. Seminiferous tubules are populated by numerous prepubertal Sertoli cells and fewer primordial germ cells. Germ cells are recognizable by their cleared cytoplasm. Within the loose mesenchyme are occasional cells recognizable as Leydig cells because of their eosinophilic to vacuolated cytoplasm.

dense and elongate nuclei with acrosomes. The entire process from spermatogonia to elongate spermatids is called spermatogenesis. The nondivisional maturation of spermatids is called spermiogenesis. Interstitial tissue exists between seminiferous tubules and contains Leydig cells, vascular structures, and connective tissue. Once the testis has acquired postpubertal qualities, it is not possible to determine the age of the patient histologically (Fig. 9-6).

CONGENITAL ABNORMALITIES

CRYPTORCHIDISM

Cryptorchidism is also known as undescended or maldescended testis. These testes may be intra-abdominal, intracanalicular, or ectopic (Fig. 9-7). Retractile testes

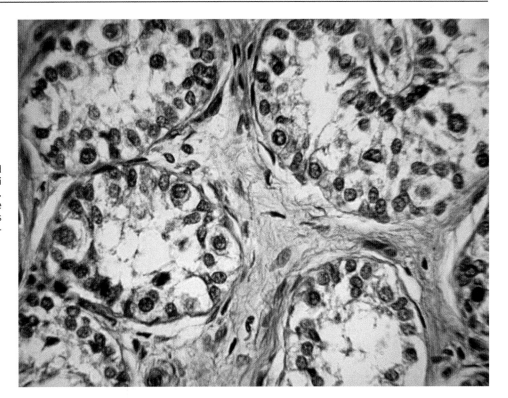

FIGURE 9-3

Mostly aluminal tubules are lined predominantly by prepubertal Sertoli cells in the testis of a 4-year-old. Spermatogonia are present along the basement membrane. No Leydig cells are identifiable within the connective tissue of the interstitium.

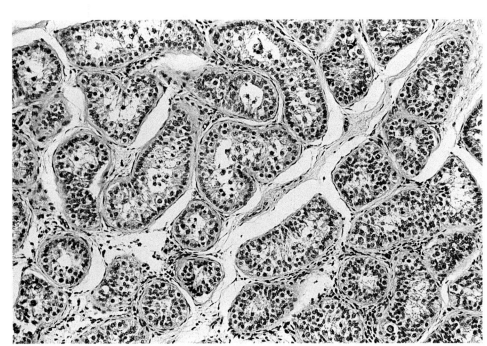

FIGURE 9-4

Early spermatogenesis has begun in an 11-year-old. Tubules have increased in size. Some tubules contain lumina. Primary spermatocytes are focally present within one tubule *(center)*. No Leydig cells are present.

are generally not considered to be cryptorchid, but the distinction can be difficult. Cryptorchidism may be discovered at any age, but it is usually discovered in children and may be discovered at the time of birth. The two major concerns in a patient with cryptorchidism are fertility and the development of a germ cell tumor. It is recognized that in cryptorchidism histologic changes occur in the testis during the first year of life, with defective maturation of primordial germ cells into spermatogonia. Fewer germ cells per tubule are present in the cryptorchid testis after the first year of life. Thickening of the tunica propria occurs during the first year of life. Surgeons generally treat cryptorchid patients before 2 years of age, sometimes after the patient has received a trial of human chorionic gonadotropin or gonadotropin-releasing hormone (GnRH). Patients with cryptorchidism have a 5.2 to 7.5 greater relative risk for the development of a malignant germ cell tumor

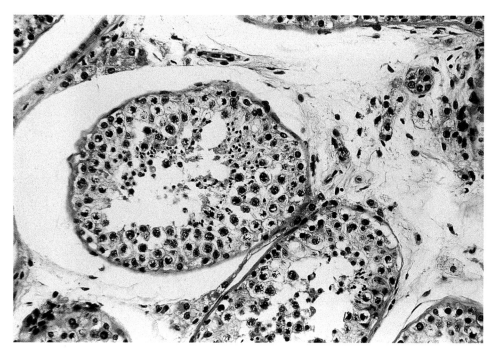

FIGURE 9-5

Seminiferous tubules are undergoing complete spermatogenesis in a 13-year-old. The least mature cells are along the basement membrane, and the most mature cells (elongate spermatids) along the luminal border. A cluster of Leydig cells with eosinophilic cytoplasm is present in the left upper corner.

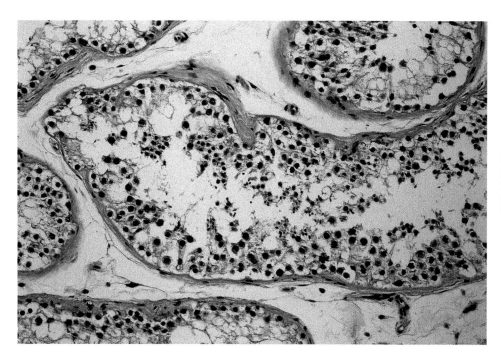

FIGURE 9-6

Spermatogenesis may persist well into old age. Complete spermatogenesis is present in the center tubule.

in adult life. Undescended testes are also susceptible to torsion and infarction. If torsion occurs in an undescended testis in an adult, the gonad may harbor a malignant tumor. Adults with unilateral cryptorchidism may be fertile, but with bilateral cryptorchidism they are unlikely to be fertile.

Cryptorchidism can be dealt with clinically in a number of ways. In infancy, hormonal therapy (Fig. 9-8) may facilitate the descent of the testis, or an orchiopexy may be performed, bringing the testis into the scrotum if this is surgically possible. Sometimes no therapy is performed in infancy and the decision to treat the condition is postponed until childhood or even adulthood. Two considerations that may determine therapy include the preservation of fertility and the risk of malignancy. Balancing these, it may be elected to perform an orchiopexy or, particularly in adulthood, to perform an orchiectomy.

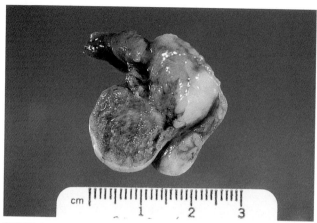

FIGURE 9-7

This intra-abdominal testis was resected incidentally in the course of abdominal aortic surgery. It is soft and shrunken, measuring 2.5 cm in maximum dimension. An area of scarring is present near the hilus.

PATHOLOGIC FEATURES

GROSS FINDINGS

In early life, the gonad appears normal. With progression of age, the cryptorchid testis is smaller than a normally descended testis.

MICROSCOPIC FINDINGS

By light microscopy in infancy, the testis may appear normal. As the patient gets older, there are reduced numbers of germ cells per tubule. In postpubertal individuals, seminiferous tubules are of reduced diameter, with increased tunica propria thickening and reduced spermatogenesis (Fig. 9-9). Some tubules are lined exclusively by Sertoli cells. There may be foci of per-

sistent immature tubules (so-called Pick's adenomas) in the adult cryptorchid testis (Fig. 9-9). These foci are suggestive but not diagnostic of cryptorchidism. A biopsy may be obtained of the testis at the time of orchiopexy. Marked dystrophic calcifications may sometimes be found (Fig. 9-10). Pathologists should assess the biopsy specimen for the presence of malignant intratubular germ cells and the presence of normal germ cells. Malignant intratubular germ cells have been identified in testes with prior orchiopexy in up to 8% of cases. Immunoperoxidase stains for CD117 and placental alkaline phosphatase (PLAP) are useful in confirming the presence of malignant intratubular germ cells in patients older than 1 year of age (Fig. 9-11). Positive immunohistochemical stains in the first year of life are not helpful in identifying malignant cells. Immunoperoxidase stain for inhibin will stain Sertoli and Leydig cells and leave germinal cells unstained (Figs. 9-12 and 9-13).

ANORCHISM

Anorchism, the absence of testis, is a diagnosis that is made after a gonad is not discovered at the time of surgical exploration. Because of the risk of development of a malignant tumor in adulthood, the surgeon attempts to discover the cryptorchid testis and bring it into the scrotum if it is viable. Surgical evaluations are often performed laparoscopically. In the absence of a defined gonad, the surgeon usually resects what is clinically interpreted as a gonadal remnant. If the gonadal remnant contains a portion of wolffian duct, then the patient had a functioning testis during prenatal development. Subsequent to the development of the wolffian duct, testicular regression may have occurred

FIGURE 9-8

This 2-year-old patient was previously given gonadotropin therapy in an attempt to encourage descent of the testis. Gonadotropic hormones have stimulated the hyperplastic Leydig cells. Seminiferous tubules are prepubertal in type.

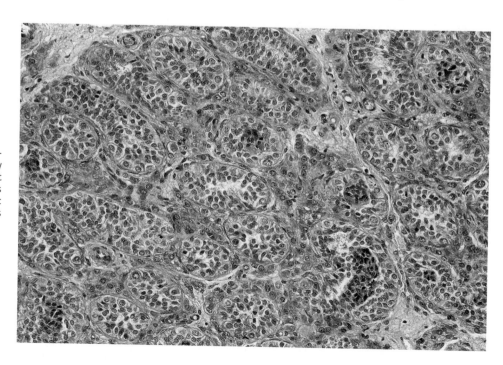

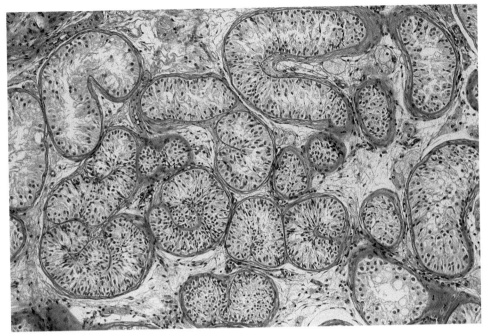

FIGURE 9-9

A nodule of persistent prepubertal-type tubules (so-called Pick's adenoma) comprises the majority of the photomicrograph. Tubules are lined by Sertoli cells having less abundant cytoplasm than would be expected in this 18-year-old. A tubule lined by postpubertal Sertoli cells is in the upper left.

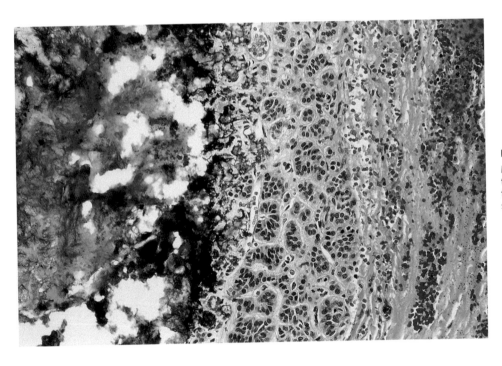

FIGURE 9-10

Marked dystrophic calcification in the cryptorchid testis of a 4-year-old that presented as a mass of the left spermatic cord.

as a result of infection, trauma, torsion, or prenatal hormone-induced atrophy. This is an example of testicular regression syndrome.

PATHOLOGIC FEATURES

The surgeon usually resects a 1-cm, cord-like structure. Microscopically, vas deferens and/or epididymis can be identified, and very often there is concomitant fibrosis, hemosiderin deposition, and/or calcification. The pathol-

ogist should examine the entire specimen histologically, searching for gonadal tissue. If wolffian duct structures are identified, particularly with evidence of fibrosis, calcification, and iron deposition, this should be reported as consistent with testicular regression syndrome.

POLYORCHISM

Polyorchism, the presence of more than two testes, is unusual. The relationship of the testes to the excurrent

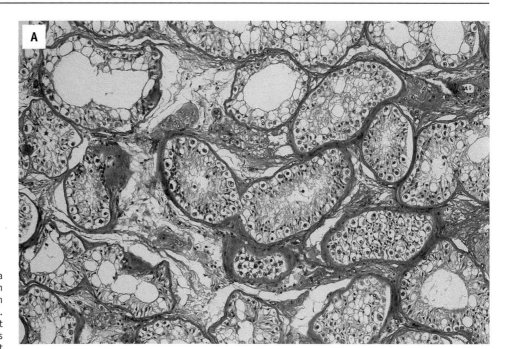

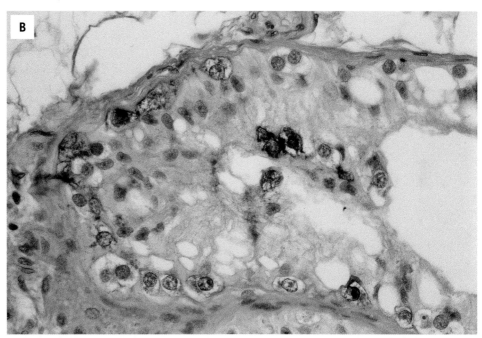

FIGURE 9-11

A, At the time of orchiopexy in a 15-year-old boy, a frozen section revealed malignant intratubular germ cells. An orchiectomy was performed. Many tubules contain malignant intratubular germ cells. These cells are predominantly along the basement membrane; they contain enlarged and somewhat irregular nuclei, prominent nucleoli, and clear cytoplasm. **B,** Immunoperoxidase stain for placental alkaline phosphatase (PLAP) demonstrates positive plasma membrane and cytoplasmic staining of malignant intratubular germ cells.

duct system is variable. There may be connection between a single epididymis and two testes, or there may be two individual testes, epididymides and vasa deferentia, that join distally. Spermatogenesis can occur in polyorchism, and tumors have been reported.

TESTICULAR-SPLENIC FUSION

Gonadal-splenic fusion, which occurs most frequently in the male (male/female ratio, approximately 9:1),

manifests as a testicular mass, rarely as a tender testicular enlargement in a male with systemic infection, or most frequently in an individual with limb defects and other anomalies including severe congenital malformations of the extremities and/or oromandibular limb hypogenesis (Fig. 9-14). Testicular-splenic fusion always occurs on the left side, and the connection of the spleen to the gonad is either continuous or discontinuous (Fig. 9-15). The coexistence of this lesion with limb-bud abnormalities suggests that it occurs during the fifth to seventh week of gestation. The testes may be either descended or cryptorchid. Rare germ cell tumors have been identified in the testis.

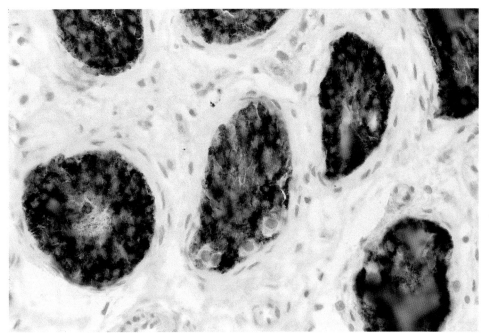

FIGURE 9-12

This biopsy specimen of a cryptorchid testis, obtained at the time of orchiopexy in a 13-year-old boy, demonstrates that seminiferous tubules are composed predominantly of Sertoli cells. Immunoperoxidase stain for inhibin demonstrates marked positivity of Sertoli cells. Occasional unstained cells along the basement membrane are spermatogonia. This biopsy has the appearance of a prepubertal testis except for the occasional, lightly staining inhibin positive Leydig cells within the interstitium *(upper center)*.

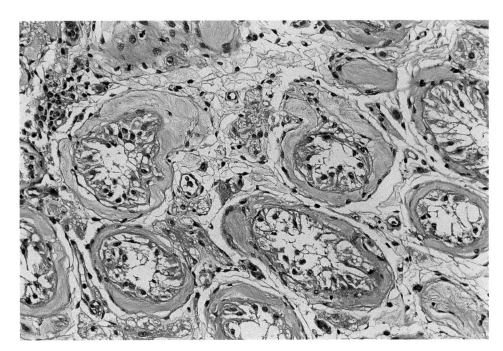

FIGURE 9-13

The seminiferous tubules are markedly reduced in diameter, with extensive tunica propria thickening, in this 41-year-old man with cryptorchidism. Seminiferous tubules contain only Sertoli cells.

PATHOLOGIC FEATURES

MICROSCOPIC FINDINGS

Encapsulated splenic tissue is present in juxtaposition to the testis. Seminiferous tubules adjacent to the splenic tissue may show germinal cell aplasia and hypoplasia. This condition has no inherent malignant potential.

ADRENAL CORTICAL RESTS

PATHOLOGIC FEATURES

The rests of adrenal cortex are generally identified along the pathway of descent of the testis at the time of

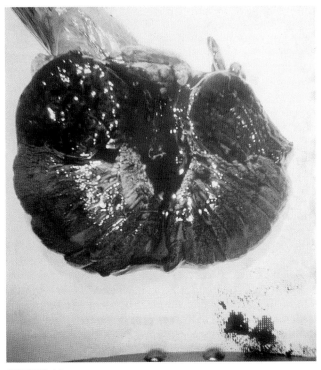

FIGURE 9-14

A 17-year-old boy with peromelia (limb bud defects identical to those seen in thalidomide embryopathy) developed an intrascrotal mass. An orchiectomy revealed a nodule of benign splenic tissue adherent to the tunica albuginea. Bivalved testis with splenic tissue (darkened) at one pole.

surgical exploration in the treatment of cryptorchidism. These have been described in 4% to 15% of males. The rests are small, rounded, and yellow. Microscopically, they are comprised of adrenal cortical tissue without adrenal medullary tissue. These rests are inconsequential except in cases where they respond to stimulation by endogenous or exogenous adrenocorticotropic hormone (ACTH). These nodules are described later in the discussion of congenital adrenal hyperplasia.

ACQUIRED ABNORMALITIES

SPERMATIC CORD TORSION AND TESTICULAR INFARCTION

CLINICAL FEATURES

Torsion of the spermatic cord refers to twisting of the cord. Depending on the extent and duration of torsion, there may be infarction of the testis. Torsion may occur within the tunica vaginalis as a result of a high insertion of the tunica vaginalis on the spermatic cord, or the torsion may be external to the tunica vaginalis (extravaginal). Extravaginal torsion usually occurs in utero or in infancy. Intravaginal torsion usually occurs in adolescence or young adulthood. Torsion is variable and may exceed 360 degrees. Torsion of less than

FIGURE 9-15

Testicular-splenic fusion. Splenic tissue *(right)* fused to and involving testicular parenchyma *(left)*.

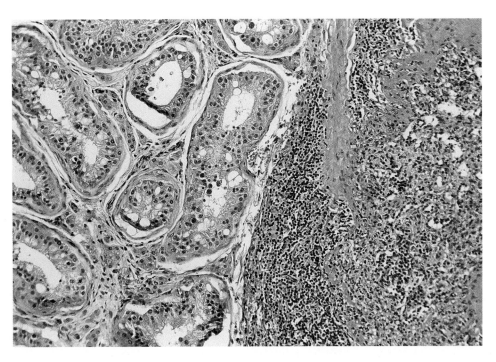

6 hours' duration probably will not cause a testicular infarct (Fig. 9-16). Torsions that last longer than 24 hours will almost certainly produce a hemorrhagic infarct. Because of the importance of early diagnosis, the "acute scrotum" should be promptly diagnosed and treated. Surgical exploration is sometimes necessary to distinguish torsion and/or infarction from other causes of intrascrotal pain.

RADIOLOGIC FEATURES

Color-flow duplex Doppler ultrasound and radionuclide scintigraphy are frequently used and may be useful in resolving cases of acute scrotal pain. Both studies have 80% to 90% sensitivity and 75% to 95% specificity. If they are immediately available, they may be of clinical value, but their use should not delay attempted manual detorsion and scrotal exploration.

PATHOLOGIC FEATURES

GROSS FINDINGS

Changes vary depending on the extent and duration of torsion. Usually, the testicle and spermatic cord are detorsed in the operating room. It is only when the urologist has determined that the testis is no longer viable that it is removed. The pathologist usually is unable to identify the site of torsion. Sometimes a part or all of the epididymis is also infarcted. The infarcted testis is swollen and dark red to blue as a result of being suffused with blood. On cut section, there may be a small preserved rim of normal testis testis and a sharp demarcation of hemorrhagic to necrotic testicular parenchyma. In cases of ancient infarct, the testis will be shrunken and whitish, without recognizable tubular architecture. In cases of more recent infarct, an intraoperative biopsy and frozen section may have taken place and a sutured biopsy site may be present.

MICROSCOPIC FINDINGS

The histologic changes may occur in a zonal distribution. A thin rim of preserved seminiferous tubules may be present beneath the tunica albuginea. Beneath this, depending on the extent and duration of torsion, the testis shows venous congestion, interstitial hemorrhage, and necrosis. A polymorphonuclear leukocyte reaction may be seen at the periphery of an infarct. I have identified viable tubules in testes 5.5, 6, and 18 hours after onset of torsion, and partial necrosis of tubules was identified 24 hours after onset. Complete tubule necrosis with lack of viable tubules was identified in a testis removed 57.5 hours after onset of torsion. Partial necrosis of epididymal tubules was noted 24 hours after onset of torsion. Focal capsular granulation tissue was first identified at 5 days. Infarct and granulation tissue become more extensive with time (Figs. 9-17 to 9-19). Remote infarction may result in mummification as well as fibrosis and calcification.

To completely study an infarct and the extent of reaction to it, it is important to adequately sample the cord, epididymis, and testis in a number of areas, including the periphery of the testis and paratesticular tissue.

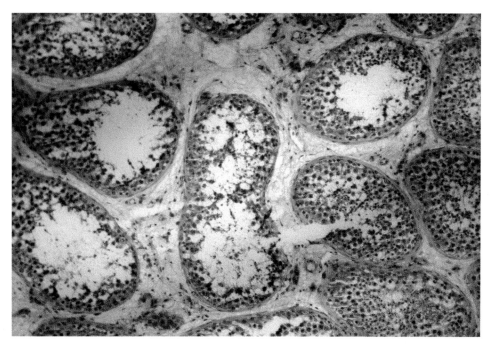

FIGURE 9-16

Frozen-section biopsy specimen $5\frac{1}{2}$ hours after the onset of torsion demonstrated a viable testis with extensive interstitial vascular congestion and hemorrhage. Seminiferous tubules are undergoing spermatogenesis, and their cells appear viable. Acetic acid, used in processing the frozen section, has caused lysis of red blood cells, so congestion and hemorrhage cannot be seen.

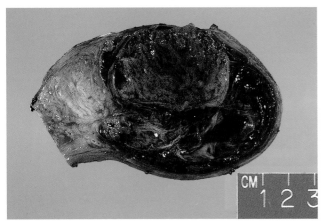

FIGURE 9-17
This 41-year-old man had a history of intermittent torsion that culminated in constant testicular pain of 2 days' duration. The specimen weighed 162 g, was completely infarcted, and was partially surrounded by a hematocele.

VARICOCELE

CLINICAL FEATURES

Varicocele consists of an abnormal dilation and tortuosity of veins in the pampiniform plexus of the spermatic cord. The entity is common, is usually left-sided, and develops during puberty. The patient may or may not know that he has an abnormality in the scrotum. Sometimes the patient feels a large varicocele, which has been described as "a bag of worms." At other times, it is only after the patient has a recognized infertility problem that the varicocele is discovered. The varicocele is the result of faulty or absent venous valves. The varicoceles tend to involve the left spermatic vein, and they may affect semen quality. They can be treated in a number of ways. The veins may be tied off, a vein segment may be removed, or the vein may be occluded by embolization.

PATHOLOGIC FEATURES

If a varicocele is treated surgically, a small segment of vein will be removed. This is usually unremarkable grossly. Microscopically, the vein shows evidence of fibrous thickening of the wall, phlebosclerosis. Testis biopsy specimens obtained at the time of therapy for varicocele are usually of the left testis and show changes of hypospermatogenesis or maturation arrest. Agger and Johnsen examined rebiopsied testes and found improvement in histology 1 year after venous ligation.

MICROLITHIASIS

In males studied with ultrasound, the presence of more than five foci of calcification less than 2 mm in diameter, randomly distributed in the testis, is classified as testicular microlithiasis. This finding has been reported in children and adults, in infertility patients, in association with testicular germ cell tumors, in descended and undescended testes (Fig. 9-20).

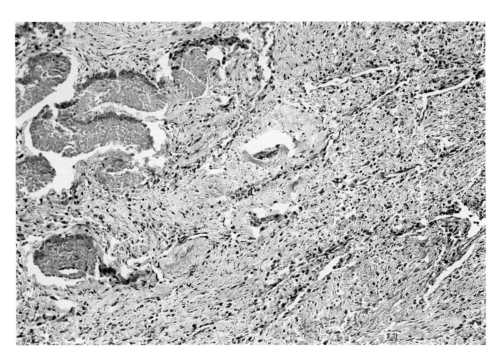

FIGURE 9-18
The patient is a 14-year-old boy who had a history of torsion and infarction for 1 month. The seminiferous tubules *(left)* are completely necrotic. Granulation tissue is present at the periphery *(right)*.

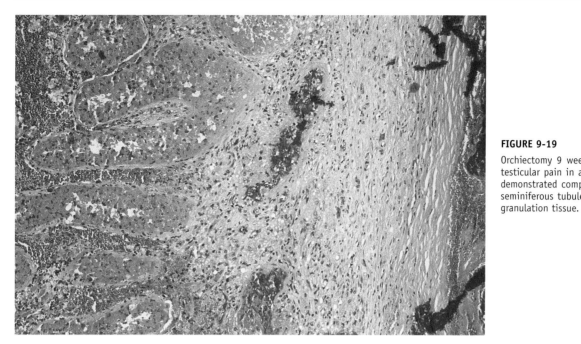

FIGURE 9-19
Orchiectomy 9 weeks after onset of testicular pain in a 19-year-old man demonstrated complete infarction of seminiferous tubules with peripheral granulation tissue.

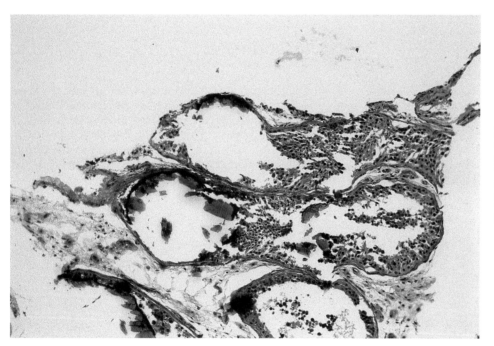

FIGURE 9-20
This intrapubertal testis contains intratubular laminated calcifications. The architecture is distorted and disrupted by tissue artefact secondary to the presence of calcification. There is no evidence of malignant intratubular germ cell neoplasia.

CLINICAL FEATURES

There are no clinical findings other than the ultrasonically discovered multiple foci of microcalcification.

PATHOLOGIC FEATURES

There are no gross pathologic features. The microscopic findings consist of laminated intratubular calcifications.

These may occur in otherwise unremarkable testes or in testes with other pathologic abnormalities, including malignant intratubular germ cell neoplasia, cryptorchidism, and testicular germ cell tumors.

PROGNOSIS AND TREATMENT

Because of the frequency of testicular microlithiasis in testes with malignant germ cell tumors, the question has arisen as to whether it is a risk factor for the development of malignant germ cell tumors. As of 2004, there have been only five reported cases of patients with known testicular microlithiasis on ultrasound examination who had no prior or coexistent tumor and who eventually developed a primary testicular germ cell tumor. There is a 2% to 6% incidence of testicular microlithiasis in asymptomatic populations. Because of the discrepancy between the incidence of testicular microlithiasis in a healthy population and the low incidence of testicular germ cell tumors in the general population, it has been suggested that patients should not be monitored solely on the basis of testicular microlithiasis. Rather, other risk factors for testicular tumors should determine follow-up. These factors are cryptorchism, testicular atrophy, infertility, malignant intratubular germ cell neoplasia, gonadal dysgenesis, the presence of a contralateral germ cell tumor of the testis, and exogenous estrogen administration to the mother when the patient was in utero.

TESTICULAR INVOLVEMENT IN SYSTEMIC DISEASES

VASCULITIS

Systemic vasculitis is associated with a variety of pathologic entities: polyarteritis nodosum, Wegener's granulomatosis (Fig. 9-21), Henoch-Schönlein's purpura, typhus, acute myelogenous leukemia, hairy cell leukemia, Goodpasture's syndrome, and necrotizing sarcoid. In addition, isolated testicular vasculitis, unassociated with systemic vasculitis, rarely occurs. A case of Buerger's disease of the spermatic cord has been reported.

CLINICAL FEATURES

Vasculitis usually occurs in adults, although I have studied a case of polyarteritis nodosum in an intrapubertal male. The testis may be enlarged and painful, or shrunken, or it may present as a mass lesion. Vasculitis may be discovered at the time of postmortem examination (Figs. 9-21 and 9-22). In cases of suspected systemic vasculitis, the pathologist may be consulted before the performance of the biopsy. The pathologist should recommend that the biopsy include the tunica albuginea, the tunica vasculosa, and underlying testicular parenchyma. Therefore, a wedge biopsy should be performed.

PATHOLOGIC FEATURES

GROSS FINDINGS

The testis may be enlarged or small. The findings may be secondary to the vasculitic lesion or the result of ischemia. Arterial lesions may occur in the parenchyma of the testis, particularly in the tunica vasculosa (the vascular layer immediately beneath the tunica albuginea) or in extratesticular tissues. Parenchymal lesions include infarcts, scars consistent with healed infarcts, diffuse fibrosis, and focal tubular hyalinization.

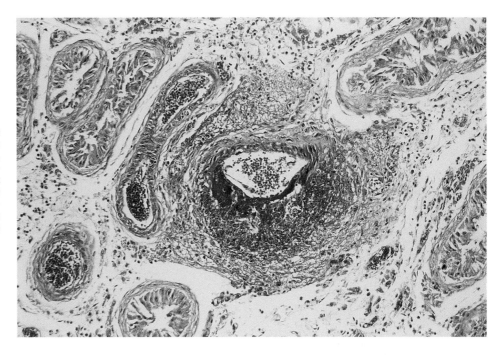

FIGURE 9-21

A 38-year-old man with Wegener's granulomatosis had multisystem involvement including arthralgias, cutaneous vasculitis, nasal ulceration, and glomerulonephritis. At autopsy, the testes were grossly unremarkable. Microscopically, segmental necrotizing arteritis with extensive fibrinoid changes is present.

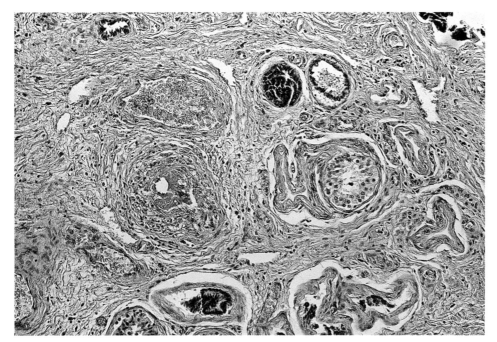

FIGURE 9-22

The patient is a 16-year-old intrapubertal male with necrotizing arteritis associated with polyarteritis nodosum. Inflammation extends throughout the arterial wall.

Hematomas and foci of interstitial hemorrhage may occur. Punctate hemorrhages, so-called "flea bites," may indicate the presence of an active vasculitis.

MICROSCOPIC FINDINGS

Active vasculitis is manifested by fibrinoid necrosis of a small or medium-sized artery. There may or may not be a cellular reaction (Fig. 9-23). The appearance of the vessels is similar to those with vasculitis elsewhere in the body. Infarcts may be of varying ages and consist of segmental necrosis of testicular parenchyma, including tubules and interstitium. In cases of older vasculitis, scars may involve testicular parenchyma and may obliterate parenchymal architecture. If vasculitis is suspected and the initial sections do not demonstrate it, the specimen should be serially sectioned, because vasculitis can be a focal phenomenon.

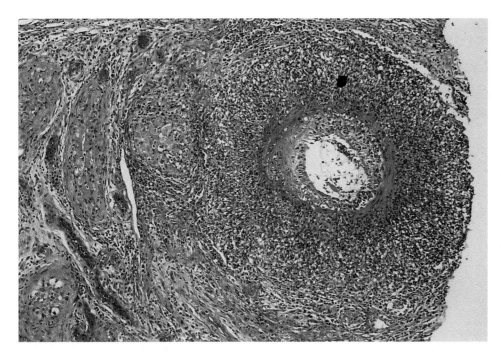

FIGURE 9-23

This 29-year-old man with necrotizing sarcoid also had non-necrotizing granulomas of mediastinal lymph nodes. In the orchiectomy specimen, there is panarteritis with numerous polymorphonuclear neutrophils involving all layers of an artery. Inflammation extends into periarterial connective tissue. A non-necrotizing granuloma is present to the left of the arteritis.

DIFFERENTIAL DIAGNOSIS

The differential diagnosis of testicular vasculitis includes systemic and isolated testicular vasculitis. These may not be distinguishable histologically. In most instances, the patient has evidence of systemic vasculitis elsewhere.

PROGNOSIS AND TREATMENT

Cases with testicular vasculitis should be clinically evaluated and the presence of systemic vasculitis ascertained. Where no evidence of systemic vasculitis is present after a thorough clinical evaluation, the patient should be clinically monitored. In some cases, there will be no evidence of systemic vasculitis.

AMYLOIDOSIS

Systemic amyloidosis frequently involves the testis. I am unaware of localized testicular amyloidosis with or without a mass lesion of the testis.

CLINICAL FEATURES

Systemic amyloidosis may manifest in a number of ways that are beyond the scope of this chapter. If the clinician suspects amyloidosis, a clinical biopsy usually renders the diagnosis. Although the testis is generally not selected as the primary biopsy site, it is more sensitive than rectal biopsy for the diagnosis of primary and secondary amyloidosis. The testis may be enlarged or firm. Only rarely, however, is infertility the chief complaint of a patient with amyloidosis.

PATHOLOGIC FEATURES

GROSS FINDINGS

In general, no gross findings have been described in systemic amyloid deposition in the testis. However, microscopic involvement may be extensive.

MICROSCOPIC FINDINGS

Amyloid deposition occurs within the blood vessels of the interstitium and, to a lesser degree, in the outer walls of the seminiferous tubules (Fig. 9-24). The extent and smudgy nature of the amyloid within the walls of the vessel and in the interstitium suggests the diagnosis of amyloid. Amyloid may also extend into the lumina of the tubules. The diagnosis of amyloid should always be confirmed with apple-green birefringence demonstrated by Congo red stain. Patients with amyloidosis involving the testis also have pathologic changes similar to those seen in infertility biopsies.

PATHOLOGY OF MALE INFERTILITY

The evaluation of infertility must involve both the male and the female. In approximately 40% of couples,

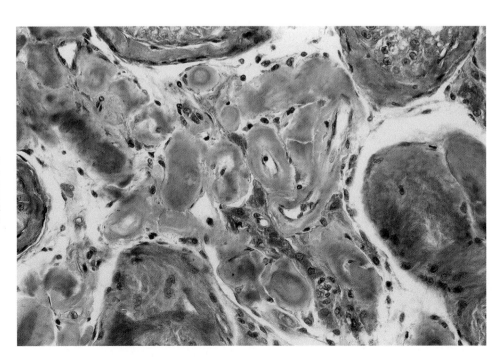

FIGURE 9-24
This 42-year-old man with systemic amyloidosis underwent an orchiectomy. Most of the amyloid is in the walls of interstitial blood vessels. A small amount of amyloid is present in the wall of a seminiferous tubule *(lower right)*.

Table 9-1
Testicular Findings Associated with Male Infertility

Normal spermatogenesis

Hypospermatogenesis

Maturation arrest

Germinal cell aplasia

Germinal cell aplasia with focal spermatogenesis

Testicular changes associated with genetic abnormalities

Tubular sclerosis and interstitial fibrosis (end-stage testis)

Active spermatogenesis compatible with excurrent duct
obstruction

infertility is caused by a problem with the male partner alone. In another 20% of couples, the infertility problems exist both in the male and female. Although relatively few testis biopsies are performed to diagnose a problem with regard to sperm production or transportation, it is important to identify the pathologic changes and distinguish between a primary testicular problem and excurrent duct obstruction. The classification that I use is principally morphologic, but I also use known or suspected clinical findings that may reflect hormonal or genetic abnormalities or excurrent duct obstruction (Table 9-1).

A testicular biopsy should never be reviewed without adequate clinical information. Ideally, there should be information regarding the previous medical history, including paternity, semen analysis, pertinent physical findings relating to testicular size, and the results of serum gonadotropin measurements. The biopsy should be read blind, but it should subsequently be interpreted in conjunction with clinical information. A biopsy should never be reported without knowing the patient's age, the serum follicle-stimulating hormone (FSH) level, and the results of semen analysis.

MALE INFERTILITY

CLINICAL FEATURES

The chief complaint that accompanies any testis biopsy for infertility is generally the same (i.e., infertility). It is important to know whether the patient has a low sperm count (oligospermia) or a zero sperm count (azoospermia). Physical findings vary. It must be established whether both testes are descended or whether one or both testes have been brought down into the scrotum and, if so, at what time in the patient's life this

MALE INFERTILITY—FACT SHEET

Definition
▶ Group of conditions affecting the testis caused by genetic, developmental, hormonal, or anatomic abnormalities resulting in decreased production or delivery of spermatozoa or production of abnormal spermatozoa

Incidence and Location
▶ Common (affects approximately 5 million men in the United States)
▶ There is a consensus that sperm counts are decreasing in the United States, although not to an alarming level
▶ Approximately 40% of infertile couples have a problem exclusively in the female, 40% exclusively in the male, and 20% in both male and female
▶ Biopsies are usually performed to distinguish between obstructive and nonobstructive causes of azoospermia, to confirm the presence of obstruction, and for sperm retrieval for assisted reproductive techniques. Biopsies are not performed in the majority of male infertility cases

Gender, Race, and Age Distribution
▶ Adult males of all races in their reproductive years

Clinical Features
▶ Asymptomatic
▶ Sometimes associated with a history of cryptorchidism, prior orchitis and/or epididymitis, environmental factors, excurrent duct obstruction, varicocele, concurrent medical conditions (e.g., diabetes mellitus), prior surgery (e.g., vasectomy, hernia repair, retroperitoneal lymph node dissection), malignancy treated with chemotherapy or irradiation, recreational drug use, or use of anabolic steroids
▶ Diagnosis of testicular biopsy should always be made in conjunction with knowledge of the sperm count and the level of serum FSH

Radiologic Features
▶ Important only in cases of excurrent duct obstruction

Prognosis and Treatment
▶ Assisted reproductive technology (intrauterine insemination, in vitro fertilization, and intracytoplasmic sperm injection) may produce pregnancy if male has available and satisfactory sperm
▶ Testis biopsy may be necessary to harvest sperm
▶ Excurrent duct obstruction may be treated surgically by vasovasostomy or vasoepididymostomy
▶ Without reproductive technology, maturation arrest, prepubertal gonadotropin deficiency, and hypospermatogenesis may be treated medically with some hope of future fertility
▶ Without reproductive technology, future fertility is unlikely in patients with germ cell aplasia, germ cell aplasia with focal spermatogenesis, Klinefelter syndrome, or diffuse tubular sclerosis and peritubular fibrosis

was done. In the presence of azoospermia, it should be known whether the vas deferens are palpable and whether the epididymes are palpable or dilated and full. The size and consistency of the testes should be known. Infertile testes may be small. For purposes of optimal morphology, fixation of testicular biopsies in Bouin's or Hollande's solution is preferable to formalin.

RADIOLOGIC FEATURES

Ultrasound evaluation may be used in the evaluation of an infertile male, to evaluate the prostate, seminal vesicles, ejaculatory ducts, testis, and epididymis. A vasogram may be performed at the time of corrective surgery for excurrent duct obstruction. In this circumstance, contrast material is injected into the vas deferens, and radiographs are taken to demonstrate their patency.

PATHOLOGIC FEATURES

GROSS FINDINGS

In the evaluation of infertility, the urologist usually obtains an incisional biopsy of the testis that measures several millimeters. Although the urologist can evaluate the consistency of the testis and may get a general idea of fibrosis, the biopsy will have been immediately placed in fixative, so that any gross changes are masked.

MICROSCOPIC FINDINGS

Normal Spermatogenesis

In these biopsies, the tubules are undergoing active spermatogenesis (Fig. 9-25). Correlations have been made between the number of elongate late spermatids per round cross-section of tubule and sperm count. Heller and Clermont pointed out that the normal testis actually has a mosaic appearance, with varied combinations of cells lining the tubules, but always with the least mature cells against the basement membrane and the most mature cells along the tubular lumen. Not all normally active seminiferous tubules culminate in elongate late spermatids. Normal spermatogenesis in the presence of azoospermia indicates the presence of excurrent duct obstruction. Histologically, normal spermatogenesis in the presence of a reduced sperm count may indicate partial excurrent duct obstruction. Histologically, normal spermatogenesis in the presence of a normal sperm count may indicate abnormalities in sperm morphology or motility.

Hypospermatogenesis

The term hypospermatogenesis indicates reduced spermatogenesis (Fig. 9-26), but not a process that stops at a particular point in the sequence of spermatogenesis or spermiogenesis. Generally, there are reduced numbers of germ cells of all types. Usually, there are other

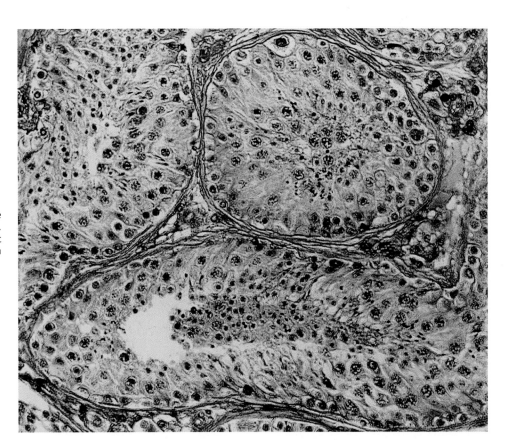

FIGURE 9-25

Three seminiferous tubules are undergoing active spermatogenesis. Elongate late spermatids are present along the luminal border of each tubule.

MALE INFERTILITY—PATHOLOGIC FEATURES

Gross Findings

▶ The pathologist only sees a 3- or 4-mm biopsy segment

Microscopic Findings

▶ Tubules may be of normal or reduced size
▶ The presence and level of germ cell maturation must be ascertained
▶ Tunica propria may be thickened, or individual tubules or groups of tubules may be sclerotic
▶ Interstitium may be fibrotic
▶ Leydig cell population may vary
▶ As tubules become atrophic, Leydig cells become more prominent
▶ Nodules of Leydig cells may occur, particularly in Klinefelter syndrome
▶ After diagnosis based on a testicular biopsy specimen, the pathologist should look for malignant intratubular germ cells, which occur in approximately 1% of testis biopsies obtained for infertility

Fine-needle Aspiration Biopsy Findings

▶ Used generally when the physician wants to know whether sperm are present in the testis or epididymis
▶ May be used to obtain sperm for associated reproductive techniques
▶ Alternative methods of biopsy for diagnosis are open biopsy and core biopsy using a spring-loaded gun
▶ Touch preparation followed by immediate spray fixation may be a useful adjunct with open or core biopsies

Differential Diagnosis

▶ Infectious diseases (e.g., schistosomiasis, leprosy)
▶ Vasculitis
▶ Amyloidosis
▶ Malignant intratubular germ cells
▶ Sarcoidosis
▶ All of these conditions are quite rare

changes, including thickening of the tunica propria with increased collagen deposition, and interstitial fibrosis. Changes in the tubules are variable. Some tubules may show complete sclerosis. Sloughing of germinal cells may occur into the lumen, resulting in a disorganized appearance. These changes are not specific. Leydig cells are usually present in adequate numbers. The pathologist should not attempt to quantify Leydig cells other than to indicate their absence or almost total absence or their presence in large numbers including nodules. Hypospermatogenesis is a frequent diagnosis, but does not indicate the cause of the changes. These changes

may occur as a result of varicocele, exposure to environmental toxins or increased heat, or hypothyroidism, among other causes.

Maturation Arrest

Spermatogenesis may be thought of in a linear fashion, beginning with a pale spermatogonium and finishing with an elongate late spermatid. Maturation arrest may be thought of as a line, drawn somewhere in this continuum, beyond which there is no further maturation. This usually occurs at the level of the primary

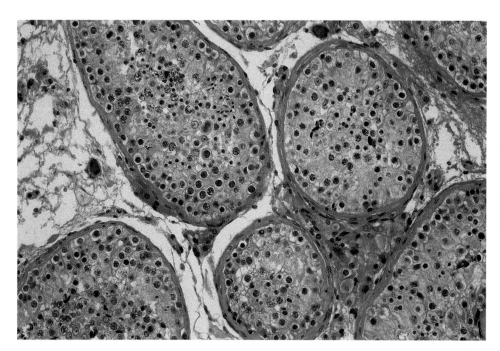

FIGURE 9-26

Testis biopsy in a 30-year-old man with a varicocele and hypospermatogenesis. Seminiferous tubules are undergoing reduced spermatogenesis. Rare elongate late spermatids are identifiable only in the two left tubules.

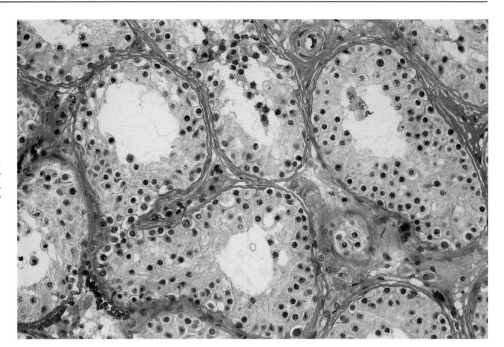

FIGURE 9-27

The patient is a 25-year-old man with azoospermia and complete naturation arrest. Spermatogenesis matures only to the level of primary spermatocytes.

spermatocyte or the spermatid (Fig. 9-27). Maturation arrest may be either complete, in which there is no maturation to elongate spermatids, or incomplete, in which elongate spermatids are microfocally present (Fig. 9-28).

The etiology of maturation arrest may be similar to that of hypospermatogenesis, or it may occur secondary to postpubertal gonadotrophin deficiency, chemotherapy, or radiation therapy. Generally, seminiferous tubules have a somewhat reduced diameter. There is usually no increase in tunica propria thickening or abnormalities of the interstitium or Leydig cells. Even if no elongate late spermatids are present in the biopsy specimen, it cannot be inferred that there is no spermatogenesis elsewhere in the testis. Morphologic changes should be correlated with the results of semen analysis.

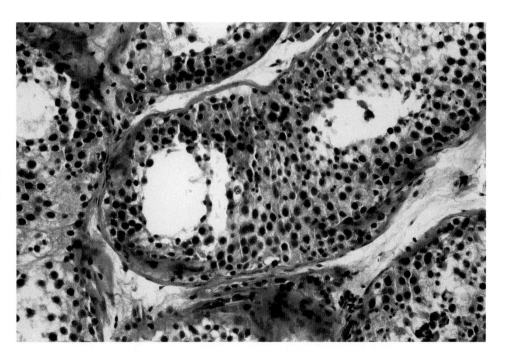

FIGURE 9-28

Testis biopsy specimen from an azoospermic 47-year-old man. Spermatogenesis matures only to the level of round spermatids.

GERMINAL CELL APLASIA (DEL CASTILLO SYNDROME, SERTOLI CELL ONLY SYNDROME)

CLINICAL FEATURES

A number of clinical scenarios are associated with germinal cell aplasia (GCA). In del Castillo syndrome, phenotypically normal men have small soft testes, normal secondary sex characteristics, normal levels of serum testosterone, azoospermia, and increased or high-normal levels of serum FSH. A similar histologic appearance may occur after chemotherapy, particularly with alkylating agents, or after irradiation in sufficient doses. GCA may also occur in patients with Y chromosome microdeletions in the azoospermia factor genes (AZF) region.

PATHOLOGIC FEATURES

Biopsies in GCA have a uniform appearance. In postpubertal men, seminiferous tubules of reduced diameter are lined exclusively by postpubertal Sertoli cells (Figs. 9-29 and 9-30). In all cases, Sertoli cells are oriented perpendicular to the seminiferous tubular basement membrane. No germinal cells are present. If the overall morphology is that of GCA and a few spermatogonia are present, this is termed "germinal cell hypoplasia." The nucleus of the Sertoli cell is variably shaped, oval and indented. The nuclear membrane has an undulating appearance. Sertoli cell nuclei contain prominent nucleoli.

Sertoli cells do not undergo mitosis. Fine filamentous structures may be seen within and sometimes outside the cytoplasm of the Sertoli cell. These are Charcot-Böttcher (CB) crystals. CB crystals are not truly crystalline; ultrastructurally, they are microfilament bundles. The pathologist should be careful in the examination of biopsy specimens having the appearance of GCA. Occasionally, tiny microfoci of spermatogenesis may be identified. Very rarely, one or several tubules are found to harbor malignant intratubular germ cells. Rarely, these coexist with malignant germ cells within the interstitium.

GERMINAL CELL APLASIA AND FOCAL SPERMATOGENESIS

CLINICAL FEATURES

Patients with GCA and focal spermatogenesis may be azoospermic or oligospermic. The contralateral testis may show GCA.

PATHOLOGIC FEATURES

In some patients, testis biopsies contain two populations of tubules. One population is undergoing spermatogenesis, and the other is lined exclusively by Sertoli cells (Fig. 9-31). Occasional tubules, cut longitudinally, may demonstrate an area of spermatogenesis leading

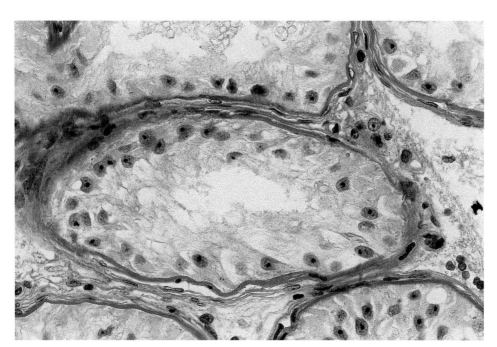

FIGURE 9-29

Testis biopsy specimen from an azoospermic 29-year-old man with germinal cell aplasia. All seminiferous tubules are lined by postpubertal-type Sertoli cells.

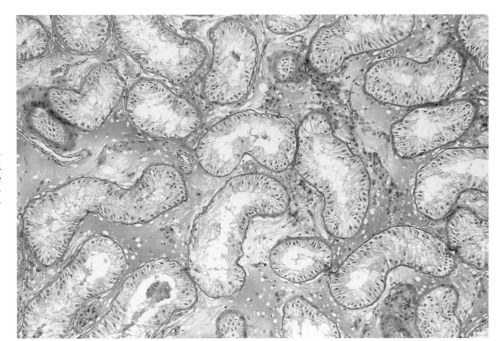

FIGURE 9-30

Testis biopsy specimen in a post-pubertal man with germinal cell aplasia after chemotherapy for acute lymphocytic leukemia. All seminiferous tubules are lined by postpubertal-type Sertoli cells.

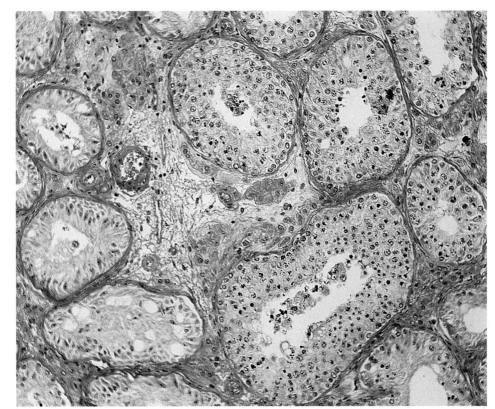

FIGURE 9-31

Two populations of seminiferous tubules are present, one lined by cells undergoing active spermatogenesis *(right)*, and the other, of smaller diameter, lined exclusively by Sertoli cells (germinal cell aplasia) *(left)*.

into a portion of the tubule lined only by Sertoli cells. Some patients with bilateral biopsies may have GCA on one side and GCA with focal spermatogenesis on the other.

TESTICULAR CHANGES ASSOCIATED WITH GENETIC ABNORMALITIES

CLINICAL FEATURES

In 1942, Klinefelter and colleagues described the phenotype of male patients that is now known as Klinefelter syndrome. These patients sometimes have a eunuchoid habitus, reduced body and pubic hair, gynecomastia, small testes, and increased serum FSH and luteinizing hormone (LH). Most of these patients have been characterized by a karyotype of 47,XXY.

PATHOLOGIC FEATURES

The testes are histologically normal after birth, but the number of intratubular germ cells diminishes with time. Some prepubertal tubules may be lined only by Sertoli cells. After puberty, the testis usually has marked tubular atrophy, with tubular sclerosis and Leydig cell nodules. Although some biopsies may show no spermatogenesis, others may show a degree of spermatogenesis, and spermatozoa may be found in the semen of 47,XXY men. These men are rarely fertile, but sperm harvested from the testes with testicular sperm extraction techniques may successfully produce a pregnancy with intracytoplasmic sperm injection procedures. Single-blastomere biopsy may be used to determine whether the embryo has a 46,XXY karyotype. Histologic changes identical to Klinefelter syndrome (Fig. 9-32) may occur in patients who do not have the genetic abnormality and also may occur in patients with a 46,XX karyotype.

Polymerase chain reaction (PCR) is being performed more frequently on biopsy specimens from patients with infertility. Microdeletions have been identified in region q11 of the Y chromosome. These have been divided into AZF regions a, b and c. Specific microdeletions are not uniformly associated with a particular testicular morphology. Biopsies may show germ cell hypoplasia, maturation arrest, hypospermatogenesis, or GCA. Patients with Y chromosome microdeletions may be either azoospermic or oligospermic. The presence of a Y chromosome microdeletion does not necessarily indicate infertility. Microdeletions may be passed from father to son. Patients with Y chromosome microdeletion may not have a stable morphology. In one patient whose first biopsy demonstrated maturation arrest, a second biopsy 1 year later was predominantly GCA with 10% maturation arrest. Therefore, some patients with Y chromosome microdeletion may undergo regression of spermatogenesis.

TUBULAR SCLEROSIS AND INTERSTITIAL FIBROSIS

Biopsies of all types may show focal tubular sclerosis and interstitial fibrosis. Occasionally, a biopsy specimen is composed exclusively of sclerotic tubules with inter-

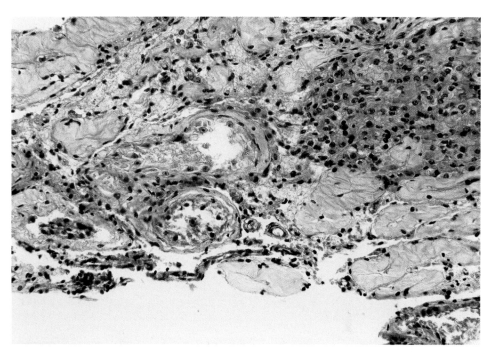

FIGURE 9-32

A nodule of Leydig cells is present on the right. Elsewhere there are completely sclerotic tubules and tubules lined exclusively by Sertoli cells in a man with Klinefelter syndrome.

stitial fibrosis, and there may be no evident Leydig cells (Fig. 9-33). Such changes may follow chronic orchitis, ischemia, acquired gonadotropin deficiency, or no known cause. It cannot be determined from examination of the biopsy specimen whether these changes involve the entire testis or both testes. Clinical findings, including semen analysis, serum testosterone and gonadotrophin levels, and physical and ultrasound findings, may indicate whether the process involves all of the testicular parenchyma. If so, the testes have no reproductive or hormonal function.

EXCURRENT DUCT OBSTRUCTION

CLINICAL FEATURES

Excurrent duct obstruction may be congenital or acquired. Congenital obstruction may occur in the cystic fibrosis syndrome, and many patients with congenital bilateral absence of the vas deferens (CBAVD) have mutations of the cystic fibrosis transmembrane receptor (CFTR) gene. These abnormalities may be associated with agenesis or atresia of any part of the excurrent duct system, from the epididymis to the vas deferens. Patients with CBAVD should have CFTR gene testing for themselves and their wives, because carriers with CFTR mutations have a 1 in 4 chance of producing an offspring with cystic fibrosis. Acquired obstruction may occur from voluntary or involuntary sterilization associated with scrotal surgery or secondary to infection, usually epididymitis.

In general, patients with excurrent duct obstruction have azoospermia, normal size testes, and active, although not necessarily normal, spermatogenesis. Occasionally, physical findings in the testes are variable because of pathology in one of the testes. In evaluating a biopsy specimen from a patient with possible excurrent duct obstruction, it is mandatory that the pathologist knows the patient's sperm count. Azoospermia in the presence of normal or active spermatogenesis indicates excurrent duct obstruction (Fig. 9-34). If the sperm count is extremely low, the degree of spermatogenesis should be correlated with the sperm count, to assess whether a partial obstruction may be present. Excurrent duct obstruction occurs after voluntary vasectomy. If a patient wishes to become fertile some years after vasectomy, the vasectomy site may be excised and the patient may undergo vasovasostomy or epididymovasostomy.

PATHOLOGIC FEATURES

MICROSCOPIC FINDINGS

A variety of the changes may occur in the testis after vasectomy. Jarow and associates found that interstitial fibrosis was the factor that most adversely affected prognosis for fertility in patients who had undergone vasovasotomy after vasectomy. Other changes were increased thickness of the seminiferous tubular wall, increased cross-sectional tubular area, and decreased numbers of Sertoli cells and spermatids. Spermatogenesis occurs in the face of obstruction. Spermatogenesis persists in patients in their 20s and older who have CBAVD. Interstitial fibrosis may be negligible in these patients.

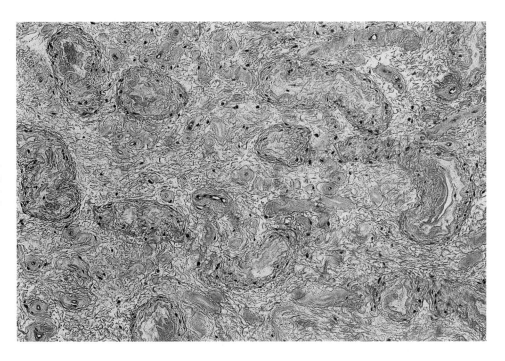

FIGURE 9-33

All seminiferous tubules are completely sclerotic. The interstitium is fibrotic. No Leydig cells are identified. The specimen is from an orchiectomy in a 32-year-old man.

A disparity between the sperm count and the degree of spermatogenesis as identified by testicular biopsy may indicate partial obstruction of the excurrent duct system. In a study of testis biopsies in men without excurrent duct obstruction, Silber and Rodriguez-Rigau correlated the number of elongate spermatids in round cross-sections of seminiferous tubules with the number of sperm per milliliter of semen. They found that counts of 45, 40, 20, and 6 to 10 elongate spermatids per tubule equated to sperm counts of approximately 85, 45, 10, and 3 million per milliliter. If the sperm count corresponds to the number of elongate spermatids in the biopsy specimen, there is no suspicion of obstruction. If the sperm count is appreciably lower than what would be expected from the biopsy, there is evidence of partial excurrent duct obstruction. Silber and Rodriguez-Rigau indicated that at least 20 tubules should be counted. In some specimens, 20 properly oriented tubules may not be present. I count as many properly oriented tubules as are available, up to 20 per testis.

Gonadotropin Deficiency

PREPUBERTAL GONADOTROPIN DEFICIENCY

CLINICAL FEATURES

Testicular development and function depend on the presence of an intact hypothalamic-pituitary-testicular axis. Anything that interferes with the release of GnRH and subsequent release of FSH leads to prepubertal gonadotropin deficiency (PPGD, also called hypogonadotropic, hypogonadism). The integrity of the system also includes the presence of hormone receptors. If gonadotropins have never been secreted in a normal manner, an adult patient is considered to have PPGD. Patients may have isolated LH, FSH, or GnRH deficiency or combined LH/FSH deficiency. PPGD may be associated with a variety of syndromes. Kallmann's syndrome is associated with a hypothalamic defect, anosmia, or hyposmia as well as PPGD. Genetic mutation in the code for an amino acid in the β subunit of LH has been reported to be the cause of hypogonadism. Testicular biopsies are usually not indicated in PPGD, because the syndrome can be identified clinically with measurements of serum gonadotropins and serum testosterone together with the results of GnRH and clomiphene administration. However, it is important that the pathologist recognize the morphology of a prepubertal testis, because some patients may be biopsied.

PATHOLOGIC FEATURES

GROSS FINDINGS

In PPGD, the testis has the appearance of a prepubertal gonad.

MICROSCOPIC FINDINGS

The structure of the testis is similar to that of an infant or prepubertal child. In the adolescent or adult, the morphology of the testis is inappropriate for the

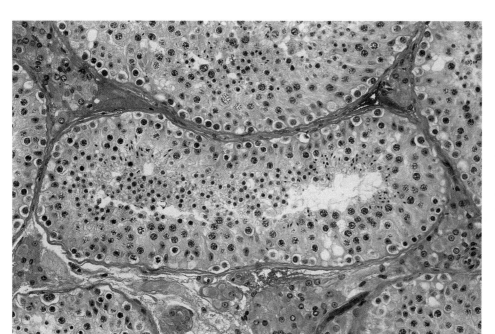

FIGURE 9-34

The biopsy specimen is from an azoospermic 34-year-old man with congenital bilateral agenesis of the vas deferens. All seminiferous tubules are undergoing active spermatogenesis.

patient's age. Seminiferous tubules are small, often aluminal, and populated by prepubertal Sertoli cells with variable numbers of spermatogonia. The interstitial connective tissue is loose, and there are no recognizable Leydig cells (Fig. 9-35). If the syndrome has been recognized clinically, the patient may be treated with hormonal combinations that have both LH and FSH activity. When this occurs, the interstitium transforms into clusters of recognizable Leydig cells with eosinophilic cytoplasm. Seminiferous tubules increase in size and complete spermatogenesis develops. If gonadotropin replacement is maintained, therapy may result in fertility (Fig. 9-36).

POSTPUBERTAL GONADOTROPIN DEFICIENCY

CLINICAL FEATURES

In patients who have undergone normal pubertal development, testicular regression may be caused by damage to the hypothalamus or pituitary through trauma, surgery, neoplasm, irradiation, or excess levels of estrogen or androgen.

PATHOLOGIC FEATURES

The histologic changes tend to be progressive. Spermatogenesis regresses, going through levels of incomplete maturation arrest, complete maturation arrest, germ cell hypoplasia, GCA, and possibly total tubular sclerosis. The walls of the seminiferous tubules become progressively thickened and fibrotic, Leydig cells become atrophic and may disappear, and the interstitium becomes fibrotic (Fig. 9-37). I have examined orchiectomy specimens from transsexual patients who had prolonged high-dose estrogen therapy. The seminiferous tubules were reduced in diameter, contained thickened tunica propria, and had seminiferous tubules lined predominantly by Sertoli cells and spermatogonia. The interstitium was devoid of Leydig cells, with only rare scattered pigment-containing cells within a loose fibrous matrix (Fig. 9-38). In the past, low-dose estrogen therapy was given for adenocarcinoma of the prostate. This produced arrested maturation of germ cells, tunica propria thickening of the seminiferous tubules, and subtotal atrophy of Leydig cells. In cases of postpubertal gonadotropin deficiency acquired as a result of pituitary surgery, if gonadotropin administration is given soon after the onset of gonadotropin deficiency, spermatogenesis may be maintained.

MACROORCHIDISM

CLINICAL FEATURES

Non-neoplastic testicular enlargement has been described in cases of fragile X syndrome (which is the most common cause of inherited mental retardation), familial mental retardation, Carney's complex, sexual precocity, congenital adrenal hyperplasia, testotoxicosis, juvenile hypothyroidism, and microadenoma of the pituitary secreting FSH.

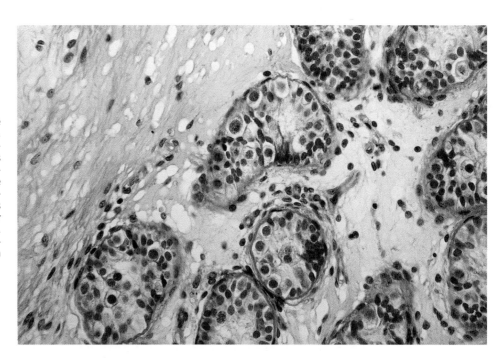

FIGURE 9-35

This biopsy specimen is from a male adolescent with Kallmann's syndrome. All seminiferous tubules are of prepubertal type. Seminiferous tubules contain predominantly prepubertal-type Sertoli cells. Spermatogonia are arranged around the basement membrane of the seminiferous tubules and have larger nuclei and clear cytoplasm. The interstitium is loose. No demonstrable Leydig cells are present. (Masson trichrome stain, high power).

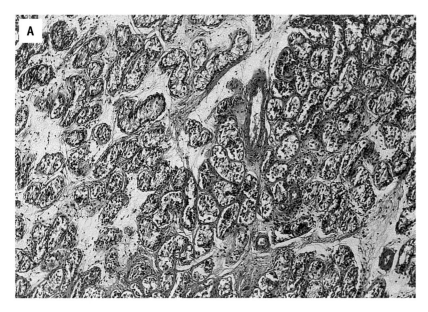

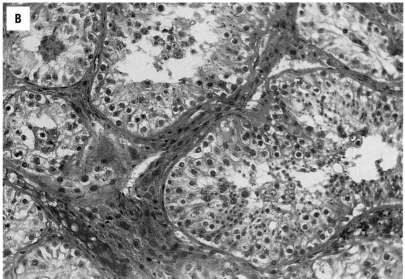

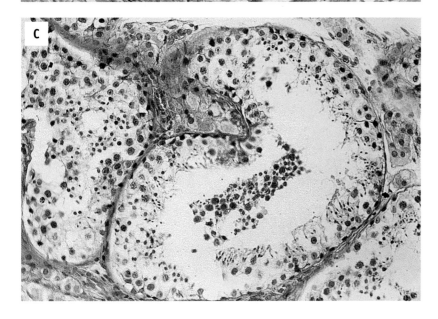

FIGURE 9-36

A, Testis biopsy specimen from a 19-year-old man with small testes and infantile genitalia. Seminiferous tubules are of prepubertal type. **B,** The patient was administered gonadotropic hormones with predominant luteinizing hormone (LH) activity. Seminiferous tubules are of postpubertal type. Round and elongate late spermatids are present in the tubule in the lower right. Numerous Leydig cells are present *(lower left)*. The patient had a sperm count of 1 million per milliliter. **C,** Testis biopsy specimen obtained after gonadotropin therapy with hormones having both follicle-stimulating hormone (FSH) and LH activity. Seminiferous tubules are essentially those of a normal male. Sperm count was 10 million per milliliter.

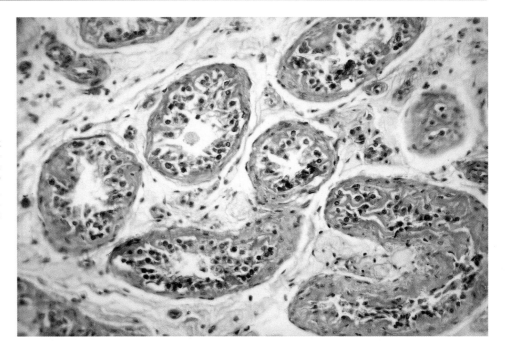

FIGURE 9-37

Orchiectomy specimen in a patient treated with estrogen for adenocarcinoma of the prostate. Seminiferous tubules are reduced in diameter. They have a thickened tunica propria. Germ cell maturation is arrested. Leydig cells are atrophic and contain increased lipochrome pigment.

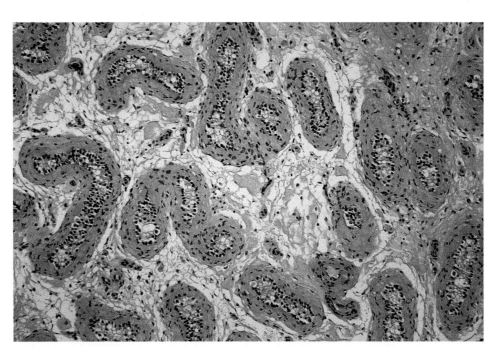

FIGURE 9-38

Bilateral orchiectomy in a 29-year-old transsexual patient who had undergone long-term estrogen therapy. Tunica propria of seminiferous tubules is markedly thickened. Tubules are lined predominantly by Sertoli cells having an immature appearance and a few spermatogonia. Leydig cells are extremely rare and atrophic.

PATHOLOGIC FEATURES

In patients with macroorchidism and fragile X syndrome, seminiferous tubules may show varying combinations of normal, dilated, and atrophic tubules, with mature or immature Sertoli cells.

INFECTIOUS DISEASES

Testes harboring infectious diseases usually are not subjected to biopsy or orchiectomy; however, when infectious diseases occur, they should be recognized, because optimal treatment may be specific to the infectious agent. When infections do occur, microbiologic studies should be performed on pathologic material to obtain the most specific diagnosis.

BACTERIAL INFECTIONS

Bacterial infections are usually associated with fever and pain in the involved testis, which is enlarged, tender, and usually accompanied by a hydrocele. The scrotal skin may be red and edematous. Acute bacterial orchitis is usually associated with epididymitis. Many bacteria have been known to cause orchitis. In addition to epididymoorchitis, organisms may reach the testis via lymphatics or blood vessels. Among the bacteria that have caused orchitis are *Escherichia coli, Pseudomonas aeruginosa, Brucella, Staphylococcus, Streptococcus, Klebsiella, Salmonella, Listeria monocytogenes,* and *Actinomyces.*

PATHOLOGIC FEATURES

GROSS FINDINGS

The morphology of the testis varies with the duration of the inflammatory process. The testis may be hyperemic in cases of acute orchitis, or they may contain microscopic or massive abscess formations.

MICROSCOPIC FINDINGS

Acute orchitis is characterized by acute inflammatory cells within interstitium and seminiferous tubules. Abscesses destroy underlying tissue (Figs. 9-39 and 9-40). Brucellosis may involve the testis and epididymis. This is a tubule-oriented inflammatory process that is accompanied by massive interstitial mononuclear inflammation. It may produce a somewhat granulomatous appearance in the testis, tunica albuginea, or spermatic cord. In many cases, the cause of chronic orchitis (Fig. 9-41) is not known. Morphologically, chronic orchitis consists of interstitial mononuclear cell infiltration by lymphocytes, plasma cells, and histiocytes. This is often accompanied by interstitial fibrosis, tubular atrophy, thickening of the tunica propria, and tubular sclerosis.

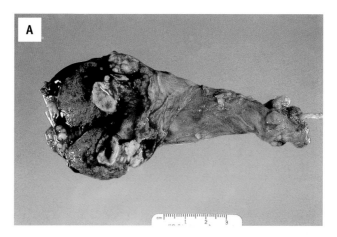

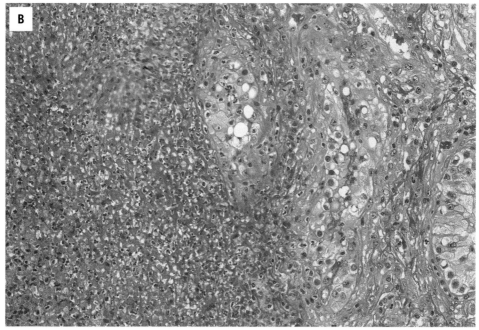

FIGURE 9-39

A, Within the bivalved testis of a 69-year-old man is a 1.2-cm abscess filled with gray-green, soft, purulent material. **B,** Abscess containing many polymorphonuclear neutrophils (PMNs). Inflammatory cells extend into surrounding testicular parenchyma.

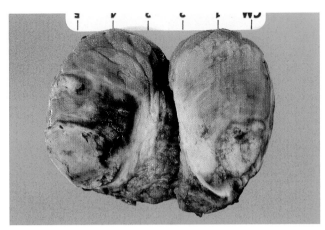

FIGURE 9-40

The specimen is from an orchiectomy in a 15-year-old boy. Approximately one third of the parenchyma was occupied by a soft, necrotic, yellow-green, circumscribed focus measuring 2 cm in diameter with contiguous hemorrhage.

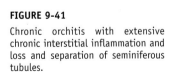

MYCOBACTERIAL DISEASES

CLINICAL FEATURES

Tuberculosis is always associated with infection elsewhere and is a relatively infrequent cause of granulomatous orchitis. Infection usually spreads directly from the epididymis or via the bloodstream. In the United States at present, tuberculosis of the testis or epididymis is rare. When tuberculosis does occur, involvement is usually bilateral. Microbiologic studies should always be performed, because nontuberculous mycobacteria,

including *Mycobacterium kansasii* and *Mycobacterium avium-intracellulare,* have also been cultured.

Leprosy is rarely seen in the United States. However, many people arrive in the United States from countries where leprosy is extant. Leprosy may manifest as a testicular mass. In Egypt, infertility patients have been reported to have the lesions of leprosy on testicular biopsy. Because of extensive involvement of the testis, some patients with leprosy present with gynecomastia.

PATHOLOGIC FEATURES

GROSS FINDINGS

In tuberculosis, enlarged, dilated epididymes are usually present and may contain necrotic, caseating material. Inflammation may extend into the testis, where necrotic foci may be present. Fistulas from testis and/or epididymis may extend to the scrotum.

MICROSCOPIC FINDINGS

In cases of tuberculous epididymoorchitis (Fig. 9-42), the inflammatory process extends from the epididymis, which is usually involved more extensively than the testis. The inflammation may be nonspecific, with mononuclear infiltration of tissues. In some instances, necrotizing caseating granulomas are present. The testis may also be involved in disseminated tuberculosis. In these cases, small nodules with granulomatous inflammation up to 3 mm may be distributed within testicular parenchyma.

Testicular leprosy occurs in three phases. In the vascular phase, histiocytic lepra cells are stuffed with acid-fast bacilli in blood vessels walls and in the

FIGURE 9-41

Chronic orchitis with extensive chronic interstitial inflammation and loss and separation of seminiferous tubules.

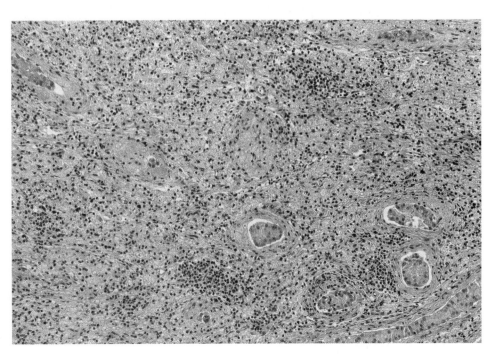

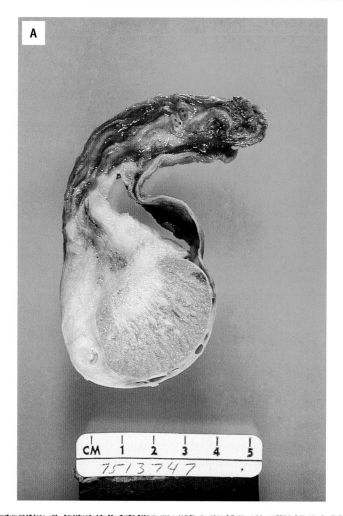

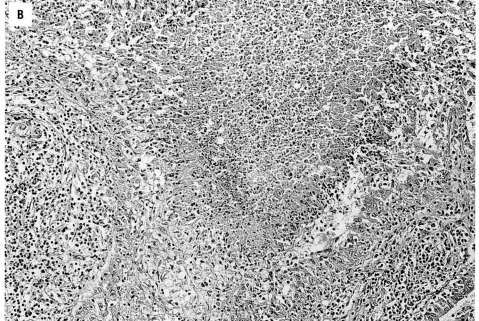

FIGURE 9-42

A, Formalin-fixed testis and epididymis with tuberculous epididymo-orchitis demonstrating whitish opacity of obliterated epididymal and testicular architecture. **B,** Marked chronic inflammation with suppurative granuloma *(upper center)*.

interstitium (Fig. 9-43). The interstitial stage is characterized by an obliterative endarteritis, clusters of Leydig cells, interstitial fibrosis, histiocytes with clear cytoplasm containing acid-fast bacilli, and reduced spermatogenesis. The obliterative phase shows a total fibrosis, absence of seminiferous tubules, diminished vascularity, and few acid-fast bacilli. The later two phases tend to merge. Histologic diagnosis should be proved with a Fite-Faroco stain. In contrast to *Mycobacterium tuberculosis*, myriad *Mycobacterium leprae* organisms are present.

FUNGAL DISEASES

Fungal organisms are generally associated with a systemic illness. The infection may be part of an epididymoorchitis. A variety of organisms have been identified in the testis, including *Candida*, *Blastomyces*, *Aspergillus*, *Histoplasma capsulatum*, *Trichophyton mentagrophytes*, and *Coccidioides immitis*.

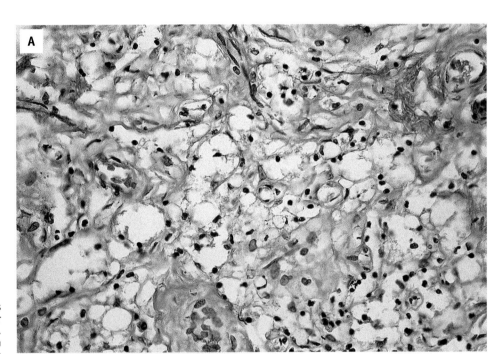

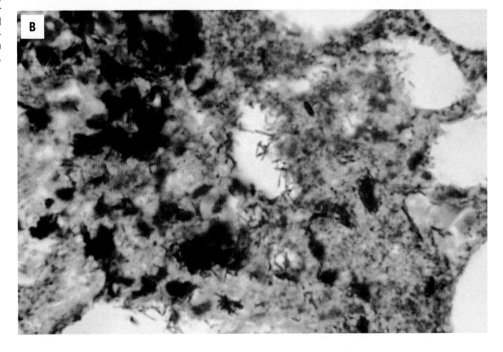

FIGURE 9-43

A, The testicular interstitium is replaced by macrophages with clear cytoplasm and a few lymphocytes. This is an orchiectomy specimen from a 19-year-old Mexican-American man with leprosy and a testicular mass. **B**, Macrophages are stuffed with numerous acid-fast bacilli (Fite-Faroco stain). Courtesy of Dr. William Hicken, St. Agnes Hospital, Baltimore, MD.

PATHOLOGIC FEATURES

MICROSCOPIC FINDINGS

As in other parts of the body, fungal organisms may not be identifiable on sections stained with hematoxylin and eosin (H&E). There may be a nonspecific, chronic active inflammatory process, as is seen in blastomycosis (Figs. 9-44 and 9-45), or there may be a granulomatous reaction, as is seen with histoplasmosis. In any case, if a fungal organism is suspected, it is mandatory to perform fungal stains in an attempt to identify the organism. Failure to treat an orchitis caused by a fungal organism may result in subsequent dissemination.

RICKETTSIAL INFECTION

Orchitis may occur in patients with typhus or Q fever.

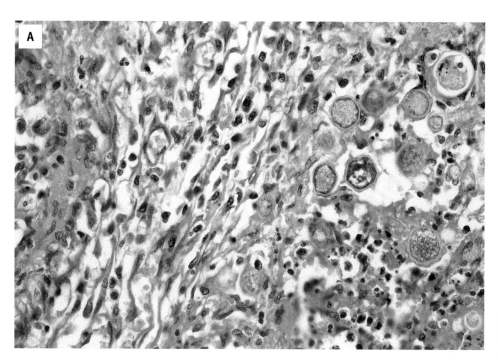

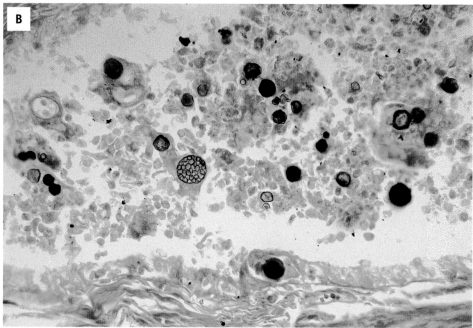

FIGURE 9-44

A, Systemic blastomycosis with multiple sporangia containing spherules with surrounding chronic active inflammation. **B,** Multiple spherules and sporangia (Gomori methenamine silver stain).

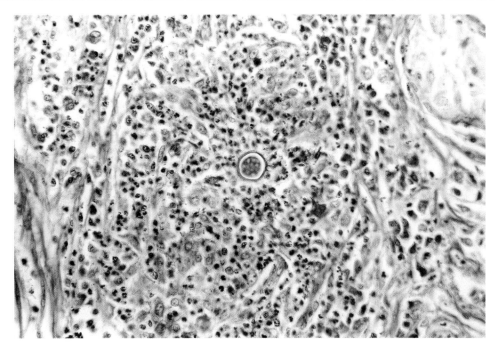

FIGURE 9-45
Blastomyces dermatitidis organism with multiple nuclei is surrounded by chronic active inflammation in a case of disseminated blastomycosis (periodic acid-Schiff stain).

PATHOLOGIC FEATURES

In typhus, large numbers or organisms are present in swollen capillary endothelial cells with accompanying vascular thrombi.

VIRAL INFECTIONS

CLINICAL FEATURES

In cases of viral orchitis, testicular swelling and pain usually occurs in the course of the disease. Viral orchitis has been demonstrated in cases of mumps, variola, varicella, ECHO, lymphocytic choriomeningitis, group E arborvirus infection, influenza, dengue fever, sandfly fever, and coxsackie B viral infections.

Mumps is caused by a paramyxovirus. In the past, it was the most common cause of viral orchitis. However, vaccination with live attenuated mumps virus protects against infection in more than 95% of cases. The virus has been well studied and may be a prototype for understanding other types of viral orchitis. The discussion of clinical and pathologic features refers to mumps orchitis.

CLINICAL FEATURES

Mumps orchitis usually follows parotitis by 2 or 3 days but may precede it. The testis is painful, tender, and enlarged. There may be accompanying fever. Bilateral clinical orchitis occurs in fewer than 15% of the cases. Orchitis rarely occurs prepubertally. Testicular atrophy develops in about one third of patients with clinical orchitis. It is estimated that fewer than 2% of all patients with mumps develop infertility as a result of orchitis.

PATHOLOGIC FEATURES

Initially the testis shows edema, congestion, interstitial lymphocytic infiltration, and hemorrhage. Subsequently, there is a progression to mixed lymphocytic-polymorphonuclear neutrophil (PMN) interstitial infiltration with hemorrhage and inflammation of the seminiferous tubules (Fig. 9-46). Intratubular inflammation may be extensive and may be composed of numerous PMNs and few histiocytes. Germinal cells may become necrotic, leaving only Sertoli cells. These may disappear from the tubules. The process becomes more intense with interstitial lymphocytic and histiocytic inflammation; tubules become filled with inflammatory debris, and tubule walls are infiltrated by

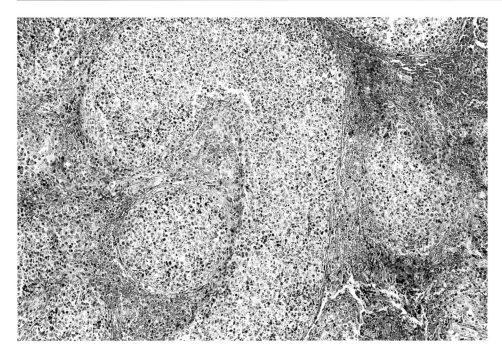

FIGURE 9-46

A patient with acute mumps had a wedge excision of the testis to relieve intratesticular pressure and pain. There are extensive intra-tubular and interstitial PMNs, as well as mononuclear inflammatory cell infiltration and hemorrhage.

lymphocytes and plasma cells. In patients who have had remote orchitis, there may be very little inflammation and considerable tubular sclerosis. I have seen a seminoma in an atrophic testis after mumps orchitis.

SPIROCHETAL INFECTIONS

CLINICAL FEATURES

Syphilitic orchitis may occur in both congenital and acquired syphilis. In acquired syphilis, the testicular enlargement is usually painless.

PATHOLOGIC FEATURES

GROSS FINDINGS

The testis may be either fibrotic or gummatous. There are no specific lesions in the fibrotic variety. In the gummatous form, the enlarged testis is irregular or nodular. Discrete gummas are identifiable grossly and contain a central area of necrosis surrounded by a fibrous capsule.

MICROSCOPIC FINDINGS

In the fibrotic form of acquired syphilis, interstitial mononuclear cells infiltrate peritubular areas (Fig. 9-47). Small seminiferous tubules contain reduced

numbers of germ cells, and peritubular fibrosis is present. In the gummatous form, gummas show central coagulative necrosis with a peripheral zone of lymphocytes, plasma cells, and occasional histiocytic giant cells which extend into surrounding testis (Figs. 9-48 and 9-49). Obliterative endarteritis with inflammation of the intima may be present. Spirochetes usually cannot be identified in the fibromatous form, but they are present in the gummatous form in secondary syphilis. In secondary syphilis, there is massive interstitial infiltration of testicular parenchyma by lymphocytes, plasma cells, and histiocytes.

ACQUIRED IMMUNODEFICIENCY SYNDROME

The testis usually is not clinically involved in patients with acquired immunodeficiency syndrome (AIDS).

PATHOLOGIC FEATURES

MICROSCOPIC FINDINGS

At autopsy, testes demonstrate markedly decreased spermatogenesis, arrested maturation, GCA with tunica propria thickening, tubular hyalinization, interstitial inflammation, reduced numbers of Leydig cells, and interstitial fibrosis. Many secondary infections have been described in testes of AIDS patients, including toxoplasmosis, tuberculosis, candidiasis, and cytomegalovirus infection. Kaposi's sarcoma has been rarely identified in

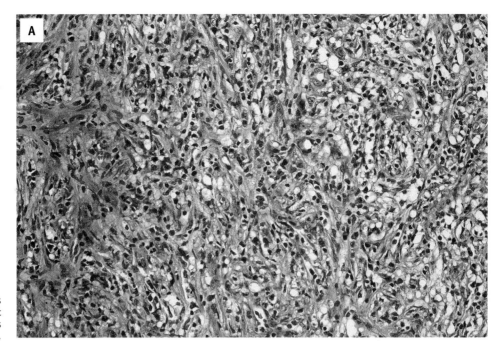

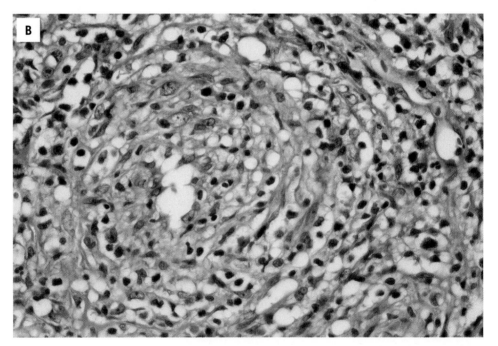

FIGURE 9-47

This patient with syphilitic orchitis presented with an enlarged left testis. **A,** The inflammatory process is interstitial, with many lymphocytes, plasma cells, and multinucleated histiocytic giant cells. **B,** Extensive, predominantly lymphocytic, interstitial inflammation and obliterative endarteritis are present.

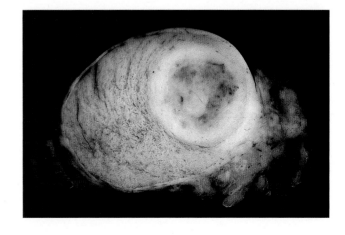

FIGURE 9-48

Syphilitic orchitis with gumma. The testis contains a rounded intratesticular discrete, white, firm mass with central necrosis.

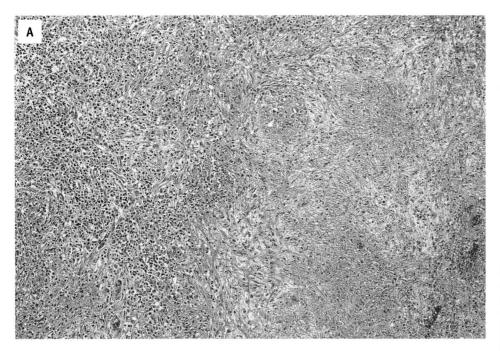

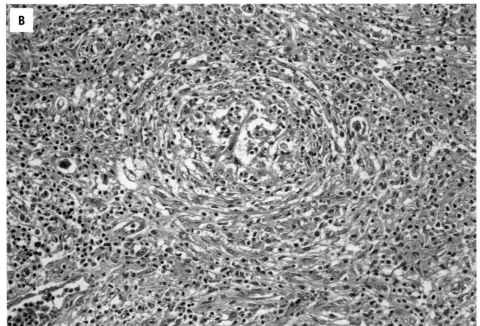

FIGURE 9-49

Syphilitic orchitis with gumma. **A,** Coagulative necrosis with degenerating cells including PMNs comprises the central portion of the gumma. Surrounding this is massive interstitial inflammation with large numbers of histiocytes, lymphocytes, and PMNs. **B,** In the tissue adjacent to gumma, there is massive interstitial inflammation with lymphocytes and histiocytes. Spirochetes were identified in the specimen.

the testis and epididymis of AIDS patients. Testicular germ cell tumors occur in AIDS patients with an increased incidence relative to the general population.

NONSPECIFIC GRANULOMATOUS ORCHITIS

Nonspecific granulomatous orchitis (NSGO) is usually unilateral. The testis is usually firm and enlarged. NSGO generally occurs in middle-aged men and may be preceded by a flu-like illness. It is probably of infectious origin.

PATHOLOGIC FEATURES

GROSS FINDINGS

On cut section, the testis is enlarged by a homogeneous, tan infiltrate that obscures testicular architecture. The differential diagnosis includes lymphoma, leukemia, and malakoplakia. The inflammatory process may involve the epididymis (Fig. 9-50A).

MICROSCOPIC FINDINGS

The inflammatory reaction is mixed and tubule oriented. Large numbers of histologically benign

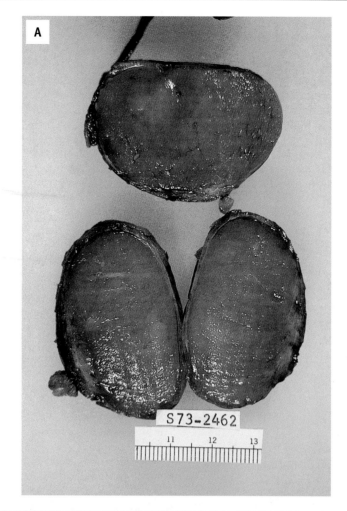

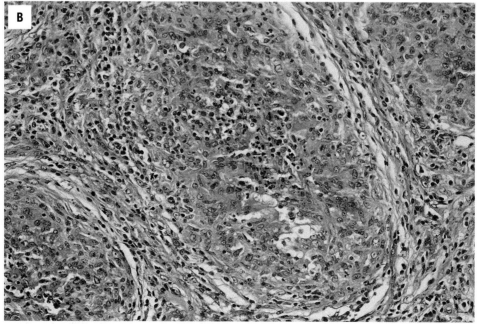

FIGURE 9-50

A, A 45-year-old man had a 6-month history of unilateral testicular enlargement and fever. The testis weighed 45 g and had a uniform, tan-colored parenchyma. **B,** The testicular architecture was obliterated by a pleomorphic, tubule-oriented and interstitial inflammatory infiltrate composed of lymphocytes, plasma cells, histiocytes, and a few PMNs. The appearance is vaguely granulomatous, but there are no discrete granulomas. (Courtesy of Dr. Gurdev Garewal, Marymount Hospital, Maples Heights, OH).

lymphocytes and plasma cells infiltrate the interstitium, surround seminiferous tubules, broaden tubular walls, and may be within tubular lumina (Fig. 9-50B). The tubular orientation of the inflammatory process and the presence of histiocytes and occasional multinucleated giant cells may give a vaguely granulomatous appearance. It is very important in these cases that the pathologist distinguish among NSGO, malignant lymphoma, and an infectious process caused by a specific organism. I believe that frozen sectioning should be performed on all testicular masses, so that malignant lymphomas and infectious processes can be identified early and optimally processed and evaluated.

MALAKOPLAKIA

CLINICAL FEATURES

Testicular malakoplakia is an inflammatory process of bacterial origin that closely resembles NSGO. It develops also in middle-aged men and manifests as testicular enlargement.

PATHOLOGIC FEATURES

GROSS FINDINGS

The testis is usually enlarged, yellow, tan or brown and may contain abscesses. The epididymis may be involved.

MICROSCOPIC FINDINGS

The process consists of a diffuse histiocytic infiltrate of testicular parenchyma including tubules and interstitium. Other inflammatory cells, including PMNs and mononuclear cells, may be present. The characteristic finding is the presence of Michaelis-Gutmann bodies, which are rounded blue, laminated, calcific structures having an owl-eye appearance. Michaelis-Gutmann bodies are positive for calcium and iron with von Kossa and Prussian blue stains as well as PAS stain. Phagolysosomes stain positively with PAS stain. Ultrastructural study demonstrates the presence of bacteria within phagolysosomes. Michaelis-Gutmann bodies have the appearance of myelin figures.

Intersex

Intersex refers to a number of syndromes in which there is a discordance among at least two of the following: genetic sex, gonadal sex, genital tract sex, pheno-

typic sex, and psychological sex. In order to obtain the correct diagnosis, the pathologist should be aware of cytogenetic, anatomic, biochemical, and clinical facts. The surgical pathologist may receive a biopsy of a gonad, potential gonad, germ cell tumor, indeterminate tissue, or a major resection specimen. If the specimen is other than a biopsy, the pathologist and the surgeon should review the gross specimen together, determine the laterality of organs, label all relevant structures, and photograph the specimen for future reference. It is important that the pathologist understand the relationship of ductal structures to gonadal tissue.

In order to understand the pathology of intersex syndromes, the pathologist must understand the development of the gonads and the wolffian and müllerian ducts. Understanding the timetable of gonadal and reproductive tract development helps to clarify the findings in intersex cases. In humans, the SRY gene on the short arm of the Y chromosome determines the formation of a testis. Germ cells migrate from the yolk sac into each genital ridge. Seminiferous tubule formation is recognizable by day 45. Wolffian duct development begins on day 25 and continues thereafter. Müllerian duct formation commences on day 43. If no SRY gene is present, the gonad becomes an ovary. In the presence of an SRY gene, testes develop. Sertoli cells secrete antimüllerian hormone (AMH) approximately 62 days after fertilization. AMH causes regression of the müllerian duct, which is usually completed by day 75 to 80. This effect is ipsilateral and depends on the proximity of a gonad to the müllerian duct. The gonad must contain competent Sertoli cells to function. If Sertoli cells are not present in one gonad or are not competent, the müllerian duct will not regress ipsilaterally, and in such a situation the fallopian tube, uterus, and upper vagina will be present in some form. During intrauterine development, Sertoli cells are easily identified histologically and can be confirmed with an immunoperoxidase stain for inhibin. Shortly after the beginning of müllerian duct regression, Leydig cells appear (at about day 64) and begin production of testosterone, which continues throughout intrauterine development. Testosterone also acts ipsilaterally and causes development of the wolffian duct into epididymis, vas deferens, and seminal vesicles if androgen receptors are present and qualitatively sufficient. Without testosterone production ipsilaterally, wolffian duct degeneration begins at about day 75 and is completed by about day 84. If androgens are administered to the mother, produced by a maternal tumor, or produced by the fetus as a result of congenital adrenal hyperplasia, there may be development of the wolffian duct system. Masculinization of the external genitalia begins after testosterone production, at about day 70. Testosterone itself will not cause complete development of the male reproductive system. The cells of the external genitalia and urogenital sinus precursors must have androgen receptors and must contain 5α-reductase, which converts testosterone to dihydrotestosterone (DHT). DHT causes development of the external genitalia, which is completed between days 121 and 140 of gestation. DHT causes elongation of the phallus. If the gonads are ovaries or if no gonads are present, the gonaducts will be female. If DHT is not present, the external genitalia will have a female phenotype. Major types of intersex involving the testis are described in the following sections.

MALE PSEUDOHERMAPHRODITISM

Male pseudohermaphroditism is a general term referring to a syndrome that exists when the patient has a 46,XY karyotype, the gonads are testes, and the phenotype is ambiguous or female.

PERSISTENT MÜLLERIAN DUCT SYNDROME

CLINICAL FEATURES

Persistent müllerian duct syndrome (PMDS) is an autosomal recessive disorder that is caused by a lack of AMH activity, usually due to a mutation in the AMH gene on the short arm of chromosome 19 or an abnormality of the end-organ receptor gene on the long arm of chromosome 12. However, in some cases, no mutation of the AMH or AMH receptor gene has been detected.

PATHOLOGIC FEATURES

GROSS FINDINGS

The patient with PMDS has a 46,XY karyotype, normal external genitalia, unilateral or bilateral cryptorchidism, and sometimes an empty hemiscrotum (Fig. 9-51). The wolffian duct derivatives are normal, but a uterus and one or two fallopian tubes are present within an inguinal hernia. This entity has been termed "hernia uteri inguinale." Cases may be identified in infants and children but have been diagnosed initially in adults as well. PMDS may be associated with testicular degeneration occurring before or after birth. It is important to examine gonadal tissue to distinguish PMDS from mixed gonadal dysgenesis (MGD); bilateral gonadectomies are usually performed in MGD because of an increased risk of germ cell neoplasia. Approximately 15% of patients with PMDS have intratesticular germ cell tumors, including intratubular germ cell neoplasia unspecified. It is very important that the pathologist understands the overall topography of the gonads and the wolffian and müllerian duct derivatives. Testicular histology by itself is not diagnostic of PMDS.

PERSISTENT MÜLLERIAN DUCT SYNDROME—FACT SHEET

Definition

▶ Intersex condition in a phenotypic male characterized by persistent müllerian duct structures and a cryptorchid testis or testes

Incidence

▶ Rare

Gender, Race, and Age Distribution

▶ All patients are phenotypic males
▶ Occurs worldwide
▶ May be discovered in infants, children, and adults

Clinical Features

▶ Normal male external genitalia
▶ Often associated with an inguinal hernia
▶ Usually associated with unilateral or bilateral cryptorchidism
▶ May be discovered at the time of vasectomy, orchiopexy, or herniorrhaphy
▶ The patient may be fertile or infertile
▶ May be sporadic or inherited in an X-linked or autosomal recessive manner
▶ Some patients have a mutation of the AMH gene on the short arm of chromosome 19 or an abnormality in the end-organ receptor gene

Prognosis and Treatment

▶ 15% of patients develop germ cell tumors of testis
▶ Tumors have not been reported in müllerian structures
▶ Surgery is performed to correct cryptorchidism and preserve fertility

---

PERSISTENT MÜLLERIAN DUCT SYNDROME—PATHOLOGIC FEATURES

Gross Findings

▶ Frequent inguinal hernia which may contain a testis
▶ Occasional transverse ectopia of cryptorchid testis
▶ Proximity of gonads to müllerian duct structures
▶ Müllerian duct structures may be in close proximity to wolffian duct structures
▶ Diagnosis is largely established on gross findings

Microscopic Findings

▶ Testis may show changes of cryptorchidism
▶ Testis may harbor a malignant germ cell tumor

Differential Diagnosis

▶ Mixed gonadal dysgenesis

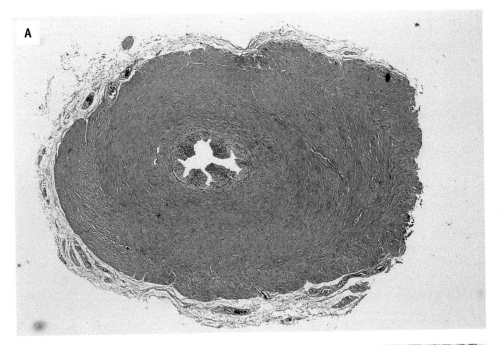

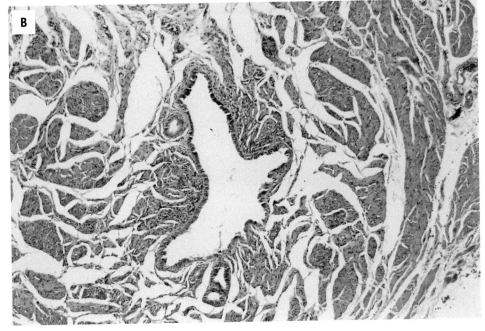

FIGURE 9-51

A 42-year-old man underwent vasectomy. The left vas deferens specimen was unremarkable (**A**). A persistent müllerian duct structure was identified on the right side, and no vas deferens was identified in the specimen (**B**). Subsequent surgery reveled a right "hernia uteri inguinale," which was resected (**C**). The right testis was biopsied (**D**). **A,** Segment of normal left vas deferens demonstrating the normal inner longitudinal smooth muscle, circular smooth muscle, and outer longitudinal smooth muscle. The mucosa contains numerous columnar cells and is unremarkable. **B,** The segment thought to be the right vas deferens consists of a müllerian remnant containing a lumen lined by cuboidal and columnar cells, some of which are ciliated. The structure lacks the dense collagenous and underlying organized smooth muscle layers of the vas deferens.

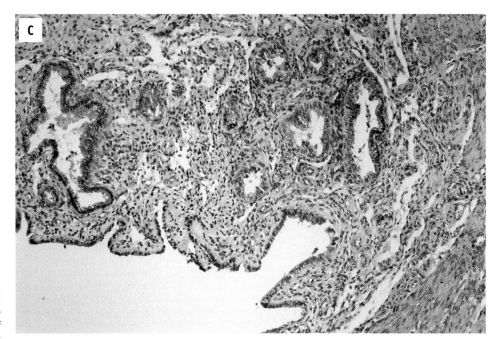

FIGURE 9-51, CONT'D

C, Müllerian remnant containing endometrial-type glands and endometrial stroma. **D,** Testicular biopsy demonstrating three populations of seminiferous tubules. Tubules on the left are undergoing spermatogenesis; those on the right are either totally sclerotic or lined exclusively by Sertoli cells. There is no evidence of intratubular germ cell neoplasia unspecified.

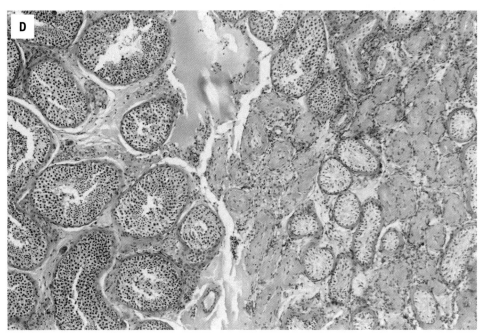

TESTICULAR REGRESSION SYNDROME

CLINICAL FEATURES

Testicular regression syndrome (TRS), also called vanishing testis syndrome, was referred to previously under the section on anorchism. The patient's phenotype may be male, female, or ambiguous. Gonads may be small or absent. The findings in the wolffian and müllerian ducts and the external genitalia phenotype depend on the extent and chronology of gonadal injury (Figs. 9-52 and 9-53). Most examples of TRS are unilateral. If the injury occurred before the development of a testis, then the absence of testosterone production eliminates the formation of epididymis, vas deferens, and seminal vesicles, and persistence of müllerian duct derivatives on that side. If damage to the testis occurs after day 75 to 80, there will be regression of müllerian duct derivatives (i.e., no fallopian tube, uterus, or upper vagina) on the side of the injury. Probably, there will not be sufficient testosterone for complete development of the ipsilateral wolffian duct. Most cases of TRS occur after the testis is formed, after the müllerian duct has completely regressed, and after at least partial formation of the wolffian duct system. Therefore, wolffian structures (epididymis and vas deferens) should be present, and often calcification, iron deposition, and fibrosis are observed.

TESTICULAR REGRESSION SYNDROME (VANISHING TESTIS SYNDROME)—FACT SHEET

Definition
▶ Intersex condition in a phenotypically normal male with absent unilateral or bilateral testes
▶ If gonadal regression occurred before the development of the testis, the external genital phenotype may be female or ambiguous

Clinical Features
▶ Unilateral or bilateral anorchism
▶ Normal male external genital phenotype

Prognosis and Treatment
▶ Infertility if testicular regression is bilateral
▶ Absence of descended testis necessitates open or laparoscopic exploration, searching for the gonad
▶ There is no risk for development of a malignant germ cell tumor if the patient has no gonadal tissue
▶ Anorchic patients have low serum testosterone and high serum gonadotropins and need testosterone supplementation beginning at puberty

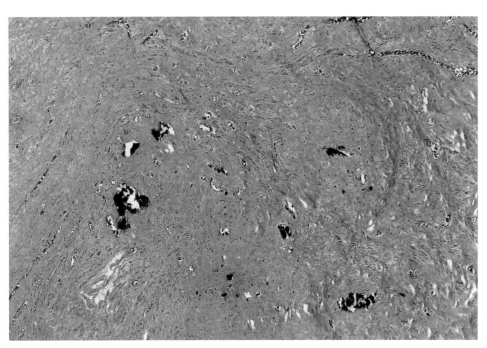

FIGURE 9-52

After scrotal exploration for a nonpalpable testis in a 1-year-old with testicular regression syndrome, a segment of vas deferens and possible testicular remnant were removed. Microscopically, this consists of fibrosis and dystrophic calcification.

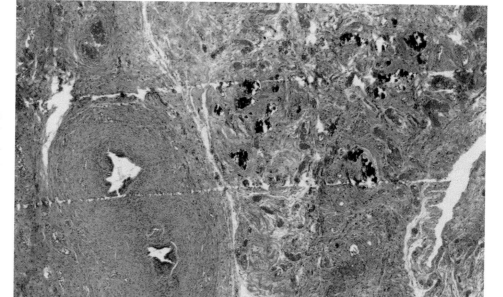

FIGURE 9-53

In the course of scrotal exploration for a nonpalpable testis in a 10-month-old with testicular regression syndrome, a possible left testicular remnant was removed. No testis was microscopically identified. However, a segment of vas deferens with adjacent hemosiderin-deposition, dystrophic calcification, and fibrosis was present.

TESTICULAR REGRESSION SYNDROME (VANISHING TESTIS SYNDROME)—PATHOLOGIC FEATURES

Gross Findings

▶ Absence of gonadal tissue
▶ Residual wolffian duct structures (epididymis and/or vas deferens), fibrosis, calcification, and hemosiderin deposition

Immunohistochemical Features

▶ Inhibin stain may be used to identify Leydig cells

Differential Diagnosis

▶ Cryptorchidism

CONGENITAL ADRENAL HYPERPLASIA

CLINICAL FEATURES

Five enzymatic defects involving steroid hormonal synthesis may be associated with male pseudohermaphroditism in congenital adrenal hyperplasia (CAH). The location and severity of the enzyme defect determines the patterns of hormone synthesis. Genetic males have cryptorchidism, variably developed wolffian duct systems, absent müllerian duct derivatives, and female or ambiguous genitalia.

PATHOLOGIC FEATURES

The morphologic changes in the testes are those found in cryptorchid testes. In some cases, 17β-hydroxysteroid dehydrogenase deficiency has been mistaken for incomplete androgen insensitivity syndrome.

The 21- and 11-hydroxylase and 17β-hydroxysteroid dehydrogenase deficiencies are occasionally associated with the development of masses that resemble Leydig cells in and adjacent to the testes. These masses are bilateral, are both intratesticular and extratesticular, and are responsive to ACTH stimulation. It has been argued that these are, in fact, Leydig cells or adrenocortical cells. In either event, they are sensitive to ACTH. If these masses are identified as part of CAH, unnecessary surgery, including orchiectomy, will be prevented, because corticosteroid therapy inhibits ACTH secretion and usually causes regression of the masses. Isosexual precocity may be associated with this form of CAH. Some testicular masses develop in patients with known CAH who have stopped steroid therapy. Testicular and paratesticular masses may develop later in life in patients who are unrecognized as having CAH (Fig. 9-54). These masses may be confused with and should be distinguished from Leydig cell tumors. Biopsies may be obtained in patients who have nodules identified clinically or by ultrasound. These nodules are multiple, dark brown, and may be lobulated.

MICROSCOPIC FINDINGS

In 21- and 11-hydroxylase and 17β-hydroxysteroid dehydrogenase deficiencies, aggregates of varying size, consisting of eosinophilic cells, are present within

CONGENITAL ADRENAL HYPERPLASIA—FACT SHEET

Definition

▶ An inborn error of metabolism of cortisol synthesis
▶ The cases discussed are limited to males who develop testicular and peritesticular nodules in childhood, adolescence, or adulthood
▶ 21-hydroxylase deficiency accounts for 95% of cases of CAH, 11β-hydroxylase deficiency accounts for 5%, and the least common deficiency is 17β-hydroxysteroid dehydrogenase deficiency
▶ Surgical pathologists rarely see cases of CAH except for previously diagnosed patients who have failed medical therapy and develop testicular nodules
▶ Rare cases of non-classic 21-hydroxylase deficiency in phenotypically normal males have been associated with infertility and treated with glucocorticoids

Incidence

▶ CAH occurs in 1 in 5,000 to 1 in 15,000 births in the United States and Europe. The highest incidence is in an Alaskan Eskimo population

Clinical Features

▶ This discussion is limited to phenotypic male adolescent or adult patients discovered and treated early in life and not the intersex situation in which symptoms of salt wasting or adrenal crisis are present at birth

▶ Patients in adolescence and early adulthood develop multiple testicular and extratesticular nodules resulting from failure to remain on glucocorticoid medication
▶ Nodules may be palpable and/or discoverable by ultrasound examination. If the clinical diagnosis is known, there may be no need for a biopsy
▶ Nodules usually regress with glucocorticoid therapy.
▶ The presence of a mass should not engender an orchiectomy
▶ Biopsy of the testis and/or peritesticular tissue may be obtained

Radiologic Features

▶ Testicular and/or peritesticular nodules may be identified unilaterally or bilaterally by ultrasound examination

Prognosis and Treatment

▶ Initial treatment is medical (glucocorticoids)
▶ Orchiectomy should not be necessary
▶ Occasional cases are refractory to medical therapy, and surgery may be needed only for cosmetic reasons
▶ There is no potential for the development of malignant tumors in CAH other than cryptorchidism

---

testicular and paratesticular parenchyma. The nuclei are round and uniform, often with a small nucleolus (Figs. 9-54 and 9-55). Cytoplasm is eosinophilic to brown. On high power magnification, the cytoplasm contains fine granular lipochrome pigment. Reinke's crystals are not present within the "tumor cells" of CAH. Native Leydig cells within the testis may be atrophic. The microscopic findings in the testis are identical to those in Nelson syndrome, in which ACTH from a pituitary tumor stimulates testicular and peritesticular ACTH-sensitive cells. This occurs following bilateral adrenalectomy.

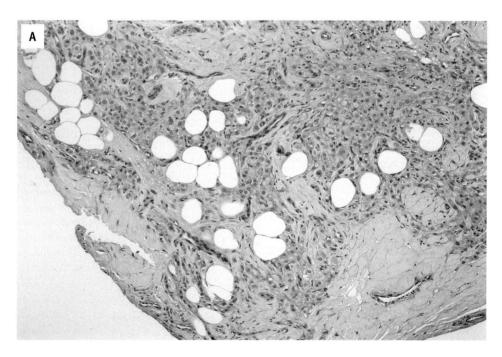

FIGURE 9-54

A, Paritesticular tissue with numerous eosinophilic cells involving fibroadipose tissue in a 21-year-old man with congenital adrenal hyperplasia.

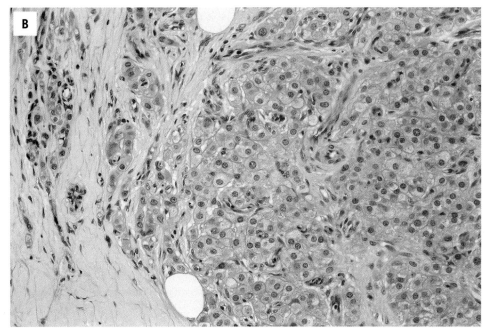

FIGURE 9-54, CONT'D

B, Aggregates of polygonal eosinophilic cells with round, uniform nuclei, some of which contain a nucleolus. The cytoplasm contains a fine brown lipochrome pigmentation.

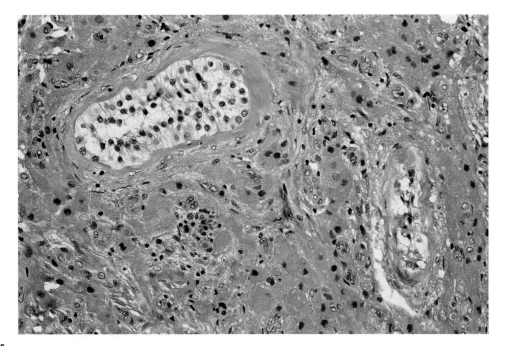

FIGURE 9-55

This 7-year-old boy with congenital adrenal hyperplasia had multiple intratesticular nodules comprised of fairly uniform polygonal cells with eosinophilic cytoplasm and round to slightly irregular nuclei. The cellular aggregates surround seminiferous tubules.

CONGENITAL ADRENAL HYPERPLASIA—PATHOLOGIC FEATURES

Gross Findings

▶ The masses may be single or multiple, are present within the testis and/or adjacent tissues, and are composed of dark brown nodules

Microscopic Findings

▶ Multiple aggregates of eosinophilic cells infiltrate testicular and/or extratesticular parenchyma
▶ Cells have eosinophilic granular cytoplasm and a fine brown background of lipochrome pigment
▶ Nuclei lack anaplastic features
▶ Native Leydig cells in the testis may be regressed
▶ Cells do not contain Reinke's crystals

Fine-needle Aspiration Biopsy Findings

▶ In the proper clinical context, the finding of a uniform population of eosinophilic cells is consistent with the diagnosis of CAH

Immunohistochemical Features

▶ Cells are positive for inhibin

Differential Diagnosis

▶ Nelson syndrome due to excessive ACTH secretion from a pituitary or nonpituitary neoplasm
▶ Leydig cell tumor—these are almost never bilateral

COMPLETE ANDROGEN INSENSITIVITY SYNDROME

CLINICAL FEATURES

Complete androgen insensitivity syndrome (AIS) is equally well-known as testicular feminization. It is the most frequent cause of male pseudohermaphroditism. AIS is caused by the lack of androgen receptor (AR). Because of this, testosterone and DHT are unable to stimulate the development of the wolffian duct system and male external genitalia. A variety of mutations in the AR gene occur at Xq11-q12. The patient with complete AIS is a tall phenotypic female with well-formed breasts, absent or scanty pubic and axillary hair, and a shallow vagina. At the time of initial presentation, it may be unrecognized that she has bilateral cryptorchidism with intra-abdominal, inguinal, or labial testes and usually absent wolffian and müllerian duct derivatives.

Complete AIS may be ascertained at birth, in adolescence, or in adulthood. Infants and children may have inguinal hernias. If the surgeon recognizes the presence of a gonad, it can be biopsied and the diagnosis made. At puberty, the absence of menarche may initiate investigation and enable the diagnosis to be made. Sometimes, however, amenorrhea is ignored and the diagnosis is made on an infertility workup. Rarely, after a sister has been diagnosed with AIS, the remaining phenotypic female siblings are evaluated. Occasionally, the presence of a pelvic mass caused by a germ cell tumor or a Sertoli cell adenoma is the presenting feature.

A number of syndromes in patients with ambiguous external genitalia, quantitatively or qualitatively abnormal androgen receptors, and variable wolffian duct development have been characterized as partial or incomplete AIS or Reifenstein syndrome. In these cases, the testes may be cryptorchid and show changes characteristic of cryptorchidism.

COMPLETE ANDROGEN INSENSITIVITY SYNDROME—FACT SHEET

Definition

▶ A syndrome characterized by a phenotypic female with a 46,XY karyotype, undescended testes, female external genitalia, breast development, diminished to absent pubic and axillary hair, shallow vagina, and absence of müllerian duct-derived organs

Incidence

▶ 1 in 20,000 to 1 in 60,000 male births

Gender and Age Distribution

▶ Complete AIS occurs in phenotypic females
▶ Incomplete AIS occurs in phenotypic males and in patients with ambiguous genitalia
▶ Complete AIS may be identified at birth, in childhood, or in adulthood

Clinical Features

▶ Physical findings as indicated in the definition
▶ 46,XY karyotype—in a prepubertal child, diagnosis can be made based on androgen receptor binding activity in cultured genital skin fibroblasts, or with PCR to characterize the androgen receptor gene in DNA from a blood sample
▶ In adults, serum testosterone and gonadotropins are elevated

Radiologic Features

▶ Pelvic ultrasonography demonstrates the absence of müllerian duct-derived organs

Prognosis and Treatment

▶ These patients are infertile
▶ Patients are at risk for the development of Sertoli cell adenomas and malignant germ cell tumors
▶ Patients need estrogen therapy beginning at puberty to cause normal female pubertal development
▶ Testes should be removed after puberty because of the risk of developing malignant germ cell tumors
▶ 30% of nongonadectomized patients develop malignant germ cell tumors by age 50 years. Few develop malignant germ cell tumors before the end of puberty

PATHOLOGIC FEATURES

GROSS FINDINGS

Cryptorchid testes have a brown appearance and may contain one to multiple white to tan nodules varying from 1 mm to 24 cm in diameter (Fig. 9-56). Often a smooth muscle mass is present medial to the testis. Cysts of wolffian or müllerian origin may be present at the lateral pole of the testis. There is a risk of development of germ cell tumors in the testes of patients with AIS. Because of this, suspicious nodules and masses should be sampled for microscopic evaluation.

MICROSCOPIC FINDINGS

Seminiferous tubules are small and comprise mostly postpubertal-type Sertoli cells. Spermatogonia are sparse, and spermatocytes have been reported. Malignant intra-tubular germ cells may be present. In the interstitium, there is marked Leydig cell hyperplasia and a variable spindle-cell proliferation that resembles ovarian-type stroma (Fig. 9-57). The nodules that are present comprise small tubules populated almost entirely by immature Sertoli cells. Germ cells are rare. The nodules are demarcated from the surrounding testicular tissue. The nodules do not show Leydig cell hyperplasia but may contain Leydig cells (Fig. 9-57). Nodules have been designated Sertoli cell adenomas based on the predominant Sertoli cell composition and their often substantial size (Fig. 9-58). They are not premalignant, are probably hamartomatous, and have not evolved into malignant tumors.

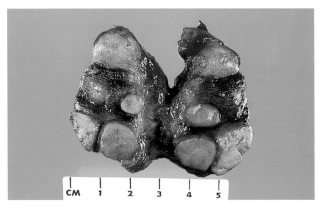

FIGURE 9-56

This is a bivalved, 5.6-cm, intra-abdominal testis in an 18-year-old phenotypic female with complete androgen insensitivity syndrome containing dark brown testicular parenchyma and multiple firm, tan nodules measuring up to 1.1 cm. The nodules are Sertoli cell adenomas.

DIFFERENTIAL DIAGNOSIS

Once a karyotype has been performed and the 46,XY karyotype has been identified, other causes of male pseudohermaphroditism should be distinguished. The phenotype of complete AIS is characteristic for the diagnosis. Androgen receptor study of a genital skin biopsy can be done for confirmation.

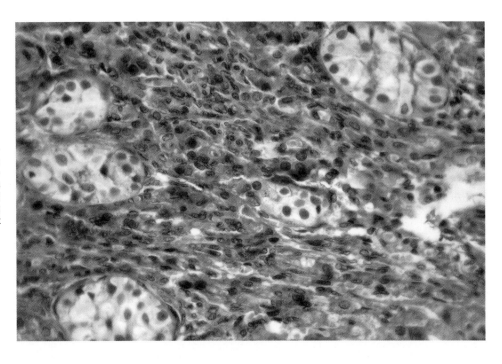

FIGURE 9-57

The patient is one of three middle-aged sisters with complete androgen insensitivity syndrome. The illustration is from a cryptorchid testis with small tubules containing Sertoli cells and germ cells. There is Leydig cell hyperplasia and prominent stromal cells.

COMPLETE ANDROGEN INSENSITIVITY SYNDROME—PATHOLOGIC FINDINGS

Gross Findings

▶ Testes are cryptorchid and usually brown; they develop white or tan nodules from 1 mm to 24 cm in size
▶ A smooth muscle mass may be present medial to the testis
▶ Cysts of müllerian or wolffian duct origin may be present bilaterally
▶ Müllerian-derived organs are absent, although rarely a tubal remnant is present

Microscopic Findings

▶ Prepubertal testes sometimes have a normal appearance
▶ In postpubertal testes, there is hyperplasia of Leydig cells, variable proliferation of ovarian-like stroma, and nodules comprised of small tubules lined by postpubertal-type Sertoli cells and sometimes spermatogonia
▶ Sertoli cell adenomas are actually hamartomatous and are discrete nodules containing small tubules lined principally by Sertoli cells of prepubertal type
▶ Spermatogonia may be present
▶ Within the interstitium there may be occasional Leydig cells
▶ Tubules may rarely contain malignant intratubular germ cells
▶ Malignant germ cell tumors increase in frequency with age, occurring in 30% of patients by age 50 years

Immunohistochemical Features

▶ CD117 and PLAP confirm the presence of malignant intratubular germ cells in patients older than 1 year
▶ Inhibin can be used to demonstrate Sertoli and Leydig cells

Differential Diagnosis

▶ 5α-reductase deficiency
▶ Mixed gonadal dysgenesis

PROGNOSIS AND TREATMENT

Because the testes are cryptorchid, there is a risk of development of malignant germ cell tumors (Fig. 9-59), most types of which have been reported. The frequency of malignant germ cell tumors has been estimated at greater than 30% by age 50 years. Because of this, bilateral gonadectomy should occur after or before completion of puberty. There is no risk of malignancy from the Sertoli cell adenomas.

GONADAL DYSGENESIS

CLINICAL FEATURES

Gonadal dysgenesis encompasses mixed gonadal dysgenesis (MGD), pure gonadal dysgenesis (PGD), and dysgenetic male pseudohermaphroditism (DMPH). Sohval described a group of intersex patients with asymmetric gonadal development. These cases included patients with (1) a testis on one side and a contralateral streak gonad, (2) a testis and contralateral gonadal dysgenesis, (3) hypoplastic gonads with rudimentary tubules in one, and (4) a streak gonad with a contralateral tumor. A germ cell tumor on one side with contralateral agenesis is also considered to be MGD (5). In MGD, various combinations of müllerian and wolffian duct-derived structures are present. Most patients have bilateral fallopian tubes. These may be present in close proximity to vas deferens and epididymis (Fig. 9-60).

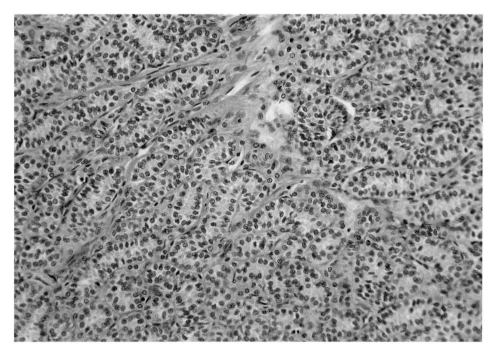

FIGURE 9-58

The adenomatous nodule is comprised of tightly packed prepubertal-type seminiferous tubules lined by Sertoli cells. Rare Leydig cells are present.

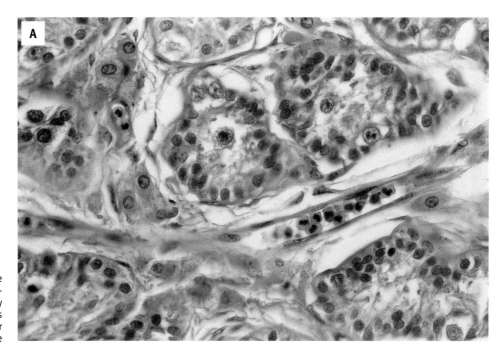

FIGURE 9-59

A, In this patient with complete androgen sensitivity syndrome, seminiferous tubules are lined mostly by Sertoli cells. Scattered larger cells with irregular chromatin and clear cytoplasm are present within some tubules. These are malignant intratubular germ cells. **B,** The plasma membranes and cytoplasm of malignant intratubular germ cells stain positively with immunoperoxidase stain for placental alkaline phosphatase (PLAP).

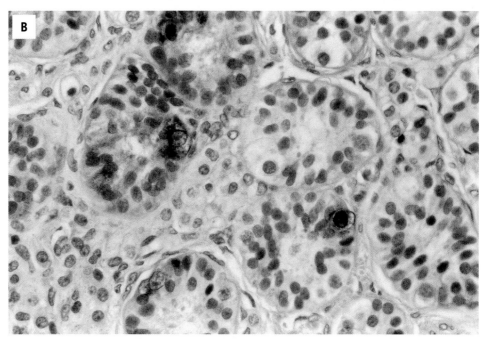

Inadequate or delayed production of testosterone by the gonad may cause incomplete masculinization of the external genitalia and poor development of ipsilateral wolffian duct structures. The majority of patients with MGD are phenotypically female, but some have ambiguous or normal external male genitalia. Phenotypic females often virilize at puberty.

PGD is characterized by bilateral streak gonads, internal müllerian structures, a 46,XY karyotype, and a female phenotype without signs of Turner syndrome.

Patients with DMPH have bilateral dysgenetic testes, persistent müllerian duct structures, cryptorchidism, and inadequate virilization. The karyotype may show 45,XO/46,XY mosaicism. Because of the overlap in syndromes with similar karyotypes, overlapping phenotypes, the susceptibility of gonads for neoplastic transformation, and often the inability to identify the type of gonad in those with germ cell tumors, PGD, DMPH, and MGD are all considered as part of the syndrome of gonadal dysgenesis.

RADIOLOGIC FEATURES

Calcification may be marked and identifiable in patients with gonadoblastoma on radiologic studies of the abdomen and pelvis.

PATHOLOGIC FEATURES

In MGD, müllerian duct derivatives occur in 95% of cases. The uterus may be infantile, rudimentary, or normal. The gonads vary considerably in MGD, and the morphology may evolve in the course of time. Streak gonads have a broad, flat appearance and are characteristically composed of spindled cells resembling ovarian stroma. Some gonads contain elements of dysgenetic testes with variable development of seminiferous tubules and stroma. In some instances, lack of differentiation is insufficient to characterize the organ as a testis or an ovary. In tissues removed in adulthood, seminiferous tubules may exhibit GCA but should be examined for the presence of malignant intratubular germ cells. There is evidence in patients who were biopsied earlier in life that there is degeneration of germ

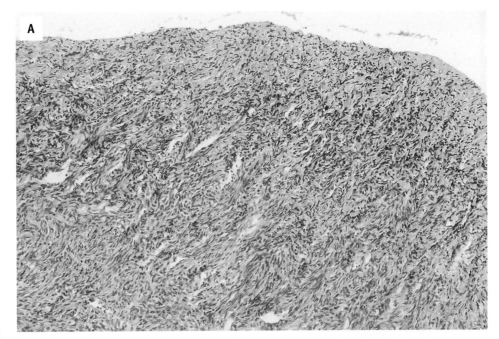

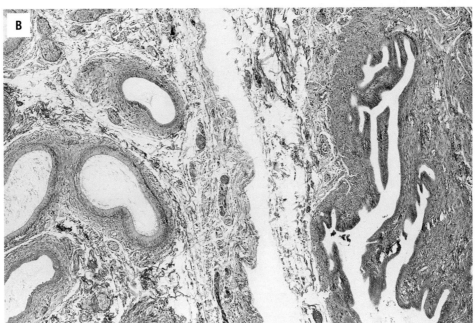

FIGURE 9-60

A, Streak gonad composed exclusively of ovarian-type stroma in a patient with mixed gonadal dysgenesis. **B**, Proximity of epididymis *(left)* and fallopian tube *(right)*.

cells. Germ cell tumors have developed in 9% to 30% of patients with MGD. The most characteristic tumor is the gonadoblastoma, a nonmetastasizing tumor composed of malignant germ cells and surrounding sex cord cells in circumscribed nests with focal or diffuse calcification. In about 50% of these cases, malignant germ cells invade the stroma and form a germinoma (seminoma) (Figs. 9-61 and 9-62). Other types of germ cell tumors may also develop in association with gonadoblastomas. Gonadoblastomas do not metastasize, but germ cell tumors occurring in association with them may metastasize. In cases that I have studied, 7 of 15 patients with MGD, all phenotypic females, had gonadal germ cell tumors. These were five gonadoblastomas, four germinomas (seminomas), and one malignant intratubular germ cell neoplasia. In addition, one patient had a gonadal stromal tumor.

ANCILLARY STUDIES

IMMUNOHISTOCHEMISTRY

Malignant germ cells may be demonstrated with immunoperoxidase stain for CK117 and PLAP.

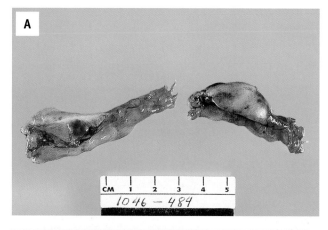

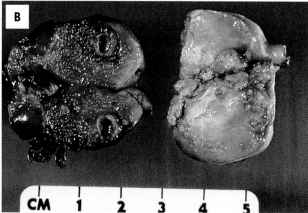

FIGURE 9-61

A, A 20-year-old woman with bilateral gonadoblastomas. The gonad on the right contains a germinoma (seminoma). The gonad on the left contains rudimentary testicular tissue. **B,** An 18-year-old woman with bilateral gonadoblastomas and germinomas (seminomas). Gonads are bivalved, measure up to 3.8 cm in maximum dimension, and weigh 6 and 6.6 g. Both gonads are firm with yellow-tan and pink-white tissue and contain flecks of calcific material.

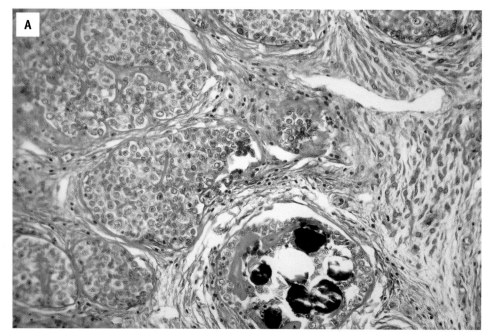

FIGURE 9-62

These micrographs are from a patient whose gross specimen is shown in Figure 9-61. **A,** A low-power micrograph demonstrates gonadoblastoma with discrete aggregates comprising gonadal stromal cells (Sertoli or granulosa cells) and malignant germ cells. A focus of laminated calcification is present.

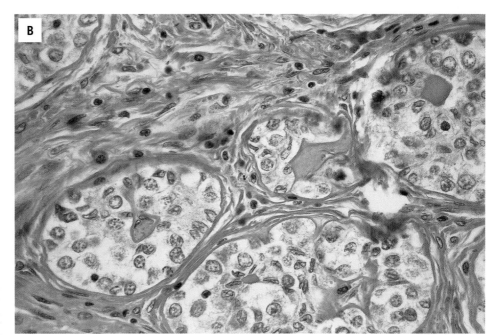

FIGURE 9-62, CONT'D

B, A high-power micrograph illustrates discrete structures containing smaller gonadal stromal-type cells (Sertoli or granulosa cells) and larger malignant germinal cells. Hyaline eosinophilic material is an extension of basement membrane. **C,** Section from the gonad illustrated in **A.** On the right is a tumor composed of seminomatous-type cells and numerous lymphocytes.

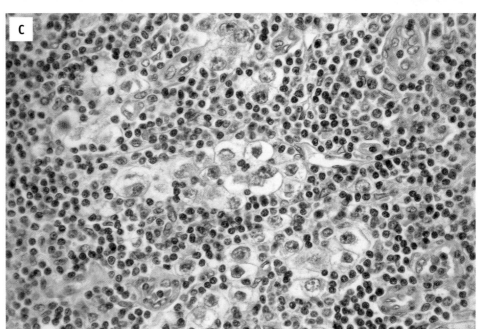

TRUE HERMAPHRODITISM

CLINICAL FEATURES

A patient with both ovarian and testicular tissue is defined as a true hermaphrodite regardless of the presence and distribution of wolffian and müllerian duct structures.

PATHOLOGIC FEATURES

The patient may have two ovotestes, an ovotestis on one side and a contralateral ovary or testis, or an ovary and a contralateral testis. The ovotestis (Fig. 9-63) is the most frequent gonad. Patients most frequently have a 46,XX karyotype, less often a 46,XY or more complex karyotype. The testicular and ovarian tissue segments of the ovotestes are end-to-end. The ovarian portion is usually histologically normal, but the testicular

TRUE HERMAPHRODITISM—FACT SHEET

Definition

▶ A patient with both ovarian and testicular tissue in any distribution

Incidence

▶ Rare

Morbidity and Mortality

▶ Some patients raised as female may virilize at puberty
▶ Germ cell tumors occur in 10% of 46,XY and 4% of 46,XX true hermaphrodites

Gender and Race

▶ 75% are raised as male, but most of these have ambiguous genitalia
▶ The incidence of true hermaphrodism is much higher in Africa

Clinical Features

▶ Most patients have ambiguous genitalia including a urogenital sinus

▶ Phenotypic males may present with gynecomastia and monthly hematuria
▶ Phenotypic females may present with amenorrhea or failure to develop secondary sex characteristics
▶ Patients have variable karyotypes, most frequently 46,XX, but 46,XY and mosaics occur
▶ Variable distribution of wolffian and müllerian duct derivatives
▶ Patients have potential for fertility if raised as females and male gonadal tissue is excised. The removal of wolffian duct-derived tissue has been suggested

Prognosis and Treatment

▶ Important considerations are gender assignment, fertility, and risk of malignancy
▶ All cryptorchid testicular tissue should be removed to eliminate the risk of germ cell tumor development
▶ If ovarian tissue remains and the müllerian duct system is intact, fertility is a possibility

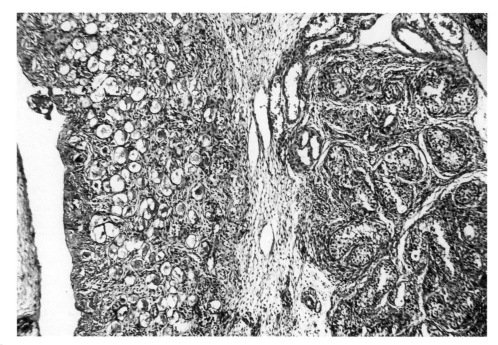

FIGURE 9-63

Gonad from 1-month-old infant with true hermaphroditism and ambiguous genitalia demonstrates both ovarian tissue with ova *(left)* and prepubertal-type seminiferous tubules *(right)*.

TRUE HERMAPHRODITISM—PATHOLOGIC FEATURES

Gross Findings

▶ Separate testis and ovary or ovotestes
▶ Testicular and ovarian segments of ovotestes are end-to-end
▶ Testicular tissue is soft, and ovarian tissue is firm
▶ Individual testes are intrascrotal in more than 50% of patients
▶ Patient usually has ambiguous genitalia with asymmetric features and combinations of müllerian and wolffian duct-derived tissues

Microscopic Findings

▶ Gonadal tissue frequently appears normal in the young
▶ Testicular tissue in an ovotestis usually has loss of germ cells and tubular sclerosis
▶ Biopsy of the gonad may not identify both testicular and ovarian tissue

Differential Diagnosis

▶ Mixed gonadal dysgenesis

---

component rarely contains spermatogonia and usually shows tubular sclerosis. In patients with scrotal testes, some degree of spermatogenesis may be present. Streak gonads are rarely found. Malignant germ cell tumors, including gonadoblastoma, have been reported in 4% to 10% of cases. Brenner tumor, mucinous cystadenoma, and endometriotic cysts have been reported in ovarian tissue. Gonadal biopsy may not identify both ovarian and testicular elements in an ovotestis.

SUGGESTED READINGS

Embryology

Moore K: The Developing Human: Clinically Oriented Embryology. Philadelphia, WB Saunders, 1982, pp 271–280.
Poulat F, Girard F, Chevron MP, et al: Nuclear localization of the testis determining gene product SRY. J Cell Biol 1995;128:737–748.

Anatomy

Muller J, Skakkebaek NE: Quantification of germ cells and seminiferous tubules by stereological examination of testicles from 50 boys who suffered from sudden death. Int J Androl 1983;6:143–156.
Prince FP: Ultrastructure of immature Leydig cells in the human prepubertal testis. Anat Rec 1984;209:165–176.

Cryptorchidism

Hadziselimovic F, Herzog B, Huff DS, Menardi G: The morphometric histopathology of undescended testes and testes associated with incarcerated inguinal hernia: A comparative study. J Urol 1991;146(2 Pt 2):627–629.
Huff DS, Hadziselimovic F, Snyder HM 3rd, et al: Postnatal testicular maldevelopment in unilateral cryptorchidism. J Urol 1989;142(2 Pt 2):546–548; discussion 572.
Krabbe S, Skakkebaek NE, Bertelsen JG, et al: High incidence of undetected neoplasia in maldescended testes. Lancet 1979;1:999–1000.
Miller KD, Coughlin MT, Lee PA: Fertility after unilateral cryptorchidism: Paternity, time to conception, pretreatment testicular location and size, hormone and sperm parameters. Horm Res 2001;55:249–253.
Mininberg DT, Rodger JC, Bedford JM: Ultrastructural evidence of the onset of testicular pathological conditions in the cryptorchid human testis within the first year of life. J Urol 1982;128:782–784.
Prener A, Engholm G, Jensen OM: Genital anomalies and risk for testicular cancer in Danish men. Epidemiology 1996;7:14–19.
Swerdlow AJ, Higgins CD, Pike MC: Risk of testicular cancer in cohort of boys with cryptorchidism. BMJ 1997;314:1507–1511.

Anorchism

Federman DD: Disorders of gonadal development: Mixed gonadal dysgenesis. Dysgenetic male pseudohermaphroditism: Agonadism. In Federman DD: Abnormal Sexual Development. Philadelphia, WB Saunders, 1968, pp 84–88.
Smith NM, Byard RW, Bourne AJ: Testicular regression syndrome: A pathological study of 77 cases. Histopathology 1991;19:269–272.

Polyorchism

Nistal M, Paniagua R: Congenital anomalies of the testis and the epididymis. In Nistal M, Paniagua R: Testicular and Epididymal Pathology. New York, Thieme-Stratton, 1984, pp 72–93.

Testicular-Splenic Fusion

Bonneau D, Roume J, Gonzalez M, et al: Splenogonadal fusion limb defect syndrome. Am J Med Gene 1999;86:347–358.
Putschar WG, Manion WC: Splenic-gonadal fusion. Am J Pathol 1956;32:15–33.

Adrenal Cortical Rests

Johnson RE, Scheithauer B: Massive hyperplasia of testicular adrenal rests in a patient with Nelson's syndrome. Am J Clin Pathol 1982;77:501–507.

Spermatic Cord Torsion and Testicular Infarction

Levin HS: Non-neoplastic diseases of the testis. In Mills SE, Carter D, Greenson JK, et al. (eds.): Sternberg's Diagnostic Surgical Pathology, Vol. 2. Philadelphia, Lippincott Williams & Wilkins, 2004, 2139–2141.
Schneck FX, Bellinger MF: Abnormalities of the testis and scrotum and their surgical management. In Campbell F, Walsh PC, Retik AB: Campbell's Urology, 8th ed. Philadelphia, WB Saunders, 2002, 2379–2384.
Schneider RE. Male genital problems. In Tintanalli JE, Kelen GD, Stapczynski JS (eds): Emergency Medicine: A Comprehensive Study Guide. New York, McGraw-Hill, 2004, pp 616–618.
Williamson RC: Torsion of the testis and allied conditions. Br J Surg 1976;63:465–476.

Varicocele

Agger P, Johnsen SG: Quantitative evaluation of testicular biopsies in varicocele. Fertil Steril 1978;29:52–57.
Turner TT: Varicocele: Still an enigma. J Urol 1983;129:695–699.

Microlithiasis

Peterson AC, Bauman JM, Light DE, et al: The prevalence of testicular microlithiasis in an asymptomatic population of men 18 to 35 years old. J Urol 2001;166:2061–2064.
Rashid HH, Cos LR, Weinberg E, Messing EM: Testicular microlithiasis: A review and its association with testicular cancer. Urol Oncol 2004;22:285–289.
Ringdahl E, Claybrook K, Teague JL, Northrup M: Testicular microlithiasis and its relation to testicular cancer on ultrasound findings of symptomatic men. J Urol 2004;172:1904–1906.

Vasculitis

Dahl EV, Baggenstoss AH, Deweerd JH: Testicular lesions of periarteritis nodosa, with special reference to diagnosis. Am J Med 1960;28:222–228.

Huisman TK, Collins WT Jr, Voulgarakis GR: Polyarteritis nodosa masquerading as a primary testicular neoplasm: A case report and review of the literature. J Urol 1990;144:1236–1238.

Kariv R, Sidi Y, Gur H: Systemic vasculitis presenting as a tumorlike lesion: Four case reports and an analysis of 79 reported cases. Medicine (Baltimore) 2000;79:349–359.

Lie JT: Isolated polyarteritis of testis in hairy-cell leukemia. Arch Pathol Lab Med 1988;112:646–647.

Shurbaji MS, Epstein JI: Testicular vasculitis: Implications for systemic disease. Hum Pathol 1988;19:186–189.

Tartakoff J, Hazard JB: Thromboangitis olibterans of the spermatic cord. N Engl J Med 1938;218:173.

Amyloidosis

Ozdemir BH, Ozdemir OG, Ozdemir FN, Ozdemir AI: Value of testis biopsy in the diagnosis of systemic amyloidosis. Urology 2002;59:201–205.

Male Infertility

Brandell RA, Mielnik A, Liotta D, et al: AZFb deletions predict the absence of spermatozoa with testicular sperm extraction: Preliminary report of a prognostic genetic test. Hum Reprod 1998;13: 2812–2815.

Calogero AE, Garofalo MR, Barone N, et al: Spontaneous regression over time of the germinal epithelium in a Y chromosome-microdeleted patient: Case report. Hum Reprod 2001;16:1845–1848.

Chang PL, Sauer MV, Brown D: Y chromosome microdeletion in a father and his four infertile sons. Hum Reprod 1999;14:2689–2694.

Del Castillo EB, Trabucco A, De la Balze FA: Syndrome produced by absence of the germinal epithelium without impairment of the Sertoli or Leydig cells. J Clin Endocrinol 1947;7:493.

Ferguson-Smith MA: Chromatin-positive Klinfelter's syndrome (primary microorchidism) in a mental-deficiency hospital. Lancet 1958;1:928.

Heller CH, Clermont Y: Kinetics of the germinal epithelium in man. Recent Prog Horm Res 1964;20:545–575.

Jarow JP, Budin RE, Dym M, et al: Quantitative pathologic changes in the human testis after vasectomy: A controlled study. N Engl J Med 1985;313:1252–1256.

Klinefelter HFJ, Reifenstein EC, Albright F: Syndrome characterized by gynecomastia, aspermatogenesis without a-Leydigism, and increased excretion of follicle stimulating hormone. J Clin Endocrinol 1942;8:615.

Levin HS: Non-neoplastic disease of the testis. In Mills SE, Carter D, Greenson JK, et al. (eds): Sternberg's Diagnostic Surgical Pathology, vol 2, 4th ed. Philadelphia, Lippincott Williams & Wilkins, 2004, pp 2142–2148.

Mak V, Zielenski J, Tsui LC, et al: Proportion of cystic fibrosis gene mutations not detected by routine testing in men with obstructive azoospermia. JAMA 1999;281:2217–2224.

Okada H, Fujioka H, Tatsumi N, et al: Klinefelter's syndrome in the male infertility clinic. Hum Reprod 1999;14:946–952.

Reubinoff BE, Abeliovich D, Werner M, et al: A birth in non-mosaic Klinefelter's syndrome after testicular fine needle aspiration, intracytoplasmic sperm injection and preimplantation genetic diagnosis. Hum Reprod 1998;13:1887–1892.

Schover LR, Thomas AJ: Congenital bilateral absence of the vas deferens (CBAVD). In Schover LR, Thomas AJ: Overcoming Male Infertility: Understanding Its Causes and Treatments. New York, John Wiley & Sons, 2000, pp 61–63.

Schover LR, Thomas AJ Jr: Getting images of your reproductive system. In Schover LR, Thomas AJ: Overcoming Male Infertility: Understanding Its Causes and Treatments. New York, John Wiley & Sons, 2000, p 43.

Silber SJ, Rodriguez-Rigau LJ: Quantitative analysis of testicle biopsy: Determination of partial obstruction and prediction of sperm count after surgery for obstruction. Fertil Steril 1981;36:480–485.

Tournaye H, Staessen C, Liebaers I, et al: Testicular sperm recovery in nine 47,XXY Klinefelter patients. Hum Reprod 1996;11:1644–1649.

Wong W, Strauss FH, Warner NE: Testicular biopsy in the study of male infertility. I. Testicular causes of infertility. II. Post-testicular causes of infertility. III. Pretesticular causes of infertility. Arch Pathol 1973;95:151,160 and 1974;98:1.

Gonadotropin Deficiency

Burris AS, Rodbard HW, Winters SJ, Sherins RJ: Gonadotropin therapy in men with isolated hypogonadotropic hypogonadism: The response to human chorionic gonadotropin is predicted by initial testicular size. J Clin Endocrinol Metab 1988;66:1144–1151.

Gemzell C, Kjessler B: Treatment of infertility after partial hypophysectomy with human pituitary gonadotrophins. Lancet 1964;15: 644.

Liu L, Bank SM, Barnes KM, Sherins RJ: Two-year comparison of testicular responses to pulsatile gonadotropin-releasing hormone and exogenous gonadotropins from the inception of therapy in men with isolated hypogonadotropic hypogonadism. J Clin Endocrinol Metab 1988;67:1140–1145.

MacLeod J, Pazianos A, Ray BS: Restoration of human spermatogenesis by menopausal gonadotropins. Lancet 1964;13:1196–1197.

Schulze C: Response of the human testis to long-term estrogen treatment: Morphology of Sertoli cells, Leydig cells and spermatogonial stem cells. Cell Tissue Res 1988;251:31–43.

Weiss J, Axelrod L, Whitcomb RW, et al: Hypogonadism caused by a single amino acid substitution in the beta subunit of luteinizing hormone. N Engl J Med 1992;326:179–183.

Macroorchidism

Heseltine D, White MC, Kendall-Taylor P, et al: Testicular enlargement and elevated serum inhibin concentrations occurring in patients with pituitary microadenomas secreting follicle stimulating hormone. Clin Endocrinol 1989;31:411–423.

Nistal M, Martinez-Garcia F, Regadera J, et al: Macro-orchidism: A clinicopathological approach. J Urol 1994;151:1155–1161.

Infectious Diseases

Craighead JE, Mahoney EM, Carver DH, et al: Orchitis due to coxsackie virus group B, type 5: Report of a case with isolation of virus from the testis. Nord Hy Tidskr 1962;267:498.

Gall EA: The histopathology of acute mumps orchitis. Am J Pathol 1947;23:637.

Grabstald H, Swann LL: Genitourinary lesions in leprosy with special reference to the problem of atrophy of the testis. JAMA 1952;145:1287.

Hepper NG, Karlson AG, Leary FJ, Soule EH: Genitourinary infection due to *Mycobacterium kansasii*. Mayo Clin 1971;46:1287.

Hunt AC, Bothwell PW: Histological findings in human brucellosis. J Clin Pathol 1967;20:267–272.

Jenkin GA, Choo M, Hosking P, Johnson PD: Candidal epididymyorchitis: Case report and review. Clin Infect Dis 1998;26:942–945.

Kahn RI, McAninch JW: Granulomatous disease of the testis. J Urol 1980;123:868–871.

Monroe M: Proceedings: Granulomatous orchitis due to *Histoplasma capsulatum* masquerading as sperm granuloma. J Clin Pathol 1974;27:929–930.

Morgan AD: Inflammation and infestation of the testis and paratesticular structures. In Pugh RC (ed): Pathology of the Testis. Oxford, England, Blackwell Scientific, 1976, pp 79–138.

Navarro-Martinez A., Solera J, Corredoira J, et al: Epididymoorchitis due to *Brucella mellitensis:* A retrospective study of 59 patients. Clin Infect Dis 2001;33:2017–2022.

Nistal M, Paniagua R: Inflammatory diseases of the epididymis and testis. In Nistal M, Paniagua R: Testicular and Epididymal Pathology. 1984, New York: Thieme-Stratton, Inc. 268–269.

Riggs S, Sanford JP: Viral orchitis. N Engl J Med 1962;266:990–993.

Schuster TG, Hollenbeck BK, Kauffman CA, et al: Testicular histoplasmosis. J Urol 2000;164:1652.

Singer AJ, Kubak B, Anders KH: Aspergillosis of the testis in a renal transplant recipient. Urology 1998;51:119–121.

Singh D, Dutta S, Kumar P, Narang A: Mixed anaerobic and aerobic testicular abscess in a neonate. Indian J Pediatr 2001;68:561–562.

von Schnakenburg C, Hinrichs B, Fuchs J, Kardorff R: Post-transplant epididymitis and orchitis following *Listeria monocytogenes* septicemia. Pediatr Transplantation 2000;4:156–158.

Werner CA: Mumps orchitis and testicular atrophy: A factor in male sterility. Ann Intern Med 1950;32:1075–1086.

Wolbach SB, Todd JC, Palfrey FW: The Etiology and Pathology of Typhus. Cambridge, MA: Harvard University Press, 1922, pp 173, 216, 222.

Acquired Immunodeficiency Syndrome

De Paepe ME, Guerrieri C, Waxman M: Opportunistic infections of the testis in the acquired immunodeficiency syndrome. Mt. Sinai J Med 1990;57:25–29.

Leibovitch I, Baniel J, Rowland RG, et al: Malignant testicular neoplasms in immunosuppressed patients. J Urol 1996;155:1938–1942.

Nistal M, Santana A, Paniagua R, Palacos J: Testicular toxoplasmosis in two men with the acquired immunodeficiency syndrome (AIDS). Arch Pathol Lab Med 1986;110:744–746.

Reichert CM, O'Leary TJ, Levens DL, et al: Autopsy pathology in the acquired immune deficiency syndrome. Am J Pathol 1983;112:357–382.

Welsh K, Finkbeiner W, Alpers CE: Autopsy findings in the acquired immune deficiency syndrome. JAMA 1984;252:1152.

Nonspecific Granulomatous Orchitis and Malacoplakia

Brown RC, Smith BH: Malacoplakia of the testis. Am J Clin Pathol 1965;43:409.

Wegner HE, Loy V, Dieckmann KP: Granulomatous orchitis: An analysis of clinical presentation, pathological anatomic features and possible etiologic factors. Eur Urol 1994;26:56–60.

Intersex

Belville C, Josso N, Picard JY: Persistence of mullerian derivatives in males. Am J Med Genet 1999;89:218–223.

Berkovitz GD, Seeherunvong T: Abnormalities of gonadal differentiation. Clin Endrocrinol Metab 1998;12:133–142.

Brinkmann AO: Molecular basis of androgen insensitivity. Mol Cell Endocrinol 2001;179:105–109.

Coulam CB: Testicular regression syndrome. Obstet Gynecol 1979;53:44–49.

Davidoff F, Federman DD: Mixed gonadal dysgenesis. Pediatrics 1973;52:725–742.

Diamond DA: Sexual differentiation: Normal and abnormal. In Campbell F, Walsh PC, Retik AB: Campbell's Urology, 8th ed. Philadelphia, WB Saunders, 2002, pp 2395–2427.

Gottlieb B, Pinsky L, BeitelLK, Trifiro M: Androgen insensitivity. Am J Med Genet 1999;89:210–217.

Imbeaud S, Rey R, Berta P, et al: Testicular degeneration in three patients with the persistent mullerian duct syndrome. Eur J Pediatr 1995;154:187–190.

Jorgensen N, Muller J, Jaubert F, et al: Heterogeneity of gonadoblastoma germ cells: Similarities with immature germ cells, spermatogonia and testicular carcinoma in situ cells. Histopathology 1997;30:177–186.

Korsch E, Peter M, Hiort O, et al: Gonadal histology with testicular carcinoma in situ in a 15-year-old 46,XY female patient with a premature termination in the steroidogenic acute regulatory protein causing congenital lipoid adrenal hyperplasia. J Clin Endocrinol Metab 1999;84:1628–1632.

Stikkelbroeck NM, Otten BJ, Pasic A, et al: High prevalence of testicular adrenal rest tumors, impaired spermatogenesis, and Leydig cell failure in adolescent and adult males with congenital adrenal hyperplasia. J Clin Endocrinol Metab 2001;86:5721–5728.

Patterson MN, McPhaul MJ, Hughes IA: Androgen insensitivity syndrome. Baillieres Clin Endocrinol Metab 1994;8:379–404.

Regadera J, Martinez-Garcia F, Paniagua R, Nistal M: Androgen insensitivity syndrome: An immunohistochemical, ultrastructural, and morphometric study. Arch Pathol Lab Med 1999;123:225–234.

Robboy SJ, Bentley RC, Russell P, et al: Embryology and disorders of sex and development. In Robboy SJ, Anderson MC, Russell P (eds.): Pathology of the Female Reproductive Tract. London, Churchill Livingstone, 2002, pp 819–860.

Rutgers JL, Scully RE: Pathology of the testis in intersex syndromes. Semin Diagn Pathol 1987;4:275–291.

Sohval AR: "Mixed" gonadal dysgenesis: A variety of hermaphroditism. Am J Hum Genet 1963;15:155–158.

Wallace TM, Levin HS: Mixed gonadal dysgenesis: A review of 15 patients reporting single cases of malignant intratubular germ cell neoplasia of the testis, endometrial adenocarcinoma, and a complex vascular anomaly. Arch Pathol Lab Med 1990;114:679–688.

Wiersma R: Management of the African child with true hermaphroditism. J Pediatr Surg 2001;36:397–399.

10 Neoplasms of the Testis

Howard S. Levin

Testicular tumors encompass a variety of types. Because of increased patient and physician awareness, new technologies, and increased incidence of germ cell tumors (GCT), pathologists are seeing more testis biopsies and orchiectomy specimens. It is important that accurate and specific diagnoses of tumors are rendered and data are generated that will enable accurate staging, so that the patient receives an accurate prognosis and the most efficacious therapy.

The two most recent classifications of testicular tumors are similar. Table 10-1 is modified from the 2004 Classification of the World Health Organization (WHO) and the 1999 Classification in the Armed Forces Institute of Pathology (AFIP) *Atlas of Tumor*

Table 10-1
Classification of Testicular and Paratesticular Tumors

GERM CELL TUMORS

Precursor lesions
Intratubular germ cell neoplasia, unclassified

Tumors of one histologic type
Seminoma
   Variant: Seminoma with syncytiotrophoblastic giant cells

Spermatocytic seminoma
   Variant: Spermatocytic seminoma with sarcoma

Embryonal carcinoma

Yolk sac tumor

Trophoblastic tumors
   Choriocarcinoma
   Others

Teratoma
   Mature teratoma
      Variants: Dermoid cyst, epidermoid cyst
   Immature teratoma
   Teratoma with a secondary malignant component
   Monodermal teratoma
      Carcinoid
      Primitive neuroectodermal tumor

Tumors of more than one histologic types
Mixed germ cell tumors (specify individual components and estimate their amounts as a percentage of the tumor)

GERM CELL-SEX CORD-STROMAL TUMORS

Gonadoblastoma

Unclassified tumors

SEX CORD-STROMAL TUMORS

Leydig cell tumor

Sertoli cell tumor
   Variants: Sclerosing Sertoli cell tumor, large cell calcifying Sertoli cell tumor

Granulosa cell tumors
   Variants: Adult-type granulosa cell tumor, juvenile granulosa cell tumor

Thecoma-fibroma group

Mixed

Unclassified

RETE TESTIS CARCINOMA

MALIGNANT MESOTHELIOMA

HEMATOPOIETIC TUMORS

Malignant lymphoma   Plasmacytoma   Leukemia

TUMORS OF OVARIAN-TYPE EPITHELIUM

METASTATIC TUMORS

PARATESTICULAR TUMORS

Adenomatoid tumor

Sarcomas
   Variants: Rhabdomyosarcoma, liposarcoma, others

Papillary cystadenoma of the epididymis

Desmoplastic small round cell tumor

Melanotic neuroectodermal tumor (retinal anlage tumor)

Modified from WHO histological classification of testis tumors. In Eble JN, Sauter G, Epstein J, Sesterhenn I (eds.): World Health Organization Classification of Tumours: Pathology and Genetics. Lyon, France, IARC Press, 2004; and Ulbright T, Amin M, Young R (eds.): AFIP Atlas of Tumor Pathology, 3rd series, Fascicle 25. Washington, DC, Armed Forces Institute of Pathology, 1999.

Pathology. In this chapter, the most common entities are discussed and illustrated. Space does not allow extensive consideration of all types of tumor. Table 10-2 is the 2002 TNMS Testicular Staging System, which incorporates serologic levels of serum tumor markers.

Germ Cell Tumors

More than 90% of testicular tumors are derived from germ cells. There is a great variation in the incidence of GCTs worldwide, with the highest incidence being in Europe. In the United States, GCTs of the testis are more frequent among Caucasian Americans and rare among African Americans. GCTs occur most frequently in postpubertal men in the third and fourth decades, but they may be found less frequently in childhood and beyond the age of 50 years. Although the cause of GCTs is not known, it is thought that malignant intratubular germ cells develop during intrauterine development and subsequently progress over decades. DNA abnormalities occur in testicular GCTs. It is thought that neoplastic germ cells undergo polyploidization in utero. Before the development of intratubular germ cell neoplasia unspecified (IGCNU), there is a selective loss

---

Table 10-2

TNMS Staging of Testis Tumors

PRIMARY TUMOR (T)

pTx	Primary tumor cannot be assessed
pT0	No evidence of primary tumor
pTis	Intratubular germ cell neoplasia unspecified
pT1	Tumor limited to testis and epididymis without vascular/lymphatic invasion; tumor may invade into tunica albuginea but not tunica vaginalis
pT2	Tumor limited to testis and epididymis with vascular/lymphatic invasion, or tumor extending through tunica albuginea with involvement of tunica vaginalis
pT3	Tumor invades spermatic cord with or without vascular/lymphatic invasion
pT4	Tumor invades scrotum with or without vascular/lymphatic invasion

REGIONAL LYMPH NODES (N)

pNX	Regional lymph nodes cannot be assessed
pN0	No regional lymph node metastasis
pN1	Metastasis with a lymph node ≤2 cm in greatest dimension and ≤5 nodes positive, none >2 cm in greatest dimension
pN2	Metastasis with a lymph node mass >2 cm but not >5 cm in greatest dimension, or >5 nodes positive, none >5 cm; or evidence of extranodal extension or tumor
pN3	Metastasis with a lymph node mass >5 cm in greatest dimension

DISTANT METASTASIS (M)

MX	Distant metastasis cannot be assessed
M0	No distant metastasis
M1	Distant metastasis
M1a	Nonregional nodal or pulmonary metastasis
M1b	Distant metastasis other than to nonregional lymph nodes and lungs

SERUM TUMOR MARKERS (S)

SX	Marker studies not available or not performed
S0	Marker study levels within normal limits
S1	LDH 1.5× normal AND hCG <5,000 mIU/mL AND AFP <1,000 ng/mL
SD2	LDH 1.5× normal OR hCG 5,000-50,000 mIU/mL OR AFP 1,000-10,000 ng/mL
SD3	LDH >10× normal OR hCG >50,000 mIU/mL OR AFP >10,000 ng/mL

STAGE GROUPING

Stage	T	N	M	S
Stage 0	pTis	N0	M0	S0
Stage I	pT1-4	N0	M0	SX
Stage IA	pT1	N0	M0	S0
Stage IB	pT2	N0	M0	S0
	pT3	N0	M0	S0
	pT4	N0	M0	S0
Stage IS	Any pT/Tx	N0	M0	S1-3
Stage II	Any pT/Tx	N1-3	M0	SX
Stage IIA	Any pT/Tx	N1	M0	S0
	Any pT/Tx	N1	M0	S1
Stage IIB	Any pT/Tx	N2	M0	S0
	Any pT/Tx	N2	M0	S1
Stage IIC	Any pT/Tx	N3	M0	S0
	Any pT/Tx	N3	M0	S1
Stage III	Any pT/Tx	Any N	M1	SX
Stage IIIA	Any pT/Tx	Any N	M1a	S0
	Any pT/Tx	Any N	M1a	S1
Stage IIIB	Any pT/Tx	N1-3	M0	S2
	Any pT/Tx	Any N	M1a	S2
Stage IIIC	Any pT/Tx	N1-3	M0	S3
	Any pT/Tx	Any N	M1a	S3
	Any pT/Tx	Any N	M1b	Any S

AFP, α-fetoprotein; hCG, human chorionic gonadotropin; LDH, lactic dehydrogenase.
From Greene FL, Page DL, Fleming ID, Balch CM (eds): AJCC Cancer Staging Manual, 6th ed. New York, Springer, 2002, pp 317–332.

of DNA. Further selective losses and gains occur in the development of seminomatous and nonseminomatous GCTs. Many malignant GCTs have an isochromosome of 12p that may be associated with the invasive capability of the tumors. Some risk factors for the development of GCTs are known. The major risk factors are cryptorchidism, which carries an approximately three-fold to fivefold increased risk of malignancy; infertility; and the presence of a contralateral GCT. There is an approximately 1% risk of IGCNU in biopsied infertile males (not 1% of the entire population of infertile males). There is an increased risk of GCTs in first-degree male relatives of patients with GCTs.

INTRATUBULAR GERM CELL NEOPLASIA UNSPECIFIED

CLINICAL FEATURES

Skakkebaek was the first to identify IGCNU in infertile men. Originally the intratubular cells were interpreted as atypical, and subsequently it was recognized that, if left alone, 90% of testes with IGCNU progressed to clinically malignant GCTs within 7 years. These tumors are seminomas or nonseminomas. IGCNU may be identified at any age. A cryptorchid testis may be biopsied at the time of orchidopexy, a testis may be biopsied in the course of an infertility workup, a gonad may be biopsied or resected in a patient with an intersex syndrome, or the contralateral testis may be biopsied in a patient with a testis tumor. IGCNU may be identified in any of these specimens. There is no specific symptomatology of IGCNU. Although testicular microlithiasis may be associated with testicular GCTs and with IGCNU, there is no definite evidence that microlithiasis leads to malignant GCTs. There is a consensus that follow-up of patients with microlithiasis should be on the basis of coexistent findings such as a mass, infertility, or pain, rather than microlithiasis itself.

PATHOLOGIC FEATURES

GROSS FINDINGS

There are no specific gross findings of IGCNU.

MICROSCOPIC FINDINGS

IGCNU initially always occurs in an abnormal testis. The coexistent findings are those associated with cryptorchidism, intersex, and male infertility. IGCNUs are randomly present within an affected testis. In adults, IGCNU is present in approximately 80% of testes with malignant GCTs. The seminiferous tubules containing IGCNU are usually reduced in diameter,

---

INTRATUBULAR GERM CELL NEOPLASIA UNSPECIFIED (IGCNU)— FACT SHEET

Definition
► Malignant, enlarged germ cells within seminiferous tubules

Incidence
► IGCNU occurs in approximately 1% of testes biopsied for infertility (not 1% of the male infertility population)
► In approximately 80% of testes with malignant GCTs
► In up to 8% of patients with contralateral GCTs
► In 2% to 8% of testes with cryptorchidism
► In some patients with intersex syndromes with a Y chromosome, most of whom are cryptorchid

Morbidity and Mortality
► Mortality is secondary to a clinical GCT that is associated with or develops in IGCNU
► Morbidity relates to the therapy used

Gender, Race, and Age Distribution
► In genetic males (with a Y chromosome) and intersex patients
► May be discovered after 1 year of age, but is usually found in men from the third to fifth decade

Clinical Features
► Asymptomatic
► Clinical findings relate to associated disease states

Radiologic Features
► Ultrasonography may identify microlithiasis or an associated mass

Prognosis and Treatment
► 90% of adults will develop a clinical GCT within 7 years
► May be cured by orchiectomy or radiation of sufficient dosage
► Chemotherapy is not curative in all cases
► Watchful waiting may allow the patient time to be fertile
► Consideration should be given for sperm banking

Differential Diagnosis
► Primordial germ cells and spermatogonia in males less than 1 year of age
► Giant spermatogonia in adults

---

with reduced spermatogenesis and thickened tubular walls. The IGCNU cells are generally against the tubular basement membrane and contain large nuclei of approximately 10 μm diameter with some nuclear irregularity, an irregular plasma membrane, and cleared cytoplasm (Figs. 10-1 and 10-2). Rarely, syncytiotrophoblastic giant cells (STGCs), embryonal carcinoma (EC), or teratoma cells are present within tubules. Occasionally, in the absence of a clinical tumor, malignant germ cells identical to those within tubules are present within the interstitium. IGCNU may be confirmed with immunohistochemical stains for CD117 or placental alkaline phosphatase (PLAP) (Fig. 10-3).

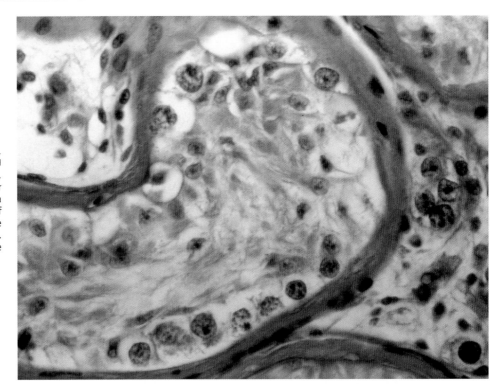

FIGURE 10-1

Intratubular germ cell neoplasia, unspecified (IGCNU). Large IGCNU cells with round to irregular nuclei, prominent nucleoli, and clear cytoplasm line the periphery of a seminiferous tubule. A cluster of similar cells is peripheral to the tunica propria in the interstitium. Cells with pink cytoplasm within the tubule are Sertoli cells.

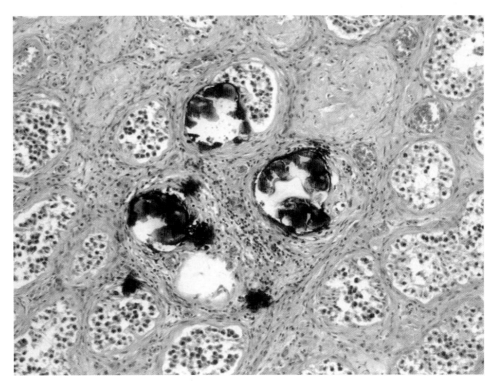

FIGURE 10-2

Intratubular germ cell neoplasia, unspecified (IGCNU) and microlithiasis. Laminated calcific bodies obliterate three tubules. IGCNU is present in surrounding tubules.

DIFFERENTIAL DIAGNOSIS

Care must be taken not to make the diagnosis of IGCNU in patients younger than 1 year of age, because the primordial germ cells and spermatogonia in the testes in this age group and their immunohistochemical reactions may be histologically identical to cells of IGCNU. It is also important that giant spermatogonia in adults not be overinterpreted as IGCNU. Giant spermatogonia occur in tubules with normal spermatogenesis, lack the histologic features of IGCNU, and do not stain with CD117 and PLAP. If the pathologist is in doubt about the diagnosis, the case should be referred to an experienced consultant.

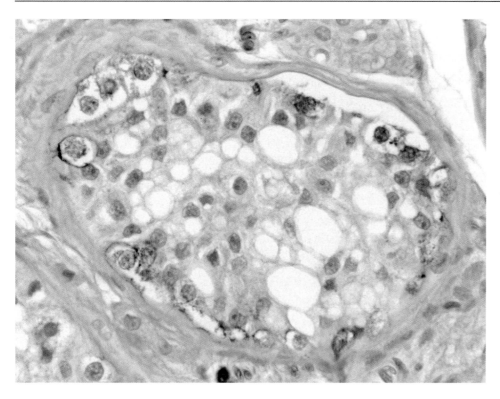

FIGURE 10-3
Intratubular germ cell neoplasia, unspecified (IGCNU). Plasma membranes of IGCNU cells are positive for placental alkaline phosphatase.

INTRATUBULAR GERM CELL NEOPLASIA UNSPECIFIED (IGCNU)—PATHOLOGIC FEATURES

Gross Findings
▶ None

Microscopic Findings
▶ Malignant cells are present in abnormal tubules with diminished diameter and diminished spermatogenesis
▶ IGCNU cells are enlarged with large nuclei, irregular nuclear borders, prominent nucleoli, and clear cytoplasm
▶ IGCNU cells may be present in biopsy or orchiectomy specimens
▶ May be associated with microlithiasis

Immunohistochemical Features
▶ Plasma membranes are positive for CD117 and PLAP
▶ IGCNU cells stain for glycogen with PAS stain

PROGNOSIS AND TREATMENT

If, after biopsy, the testis is left in situ, approximately 90% of patients with IGCNU discovered in adulthood will develop a clinical malignancy within 7 years. Therapy consists of orchiectomy, irradiation, or watchful waiting. Chemotherapy may not be curative.

SEMINOMA

CLINICAL FEATURES

Seminoma is the most common pure GCT of the testis and accounts for approximately 35% to 50% of all testicular tumors. The mean age at discovery of seminoma is approximately 40 years, 5 to 10 years later than in patients with nonseminomatous GCTs. Most seminomas are discovered as masses, and only about 10% are associated with scrotal pain. Rarely, discovery of testicular seminoma is preceded by a clinical metastasis to a peripheral lymph node, retroperitoneal lymph node, retroperitoneum, or parenchymal organ. It is important to distinguish metastatic seminoma from other tumors because of the excellent response of seminoma to irradiation or chemotherapy. Seminomas are only rarely bilateral. Because of the cure rate of seminoma, there is an approximately 2% to 5% risk for development of a GCT in the opposite testis. Serum human chorionic gonadotropin (hCG) and lactic dehydrogenase (LDH) levels may be elevated in patients with seminoma. These elevations are not specific indications of seminoma. Mild hCG elevations (in the hundreds of mIU/mL) may be associated with STGCs in seminoma. If hCG elevations are markedly elevated (in the thousands or tens of thousands of mIU/mL), an associated choriocarcinoma should be suspected. An elevated α-fetoprotein (AFP) concentration is strongly

PATHOLOGIC FEATURES

GROSS FINDINGS

The testis with a seminoma is usually enlarged and contains a palpable mass. Seminomas have a mean diameter of 5 cm but may be considerably larger. Most tumors are composed of a single gray to tan mass, but some are multinodular and some have discrete additional nodules that may or may not connect with the main tumor mass grossly or microscopically (Fig. 10-4). Most tumors are confined to the testis. Occasionally, tumors originate in the retroperitoneum (Fig. 10-5).

MICROSCOPIC FINDINGS

Seminomas comprise sheets or lobules of seminoma cells in various configurations. Seminoma cells are usually round or polygonal, with sharp plasma membranes (Fig. 10-6). The nucleus is enlarged and often vesicular, with prominent nucleoli. Mitoses are usually

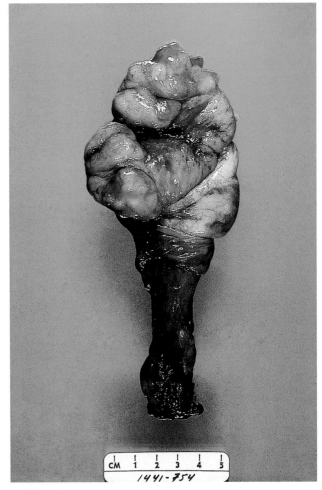

FIGURE 10-4

Seminoma: Gross Findings
Incision of testis demonstrates lobules of tan, uniform seminoma replacing the testicular parenchyma.

suspicious for yolk sac tumor (YST) in the primary tumor or a metastasis. LDH elevation in the serum may reflect the presence of bulky seminoma, but it is not a specific marker for seminoma. Metastases occur initially to para-aortic and paracaval lymph nodes, and afterward to other lymph nodes and parenchymal organs.

RADIOLOGIC FEATURES

Ultrasound examination demonstrates the presence of a well-defined and hypoechoic mass. Microlithiasis may be demonstrated.

SEMINOMA—PATHOLOGIC FEATURES

Gross Findings

► Single or multinodular gray-tan mass
► Mean diameter is 5 cm

Microscopic Findings

► Sheets or lobules of seminoma cells divided by fibrous trabeculae
► Frequently associated with aggregates of lymphocytes
► Aggregates of histiocytes are frequent
► Seminoma cells are usually round or polygonal with sharp plasma membranes. Large, often vesicular nuclei with prominent nucleoli. Frequent mitoses. Cytoplasm varies from clear to eosinophilic.
► Necrosis may be present
► May be associated with microlithiasis
► Fibrosis may be marked
► Seminoma may have a tubular growth pattern
► Seminoma may contain multinucleated STGCs

Immunohistochemical Features

► Plasma membranes of seminoma cells are positive for CD117 and PLAP
► A rare cell may be positive for CD30
► STGCs are positive for hCG

Differential Diagnosis

► IGCNU
► Embryonal carcinoma
► Yolk sac tumor
► Malignant lymphoma
► Leydig cell tumor
► Sertoli cell tumor
► Spermatocytic seminoma
► Metastatic carcinoma
► Granulomatous inflammatory disease

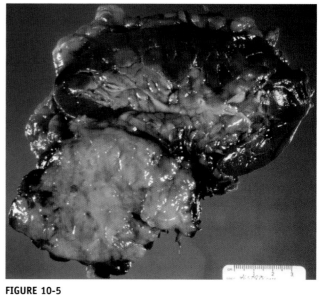

FIGURE 10-5

A 9-cm retroperitoneal (perirenal) seminoma was removed surgically with the adjacent kidney.

present within a seminoma. The cytoplasm is usually clear and stains for glycogen, but sometimes the cytoplasm is eosinophilic. The usual seminoma contains fibrous trabeculae. Most seminomas contain aggregates of lymphocytes, and they may contain plasma cells and eosinophils. There may be an exceedingly large number of lymphocytes. Necrosis may be present. There may be associated microlithiasis (Fig. 10-7). Variations in morphology can occur. Aggregates of histiocytes and sarcoidal-type granulomas are often present. Extensive

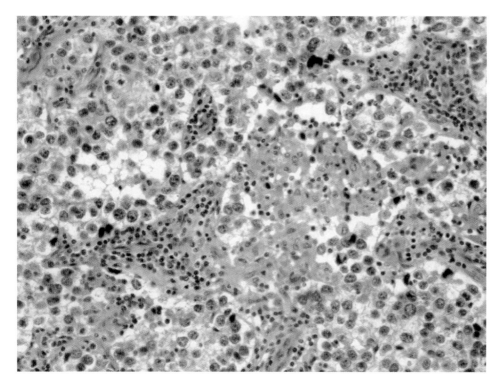

FIGURE 10-6

Aggregates of histiocytes and foci of lymphocytes separate lobules of seminoma cells. Seminoma cells contain round nuclei with one or two nucleoli, clear to eosinophilic cytoplasm, and discrete cell borders.

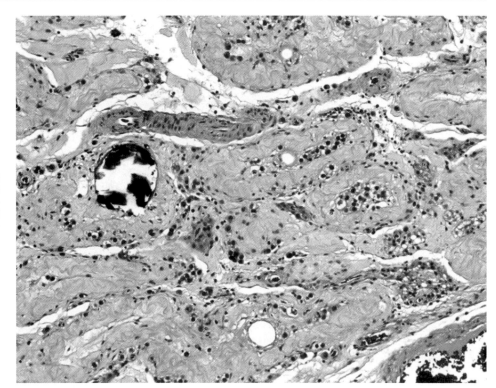

FIGURE 10-7

From a case in which seminoma was identified in other sections of the biopsy specimen, this photomicrograph illustrates microlithiasis and tunica propria thickening of surrounding tubules.

scar formation can make the recognition of a malignant process difficult, particularly in a patient with metastases and an occult primary tumor. Fibrosis may be marked (Fig. 10-8). Sometimes seminoma has a tubular pattern, but always the cells comprising the cords of cells or tubules are characteristic of seminoma (Fig. 10-9).

A recognized variant is seminoma with STGC, which may be associated with a modest elevation in serum hCG. The STGCs may resemble STGCs seen in choriocarcinoma, but without an accompanying cytotrophoblastic element. STGCs may also have clusters of seminoma-like nuclei in a cell with eosinophilic

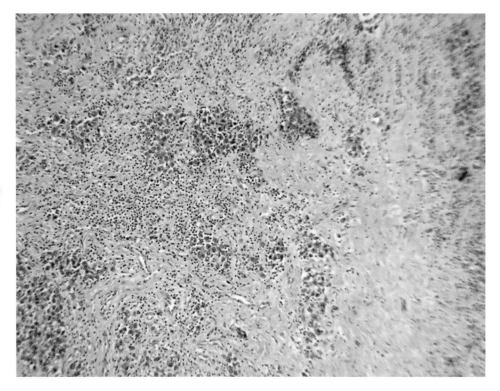

FIGURE 10-8

Dense fibrous scar tissue entraps nests of seminoma cells and surrounding lymphocytes.

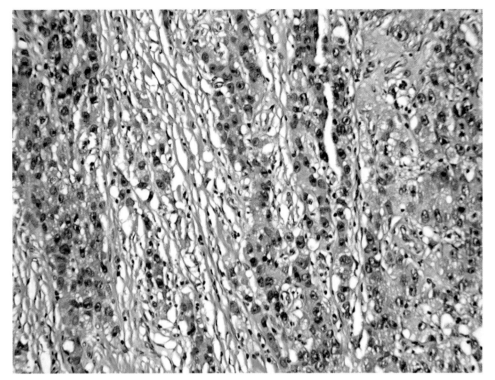

FIGURE 10-9

Dense fibrous tissue surrounds cords and solid tubules of seminoma cells.

cytoplasm. STGCs may be mononuclear and may not be evident on slides stained with hematoxylin and eosin (H&E); they are identified with immunohistochemical stain for hCG (Figs. 10-10 and 10-11). Cribriform and pseudoglandular forms may be disconcerting because of their architecture, but they contain seminoma-type nuclei.

Seminoma cells may invade blood vessels. The large majority of seminomas are associated with IGCNU cells that may extend into the rete testis. Initially, this may present a confounding appearance because of the cystic architecture and malignant-looking cells.

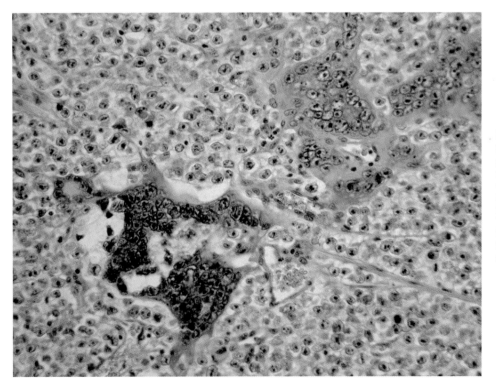

FIGURE 10-10

Seminoma with syncytiotrophoblastic giant cells (STGCs). Large, multinucleated giant cells are packed with vesicular nuclei containing prominent nucleoli. The nuclei resemble those of surrounding seminoma cells. The multinucleated cells stained positively for human chorionic gonadotropin (hCG). No cytotrophoblastic cells were present in the specimen.

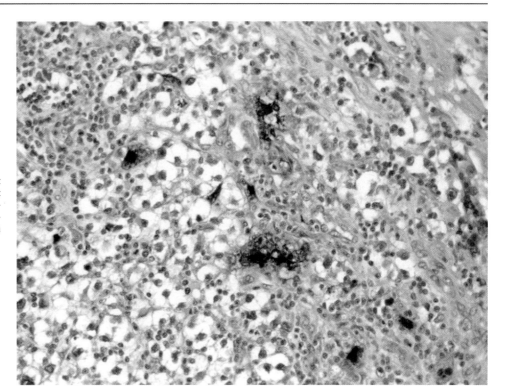

FIGURE 10-11

Seminoma with syncytiotrophoblastic giant cells (STGC). Human chorionic gonadotropin (hCG)-positive mononucleate and multinucleated trophoblastic cells are present within a seminoma.

ANCILLARY STUDIES

FINE-NEEDLE ASPIRATION BIOPSY

Fine-needle aspiration demonstrates clusters, sheets, and single cells with or without accompanying lymphocytes. There may be interspersed cytoplasmic debris. Individual cells are 15 to 20 µm in diameter in air-dried preparations, with round to oval nuclei and one or more prominent nucleoli. Fine-needle aspiration is usually done on metastatic sites rather than on primary tumors.

IMMUNOHISTOCHEMISTRY

Plasma membranes of seminoma cells are characteristically positive for CD117 and PLAP, which are the most commonly used markers (Fig. 10-12). PLAP may also stain cytoplasm. STGCs are positive for hCG. Seminoma may be focally positive for keratin, and a rare cell may be positive for CD30. If cells are positive for AFP, the pathologist should strongly consider that the focus might represent a solid growth pattern of YST.

DIFFERENTIAL DIAGNOSIS

Seminoma often comes into the differential diagnosis of other testicular tumors. Because of the many variations of seminoma morphology, it may be necessary to obtain additional sections to identify a characteristic seminomatous area. In cases of IGCNU, early microscopic infiltration of the interstitium raises the possibility of seminoma but should be considered IGCNU. Atypia in seminoma cells raises the differential diagnosis of EC. Occasional histologically atypical cells in an otherwise typical seminoma should still be considered a seminoma but should engender a search for EC in other sections. Some seminomas have a heavy lymphocytic infiltration. Additional sections demonstrating seminoma should enable the distinction between seminoma and malignant lymphoma.

Leydig cell tumors (LCTs), particularly the vacuolated cell variant, may enter the differential diagnosis of seminoma. This may be particularly difficult in the evaluation of a frozen-section slide. Seminoma cells are positive for PLAP and CD117, and LCTs are often positive for inhibin. Sertoli cell tumors (SCTs) may resemble tubular seminoma. In the differential diagnosis of SCTs and LCTs, the finding of characteristically seminomatous nuclear changes and IGCNU should clarify the diagnosis. Spermatocytic seminoma can be confused with seminoma in several respects. The larger and intermediate-size germ cells can be confused with seminoma cells, and the smaller cells can be mistaken for lymphocytes. Almost all seminomas have foci of IGCNU at the periphery of the tumor. This occurs within tubules of diminished diameter, whereas spermatocytic seminoma in situ contains all three types of spermatocytic seminomatous tumor cells in tubules of expanded diameter. Spermatocytic seminoma does not have a lymphocytic component.

Two other types of GCT may enter the differential diagnosis of seminoma. In seminoma-looking areas in a patient with elevated serum AFP, the possibility of a

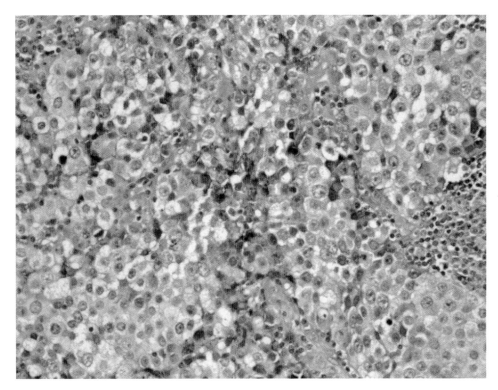

FIGURE 10-12
The plasma membranes of numerous seminoma cells are positive for placental alkaline phosphatase (PLAP).

seminoma evolving to a YST should be considered. Indeed, AFP mRNA has been found in seminoma.

Occasionally, the distinction between EC and seminoma is difficult. EC cells have larger, more irregular nuclei, indistinct plasma membranes, and overlapping nuclei. EC grows in papillary, embryoid body-like, glandular, and solid configurations; lacks a lymphoid reaction; and tends to have more necrosis than seminoma. The use of immunohistochemical stains may be useful in distinguishing seminoma from EC. EC cells often stain for CD30 in a membranous pattern, and seminoma cells are usually negative or only very focally positive for this marker. The presence of non-necrotizing granulomas should not push the pathologist to the diagnosis of an inflammatory process if other findings of seminoma are present. Very rarely, a metastatic clear cell carcinoma may mimic a seminoma. Renal cell carcinoma, clear cell type, is notorious for metastasis with an occult primary tumor. Renal cell carcinoma, clear cell type, lacks IGCNU, has a rich vascularity, has no lymphocytic or granulomatous reaction, is usually within vascular spaces, and does not stain for PLAP or CD117. Although neither PLAP nor CD117 is specific for seminoma, one should not diagnose seminoma without other excellent evidence if the cells are negative for these markers.

PROGNOSIS AND TREATMENT

Seminoma of the testis is usually treated by radical orchiectomy followed by retroperitoneal irradiation involving ipsilateral inguinal, para-aortic, and paracaval lymph nodes. The usual dose is 25 to 30 Gy in 15 to 20 daily fractions, but dosage and fields are modified in the presence of large tumors, vascular invasion in the primary tumor, or involvement of lymph nodes. Bulky retroperitoneal tumors are now treated with platinum-based chemotherapy regimens. The overall survival rate for seminoma in all stages is greater than 95%.

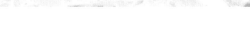

SPERMATOCYTIC SEMINOMA

CLINICAL FEATURES

Spermatocytic seminoma accounts for fewer than 5% of all testicular tumors. It is usually found in older men, with a median age at onset of 52 years, about 12 years later than for the usual seminoma. More than 100 cases of spermatocytic seminoma have been reported. Spermatocytic seminoma is more frequently bilateral than seminoma and may be multifocal. The tumor involves only the testes and is not found in other locations where GCTs may occur in the male, or in the ovary in a female. The tumor usually manifests as a painless mass. Only one case of metastatic pure spermatocytic seminoma has been reported, but approximately 12 patients with spermatocytic seminoma with sarcomatous change have been reported, all but 2 of whom died within 12 months after diagnosis.

SPERMATOCYTIC SEMINOMA—FACT SHEET

Definition

▶ Primary testicular tumor comprised of germ cells with large, medium, and small-sized nuclei resembling spermatogonia, primary spermatocytes, and spermatids

---

Incidence and Location

▶ Rare (<5% of all testicular tumors)
▶ Involve descended testes

Morbidity and Mortality

▶ Only one case of documented pure spermatocytic seminoma has metastasized
▶ Approximately 12 cases of spermatocytic seminoma with sarcomatous have been reported, and only 2 of those patients survived 1 year without metastases

---

Gender, Race, and Age Distribution

▶ Occur only in males (there is no ovarian homolog)
▶ Most occur in older men, with a mean age of 52 years

Clinical Features

▶ Tend to occur as painless testicular masses
▶ Bilateral in approximately 8% of cases
▶ Extratesticular manifestations: spermatocytic seminoma with sarcomatous may be widely metastatic and symptomatic as a result of metastases

---

Prognosis and Treatment

▶ Pure spermatocytic seminoma has an excellent prognosis and is treated with radical orchiectomy alone
▶ Majority of patients with spermatocytic seminoma with sarcomatous die within 1 year
▶ There is no satisfactory therapy for spermatocytic seminoma with sarcomatous

---

PATHOLOGIC FEATURES

GROSS FINDINGS

Spermatocytic seminoma may be bulky (up to 20 cm), multifocal, and bilateral. The tumor may be gelatinous, partially necrotic, and with cysts as a result of degeneration. Spermatocytic seminomas are generally confined to the testis.

MICROSCOPIC FINDINGS

The finding of three cell types is a sine qua non for diagnosis. The majority of cells are uniform and approximately 15 to 18 μm in diameter, with fine chromatin and with eosinophilic, not clear, cytoplasm (Fig. 10-13). Smaller cells have dense, round nucleoli and are similar in size to round spermatids or lymphocytes. The largest cells may be larger than 100 μm in diameter and have a dense, cord-like, filamentous chromatin pattern. Mitotic

figures may be present and may be atypical. There is generally no lymphocytic or granulomatous reaction. Adjacent or apart from the tumor, expanded seminiferous tubules contain the same types of cells as the tumor mass (Fig. 10-14). The tumor may invade endothelial-lined spaces. There may be considerable edema within the stroma of a spermatocytic seminoma, producing a pseudocystic appearance.

Approximately 12 cases of spermatocytic seminoma with sarcomatous change have been reported. The majority of the tumors contained undifferentiated sarcoma, but rhabdomyosarcoma and chondrosarcoma have been reported (Figs. 10-15 and 10-16).

ANCILLARY STUDIES

FLOW CYTOMETRY

Studies have demonstrated variable DNA content without a haploid cell population.

IMMUNOHISTOCHEMISTRY

Studies have yielded variable results. There are some reports of CD117 and PLAP positivity, but not the consistent cell membrane positivity of seminoma.

SPERMATOCYTIC SEMINOMA—PATHOLOGIC FEATURES

Gross Findings

▶ Large, gray, soft, friable, and gelatinous
▶ May be multifocal
▶ May be bilateral

Microscopic Findings

▶ Cells arranged in sheets in an edematous stroma
▶ Cells are of three sizes. Most are similar in size to the usual seminoma cell, but without clear cytoplasm and with a dense nucleus
▶ Small cells have dense nuclei with scant cytoplasm; larger cells are rarer than the other types and may have nuclei larger than 100 μm containing filamentous dense chromatin
▶ Accompanying spermatocytic seminoma in situ
▶ Absence of a lymphocytic component

Immunohistochemical Features

▶ CD117 and PLAP have been reported to be positive, but immunohistochemical features are not helpful in general

---

Differential Diagnosis

▶ Malignant lymphoma
▶ Plasmacytoma
▶ Seminoma
▶ Metastatic prostatic adenocarcinoma

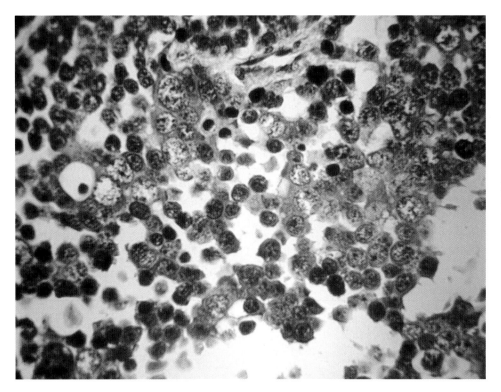

FIGURE 10-13

Spermatocytic seminoma. Large and intermediate-size cells with prominent chromatin and smaller cells with dense nuclei are present within a loose stroma.

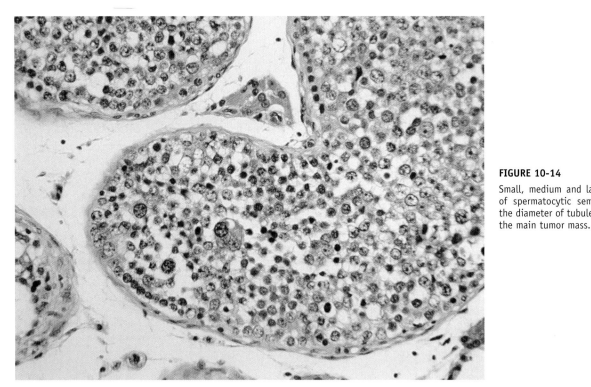

FIGURE 10-14

Small, medium and large-sized cells of spermatocytic seminoma expand the diameter of tubules peripheral to the main tumor mass.

DIFFERENTIAL DIAGNOSIS

Errors in the diagnosis of spermatocytic seminoma may occur because many pathologists are unfamiliar with the morphology of the tumor. Because of a resemblance to seminoma and the high frequency of seminoma among testicular tumors, pathologists may favor the diagnosis of seminoma. However, in addition to the required three types of cells, spermatocytic seminoma lacks the nuclear appearance of seminoma, the fibrous trabeculae, the striking granulomatous and lymphoid reaction, and the IGCNU. Spermatocytic seminoma is a

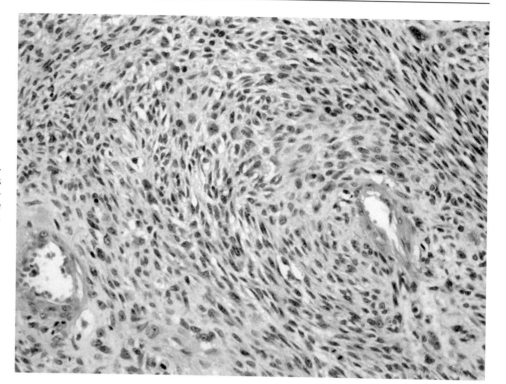

FIGURE 10-15

Spermatocytic seminoma with sarcomatous. Spindle-cell sarcoma was associated with spermatocytic seminoma which was present elsewhere in the specimen. (Courtesy of Dr. Alberto Ayala, Houston, TX).

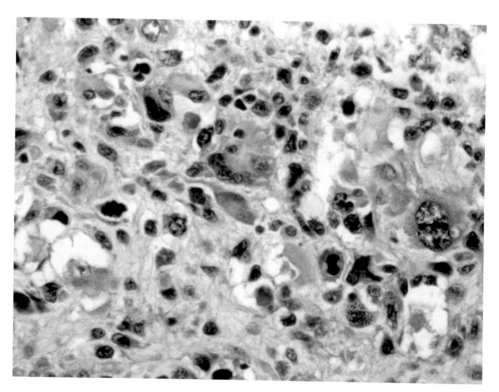

FIGURE 10-16

Rhabdomyosarcoma associated with spermatocytic seminoma. The neoplastic cells contain variably shaped anaplastic nuclei with eosinophilic cytoplasm compatible with rhabdomyoblasts. (Courtesy of Dr. Alberto Ayala, Houston, TX.)

very cellular neoplasm and may be mistaken for lymphoma and plasmacytoma in the more cellular fields. All three of these tumors occur in an older population. Both plasmacytoma and lymphoma occurring in the testis tend to present there. Plasmacytoma has a distinct eccentric nuclear location and may have peripheral clumped chromatin. Neither lymphoma nor plasmacytoma has associated IGCNU. Immunohistochemical stains can confirm the presence and type of lymphoma. Prostatic adenocarcinoma may rarely metastasize to the testis or to paratesticular tissue. Poorly differentiated prostatic adenocarcinoma may be quite cellular and lack glandular differentiation. In this circumstance, the patient should have a history of prostatic adenocarcinoma. Prostate markers should be helpful in distinguishing the two entities.

Prognosis and Treatment

Radical orchiectomy without irradiation should be curative for pure spermatocytic seminoma, and systemic chemotherapy has not cured metastatic spermatocytic seminoma with sarcomatous change.

EMBRYONAL CARCINOMA

Clinical Features

Pure EC is a rarity, occurring in about 2.7% of testicular GCTs. Earlier studies reported higher percentages of pure EC among testicular tumors. Much of what was formerly interpreted as EC is now recognized as YST. Nevertheless, EC is a frequent component of mixed GCTs of the testis. Pure ECs and mixed GCTs occur after puberty, mostly in the second through fourth decades. EC may manifest as a primary testicular tumor, or it may be symptomatic from a metastasis. Survival is dependent on the stage of the tumor, including the level of serum tumor markers. EC may occur in descended or undescended testes, retroperitoneum, the anterior mediastinum, or the pineal region.

Extratesticular specimens may be submitted to the pathologist. The most common specimen is the result of retroperitoneal lymph node dissection (RPLND). These specimens usually arrive in several parts, labeled as to where in the retroperitoneum they have come from. It is often impossible to sort out individual lymph nodes, but the pathologist should carefully describe and measure each separate part and select specimens from every type of tissue such as soft, gelatinous, solid, cystic, necrotic, hemorrhagic, red, tan, and white tissues.

Radiologic Features

Small tumors may be discovered or confirmed with ultrasound examination. Radiologic studies can be used to determine the size and number of enlarged retroperitoneal lymph nodes.

Pathologic Features

Gross Findings

It is easier to recognize a seminoma than an EC. ECs are often smaller and less homogeneous than seminomas, and they tend to have a variegated appearance. There are firm, soft, necrotic, and hemorrhagic foci (Fig. 10-17). Tumor colors are variable and may be tan, pink,

EMBRYONAL CARCINOMA—FACT SHEET

Definition
▶ Carcinomatous neoplasm lacking somatic tissue, trophoblastic, or yolk sac differentiation

Incidence and Location
▶ Pure EC is rare (approximately 2.7% of germ cell tumors)
▶ Frequent as a component of mixed GCT (up to 87%)
▶ Occurs in descended and undescended testes, retroperitoneum, mediastinum, and pineal region

Morbidity and Mortality
▶ The percentage of EC in a mixed GCT influences the prognosis

Gender, Race, and Age Distribution
▶ Occurs in males and in the ovary in females
▶ Average age at onset is approximately 10 years earlier than for seminoma (approximately 30 years)
▶ More frequent in Caucasian Americans, as are all GCTs

Clinical Features
▶ Most tumors manifest initially in the testis, but some manifest with signs and symptoms due to metastasis
▶ Testicular masses may be associated with pain

Radiologic Features
▶ Ultrasound examination demonstrates the presence of a mass
▶ Lymph node enlargement may indicate metastatic neoplasm

Prognosis and Treatment
▶ Prognosis and treatment depends on tumor stage
▶ Staging of testicular tumors includes not only the primary tumor, nodal status, and presence of lymph node or parenchymal metastases, but also the level of serum tumor markers hCG, AFP, and LDH
▶ Prognosis of ECs and nonseminomatous GCTs has improved remarkably since the prechemotherapy era. Almost 100% of stage I GCTs of the testis are cured. Approximately 98% of patients with nonbulky retroperitoneal lymph node involvement survive. Patients with bulky stage II or stage III GCTs have survival rates of 70% to 87%
▶ Therapy consists of primary orchiectomy with vigilant surveillance and/or RPLND and/or platinum-based multidrug chemotherapy
▶ Prognosis depends on the presence of angiolymphatic invasion and the presence of viable tumor in lymph nodes

or white. The tumor may appear confined to the testis, or it may extend into the tunica vaginalis or paratesticular tissue.

Microscopic Findings

ECs tend to have four main patterns: solid, tubulopapillary, glandular, or forming embryoid bodies (Figs. 10-18 through 10-21). The individual cells are generally larger than those of seminoma. Nuclei tend to be irregular and are sometimes vesicular, with prominent nucleoli. Nuclei may overlap one another. Cytoplasmic borders are often indistinct. There may be foci of undif-

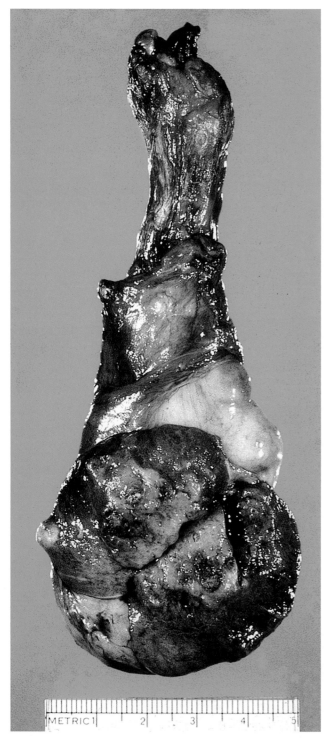

FIGURE 10-17
Embryonal carcinoma. There is extensive replacement of testicular parenchyma by variegated, focally necrotic firm tissue.

EMBRYONAL CARCINOMA—PATHOLOGIC FEATURES

Gross Findings

▶ Mean tumor diameter, about 2.5 cm
▶ Tumors are variegated with firm, soft, hemorrhagic, and necrotic foci

Microscopic Findings

▶ Four main patterns: tubulopapillary, glandular, solid, and embryoid bodies
▶ EC cells generally have pleomorphic nuclei larger than those of seminoma, with prominent nucleoli
▶ Nuclei often overlap
▶ Cytoplasm varies from eosinophilic to basophilic. Cytoplasmic borders are indistinct
▶ Mitoses are frequent
▶ Lymphocytic infiltration and granulomatous reaction may occur but are rare
▶ Vascular invasion common in pure ECs and mixed GCTs
▶ Hemorrhage and necrosis are frequent

Immunohistochemical Findings

▶ PLAP is positive in 86% to 97% of tumors
▶ Occasional cells are AFP positive. However, small foci of yolk sac tumor may be difficult to identify on H&E slides in large foci of EC
▶ CK7 is 100% positive; CAM5.2, 88%; AE1-AE3, 99%; CD30, 100%; and EMA, 12%. CK20 and high-molecular-weight keratin are 100% negative

Differential Diagnosis

▶ Seminoma
▶ Yolk sac tumor
▶ Choriocarcinoma
▶ Immature teratoma

---

bodies are discrete structures containing a central core of EC with spaces resembling amniotic cavity and with YST. When the tumor is comprised of numerous embryoid bodies, it is called polyembryoma. Some pathologists interpret these tumors as mixed GCTs composed of EC and YST, whereas others consider them to be a unique tumor type. In an EC, adjacent seminiferous tubules usually contain IGCNU or, rarely, intratubular EC. Many ECs demonstrate angiolymphatic invasion. There is often tumor hemorrhage and necrosis.

ANCILLARY STUDIES

IMMUNOHISTOCHEMISTRY

Immunohistochemical stains are useful in the diagnosis of EC and its distinction from other tumors. Most ECs are positive for PLAP, CK7, CAM5.2, AE1-AE3, and CD30. ECs are only rarely positive for CK20, are not positive for high-molecular-weight keratin, and are only rarely positive for epithelial membrane antigen (EMA) (Figs. 10-22 and 10-23).

ferentiated stroma. In the context of EC and in the absence of recognizable teratomatous foci, these areas are considered to be EC. Papillary areas may or may not have vascular cores. Glandular structures appear well formed. Solid areas may be composed of central light cells and apposed peripheral dark cells, raising the question of the presence of choriocarcinoma. Embryoid

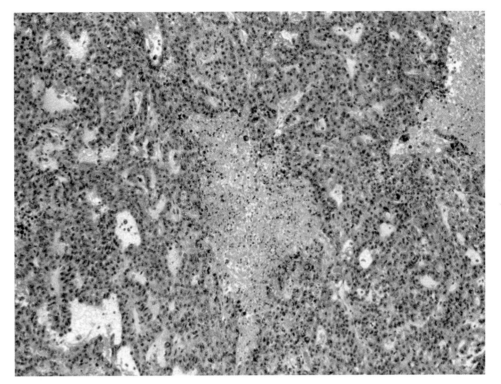

FIGURE 10-18
Embryonal carcinoma, showing well-formed glands with extensive necrosis.

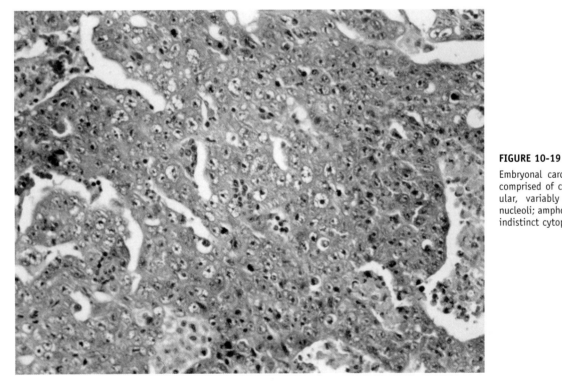

FIGURE 10-19
Embryonal carcinoma. Solid pattern comprised of cells with large, vesicular, variably sized nuclei; large nucleoli; amphophilic cytoplasm; and indistinct cytoplasmic borders.

DIFFERENTIAL DIAGNOSIS

The differential diagnosis between seminoma and EC has been discussed previously (Fig. 10-24). Foci of YST frequently occur with EC. The organoid mixtures of EC and YST resulting in double-layered structures have been characterized by some as diffuse embryoma. I prefer to consider the pattern as a juxtaposition of EC and YST. Immunohistochemical staining for AFP may demonstrate foci of recognizable YST or individual cells consistent with EC cells. If the cells on H&E section resemble EC cells, they should be considered part of

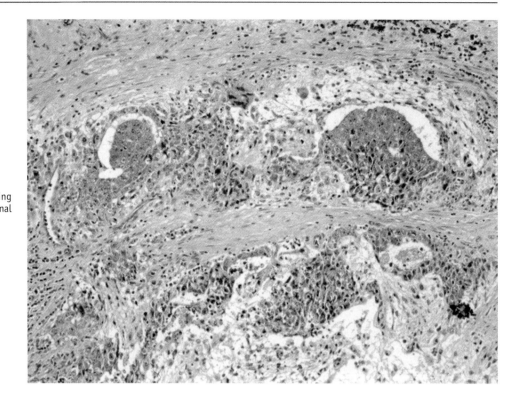

FIGURE 10-20

Two embryoid bodies containing cavities and solid areas of embryonal carcinoma.

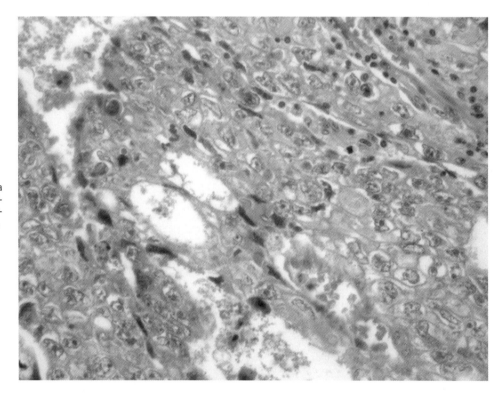

FIGURE 10-21

Embryonal carcinoma growing in a solid pattern with occasional hyperchromatic nuclei. raising the differential diagnosis of choriocarcinoma.

the EC. If the AFP-positive cells have one of the recognizable appearances of YST, they should be considered YST. Some ECs contain solid areas of apposed light and dark tumor cells, raising the question of choriocarcinoma. The dark cells are probably degenerate. They are negative for hCG. Immature stroma in some ECs can be interpreted as immature teratoma or part of an EC. There is no way to resolve the question at present. The distinction has no therapeutic implication at this time. It is best considered part of the EC.

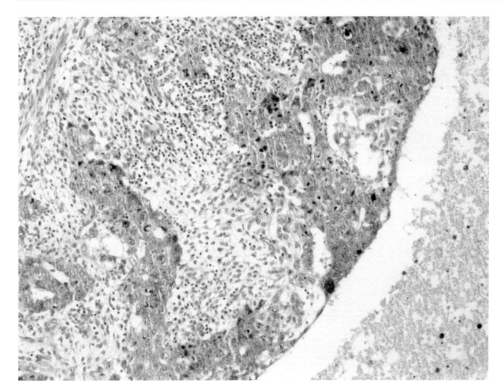

FIGURE 10-22

Embryonal carcinoma. Numerous cells are positive for placental alkaline phosphatase (PLAP).

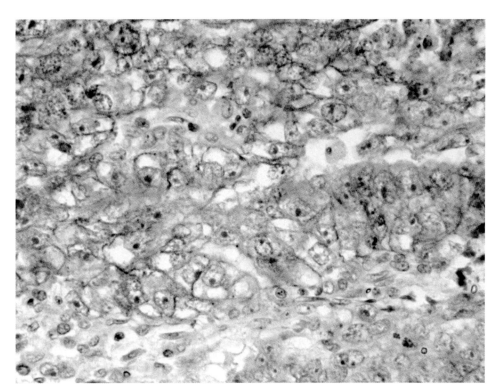

FIGURE 10-23

Marked membranous positivity for CD30 in embryonal carcinoma cells.

PROGNOSIS AND TREATMENT

Treatment of EC depends on the stage of the tumor and the presence of angiolymphatic invasion. Almost all testicular tumors are initially treated by radical orchiectomy. Exceptions to primary treatment with radical orchiectomy are patients with bulky stage II disease or stage III tumors, for whom a course of chemotherapy may precede orchiectomy. In the usual case, after orchiectomy, and depending on the extent of the disease, the patient undergoes careful observation with radiologic and serum tumor marker studies, RPLND, and possibly subsequent chemotherapy. The details of

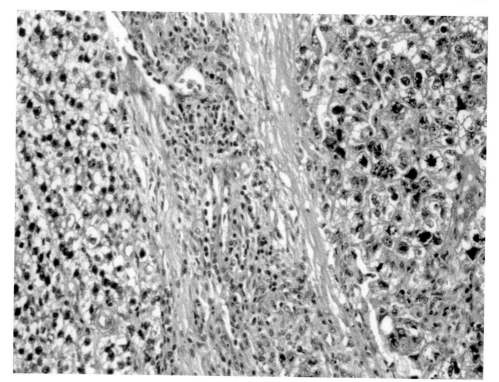

FIGURE 10-24

Side-by-side comparison of seminoma and embryonal carcinoma (EC) in a mixed germ cell tumor. Seminoma cells, on the left, contain smaller, more uniform nuclei and clear cytoplasm. EC cells, on the right, have larger, pleomorphic nuclei with some overlap.

therapy are beyond the scope of this chapter. The prognosis of ECs and nonseminomatous mixed GCTs has improved remarkably since the prechemotherapy era. Almost 100% of stage I GCTs of the testis are cured. Approximately 98% of patients with nonbulky retroperitoneal lymph node involvement survive. Patients with bulky stage II or stage III GCTs have survival rates of 70% to 87%.

YOLK SAC TUMOR

CLINICAL FEATURES

Pure YST occurs almost exclusively in infants and young children, with a mean age at onset of 16 to 18 months. In the first 6 months of life, YST is less frequent than juvenile granulosa cell tumor. Most pure YSTs occur by age 4 years. Pure YSTs rarely occur in adults, and most YSTs in adults are part of mixed GCTs. Pure YSTs occur in descended and undescended testes and in extratesticular foci where GCTs occur. Serum AFP elevation is usually associated with YST.

Before the age of chemotherapy, children younger than 2 years of age had better survival than older children. Since chemotherapy became available, age at onset does not influence survival. In mixed GCTs, the presence of YST may ameliorate the prognosis in local-

ized testicular tumors, whereas, YST may diminish survival in metastatic mixed GCTs.

PATHOLOGIC FEATURES

GROSS FINDINGS

Testicular masses are solid, tan-yellow or gray-white in color, and may have a moist, glistening surface (Fig. 10-25).

MICROSCOPIC FINDINGS

YSTs are generally composed of several patterns, which often merge from one to another (Figs. 10-26 through 10-30). The most common pattern is microvesicular, composed of microcysts. This pattern is also called the reticular pattern, because it is comprised of numerous small, thin-walled cysts lined by flattened cells with little cytoplasm. Although the cells are epithelial, some are so flattened that they resemble endothelial cells. When the cysts coalesce, they form larger cysts and may create a macrocystic appearance. Schiller-Duval bodies characterize the endodermal sinus pattern. Although these structures are characteristic of YST, they are not invariably present. Schiller-Duval bodies are papillary formations within cystic structures. The papillary formations contain a central blood vessel, often surrounded by an edematous space and lined by cuboidal to columnar cells with prominent nuclei

YOLK SAC TUMOR—FACT SHEET

Definition
▶ Tumor with many morphologic patterns that resembles embryonic yolk sac, allantois, and extraembryonic mesenchyme

Incidence and Location
▶ Pure YST is the most common testicular tumor in childhood
▶ Pure tumors occur mostly in infants and children from 6 months to 4 years of age and only rarely in adults
▶ Frequent component of mixed GCTs in adults (approximately 44%)
▶ Increased frequency is due to increased recognition of the multiple forms of YST and increased use of serum and immunohistochemical markers for AFP
▶ In descended and undescended testes and in locations where extratesticular GCTs occur
▶ In the ovary in females

Morbidity and Mortality
▶ In prechemotherapy era, children younger than 2 years of age with pure YST had a better prognosis (11% mortality) than older children (77%)
▶ In chemotherapy era, 5-year survival rate of pure YST is 91% with no difference between age groups
▶ In mixed GCTs in adults, YST in a stage I tumor may convey a better prognosis
▶ In adults with metastatic mixed GCTs, YST may confer a less favorable prognosis

Gender, Race, and Age Distribution
▶ Mean age at onset of pure YST is 16 to 18 months
▶ Rare pure YSTs may occur in children as late as 11 years and even more rarely in adults
▶ Incidence of pure YST in childhood has been described both as equal in African Americans and Caucasian Americans and as greater in Caucasian Americans

Clinical Features
▶ In childhood, tumors usually manifest as an asymptomatic mass that may be discovered by a parent or doctor in younger children and by the child if older
▶ In mixed GCTs, tumors usually manifest as scrotal masses
▶ Pure YST or YST in mixed GCTs usually have associated elevations of serum AFP
▶ Pure YST metastasizes, via lymphatics and blood vessels, to retroperitoneal lymph nodes and lungs

Radiologic Features
▶ YSTs are identifiable on ultrasound

Prognosis and Treatment
▶ Therapy depends on tumor stage
▶ In infants and children with clinical stage I tumors, patients undergo radical orchiectomy and vigilant surveillance with chemotherapy for those who relapse
▶ Adult patients with YST in mixed GCTs are treated the same as for mixed GCTs without YST
▶ In pure YST in children, chemotherapy is generally used for advanced or recurrent tumors
▶ In patients with YST in mixed GCTs, treatment and prognosis are the same as for mixed GCTs without YST and are based on tumor stage

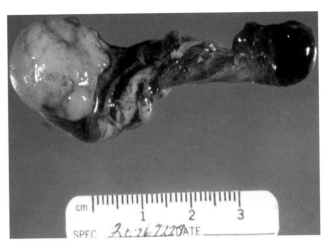

FIGURE 10-25

Yolk sac tumor. Uniform, tan, 2.5-cm tumor with a moist cut surface replaces parenchyma of child's testis.

and clear cytoplasm. These glomeruloid structures occur within a cystic space that is lined by epithelial cells. Schiller-Duval bodies may be sectioned so that they appear in cross-, longitudinal, and oblique sections. The papillary pattern contains epithelial-lined papillary structures with fibrovascular cores. These structures lack the definitive morphology of Schiller-Duval bodies of the endodermal sinus pattern.

In the alveolar-glandular pattern, there are structures of glands and papillary formations. Cells lining the spaces may be hobnail, cuboidal, polygonal, or flattened. Some glands resemble intestinal-type glands, and others have a more endometrioid appearance, with vacuolated cytoplasm. The solid pattern contains sheets of polygonal epithelial cells with clear to eosinophilic cytoplasm and mostly uniform nuclei. Blood vessels are present within the solid sheets. Pleomorphic nuclei may be present within solid areas. In the polyvesicular-vitelline pattern, pear-shaped epithelial-lined structures, often with constrictions, resemble the cartoon character, the Schmoo. These structures are lined by columnar to flattened, sometimes vacuolated, epithelium. The hepatoid pattern is relatively rare and usually comprises small aggregates of cells with bright eosinophilic cytoplasm resembling liver cells. Bile canaliculi may be present. In the myxomatous pattern, there is prominent myxoid stroma supported by spindled and stellate cells. Focally, spindled epithelial cells may occur in a tumor that is otherwise a characteristic YST. The parietal pattern consists of bands of eosinophilic basement membrane-like material among epithelial cells. Hyaline droplet or globule formation may occur in epithelial cells, principally in hepatoid or microvesicular areas. These eosinophilic droplets vary in size and appear to be mostly intracellular on H&E stains. Hyaline droplets occur in some nontesticular tumors, but not in other types of GCT. IGCNU generally does not occur in pure YSTs in children, but it occurs adjacent to mixed GCTs in adults.

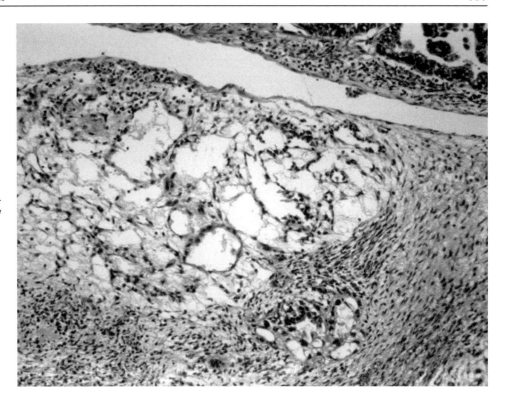

FIGURE 10-26

Yolk sac tumor. Microvesicular pattern with small cysts lined by flattened epithelium.

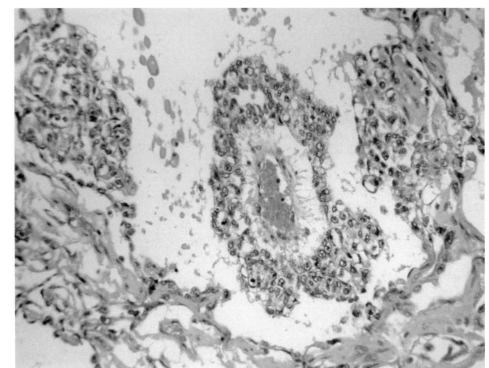

FIGURE 10-27

Yolk sac tumor. Schiller-Duval body characterized by a glomeruloid structure with a central blood vessel, edematous perivascular space, and peripheral epithelial lining, projecting into a cystic space.

ANCILLARY STUDIES

IMMUNOHISTOCHEMICAL FEATURES

AFP stains most tumors, but in a variable manner (Fig. 10-31). Often, only a few cells stain in a focus of YST. Generally, hyaline droplets do not stain for AFP, but they may stain for α-1-antitrypsin. Half of YSTs stain for α-1-antitrypsin, and 39% to 85% stain for PLAP. Almost all YSTs are positive for low-molecular-weight cytokeratin. CD30 does not stain YSTs, and EMA is usually negative.

YOLK SAC TUMOR—PATHOLOGIC FEATURES

Gross Findings

▶ Solid, tan to yellow to gray-white tumors, often with a mucoid, moist cut surface

Microscopic Findings

▶ Multiple patterns as follows:
▶ Reticular (microcystic)—most frequent pattern
▶ Macrocystic—due to coalesced microcysts
▶ Endodermal sinus—most characteristic pattern; contains Schiller-Duval bodies
▶ Papillary—lacks classic appearance of Schiller-Duval bodies
▶ Solid—some resemblance to seminoma
▶ Glandular-alveolar—may resemble intestinal or endometrial glands
▶ Myxomatous—large amounts of myxoid stroma with spindled epithelial cells and prominent blood vessels; spindle cells may undergo mesenchymal differentiation
▶ Sarcomatoid—rare; retains keratin positivity
▶ Polyvesicular vitelline—contains pear-shaped "Schmoo" bodies, said to resemble subdivision of primary into secondary yolk sac
▶ Hepatoid—stains intensely for AFP
▶ Parietal—pink bands of basement membrane material among epithelial cells

▶ Hyaline droplet formation—probably intracellular (seen also in nontesticular tumors, but not in other testicular germ cell tumors), PAS-positive, diastase resistant
▶ Most tumors have combinations of patterns
▶ Pure YST is rarely associated with IGCNU

Immunohistochemical Features

▶ Almost all YSTs stain positively for AFP
▶ AFP staining may be focal
▶ Staining of hepatoid foci most intense for AFP
▶ Hyaline droplets usually negative for AFP
▶ Hyaline droplets stain positively for α-1-antitrypsin in 50% of YSTs
▶ Cytokeratin stains cells in almost all cases
▶ EMA stain is usually negative
▶ CD30 stain is negative

Differential Diagnosis

▶ Seminoma
▶ Embryonal carcinoma
▶ Juvenile granulosa cell tumor

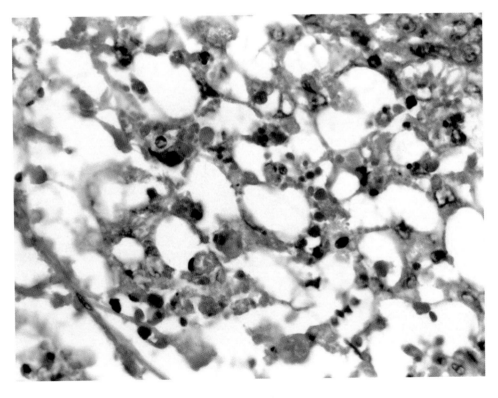

FIGURE 10-28
Yolk sac tumor, showing numerous hyaline droplets of varying size.

DIFFERENTIAL DIAGNOSIS

Although there is a resemblance between the solid patterns of YST and seminoma, and between the glandular-alveolar and papillary patterns of YST and EC, EC and seminoma do not occur in the pediatric age group in which pure YST occurs. Juvenile granulosa cell tumor may pose a significant differential diagnostic problem. This tumor typically occurs during the first 6 months of life and has both solid and cystic patterns. To confound the diagnostic problem, serum AFP levels are usually markedly elevated relative to adult concentrations. This is not an abnormal finding, because levels

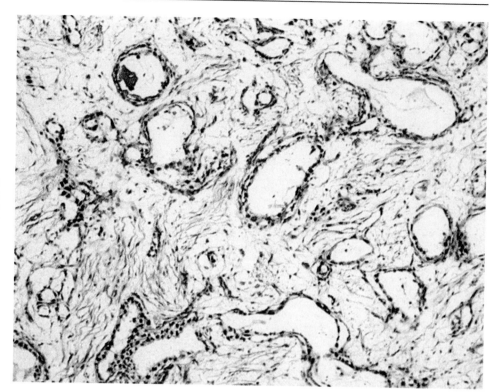

FIGURE 10-29

Yolk sac tumor. Numerous cyst-like structures with flattened epithelium and constrictions within loose mesenchyme characterize the polyvesicular vitelline pattern.

of AFP in normal neonates and infants are markedly elevated relative to the levels in adults. Although solid areas and microcysts in juvenile granulosa cell tumor can be confused with YST, other patterns similar to YST are not present, and the follicular cysts of juvenile granulosa cell tumor have no counterpart in YST. YST

tumors should stain for AFP, and juvenile granulosa cell tumors do not. On the other hand, juvenile granulosa cell tumors should be positive for inhibin, whereas YST should be negative.

In adults, the distinction between solid pattern YST and seminoma can be difficult. At least some of the

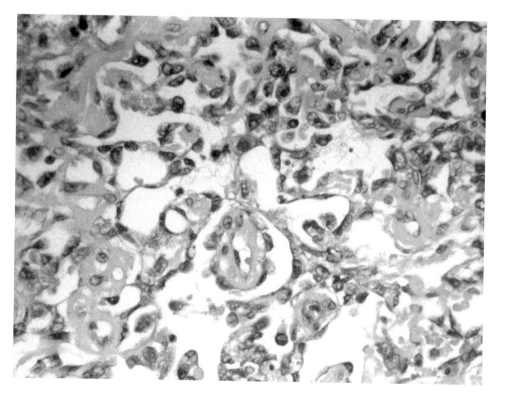

FIGURE 10-30

Yolk sac tumor. Microcystic pattern with intercystic eosinophilic material that characterizes the parietal pattern.

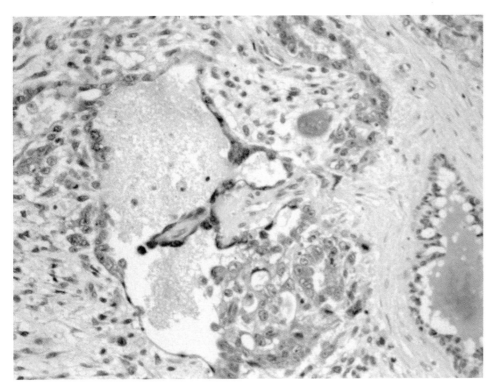

FIGURE 10-31

Yolk sac tumor. Microcystic structures with cytoplasmic positivity for α-fetoprotein (AFP).

seminomas with elevated serum AFP may represent YST. Solid YSTs lack the granulomatous and lymphoid component of seminoma, as well as the fibrous trabeculae that divide seminoma cells into groups. Scattered pleomorphic nuclei in solid areas are characteristic of solid YST, not seminoma. AFP should stain YST, but not seminoma.

At times, the distinction between glandular-alveolar or papillary patterns of YST and EC can be problematic, particularly because both tumor types may be present in mixed GCTs. The distinction tends to be important only in determining the percentage of EC within a tumor. CD30 stains EC cells but not YST cells. AFP stains YST cells but usually not EC cells.

TERATOMA

CLINICAL FEATURES

Teratomas usually manifest as masses in descended or undescended testes and in extratesticular tissues where GCTs occur. They occur as pure tumors in infants and young children, in whom they are universally benign, and in adults, in whom they carry an approximately 25% risk of metastasis. For this reason, teratomas in adults should not be designated as benign. Teratomatous foci occur in about 50% of mixed GCTs in adults.

Mixed GCTs containing teratoma have a more favorable prognosis than mixed GCTs without teratoma. Three varieties of neoplasm are considered monodermal teratomas: dermoid cyst (D cyst), primitive neuroectodermal tumor (PNET), and carcinoid. Epidermoid cyst (E cyst) is not considered by all to be a monodermal teratoma, but because it has most of the features of the D cyst, it is discussed with teratomas here.

An E cyst is a cyst that is lined exclusively by squamous epithelium and contains keratinous debris. It accounts for 1% to 2% of testis tumors. E cyst usually occurs in adults, but a few have occurred in prepubertal boys. The tumor generally manifests as a painless intratesticular nodule. Ultrasound demonstrates its cystic nature. It has not been shown to have malignant potential.

The D cyst is a cyst lined by squamous epithelium with skin appendages within the cyst wall. Most D cysts are intratesticular, but they have been reported in paratesticular tissue. All D cysts have behaved in a benign fashion. They are rarer than E cysts. Ultrasound examination should demonstrate their cystic nature. As with E cysts, orchiectomy or partial orchiectomy, with complete excision of the tumor, should be curative. In both E cyst and D cyst, if partial orchiectomy is undertaken, it is important that the pathologist does not find other teratomatous tissues or IGCNU and that the E cyst or D cyst is not present at the tissue margin.

PNET is a teratoma composed of malignant small cells, usually with neural differentiation. Pure PNET tumors of the testis have been reported, but most are part of mixed GCTs. Tumors occur in young adults, are

TERATOMA—FACT SHEET

Definition

▶ Germ cell neoplasm derived from combinations of ectoderm, mesoderm, and endoderm forming embryonic or mature tissues

Incidence and Location

▶ Pure teratoma represents 2.7% to 7% of GCTs
▶ Teratoma is present in about 50% of mixed GCTs
▶ Teratomas occur in descended and undescended testes, in extratesticular locations where GCTs occur, and in the ovary in females

Morbidity and Mortality

▶ Teratomas occurring prepubertally are benign
▸ Incidence of teratoma in children is 20% to 36% of testicular tumors
▶ In adults, in pure teratomas, there is an approximately 25% risk of metastasis after radical orchiectomy
▶ In mixed GCTs, the presence of teratoma may confer a somewhat better prognosis

Clinical Features

▶ Tumor usually manifests as a painless testicular mass

Radiologic Features

▶ Ultrasonography demonstrates a mass and whether it has a cystic component
▶ Radiologic studies identify retroperitoneal lymph node enlargement

Prognosis and Treatment

▶ Teratomas in children need no therapy beyond orchiectomy
▶ Pure teratoma and teratoma as part of a mixed GCT in adults are treated as nonseminomatous GCTs
▶ Teratoma occurring in RPLND is considered a favorable finding
▶ Teratomas may be bulky and may grow but are not treated by chemotherapy
▶ Teratoma with associated somatic malignancy in the primary testicular tumor does not confer an unfavorable prognosis
▶ Teratoma with associated somatic malignancy in a metastasis has an unfavorable prognosis
▶ Metastases from teratoma occur in retroperitoneal lymph nodes and parenchymal organs

PATHOLOGIC FEATURES

GROSS FINDINGS

Teratomas are solid and/or cystic and of varying size (Fig. 10-32). The gross appearance reflects the histologic composition. Tissues that may readily be recognized include bone and cartilage, as well as keratin debris and pigmented areas.

MICROSCOPIC FINDINGS

All manner of tissues are present in teratomas and may be mature or immature (Figs. 10-33 through 10-35). Prepubertal teratomas are usually pure. Postpubertally, teratomas may be part of a mixed GCT. Cystic structures are often present and may be lined by gastrointestinal or respiratory epithelium. Some cysts may be cuffed by smooth muscle. Immature tissues are those that resemble embryonic tissues. A mature teratoma can be described and reported, but this does not confer any information regarding malignancy. In some teratomas, there are foci of non-germ cell malignancy (Figs. 10-36 and 10-37). These are presently designated as teratoma with somatic-type malignancies and were formerly designated as teratoma with malignant transformation. These foci are defined as being of non-germ cell type, histologically malignant, invasive, and at least as large as one-half of a 4× microscopic field. If these foci are present in a primary tumor, they do not confer a poorer prognosis than teratoma itself. If teratoma with associated somatic malignancy occurs in a metastatic site, there is a worsened prognosis. Most somatic malignancies are sarcomas, although carcinomas can occur. Teratoma with associated somatic malignancy usually occurs in foci of teratoma within a nonseminomatous GCT.

In E cyst, the lining is entirely squamous, although much of the lining may be desquamated. Keratin adjacent to a partially ruptured cyst may elicit a granulomatous reaction (Figs. 10-38 and 10-39). The gross appearance and the lining of a D cyst are identical to

malignant, and are treated as nonseminomatous GCTs. The differential diagnosis consists of the gamut of small cell malignant tumors.

Primary carcinoid tumors are either pure or associated with teratomas. Sixty-two testicular carcinoids had been reported by 1992. Presenting symptoms are mass, possibly with pain and tenderness. The majority of tumors are unilateral, are unassociated with carcinoid syndrome, and behave in a benign fashion. The differential diagnosis includes sertoli cell tumor (SCT), metastatic prostatic adenocarcinoma, and metastatic carcinoid tumor.

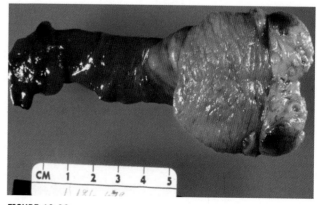

FIGURE 10-32
Bivalved testis with a 3-cm, partly cystic, partly solid teratoma, right.

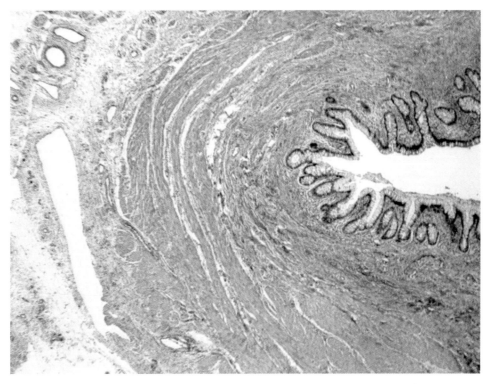

FIGURE 10-33

Mature teratoma. Cystic structures with mature gastrointestinal epithelium and surrounding muscularis propria.

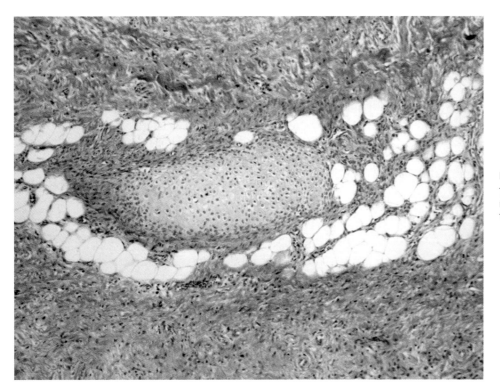

FIGURE 10-34

Teratoma. Immature cartilage and mature adipose and collagenous tissue.

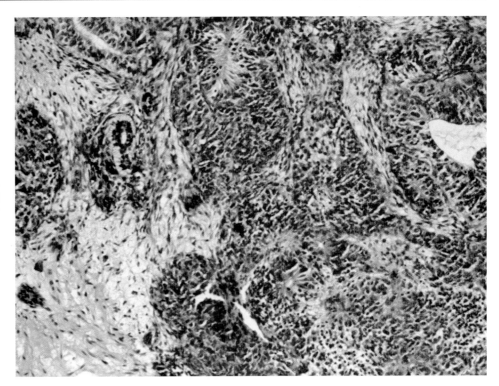

FIGURE 10-35

Immature teratoma. Scattered immature glands and neuroepithelial structures surrounded by primitive-appearing small cells.

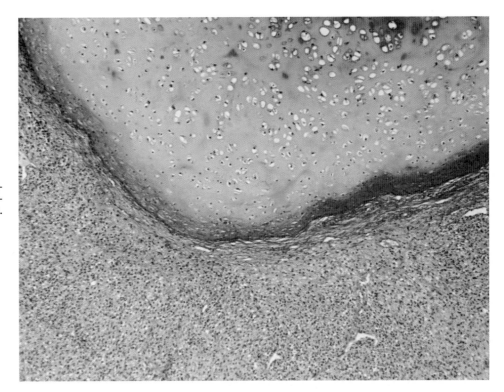

FIGURE 10-36

Teratoma with somatic-type malignancy. Cartilaginous tissue surrounded by malignant small cells. (Low-power magnification.)

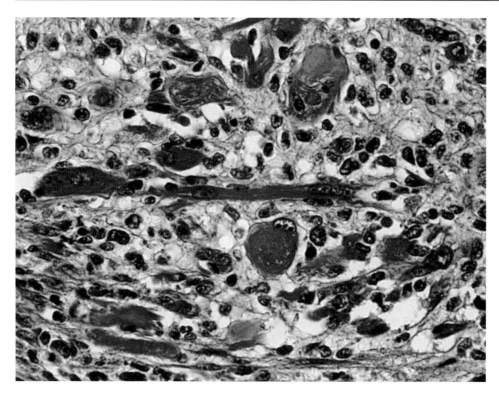

FIGURE 10-37

Teratoma with somatic-type malignancy. Rhabdomyoblasts in a large invasive focus. Same case as in Figure 10-36. (High-power magnification.)

those of an E cyst (Fig. 10-40). In addition, there are skin appendages, and cartilage, fibrous tissue, and glial cells may be present within the cyst wall. IGCNU is not associated with either tumor.

PNET tumors are histologically similar to PNET tumors elsewhere and consist of aggregated, poorly differentiated small cells, usually with differentiation into primitive neural-type tubules, neuroblastic-type tissue, or ependymal rosettes. Tumor cells stain positively for CD99, HBA-71, and vimentin.

Carcinoid tumors may or may not be associated with other teratomatous structures. Aggregates of carcinoid tumor may grow in insular or acinar patterns within a fibrous stroma. (Fig. 10-41A). The individual cells have round, uniform nuclei with dispersed chromatin and abundant eosinophilic cytoplasm. Granularity of the cytoplasm is particularly evident peripherally. Carcinoid tumors stain positively with argentaffin and argyrophil stains, giving a punctate black cytoplasmic positivity (Fig. 10-41C).

ANCILLARY STUDIES

IMMUNOHISTOCHEMISTRY

There are no specific markers for teratoma per se, but individual antibodies can be used to identify particular tissues. Intestinal-type glands and cysts may be positive for AFP. In cases of D cyst and E cyst, CD117 and PLAP can be used to identify or exclude IGCNU if there are atypical cells in seminiferous tubules at the periphery of the cysts. CD99 and vimentin can be used to aid in the diagnosis of PNET. Carcinoid tumors should stain with neuroendocrine markers, particularly chromogranin and synaptophysin (Fig. 10-41D).

MOLECULAR STUDIES

Confirmation of the diagnosis of a PNET tumor should be made with studies demonstrating a t(11,22)(q24; q12) translocation.

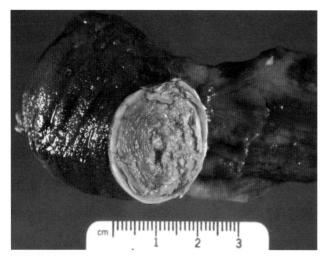

FIGURE 10-38

Epidermoid cyst. Discrete, 3-cm, intratesticular cyst filled with keratinous material.

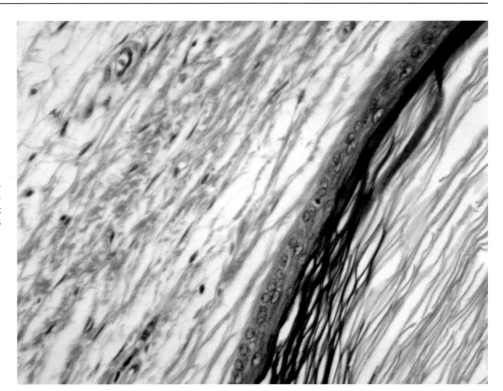

FIGURE 10-39

Epidermoid cyst. Cyst wall is composed of mature squamous epithelium. Laminated keratin is present within the lumen. Mature collagen is present adjacent to cyst.

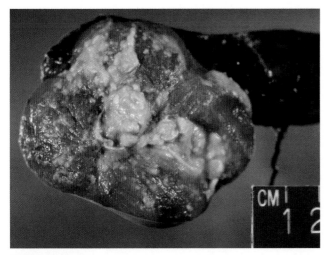

FIGURE 10-40

Dermoid cyst. Bivalved testis contains cyst filled with sebaceous-like material.

DIFFERENTIAL DIAGNOSIS

Problems that arise in the diagnosis of teratoma include the distinction between immature teratoma and teratoma with associated somatic malignancy. Before diagnosing the latter, the criteria of associated somatic malignancy should be adhered to. If carcinoma or sarcoma is identified in the testis, the pathologist must be sure that the sarcoma or carcinoma is in the appro-priate milieu (i.e., in the background of a teratoma). The two cystic tumors, E cyst and D cyst, are benign. Teratoma in a postpubertal man carries a risk of metastasis, and some areas within the teratoma may be identical to E cyst or D cyst. E cyst and D cyst are both cystic grossly and do not have a solid component. E cyst has no other components, and in D cyst, any non-skin appendage tissues, such as cartilage or intestinal tissue, should be in the fibrous wall. Neither cystic entity can have IGCNU. PNET tumors must be distinguished from other small cell malignant tumors, because therapy is specific for each of them. The small cell tumors include malignant lymphoma, embryonal rhabdomyosarcoma, neuroblastoma, nephroblastoma, neuroendocrine carcinoma, and desmoplastic small round cell tumor. Cases of PNET in other organs have had a t(11; 22) (q24; q12) translocation. Of the other small cell neoplasms in the differential diagnosis, only lymphoblastic lymphoma should also stain for CD99. Lymphoblastic lymphoma should also stain for CD45RB. Other immunohistochemical stains can be used to identify the other small cell tumors.

Desmoplastic small round cell tumors are generally paratesticular as well as in pelvic and peritoneal cavities. They stain positively with desmin in a paranuclear dot pattern, and they stain positively for EMA and vimentin. Ninety-one percent of tumors express *EWS-WT1* gene fusion transcript.

Carcinoid tumors usually are not difficult to diagnose. However, it may be difficult to determine whether the carcinoid is primary or metastatic. Factors that favor a metastatic origin are bilateral involvement of testes, involvement of paratesticular structures, and the

TERATOMA—PATHOLOGIC FEATURES

Gross Findings

▶ Tumors are combinations of solid and cystic masses
▶ Gross morphology reflects tumor composition and varies with the mesenchymal, epithelial, and pigmented components
▶ Tumors are variable in size

Microscopic Findings

▶ Teratomas may be derived from one or more than one germ cell layer
▶ May comprise mature and/or immature tissues
▶ Teratomatous tissues may be associated with a focus or foci of somatic malignancy
▶ May invade blood vessels
▶ Mixed GCTs contain teratoma in approximately 50% of cases
▶ Carcinoid tumor, primitive neuroectodermal tumor, dermoid cysts, and epidermoid cysts are considered monodermal teratomas and are discussed separately in the text

▶ Teratoma is considered as having associated somatic malignancy if the focus is not a focus of GCT, is histologically malignant, is invasive, and involves at least half of a 4× microscopic field

Immunohistochemical Features

▶ There is no specific marker for teratoma
▶ Markers of mesenchymal and epithelial tissues are positive in those tissues
▶ AFP may be present in enteric glands or cysts

Differential Diagnosis

▶ Immature teratoma versus a secondary malignant component
▶ Metastatic carcinoma or sarcoma
▶ Epidermoid and dermoid cysts versus teratoma
▶ Primitive neuroectodermal tumor versus other small cell tumors
▶ Primary versus secondary carcinoid tumor
▶ Carcinoid tumor versus Sertoli cell tumor or metastatic prostatic adenocarcinoma

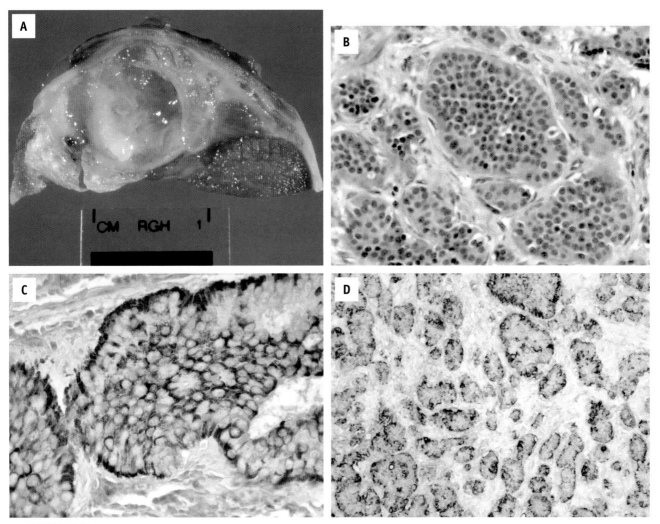

FIGURE 10-41

Teratoma with carcinoid. **A,** Cystic and solid, 2-cm intratesticular mass. **B,** Insular nests of epithelial cells with uniform nuclei containing nucleoli and eosinophilic cytoplasm. **C,** Marked cytoplasmic positivity with Grimelius stain. **D,** Marked cytoplasmic positivity with immunoperoxidase stain for chromogranin.

presence of carcinoid syndrome symptomatology. Carcinoid tumor, in rare instances, must be distinguished from SCT. Additional sections may be useful in demonstrating the stromal component of a SCT. The presence of a teratomatous component would indicate that the tumor is a carcinoid. Inhibin positivity of tumor cells is consistent with a SCT. Chromogranin positivity has been reported in both Sertoli cell and carcinoid tumors and would not definitively distinguish between them.

In an older patient, the possibility of a metastatic prostatic adenocarcinoma might be in the differential diagnosis of a carcinoid. This would be a likely consideration only in a patient with known prostatic adenocarcinoma. A carcinoid tumor should be chromogranin positive, and a prostatic adenocarcinoma should be prostate specific antigen (PSA) positive. Both could be positive for prostate-specific acid phosphatase (PSAP). Prostatic tissue has also been described in a mixed GCT of the sacrum comprised predominantly of prostatic tissue; therefore, the possibility of prostatic carcinoma within a teratoma is a remote consideration. This would be a diagnostic consideration only in the absence of clinical prostatic carcinoma.

PROGNOSIS AND TREATMENT

The therapy for teratoma in children is radical orchiectomy alone. However, in adults, there is a 25% risk of metastasis after orchiectomy, and pure teratoma and teratoma within a mixed GCT are treated as nonseminomatous GCTs.

CHORIOCARCINOMA

CLINICAL FEATURES

Because of the differences in prognosis of tumors with trophoblastic elements, diagnosis must be precise. Pure choriocarcinomas occur in 0.1% to 0.3 % of patients with testis tumors. Choriocarcinoma occurs in about 15% of mixed GCTs and can occur in the male in extratesticular sites where GCTs occur. Pure choriocarcinoma has a high mortality rate. High serum hCG levels also correlate with a worsened prognosis. Choriocarcinomas and mixed GCTs are treated as nonseminomatous GCTs. Pure choriocarcinomas occur in postpubertal men from the second into the sixth decade. Testicular choriocarcinoma usually manifests with metastatic disease and/or symptoms of hCG production such as gynecomastia or hyperthyroidism. Pulmonary symptomatology may be associated with massive neoplastic infiltration of the lungs and hemoptysis. Other symptomatology depends on the sites of metastasis. Even with extensive metastasis with marked serum hCG elevation, the testicular mass may be impalpable or palpated with difficulty.

RADIOLOGIC FEATURES

On chest radiography, a patient with choriocarcinoma may have multiple metastases or a virtual whiteout. Ultrasound demonstrates hypoechoic, isoechoic, or hyperechoic foci in the testis.

CHORIOCARCINOMA—FACT SHEET

Definition
- ▶ Malignant trophoblastic tumor, usually an admixture of syncytiotrophoblastic and cytotrophoblastic cells in juxtaposition

Incidence and Location
- ▶ Pure choriocarcinoma is rare, occurring in 0.1% to 0.3% of testicular tumors
- ▶ Approximately 15% of mixed GCTs contain choriocarcinoma
- ▶ Occurs in descended and undescended testes and in extratesticular locations where GCTs occur

Morbidity and Mortality
- ▶ May be associated with choriocarcinoma syndrome, in which hemorrhagic metastases are associated with a poor prognosis
- ▶ Some patients with metastatic pure choriocarcinoma have survived

Gender, Race, and Age Distribution
- ▶ Occurs in postpubertal men through the sixth decade

Clinical Features
- ▶ Pure choriocarcinoma usually manifests with metastases
- ▶ May initially manifest with hemoptysis, "white-out" on chest radiographs, hyperthyroidism, or gynecomastia
- ▶ Testicular mass may not be palpable

Radiologic Features
- ▶ Pulmonary "white-out"
- ▶ Ultrasonography may demonstrate mass and hemorrhage
- ▶ Masses may be hypoechoic, isoechoic, or hyperechoic

Prognosis and Treatment
- ▶ Choriocarcinoma has the worst prognosis of any GCT
- ▶ Prognosis is worsened with increased amounts of choriocarcinoma in mixed GCTs
- ▶ Prognosis is worsened with elevated serum concentrations of hCG
- ▶ Pure choriocarcinoma and choriocarcinoma as part of a mixed GCT are treated with chemotherapy

PATHOLOGIC FEATURES

GROSS FINDINGS

The tumors are often quite small and hemorrhagic. Hemorrhage can be massive. Sometimes there is a tan to gray rim of tumor. At other times, definite tumor is not grossly identifiable. Occasionally, even in the face of massive metastasis, there is only a scar with hemosiderin deposition in the testis. Metastases are usually hemorrhagic and can occur in virtually any parenchymal organ or lymph node.

MICROSCOPIC FINDINGS

Choriocarcinoma is a tumor that demonstrates trophoblastic differentiation. Almost always this consists of syncytiotrophoblastic and cytotrophoblastic cells in juxtaposition (Figs. 10-42 and 10-43). Syncytiotrophoblasts usually cap sheets of cytotrophoblasts. Syncytiotrophoblasts may have round, nucleolated nuclei, or they may be elongated spindled cells with smudgy nuclei. Some syncytiotrophoblastic cells contain red blood cells within vacuoles. Cytotrophoblasts typically grow in sheets or aggregates and are composed of cells with single, irregularly shaped nuclei and one or two nucleoli. The cytoplasm is usually clear to pale. Cytotrophoblasts may resemble a solid form of YST. Intermediate trophoblasts are larger than cytotrophoblasts with irregular and smudged nuclei and eosinophilic cytoplasm. They grow in an infiltrating pattern.

ANCILLARY STUDIES

IMMUNOHISTOCHEMISTRY

Syncytiotrophoblasts are positive for hCG, EMA, the α subunit of inhibin, human placental lactogen (HPL), and pregnancy-specific β-1-glycoprotein (SP1) (Fig. 10-44). Cytotrophoblasts are usually negative or weakly positive for hCG and negative for SP1 and HPL. Intermediate trophoblasts are positive for HPL and SP1. About 50% of trophoblasts are positive for cytokeratin and PLAP. Inhibin stains cells that are intermediate between mononuclear trophoblasts and syncytiotrophoblasts.

DIFFERENTIAL DIAGNOSIS

The differential diagnosis of choriocarcinoma is important because of therapeutic and prognostic implications. Seminoma with STGC has the same prognosis and therapy as seminoma. Rare cases of seminoma with choriocarcinoma do occur and must be treated as nonseminomatous GCTs. In mixed GCTs, it can be extremely difficult to distinguish EC with light and dark cells from choriocarcinoma. Although accurate distinction will allow evaluation of the relative amounts of EC and choriocarcinoma, the therapy will probably be similar. Increased amounts of choriocarcinoma and EC both

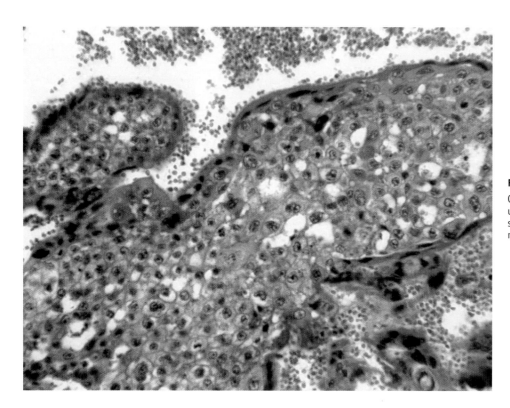

FIGURE 10-42

Choriocarcinoma, showing abundant uniform cytotrophoblasts capped by syncytiotrophoblasts with hyperchromatic nuclei.

CHORIOCARCINOMA—PATHOLOGIC FEATURES

Gross Findings

- ▶ Tumors are often quite small and hemorrhagic
- ▶ Hemorrhage may be considerable
- ▶ May have a rim of gray-tan tumor
- ▶ Occasionally a scar with hemosiderin is the only gross finding
- ▶ Metastases may be present in many parenchymal organs, including brain, lungs, gastrointestinal tract, spleen, adrenal glands, and retroperitoneal lymph nodes

Microscopic Findings

- ▶ Must have juxtaposition of syncytiotrophoblastic and cytotrophoblastic cells
- ▶ Syncytiotrophoblasts often cap cytotrophoblasts
- ▶ Often associated with hemorrhage and necrosis
- ▶ Syncytiotrophoblasts may have round nucleolated nuclei with eosinophilic cytoplasm or elongate spindled smudged nuclei
- ▶ Some syncytiotrophoblastic giant cells are vacuolated and contain red blood cells
- ▶ Cytotrophoblasts are generally uniform with clear to pale cytoplasm, a single irregularly shaped nucleus, and one or two nucleoli

- ▶ Intermediate trophoblasts are larger than cytotrophoblasts, with irregular hyperchromatic and smudged nuclei and eosinophilic cytoplasm

Immunohistochemical Features

- ▶ Syncytiotrophoblasts are positive for hCG, EMA, α subunit of inhibin, HPL, and SP1
- ▶ Inhibin also stains cells intermediate between mononuclear trophoblasts and syncytiotrophoblasts
- ▶ Intermediate-sized trophoblasts are positive for HPL and SP1
- ▶ All cell types are positive for cytokeratin and PLAP, with positivity in about half of the cases
- ▶ Cytotrophoblasts are weakly positive or negative for hCG
- ▶ Cytotrophoblasts are negative for SP1 and HPL

Differential Diagnosis

- ▶ Seminoma with STGC
- ▶ EC
- ▶ Placental site trophoblastic tumor
- ▶ Cystic trophoblastic tumor

worsen the prognosis. Rare cases of placental site trophoblastic tumor have been described. These are similar to uterine tumors of the same name and are comprised of infiltrating intermediate trophoblasts without accompanying cytotrophoblasts or syncytiotrophoblasts. Monophasic choriocarcinoma is composed mostly of mononucleated cytotrophoblasts, with rare syncytiotro-

phoblasts. These tumors are exceedingly rare, but they have not had an adverse prognosis. A favorable prognostic lesion called cystic trophoblastic tumor has occurred in retroperitoneal tumors after chemotherapy. These tumors have also been identified in microscopic foci in testes that have not been treated with chemotherapy. The cysts are lined by eosinophilic mono-

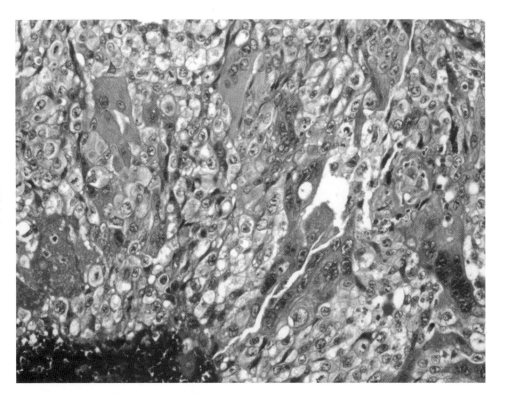

FIGURE 10-43

Choriocarcinoma. Intermixed uniform cytotrophoblast and multinucleated hyperchromatic syncytial trophoblasts with eosinophilic, focally vacuolated cytoplasm.

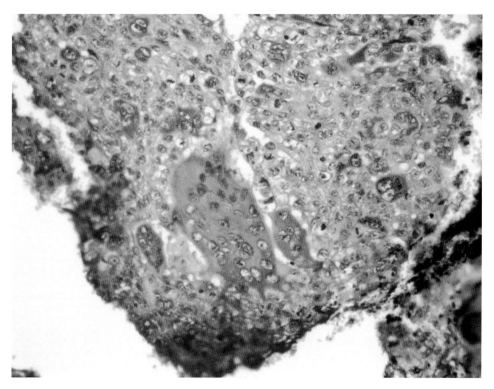

FIGURE 10-44
Choriocarcinoma. Syncytiotrophoblasts are markedly positive for
human chorionic gonadotropin.

nuclear trophoblastic cells with occasional cells that
stain positively for hCG.

PROGNOSIS AND TREATMENT

Choriocarcinoma and mixed GCTs are treated as nonseminomatous GCTs. The prognosis of choriocarcinoma as part of a mixed GCT is dependent on the tumor
stage, including the serum level of hCG. All pure
choriocarcinomas are stage III and are treated as
nonseminomatous GCTs with high levels of hCG.

MIXED GERM CELL TUMORS

CLINICAL FEATURES

Mixed germ cell tumors occur in descended or undescended testes and may occur in extratesticular sites
where GCTs occur. Approximately 40% to 60% of
testicular tumors are mixed GCTs. The highest mortality occurs in patients with high-stage tumors, in those
with 45% or more EC, and in those with angiolymphatic invasion. Mixed GCTs occur from puberty
through the fifth decade, with an average age at onset of
30 years. They rarely occur in prepubertal males. Mixed
GCTs are more frequent in Caucasian Americans and

less frequent in African Americans. These neoplasms
usually are discovered as testicular enlargement with or
without pain, but they may be discovered as the result
of signs or symptoms produced by metastases.

RADIOLOGIC FEATURES

Mixed GCTs are identifiable on scrotal ultrasound
examination, and radiologic studies identify enlarged
retroperitoneal lymph nodes.

PATHOLOGIC FEATURES

GROSS FINDINGS

Most patients have testicular enlargement, but tumors
may be 1 cm or less in diameter. The tumor may
or may not be confined to the testis. On cut section,
the appearance reflects the tumor composition. There
is usually a variegated appearance unless some GCT
components are extremely small. There may be gross
cystic, solid, soft, firm, hemorrhagic, and necrotic areas
(Fig. 10-45).

MICROSCOPIC FINDINGS

Any type of GCT may occur in variable combinations. Foci resembling early embryos with amniotic
sacs, germ disks, YST, and extraembryonic mesenchyme

MIXED GERM CELL TUMORS—FACT SHEET

Definition

▶ Mixed GCT comprises at least two types of germ cell tumors with or without IGCNU

Incidence and Location

▶ In testes and extratesticular sites in males
▶ Occurs in 32% to 60% of all testicular tumors

Morbidity and Mortality

▶ Mixed GCTs are considered nonseminomatous GCTs

Gender, Race, and Age Distribution

▶ More frequent in Caucasian Americans and less frequent in African Americans
▶ Occurs in postpubertal men, with average age at onset of 30 years

Clinical Features

▶ Usually develops as testicular enlargement with or without pain
▶ May be discovered as a result of metastasis

Radiologic Features

▶ Testicular ultrasound examination demonstrates tumor
▶ Radiologic studies demonstrate enlarged retroperitoneal lymph nodes

Prognosis and Treatment

▶ Primary treatment consists of radical orchiectomy
▶ Prognosis after orchiectomy depends on tumor stage, including the levels of serum tumor markers, vascular invasion, percentage of EC and choriocarcinoma, and the presence of teratoma and YST in the primary tumor
▶ Therapy after radical orchiectomy depends on the presence and percentage of EC, blood vessel invasion, and tumor stage including levels of serum tumor markers.
▶ In cases where the patient was treated with chemotherapy and had RPLND, prognosis and further therapy depend on the presence of viable tumor in the lymph node resection
▶ Viable tumor is considered to be seminoma, YST, EC, or choriocarcinoma, as well as teratoma with associated somatic malignancy

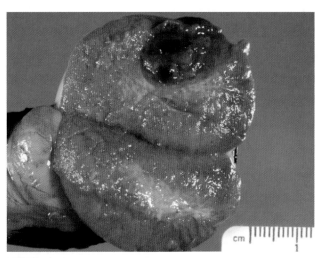

FIGURE 10-45

Mixed germ cell tumor: 2-cm subcapsular tumor containing embryonal carcinoma and yolk sac tumor.

ANCILLARY STUDIES

IMMUNOHISTOCHEMISTRY

All elements of a mixed GCT react to immunohistochemical antibodies in the same way as a pure tumor of a similar histologic type (Fig. 10-50). AFP stains are useful in identifying YST, and hCG is useful in identifying trophoblasts.

MIXED GERM CELL TUMOR—PATHOLOGIC FEATURES

Gross Findings

▶ Morphology reflects the histologic composition of the tumor and may include necrosis and hemorrhage
▶ Tumors often extend into extratesticular structures

Microscopic Findings

▶ Any type of GCT may occur in primary testicular tumor or metastasis
▶ Important to identify components and their relative amounts for reasons of prognosis and additional therapy
▶ Advanced stage of primary tumor and presence of EC, choriocarcinoma, and angiolymphatic invasion have adverse prognostic influence and may dictate further therapy
▶ Histologic findings in RPLND specimens determine further prognosis and therapy

Immunohistochemical Features

▶ Identical to findings in pure GCTs

Differential Diagnosis

▶ Distinguishing teratoma with associated somatic malignancy from immature teratoma
▶ Recognizing small foci of EC in a mixed GCT

have been termed embryoid bodies. Tumors with many embryoid bodies have been termed polyembryomas. Diffuse embryomas have formations of EC surrounded by YST. Both of these morphologies could also be considered as mixed GCTs. It is important that the tumor be evaluated carefully, because the presence of nonseminomatous components engenders different therapy than seminoma alone. In addition, identification of tumor types and their relative amounts may influence the clinician as to further therapy. The finding of EC and choriocarcinoma in large amounts worsens the prognosis, as does advanced tumor stage and angiolymphatic invasion (Fig. 10-46).

In specimens from RPLNDs, favorable findings are fibrosis, necrosis, and mature teratoma. Unfavorable findings are viable seminoma, EC, YST, choriocarcinoma, and mixed GCT (Figs. 10-47 through 10-49).

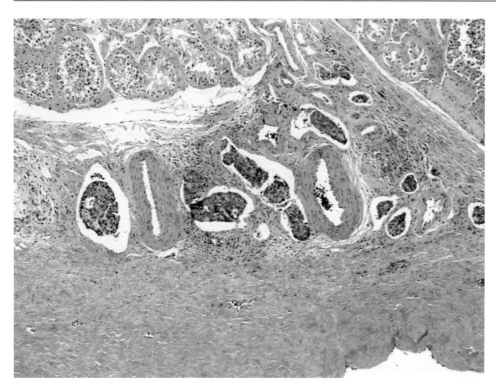

FIGURE 10-46

Mixed germ cell tumor. Embryonal carcinoma extensively invades lymphovascular spaces within tunica vasculosa (same case as in Figure 10-45).

DIFFERENTIAL DIAGNOSIS

Particularly in lymph node metastases, it is important to distinguish teratoma with associated somatic malignancy from immature teratoma for prognostic and therapeutic reasons.

PROGNOSIS AND TREATMENT

Mixed GCTs are treated as nonseminomatous GCTs, and their therapy depends on tumor stage, percentage of EC, and presence or absence of angiolymphatic invasion.

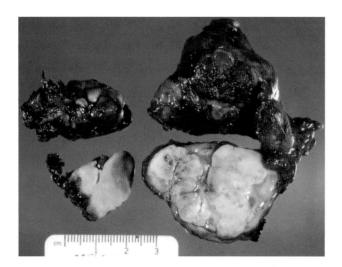

FIGURE 10-47

Tissue from retroperitoneal lymph node dissection (RPLND) demonstrates marked fat necrosis.

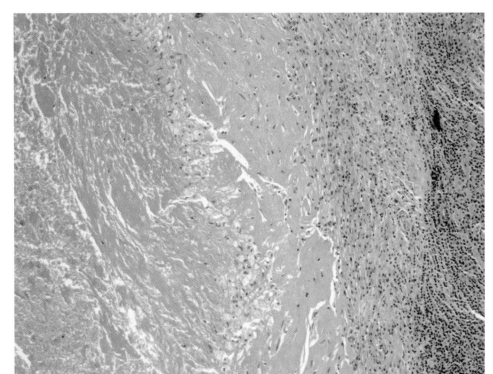

FIGURE 10-48

Retroperitoneal lymph node dissection (RPLND), showing extensive necrosis. No neoplasm was identified. This is a favorable finding.

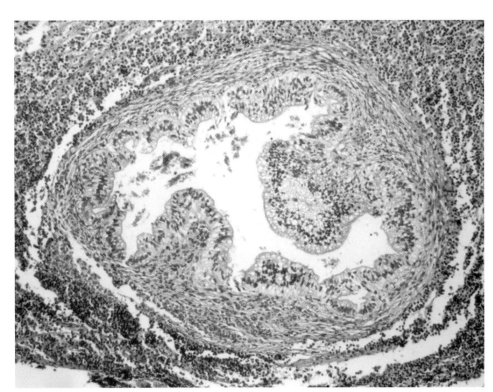

FIGURE 10-49

Retroperitoneal lymph node dissection. A metastatic, teratomatous glandular structure is present within a lymph node. This is a favorable finding.

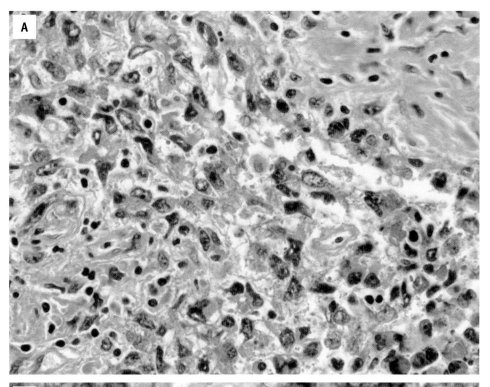

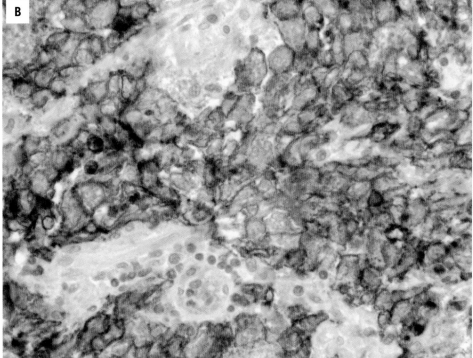

FIGURE 10-50
Retroperitoneal lymph node dissection (RPLND). **A,** A small focus of metastatic embryonal carcinoma was identified on frozen section. This image is from a permanent section made from the frozen section block. **B,** Immunoperoxidase stain is markedly positive for CD30. Embryonal carcinoma in an RPLND specimen is an unfavorable finding.

GONADOBLASTOMA

CLINICAL FEATURES

Gonadoblastoma is a nonmetastasizing tumor that almost always occurs in patients with mixed gonadal dysgenesis (MGD); but a gonadoblastoma may be associated with GCT that is capable of metastasizing. Most patients have MGD with combinations of müllerian and wolffian duct-derived organs. The patients are mostly phenotypic females, but they may be phenotypic males or have ambiguous genitalia. Patients with MGD usually have a 46,XY or mosaic karyotype containing a Y chromosome. Tumors are usually discovered in the evaluation of a young patient with

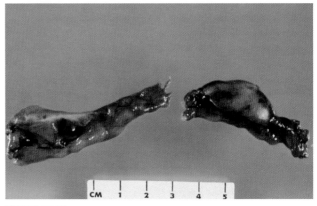

FIGURE 10-51
Bilateral gonads in a patient with mixed gonadal dysgenesis. Both gonads contained gonadoblastoma with seminoma on the right.

mass. Gonadoblastomas have been recorded up to 8 cm in diameter. They may be firm or soft, brown to yellow to gray, and may have focal flecks of calcium or extensive calcification. There may be an associated GCT that is smaller or larger than the gonadoblastoma (Figs. 10-51 and 10-52).

MICROSCOPIC FINDINGS

Gonadoblastoma is a tumor growing in organoid aggregates composed of germ cells and sex cord-stromal cells (Figs. 10-53 and 10-54). The germ cells within the nests have germ cell-type nuclei, some of which resemble IGCNU surrounded by cleared cytoplasm. Smaller cells with smaller nuclei, resembling Sertoli or granulosa cells, surround germ cells or calcified or uncalcified basement membrane-like material. Hyaline basement membrane extends from the periphery of the nests into

intersex features, a virilizing phenotypic female, or a female with a pelvic tumor.

RADIOLOGIC FEATURES

Studies may demonstrate calcifications in intra-abdominal masses.

PATHOLOGIC FEATURES

GROSS FINDINGS

Gonadoblastoma occurs in a testis or streak gonad and may be a microscopic finding or a macroscopic

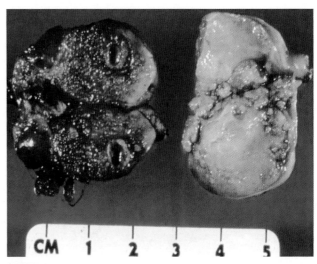

FIGURE 10-52
Bilateral, bivalved gonads in a patient with mixed gonadal dysgenesis. Both gonads contained gonadoblastoma and seminoma. Light reflections may identify flecks of calcium.

GONADOBLASTOMA—PATHOLOGIC FEATURES

Gross Findings

▶ Pure gonadoblastoma ranges from microscopic size to 8 cm in diameter
▶ Tumors may be soft or firm and brown to yellow to gray
▶ Amount of calcification is variable

Microscopic Findings

▶ Composed of aggregates of germ cells, cells of gonadal stroma-sex cord origin, basement membrane material, and, usually, calcification
▶ Gonadoblastoma has a nested appearance
▶ Germ cells resemble IGCNU
▶ Hyaline structures are extensions of basement membranes surrounding the nests and may be calcified
▶ Laminated calcifications may be microscopic or extensive

Immunohistochemical Features

▶ Many germ cells stain positive for PLAP and CD117
▶ Sex cord-stromal cells are positive for inhibin

Differential Diagnosis

▶ Foci of persistent immature tubules with IGCNU
▶ Unclassified sex cord-gonadal stromal tumor

---

cellular gonadoblastoma aggregates. Between the cellular aggregates, nests of cells with eosinophilic cytoplasm that resemble Leydig cells are present in about two thirds of patients. These cells may produce the hormones responsible for virilization, which often occurs in phenotypic females with gonadoblastoma at the time of puberty.

ANCILLARY STUDIES

IMMUNOHISTOCHEMISTRY

The malignant germ cells within gonadoblastoma aggregates are positive for PLAP and CD117. The stromal cells are positive for inhibin.

DIFFERENTIAL DIAGNOSIS

Occasionally, microscopic foci occur in testes that raise the differential diagnosis of gonadoblastoma or persistent immature tubules with or without IGCNU. In these, some germ cell nuclei are histologically malignant and the cells are positive for PLAP and CD117. These cases usually occur in phenotypically normal males with no stigmata of MGD. They may occur in cryptorchid males and probably represent IGCNU secondarily involving foci of persistent immature tubules (Pick's adenomas). There are also tumors with sex cord-stromal morphology and germ cells in varying arrangements. Questions have arisen as to the malignancy of the germ cell components in these tumors. Immunohistochemistry for CD117 and PLAP have been negative in these tumors, which reportedly have behaved in a benign manner.

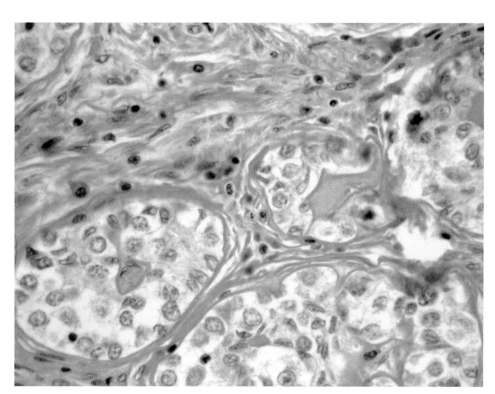

FIGURE 10-53

Nests of gonadoblastoma are composed of germ cells that have more chromatin and sex cord-stromal cells that are smaller and have more elongate nuclei. Hyaline basement membrane material extends into the nests from the periphery.

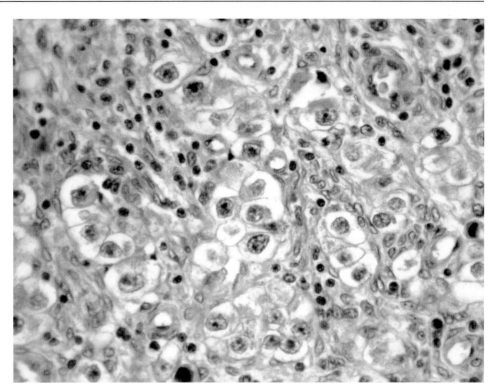

FIGURE 10-54
Gonadoblastoma and seminoma. Seminoma cells are intermixed with lymphocytes. This is from the same case as in Figure 10-53.

PROGNOSIS AND TREATMENT

Prognosis of gonadoblastoma depends on the type and stage of an accompanying GCT. Because of the frequency of gonadoblastoma bilaterally, with or without GCTs, both gonads should be resected when the diagnosis of MGD is made. Approximately 25% of patients with MGD and a Y chromosome will develop gonadoblastoma associated with GCT by age 30 years. The uterus should be resected at the time of bilateral gonadectomy because of the risk of developing an endometrial adenocarcinoma stimulated by exogenous hormone administration.

Sex Cord-Stromal Tumors

LEYDIG CELL TUMOR

CLINICAL FEATURES

LTCs are the most common sex cord-stromal tumor of the testis and account for 1% to 3% of all testicular tumors. They occur in descended and undescended testes but do not occur in extratesticular locations where GCTs may occur. LCTs occur from childhood to old age and are most common between 10 and 50 years of age. Approximately 10% to 15% of LCTs are malignant, and most patients with malignant LCTs die with metastases within 5 years after diagnosis.

The clinical presentation differs in prepubertal and postpubertal males. In the former group, symptoms and signs of isosexual precocity often precede the discovery of a painless mass. The patient may demonstrate hair loss, deep voice, maturation of external genitalia, bone growth, and aggressive behavior. Postpubertal patients are usually discovered with a testicular mass, although a functioning tumor may be associated with impotence and gynecomastia before the discovery of a palpable tumor. In adults, there may be elevation of serum androgens, estrogens, and progestins and decreased levels of serum gonadotropins. Increased libido and muscle mass are not signs of a functioning Leydig cell tumor in an adult.

LCTs have been reported in patients with Klinefelter syndrome, tuberous sclerosis, and Reifenstein syndrome (incomplete androgen insensitivity syndrome).

RADIOLOGIC FEATURES

Ultrasonography usually identifies a mass, the features of which are not diagnostic of LCT. Ultrasound is particularly valuable for the discovery of functioning impalpable tumors in children and adults.

LEYDIG CELL TUMOR—FACT SHEET

Definition

▶ Tumor composed of Leydig cells with varying degrees of differentiation

Incidence and Location

▶ Comprises 1% to 3% of testicular tumors
▶ Occurs in descended and rarely in undescended testes

Morbidity and Mortality

▶ Approximately 10% of LCTs are malignant
▶ Most patients with a clinically malignant LCT die within 5 years

Gender, Race, and Age Distribution

▶ May affect patients in all decades
▶ Equal incidence in Caucasian Americans and African Americans
▶ Analogous tumors are present in the ovary of females

Clinical Features

▶ In prepubertal males, LCTs cause isosexual precocity, with clinical signs and symptoms usually preceding the discovery of a mass
▶ In postpubertal males, LCTs usually manifest with painless enlargement
▶ 30% of postpubertal males with LCT have signs of increased hormonal function, with unilateral, bilateral, or fluctuating gynecomastia; impotence; decreased libido; and hair loss
▶ LCTs have been reported in association with Klinefelter syndrome, tuberous sclerosis, and Reifenstein syndrome
▶ May be associated with increased levels of serum androgens, estrogens, and progesterone, and decreased levels of gonadotropins

Radiologic Features

▶ Usually are identified on ultrasound examination

Prognosis and Treatment

▶ Prepubertal tumors are benign
▶ Malignant tumors in adults may metastasize to retroperitoneal lymph nodes, liver, lungs, and bone
▶ Initial treatment of LCT consists of radical orchiectomy
▶ In prepubertal patients and patients with a compromised or absent contralateral testis, local excision of the tumor may be considered
▶ In malignant tumors, RPLND may be considered
▶ There is no proven therapy for metastatic LCT involving parenchymal organs

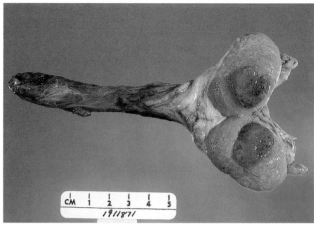

FIGURE 10-55

Leydig cell tumor in a 29-year-old with gynecomastia. Bivalved testis contains an intratesticular, unencapsulated, tan, 1.8-cm tumor.

tumors tend to be large, firm, and variegated with hemorrhage and necrosis.

MICROSCOPIC FINDINGS

Tumor cells have a variable appearance. The classic LCT comprises sheets or aggregates of polygonal cells with round nuclei, a single nucleolus, and eosinophilic cytoplasm within scant, fibrous, or edematous stroma (Figs. 10-57 and 10-58). Rarely, spindled epithelial cells may be present. Occasional cells contain two or more nuclei, and there may be some nuclear atypia. Mitoses are usually rare. Leydig cell cytoplasm may be granular, ground-glass, or vacuolated. Cells with very large vacuoles have the appearance of adipose metaplasia

PATHOLOGIC FEATURES

GROSS FINDINGS

LCTs may be less than 1 cm to more than 10 cm in diameter. Most are 3 to 5 cm in diameter (Figs. 10-55 and 10-56). They are discrete but unencapsulated and are usually yellow, tan, or mahogany, depending on their lipid and lipochrome content. LCTs are rarely bilateral. Tumors may extend into paratesticular tissues. Necrosis and hemorrhage may occur. Malignant

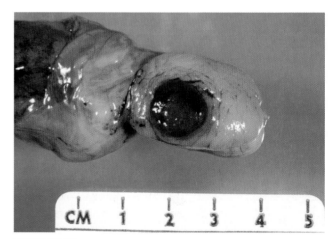

FIGURE 10-56

Leydig cell tumor in a prepubertal boy. This is a 1.1-cm, dark brown, intratesticular tumor.

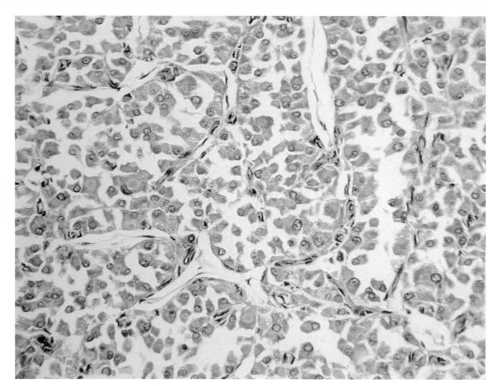

FIGURE 10-57

Leydig cell tumor. Alveolar arrangement of similar-appearing Leydig cells with round to oval nuclei, small nucleoli, no mitoses, and eosinophilic cytoplasm.

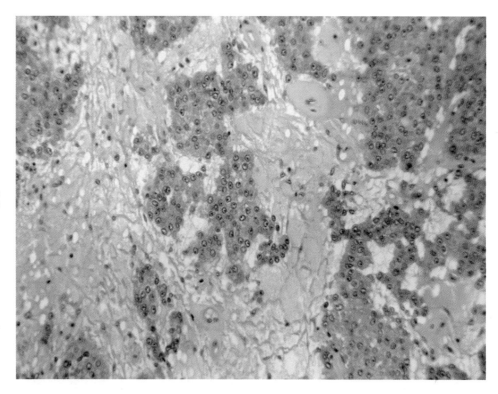

FIGURE 10-58

Leydig cell tumor. Cellular aggregates of uniform cells in an edematous stroma.

(Fig. 10-59). Within the cytoplasm, there is a variable amount of lipochrome pigmentation, which may confer a brown color to the tumor. Reinke's crystals are rhomboid-shaped, intracytoplasmic crystals of varying length and number (Fig. 10-60). They are red on H&E and Masson trichrome stains but may be chipped out by the microtome, leaving an empty space. Reinke's crystals occur in up to 40% of LCTs. At the time of frozen sectioning, a touch preparation stained with H&E may demonstrate Reinke's crystals, thereby confirming the diagnosis of LCT. LCTs may extend between seminiferous tubules at the periphery of the tumor and, in a prepubertal male, may stimulate spermatogenesis within the seminiferous tubules (Fig. 10-61). These

LEYDIG CELL TUMOR—PATHOLOGIC FEATURES

Gross Findings

▶ LCT may be quite small, particularly in prepubertal males. In adults they are usually 3 to 5 cm in diameter and may be more than 10 cm

▶ Are usually solid, tan, yellow, or mahogany

▶ Circumscribed, not encapsulated

▶ Hemorrhage and necrosis may be present

▶ May extend into extratesticular structures in 10% to 15% of cases

Microscopic Findings

▶ Leydig cell nuclei are generally round and nucleolated

▶ Cell shapes vary from polygonal to spindled

▶ Cell cytoplasm is generally eosinophilic, sometimes ground-glass, may be vacuolated to the point of adipose cell differentiation, and may contain lipid or lipochrome pigment

▶ Mitotic figures are usually sparse

▶ Up to 40% of LCTs contain Reinke's crystals

▶ Growth patterns include sheets, cords, and clusters of cells in scant or edematous stroma

▶ Changes raising suspicion of malignancy are necrosis, blood vessel invasion, cellular anaplasia, and more than 3 mitoses per 10 high-power microscopic fields

Ultrastructural Features

▶ Cells contain abundant smooth endoplasmic reticulum, mitochondria with tubular or lamellar cristae, and Reinke's crystals which show periodicity and are hexagonal

Immunohistochemical Features

▶ Cells are positive for inhibin, melan A, calretinin, cytokeratin, and S-100 protein

Differential Diagnosis

▶ Leydig cell hyperplasia

▶ Malakoplakia

▶ "Adrenal tumors" of CAH and Nelson syndrome

▶ Metastatic carcinoma

▶ Large cell calcifying Sertoli cell tumor (LCCSCT)

▶ Sertoli cell tumor with lipid vacuolization

▶ Plasmacytoma

tubules histologically resemble those of an older child. This appears to be the effect of locally produced testosterone, because these changes are not observed in the contralateral testis (Fig. 10-62). In postpubertal men, seminiferous tubules adjacent to LCT show reduced spermatogenesis. The microscopic findings of necrosis, blood vessel invasion, significant cellular anaplasia, more than 3 mitoses per 10 high-power microscopic fields, and a size greater than 5 cm are suspicious for malignancy (Figs. 10-63 and 10-64). Malignant tumors usually have four or more of these findings, and benign tumors generally have none of them.

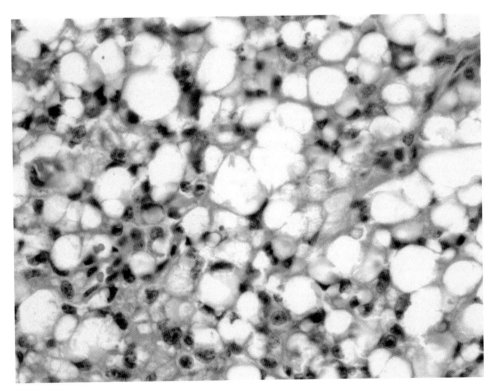

FIGURE 10-59

Leydig cell tumor. Marked cytoplasmic vacuolation and focally fatty metaplasia.

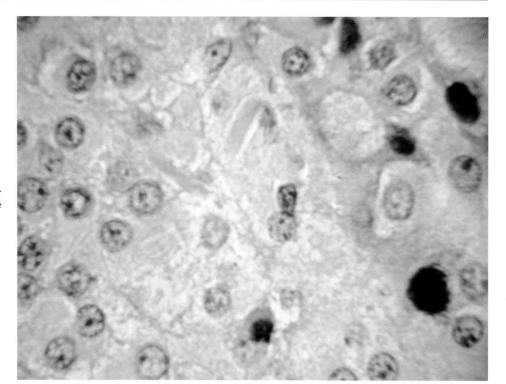

FIGURE 10-60

Leydig cell tumor. Two rectangular eosinophilic Reinke's crystals are present. (High-power magnification.)

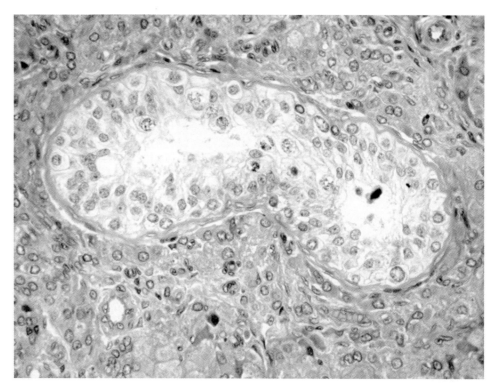

FIGURE 10-61

Leydig cell tumor (LCT) in a prepubertal boy. Image is from the periphery of a benign LCT at its interface with surrounding testicular parenchyma. Testosterone has locally stimulated germinal epithelium. Rare primary spermatocytes are present.

ANCILLARY STUDIES

IMMUNOHISTOCHEMICAL FEATURES

The parenchymal cells of LCT are positive for inhibin, melanin A, and calretinin in 87% to 96% of cases. None of these findings are specific for the diagnosis of LCT.

DIFFERENTIAL DIAGNOSIS

Although the diagnosis of most LCTs is clearcut, the differential diagnosis is large and consists of benign and malignant entities. As always, clinical information is very important. Occasional nodules of Leydig cell hyperplasia are quite large. The finding of multiple small

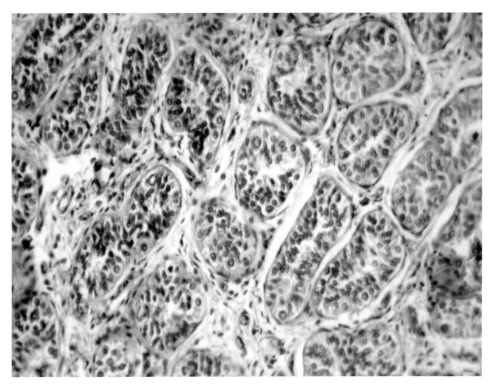

FIGURE 10-62

Biopsy of contralateral testis in a prepubertal boy with Leydig cell tumor (LCT). Prepubertal seminiferous tubules are unstimulated by testosterone produced by an LCT in the contralateral testis.

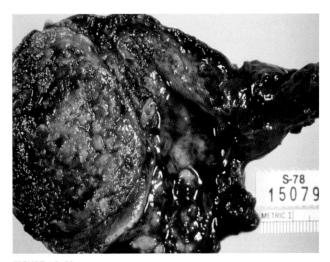

FIGURE 10-63

Malignant Leydig cell tumor.6-cm irregular, tan, firm, focally hemorrhagic mass.

nodules, usually in the presence of sclerotic tubules and tubules with regressed spermatogenesis, is helpful in reaching the diagnosis of Leydig cell hyperplasia.

Malakoplakia is extremely rare in the testis but may be composed of sheets of eosinophilic epithelioid histiocytes. The medical history should indicate a preexisting or current febrile or infectious status. CD68 and other histiocyte-marking antibodies may be helpful in rendering the diagnosis. The finding of Michaelis-Gutmann bodies is a sine qua non for the diagnosis of malakoplakia.

Proliferations of ACTH-sensitive cells in congenital adrenal hyperplasia (CAH) and Nelson syndrome may resemble Leydig cells (Fig. 10-65). These clinical entities tend to be seen initially in biopsies rather than orchiectomy specimens. The clinical histories should direct the clinician to the correct diagnosis. Some of these aggregates may be palpable, and they tend to be multifocal within both testicular and paratesticular tissue. The cytoplasm of the cells tends to have more fine lipochrome pigment than a LCT. LCTs usually are not bilateral or multifocal. The "tumor" cells of CAH and Nelson syndrome are positive for inhibin, as are the cells of LCT.

In isolated cases, metastatic carcinoma, particularly renal cell carcinoma, adrenocortical carcinoma, or prostatic adenocarcinoma may mimic LCT. Renal cell carcinoma may have either eosinophilic or clear cytoplasm and may manifest as a metastatic tumor. Renal cell carcinoma should not be positive for inhibin. In cases of suspected renal cell carcinoma, radiologic study can be recommended and may show the primary renal tumor. Adrenocortical carcinoma is usually discovered as a primary tumor before it metastasizes. Inhibin stain is not useful, because both adrenocortical cells and Leydig cells are positive for inhibin. Prostatic carcinoma is the most frequent metastatic malignancy identified in the testis. These lesions occur in patients with known prostatic adenocarcinoma who usually have been treated with androgen deprivation therapy. Immunohistochemical PSAP or prostate-specific antigen (PSA) positivity is useful in diagnosing prostatic adenocarcinoma. A history of prostatic adenocarcinoma should be obtained.

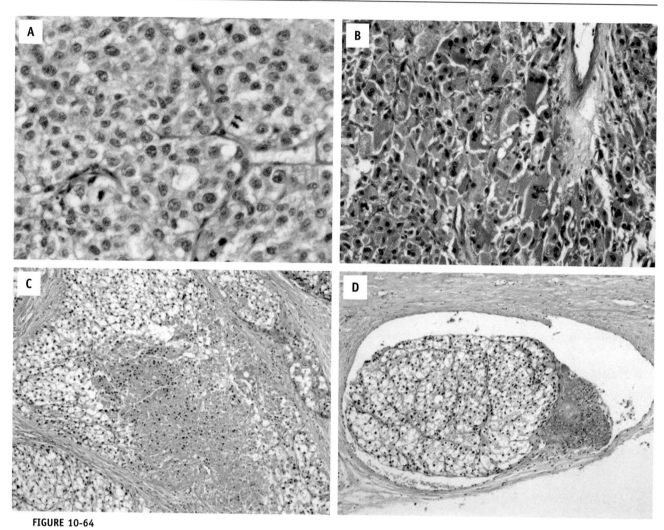

FIGURE 10-64

Malignant Leydig cell tumor. **A,** Solid arrangement of Leydig cells. Two mitotic figures are present in the field. **B,** Anaplasia of nuclei with considerable variation of nuclear shape and chromasia. **C,** Focus of necrosis within the tumor. **D,** Intratesticular vascular invasion with tumor attachment to vein wall. All images are from the same case as in Figure 10-63.

Large cell calcifying Sertoli cell tumor (LCCSCT) can be a difficult differential diagnosis. However, these tumors usually occur with a background of unique clinical findings, those of Carney syndrome or Peutz-Jeghers syndrome. These tumors are usually multifocal and bilateral. LCCSCTs contain eosinophilic cells with granular cytoplasm within both seminiferous tubules and stroma, and they also contain calcifications. LCTs are usually unilateral, virtually never intratubular, and usually without calcification.

Foci of SCT, not otherwise specified (NOS) with a solid growth pattern or extensive cytoplasmic lipid vacuolization resemble LCT. Foci of tubular differentiation favor the diagnosis of Sertoli cell tumor. Inhibin stain is more intense in LCT than in SCT. If no malignant features are present within the tumor, the consequence of misdiagnosis is negligible. Plasmacytoma may superficially resemble an LCT, but plasmacytoma lacks the cellular cohesion that is present in LCT and usually the cells of LCT have more central nuclei, are without a perinuclear hof, and lack the characteristic nuclear appearance of plasma cells. Testicular plasmacytoma may precede systemic myeloma. The identification of inhibin with immunohistochemical staining should confirm the diagnosis of LCT.

PROGNOSIS AND TREATMENT

Malignant LCTs occur in older patients, with a mean age of 63 years, compared with 40 years in benign LCTs. Malignant tumors have a shorter period of clinical symptoms and are larger than benign tumors. The majority of malignant tumors metastasize to retroperitoneal lymph nodes and subsequently to the liver, lungs, and brain. After initial radical orchiectomy, RPLND may be performed. There is no successful therapy for metastasis to parenchymal organs.

For tumors not suspected of being malignant, radical orchiectomy is the usual therapy. However, conservative

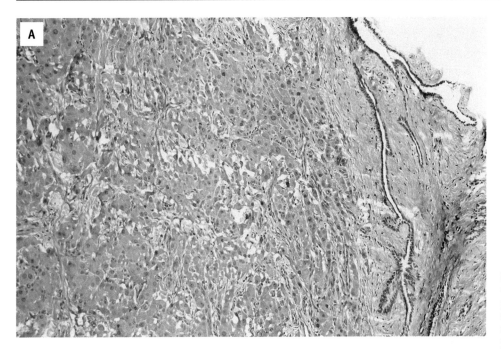

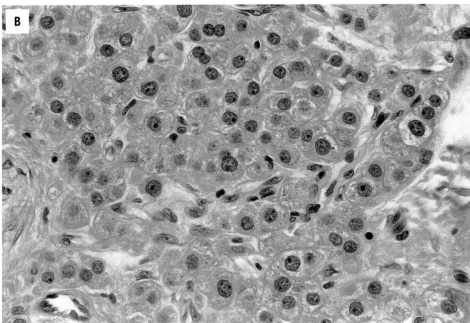

FIGURE 10-65

"Tumor" of congenital adrenal hyperplasia. **A,** Intratesticular nodule of eosinophilic cells compressing the rete testis. **B,** Extratesticular nodule composed of eosinophilic cells with fine granular cytoplasmic lipochrome pigment. These cells have a similar appearance to Leydig cells, but they are bilateral, intratesticular and extratesticular. Reinke's crystals have not been described in these cells.

therapy may be considered if the contralateral testis is absent or damaged.

SERTOLI CELL TUMOR

Five varieties of Sertoli cell tumors have been defined: SCT NOS (the classic Sertoli cell tumor), sclerosing SCT (SSCT), large cell calcifying Sertoli cell tumor (LCCSCT), Sertoli cell adenoma, and Sertoli-Leydig cell tumor. Sertoli cell adenoma was discussed in the chapter on non-neoplastic diseases of the testis under the heading of androgen insensitivity syndrome. SCT NOS and SSCT are discussed in this section, and LCCSCT is discussed in a separate section. Sertoli-Leydig cell tumor is extremely rare. It is discussed as part of the differential diagnosis of SCT NOS.

CLINICAL FEATURE

Fewer than 1% of testis tumors are SCT NOS. With refinement of diagnostic criteria, they rarely occur in men younger than 20 years of age, and they do not occur

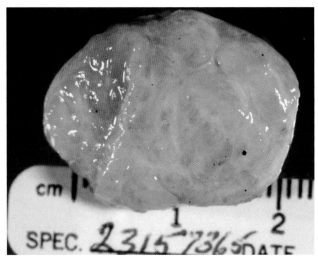

FIGURE 10-66

Sertoli cell tumor, not otherwise specified. Locally excised 2.5-cm tan tumor with fibrous trabeculae. An orchiectomy was performed after frozen section.

in extratesticular locations, as GCTs may. Approximately 10% are malignant. Most tumors are discovered as painless testicular masses, but malignant SCT NOS may manifest with lymph node metastasis.

Approximately 20 SSCTs have been reported in patients from 18 to 80 years of age. They have all behaved in a benign fashion. The tumor may occur in a cryptorchid testis or in one with a history of treated cryptorchidism.

RADIOLOGIC FEATURES

Ultrasound identifies solid and cystic intratesticular tumors.

PATHOLOGIC FEATURES

GROSS FINDINGS

SCT NOSs are circumscribed but unencapsulated, solid and cystic, yellow-tan or white, sometimes hemorrhagic masses (Fig. 10-66) Almost all tumors are unilateral. SSCTs tend to be smaller, with a mean diameter of 1.5 cm; they are well-demarcated, firm, and yellow-white to tan.

MICROSCOPIC FINDINGS

SCT NOS has a variety of growth patterns. The tumors may produce solid or hollow tubular structures, cords, sheets, cellular aggregates, or retiform structures (Fig. 10-67 and 10-68). Tubular structures may merge with spindled stromal cells. Epithelial aggregates may be separated by fibrovascular septa. Tumor cytoplasm may be pale, eosinophilic, or lipid rich. Sertoli cell nuclei are round to oval and may contain nucleoli. Charcot-Böttcher crystals should not be depended upon to render a diagnosis of SCT NOS.

SSCT is a sharply demarcated, unencapsulated tumor with anastomosing tubules, large cellular aggregates, and cords of epithelial cells. Tumor cells are of medium size, with round, vesicular to dark nuclei. Within the bounds of the tumor are entrapped tubules that have a somewhat prepubertal look (Fig. 10-69). Although most SSCTs are confined to the testis, epithelial structures have invaded blood vessels and paratesticular tissue in one case.

ANCILLARY STUDIES

ULTRASTRUCTURAL EXAMINATION

Charcot-Böttcher crystals (microfilament bundles) have not been found in SCT NOS tumors examined ultrastructurally.

IMMUNOHISTOCHEMISTRY

SCT NOS tumors have been positive for cytokeratin in 80% of cases, vimentin in 90%, inhibin in 40%, and S100 protein focally in 30%. The tumors are negative for EMA, PLAP, AFP, and hCG.

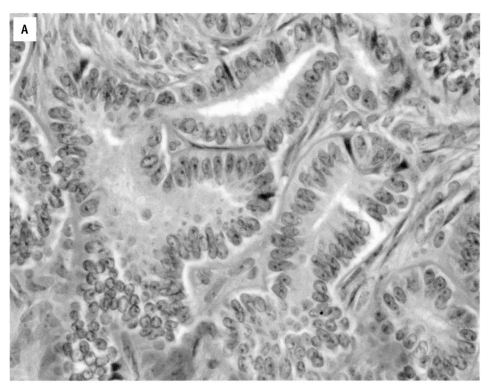

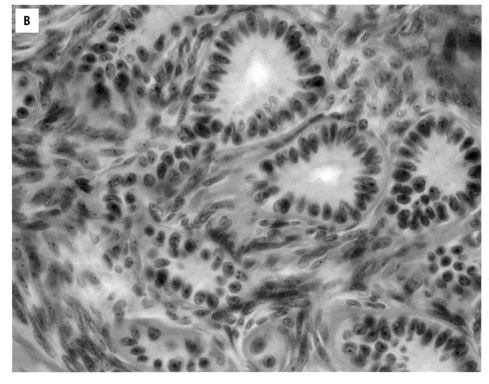

FIGURE 10-67
Sertoli cell tumor, not otherwise specified. **A,** Basement membrane-bound tubular structures lined by columnar cells with round to oval nuclei and small nucleoli. **B,** Elongate stromal cells adjacent to tubules.

DIFFERENTIAL DIAGNOSIS

Seminoma enters the differential diagnosis when SCT NOS is growing in a sheet-like pattern and the cells are lipid rich. Other aspects of seminoma, such as lymphoid reaction, granulomas, and IGCNU, are absent. Immunohistochemical stains should be negative for PLAP and CD117, and they are often positive for inhibin in SCT NOS. LCT may mimic SCT NOS if the LCT forms pseudotubules or if cell cytoplasm of the LCT is lipid rich. Additional sections may demonstrate classic areas of SCT. The finding of unequivocal tubular structures indicates SCT rather than LCT. LCTs stain much more diffusely and intensely for inhibin than do SCTs. There have been rare reported cases of Sertoli-Leydig

SERTOLI CELL TUMOR—PATHOLOGIC FEATURES

Gross Findings

- ▶ Generally solid, occasionally cystic; circumscribed; yellow, tan, or white; and may be hemorrhagic
- ▶ Most tumors are unilateral
- ▶ Sclerosing SCTs are usually 1.5 cm or less in diameter, well demarcated, hard, and yellow

Microscopic Findings

- ▶ SCT NOS comprises hollow or solid tubules, cords, sheets, aggregates, and retiform configurations separated by fibrovascular septae
- ▶ Tumor cell cytoplasm may be pale or pink and may contain lipid vacuoles
- ▶ SCT NOS nuclei are round and may contain nucleoli
- ▶ Sclerosing SCTs contain simple and anastomosing tubules, large cellular aggregates, and cords of epithelial cells. Cells are medium sized, with round vesicular to dark nuclei
- ▶ In sclerosing SCT, epithelial cells are within a dense hyalin stroma
- ▶ SCTs NOS behaving in a malignant fashion are greater than 5 cm in diameter, have vascular invasion, exhibit necrosis, have grade II or III nuclei, and have more than 5 mitoses per 10 high-power fields

Ultrastructural Features

- ▶ Charcot-Böttcher crystals have not been identified in SCTs NOS that have been examined ultrastructurally

Immunohistochemical Features

- ▶ Cytokeratin staining is present in 80%, vimentin in 90%, inhibin in 40%, and S-100 protein focally in 30% of SCTs NOS
- ▶ Staining is negative for EMA, PLAP, AFP, and hCG in SCT NOS

Differential Diagnosis

- ▶ Seminoma, particularly tubular seminoma
- ▶ LCT with cytoplasmic vacuolation
- ▶ Rete testis carcinoma
- ▶ Foci of persistent immature tubules
- ▶ Carcinoid tumor
- ▶ Metastatic carcinoma
- ▶ Adenomatoid tumor

cell tumors. These consist of tubules and cords within a cellular neoplastic stroma. These tumors may or may not contain Leydig cells. Because of their rarity, gynecologic pathologists with experience in this area should best evaluate them.

Some SCTs NOS grow in a retiform pattern, raising the differential diagnosis of rete testis carcinoma. The latter must fulfill the criteria that the tumor is at the testicular hilus with a transition from normal rete testis to rete testis carcinoma. The nuclei of rete testis carcinoma are generally larger, more pleomorphic, and with coarser chromatin than in SCT. Rete testis carcinoma is negative for inhibin. Rete testis carcinoma is positive for EMA, and SCT NOS is negative. Foci of persistent

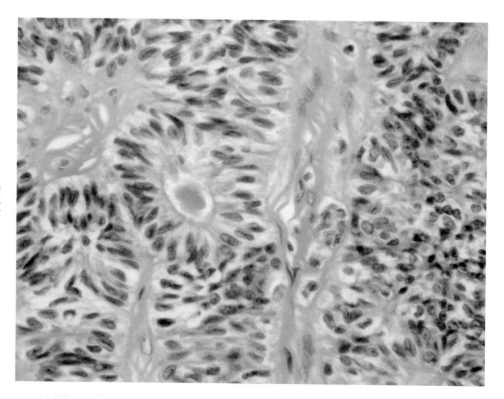

FIGURE 10-68

Sertoli cell tumor, not otherwise specified. Mostly solid epithelial nests with focal hollow tubular structures.

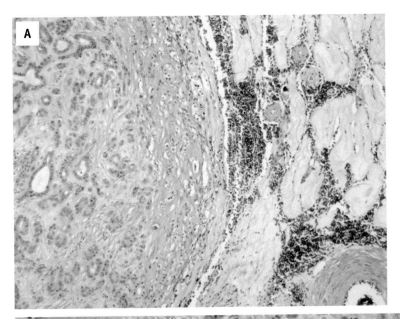

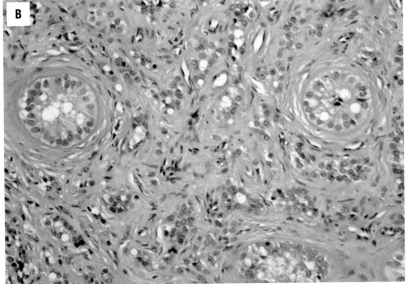

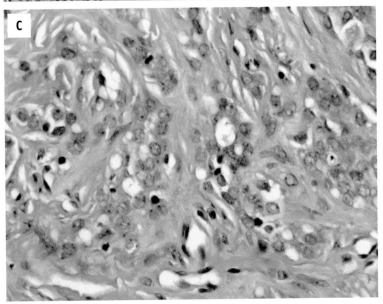

FIGURE 10-69

Sclerosing Sertoli cell tumor. **A,** Sharply defined, unencapsulated mass composed of tubules of various sizes within a dense fibrous matrix. (Low-power magnification.) **B,** Cords and small tubular structures within a dense fibrous matrix infiltrating between two seminiferous tubules lined exclusively by Sertoli cells. (Intermediate magnification.) **C,** Cords and tubules are composed of cells with vesicular nuclei and indistinct cytoplasmic borders. (High-power magnification.)

immature tubules are generally microscopic in size but may measure 1 mm or slightly more in maximum dimension. They usually occur in cryptorchid or previously cryptorchid testes and are not neoplastic. The Sertoli cells in these foci have a prepubertal appearance. Spermatogonia are usually present, and occasionally IGCNU is present in foci of persistent immature tubules along with hyalinized or calcified bodies. The presence of ICGNU may be confirmed with immunohistochemical stains for CD117 and PLAP. Foci of persistent immature tubules are usually surrounded by testicular parenchyma with some degree of atrophy. Pure carcinoid tumors may grow in an insular or cystic pattern. Carcinoid tumors are positive for chromogranin and synaptophysin.

Metastatic carcinoma forming tubular glands, or a solidly growing tumor such as prostatic adenocarcinoma, might mimic SCT NOS. The presence of intravascular tumor, multiple tumor foci, and the history of a primary carcinoma elsewhere would strongly favor metastasis. The use of inhibin, which is frequently positive in SCT NOS, might help to distinguish SCT NOS from some tumors. Some histologic foci of adenomatoid tumor whose cells have extensive eosinophilic cytoplasm might resemble SCT NOS. Although adenomatoid tumor may involve the testis, it is predominantly extratesticular, in contrast to the location of SCT NOS. Additional sections of tumor might well identify classic foci of adenomatoid tumor with large intracytoplasmic vacuoles. The adenomatoid tumor cells should stain positive for calretinin and negative for inhibin.

PROGNOSIS AND TREATMENT

Ninety percent of SCTs NOS are benign and are treated by radical orchiectomy. Malignant tumors may be treated by RPLND if there is evidence of retroperitoneal lymph node involvement. There is no consistently satisfactory therapy for advanced-stage tumor.

LARGE CELL CALCIFYING SERTOLI CELL TUMOR

CLINICAL FEATURES

More than 50 cases of LCCSCT have been reported from throughout the world. They occur in testes and not in extratesticular locations. By 1999, 8 of 47 cases were found to be malignant. The benign tumors themselves are not associated with morbidity or mortality. However, 40% of patients with benign tumors had associated Carney syndrome or Peutz-Jeghers syndrome (PJS). Patients with PJS and LCCSCT may have

associated gynecomastia. Both of these syndromes have significant components, some of which are potentially lethal and must be investigated clinically. Benign tumors occur in younger patients, with a mean age of 17 years. Malignant tumors occur in older patients, with a mean age of 39 years. Only one reported malignant tumor has been associated with the features of Carney syndrome.

LARGE CELL CALCIFYING SERTOLI CELL TUMOR—FACT SHEET

Definition
▶ Tumors composed of interstitial and intratubular aggregates of large eosinophilic cells of probable Sertoli cell origin

Incidence and Location
▶ Approximately 50 cases reported by 1999
▶ Tumors reported from all over the world
▶ Occur in testes, not in extratesticular tissues

Morbidity and Mortality
▶ 8 of 47 cases reported by 1999 were malignant
▶ Morbidity occurs in patients with benign tumors and relates to the manifestations of associated Carney syndrome or Peutz-Jeghers syndrome (PJS)

Gender, Race, and Age Distribution
▶ Benign tumors occur in males averaging 17 years of age
▶ Malignant tumors occur in males averaging 39 years of age
▶ Analogous tumors have not been reported in the ovaries of females, although females with PJS may have sex cord tumors with annular tubules

Clinical Features
▶ About 40% of cases are associated with Carney syndrome or PJS
▶ Syndrome-associated cases have findings of these syndromes
▶ Malignancy occurs in about 20% of cases
▶ Only 1 of 8 malignant cases has had findings of either Carney syndrome or PJS
▶ Patients with PJS may have associated gynecomastia

Radiologic Features
▶ Ultrasound demonstrates the presence of tumors, calcification, bilaterality, and multiplicity
▶ Ultrasound findings strongly suggest the diagnosis in patients of appropriate age and with appropriate clinical findings

Prognosis and Treatment
▶ Malignant tumors may metastasize
▶ Prognosis of benign tumors relates to other manifestations of the syndrome
▶ Treatment of benign tumors can be limited, attempting to conserve testicular parenchyma
▶ Treatment of patients with retroperitoneal lymph node involvement may include RPLND
▶ No specific accepted therapy for metastatic LCCSCT involving parenchymal organs

RADIOLOGIC FEATURES

If the clinician recognizes that the patient has either PJS or Carney syndrome, ultrasound findings consisting of a solid tumor or tumors, multifocality, bilaterality, and calcification may be virtually diagnostic of LCCSCT.

PATHOLOGIC FEATURES

GROSS FINDINGS

Benign tumors are less than 4 cm in diameter, with a mean diameter of 1.4 cm. They are confined to the testis, are often multifocal, are bilateral in 40% of the cases, are composed of firm yellow-tan tissue, and may contain calcific foci. Malignant tumors are unilateral, typically larger than 4 cm with a mean diameter of 5.4 cm, and possibly with hemorrhage and necrosis.

MICROSCOPIC FINDINGS

The tumor grows in sheets, nests, trabeculae, and cellular clusters. About 50% of tumors also grow within seminiferous tubules. The stroma is loose, myxoid, or densely collagenous. There is focal or extensive laminated calcification. Tumor cells are large and round, or occasionally cuboidal or columnar, with eosinophilic, occasionally amphophilic, vacuolated cytoplasm (Fig. 10-70). Some cases associated with PJS may lack calcification and may show features of sex cord tumor with annular tubules (Fig. 10-71). These patients may also have intratubular Sertoli cell proliferations. Malignant tumors contain two or more of the following: extratesticular spread, greater than 4 cm in diameter, greater than 3 mitoses per 10 high-power microscopic fields, significant nuclear atypia, necrosis, and vascular invasion.

ANCILLARY STUDIES

ULTRASTRUCTURAL EXAMINATION

Tumor cells may contain Charcot-Böttcher crystals (microfilament bundles).

IMMUNOHISTOCHEMISTRY

Tumor cells stain positively for low-molecular-weight cytokeratin, vimentin, and S-100 protein.

DIFFERENTIAL DIAGNOSIS

Because of the pink cytoplasm of the tumor cells, some LCCSCTs have been misdiagnosed as LCT. The pres-

---

LARGE CELL CALCIFYING SERTOLI CELL TUMOR— PATHOLOGIC FEATURES

Gross Findings

→ Benign tumors are usually 4 cm or less in diameter, confined to the testis, often multifocal, bilateral in 40%, composed of yellow-tan tissue, and may contain calcific foci

→ Malignant tumors are unilateral and larger than 4 cm in diameter with a mean size of 5.4 cm, with hemorrhage and necrosis

Microscopic Findings

▶ Grows in sheets, nests, trabeculae, cellular clusters, and solid tubules

▶ Intratubular in 50% of cases

▶ Stroma is loose, myxoid, or densely collagenous

▶ Focal to extensive laminated calcification

▶ Tumor cells are large, round, or occasionally cuboidal or columnar with eosinophilic, granular, or occasionally amphophilic vacuolated cytoplasm

▶ Malignant tumors contain two or more of the following: extratesticular spread, size greater than 4 cm, more than 3 mitoses per 10 high-power fields, significant nuclear atypia, necrosis, and blood vessel invasion

▶ Some tumors associated with PJS have intratubular Sertoli cell proliferations with or without associated LCCSCT

▶ Tumors associated with PJS may be hybrids of LCCSCT, lack calcification, and show features of sex cord tumor with annular tubules

Ultrastructural Features

▶ Some benign LCCSCTs have Charcot-Böttcher crystals (microfilament bundles)

Immunohistochemical Features

▶ Tumor cells are positive for low-molecular-weight cytokeratin, vimentin, and S-100 protein

Differential Diagnosis

▶ LCT

▶ Sex cord tumor with annular tubules

---

ence of multifocality, intratubular growth, absence of Reinke's crystals, the presence of calcification, and bilaterality all favor the diagnosis of LCCSCT.

PROGNOSIS AND TREATMENT

Benign tumors may be treated conservatively, preserving testicular parenchyma. Malignant tumors should be treated by radical orchiectomy. If lymph node involvement is suspected, RPLND may be performed. There is no definitive treatment for malignant LCCSCT involving parenchymal organs. The tumors of patients with PJS have all been benign.

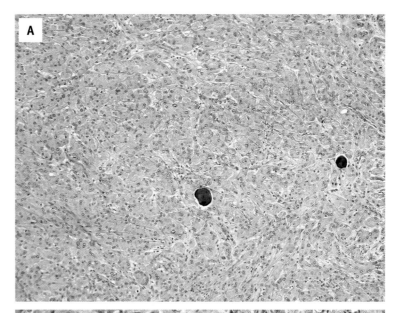

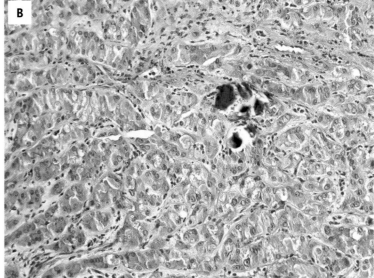

FIGURE 10-70

Large cell calcifying Sertoli cell tumor. **A,** Sheets of epithelial cells with abundant eosinophilic cytoplasm, round nuclei, and prominent nucleoli. A laminated calcification (psammoma body) is present. **B,** Sheets of cells with round nuclei, eosinophilic to amphophilic cytoplasm, and calcific fragments. **C,** Intratubular neoplasm composed of large eosinophilic Sertoli cells and small papillary proliferations, laminated calcification, and increased basement membrane-like material. (Courtesy of Dr. Isabell Sesterhenn, AFIP, Washington, DC.)

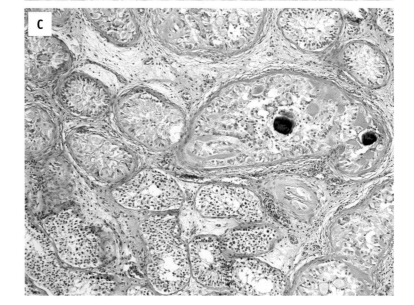

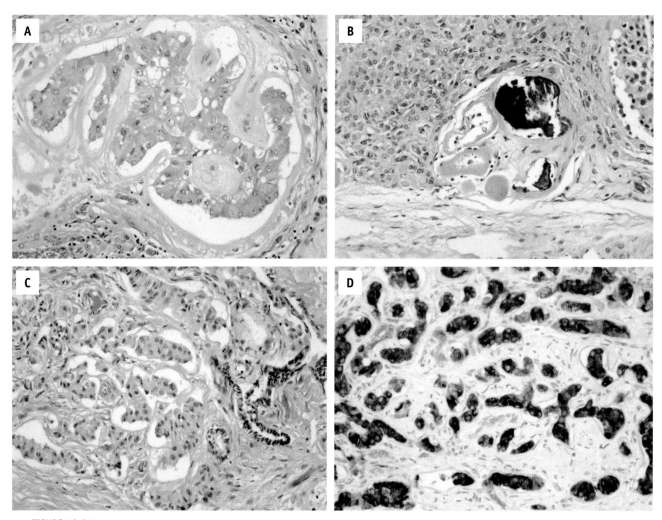

FIGURE 10-71
Large cell calcifying Sertoli cell tumor associated with Peutz-Jeghers syndrome. **A,** Intratubular proliferation of enlarged eosinophilic Sertoli cells with vesicular nuclei and prominent nucleoli surrounded by hyaline basement membrane-like material. **B,** Proliferation of interstitial eosinophilic cells. Hyaline thickening of tubular walls with intratubular calcification. **C,** Tubular Sertoli cell proliferations invading rete testis. **D,** Positive inhibin stain of Sertoli cells. These foci were present multifocally and bilaterally and were identified at autopsy.

Granulosa Cell Tumors

Granulosa cell tumors occur both in pediatric and adult populations. They are clinically and pathologically distinct in these two populations and therefore are discussed separately.

ADULT GRANULOSA CELL TUMOR

CLINICAL FEATURES

These tumors are quite rare and have been reported in adults from ages 16 to 76 years. However, some of these tumors may be interpreted as unclassified sex cord-stromal tumors. Tumors usually manifest with testic-

ular enlargement. Adult patients may have associated gynecomastia. Elevated serum levels of inhibin and anti-müllerian hormone have been reported.

PATHOLOGIC FEATURES

GROSS FINDINGS

Tumors measure up to 13 cm in diameter, are solid and may be cystic, yellow-tan to white, firm and lobulated.

MICROSCOPIC FINDINGS

Tumors resemble their ovarian counterparts (Fig. 10-72). The microfollicular pattern is most frequent, but diffuse and other patterns may be present. Nuclei are round, oval, or elongate and contain nuclear groves.

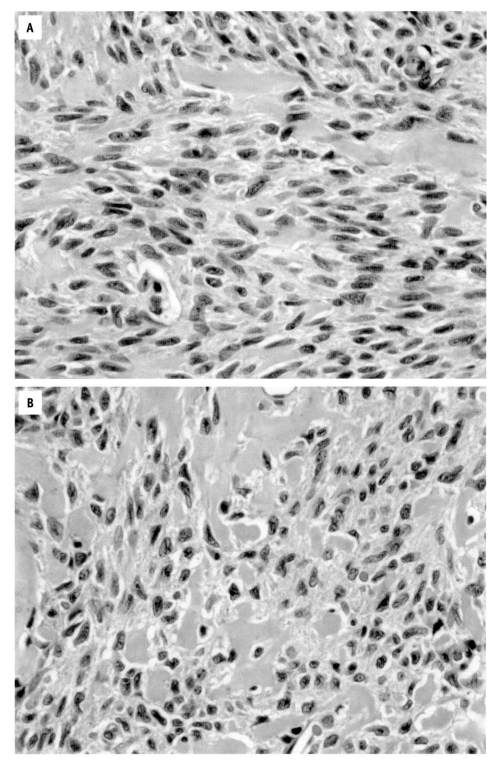

FIGURE 10-72
Adult Granulosa Cell Tumor. **A,** Diffuse proliferation of spindled cells with ovoid to spindled, sometimes grooved nuclei and scant cytoplasm. **B,** Granulosa cells intermixed with abundant hyaline basement membrane-like material. The tumor was present in a 50-year-old male.

Cytoplasm is scant and mitoses are rare. Stroma may be fibrous and thecomatous and may contain smooth muscle.

ANCILLARY STUDIES

IMMUNOHISTOCHEMISTRY

Tumor cells are positive for vimentin, inhibin, smooth muscle actin, MIC2, and focally for cytokeratin.

DIFFERENTIAL DIAGNOSIS

The diagnosis of adult granulosa cell tumor should be made when the tumor has the morphology of a granulosa cell tumor in its entirety or almost so. Some pathologists may interpret the tumor as an undifferentiated sex cord-stromal tumor with granulosa cell features. The presence of lutein-type cells in juxtaposition with stromal cells may raise the question of a tumor with both germ cell and sex cord-stromal elements. Negative CD117 or PLAP staining of these cells militates against the diagnosis of a malignant germ cell component.

PROGNOSIS AND TREATMENT

Approximately 15% to 20% of adult granulosa cell tumors are malignant. Metastasis may occur several years after diagnosis. Retroperitoneal lymph node involvement may be present at diagnosis. Survival may be prolonged, but some patients have died of metastatic neoplasm. The treatment of the primary tumor is radical orchiectomy. If there is evidence of retroperitoneal lymph node metastasis, RPLND can be performed. There is no definite therapy for higher-stage malignancy.

JUVENILE GRANULOSA CELL TUMOR

CLINICAL FEATURES

Juvenile granulosa cell tumor (JGCT) is the most common testicular neoplasm in boys during the first 6 months of life. It occurs in children with ambiguous genitalia, intersex syndromes, or sex chromosomal mosaicism, including 45,XO/46,XY and 45,XO/46,X iso Yq), but it is not associated with isosexual precocity. The tumors are usually found in descended testes,

---

JUVENILE GRANULOSA CELL TUMOR—FACT SHEET

Definition
▶ A mixed solid and cystic neoplasm resembling Graafian follicles

Incidence and Location
▶ The most frequent tumor in the first 6 months of life and often detected at birth
▶ About 7% of prepubertal testicular tumors
▶ Occurs in descended and undescended testis

Morbidity and Mortality
▶ All testicular JGCTs have been benign without recurrence

Gender, Race, and Age Distribution
▶ Most frequently occurs in the first 6 months of life, with a few tumors in children and adults

Clinical Features
▶ May occur in children with ambiguous genitalia, intersex disorders, and sex chromosome mosaicism
▶ Often detected at birth as a testicular mass
▶ Not associated with isosexual precocity

Radiologic Features
▶ Ultrasound demonstrates a complex, multiseptate, hypoechoic mass

Diagnosis and Treatment
▶ Treatment has been radical orchiectomy
▶ Recently, testis-sparing enucleation has been performed successfully

---

although they have been found in undescended and torsed testes.

RADIOLOGIC FEATURES

Ultrasonography demonstrates a complex, multiseptate, hypoechoic mass.

PATHOLOGIC FEATURES

GROSS FINDINGS

The testis is usually enlarged with a solid and cystic mass. Cysts may bulge the tunica albugineal surface, but they are better seen on cross-section (Fig. 10-73). Solid areas vary from yellow to tan. Tumors range from four microscopic lobules to 13 cm in diameter.

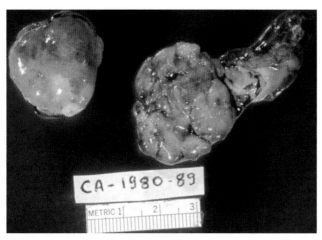

FIGURE 10-73
Juvenile granulosa cell tumor. Surface and cross-section of solid and cystic 3-cm tumor. Cysts bulge the capsule and are visible on the cut surface.

JUVENILE GRANULOSA CELL TUMOR—PATHOLOGIC FEATURES

Gross Findings

▶ Testis is usually enlarged with a solid and cystic mass
▶ Tumors range from four microscopic lobules to 13 cm in diameter

Microscopic Findings

▶ Follicular structures of varying size are lined by one to multiple cell layers with pale intracystic eosinophilic or basophilic material
▶ Smaller cysts may be lined by attenuated cells
▶ Stroma is fibrous
▶ Only rare cells with grooved nuclei resemble adult granulosa cells
▶ In solid areas, cells grow in sheets, nodules, and cellular aggregates
▶ Nuclei are round to oval with inconspicuous nucleoli
▶ Mitoses are frequent

Immunohistochemical Features

▶ Tumor cells are positive for vimentin, inhibin, S-100 protein, smooth muscle actin, and desmin, and focally for low-molecular-weight keratin

Differential Diagnosis

▶ Yolk sac tumor

MICROSCOPIC FINDINGS

Both solid and cystic areas are present, with prepubertal testis at the periphery. Cysts are usually follicular, with multiple cell layers surrounding a lumen containing eosinophilic to basophilic material that may stain for mucin (Fig. 10-74). Microcysts are small and lined by flattened epithelial cells with attenuated nuclei. Sheets, nodules, and aggregates of epithelial cells with round to oval nuclei and small nucleoli comprise the solid areas. Nuclei are not grooved in the majority of cells. Cytoplasm is pale to eosinophilic. Mitoses are frequent (Fig. 10-75).

ANCILLARY STUDIES

IMMUNOHISTOCHEMISTRY

Tumor cells are positive for vimentin, inhibin, S-100 protein, smooth muscle actin, desmin, and, focally, low-molecular-weight keratin.

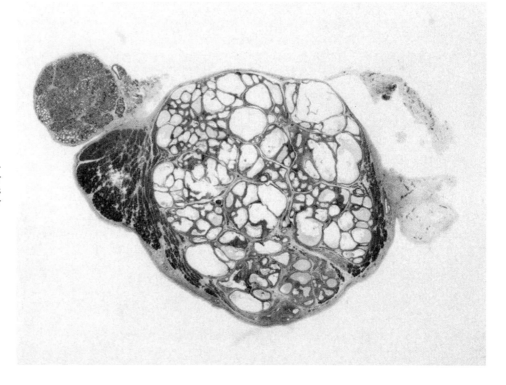

FIGURE 10-74
Juvenile granulosa cell tumor, showing multiple follicular cysts. Tumor compresses prepubertal seminiferous tubules on the left. (Low-power magnification.)

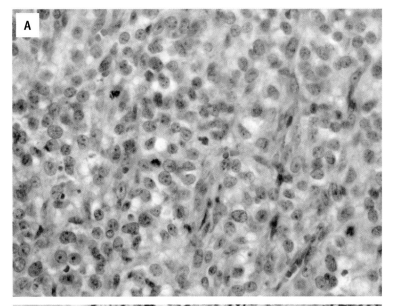

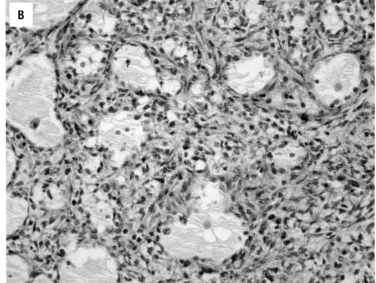

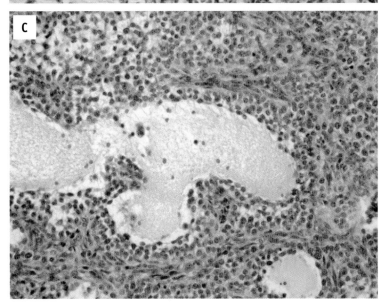

FIGURE 10-75

Juvenile granulosa cell tumor. **A,** Solid proliferation of cells with large round nuclei, nucleoli, multiple mitoses, pale cytoplasm, and indistinct cell borders. **B,** Multiple small cysts lined by flattened epithelium and containing pale basophilic intraluminal content. Cells with rounded and spindled nuclei, indistinct cytoplasmic borders, and a basophilic edematous stroma are present adjacent to and between cysts. **C,** Follicular cysts are lined by layers of cells and contain intraluminal basophilic material. Sheets of similar cells are adjacent to cysts.

Differential Diagnosis

The distinction between JGCT and YST is an important one. JGCT usually occurs during the first 6 months of life. YST usually occurs after that. JGCT may occur in a patient with ambiguous genitalia and an intersex syndrome. The finding of an elevated serum AFP level relative to normal adult levels is a dangerous red herring. Infants normally have elevated serum AFP levels compared with adults. Serum levels generally fall to normal adult levels by 8 months of age. From a histologic viewpoint, both tumors contain cysts. However, YST does not contain follicular cysts. Microcysts in JGCT may resemble microcysts in YST. However, staining of the tumor for AFP and inhibin should resolve the diagnosis: YST stains positive for AFP, and JGCT does not.

Prognosis and Treatment

All JGCTs of the testis have been benign without recurrence. Most cases have been treated with radical orchiectomy, although one case has been reported in which testis-sparing enucleation was performed with a 5-year recurrence-free survival.

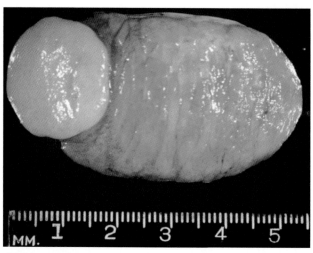

FIGURE 10-76
Fibroma. Unencapsulated, intratesticular, gray-tan, firm 2.1 cm mass.

FIBROMA-THECOMA

Fibroma-thecoma tumors resemble similarly named tumors of the ovary.

Clinical Features

These are very rare tumors. Experts suggest that thecomas of the testis may not exist. Tumors manifest as unilateral, sometimes painful, intratesticular masses. They are unassociated with increased hormonal function. The age range is 5 to 52 years, with a mean of 30 years.

Pathologic Features

Gross Findings

Tumors vary from 0.5 to 7 cm in diameter. They are firm, yellow to white, and not encapsulated (Fig. 10-76). Tumors have no evidence of hemorrhage or necrosis.

Microscopic Findings

Fibroma-thecoma tumors are composed of fusiform fibroblastic cells growing in fascicles and storiform patterns (Fig. 10-77). Connective tissue contains collagen and numerous small blood vessels. Spindle cells resemble ovarian stromal cells. Mitoses may be present, although they usually are not frequent. Up to 4 mitoses per high-power field have been recorded.

Ancillary Studies

Immunohistochemistry

Tumor cells stain positively for vimentin, for smooth muscle actin, and occasionally for cytokeratin and desmin.

Differential Diagnosis

The most important tumors in the differential diagnosis of fibroma-thecoma are primary testicular sarcomas, extratesticular sarcomas, and unclassified sex cord-stromal tumors, because all fibromas are benign and some unclassified sex cord-stroma tumors are malignant. It is important to adequately sample a fibroma, to look for epithelial areas that would place the tumor in a sex cord-stroma unclassified category, and to verify that the tumor is completely intratesticular, so that the possibility of an extratesticular sarcoma is excluded.

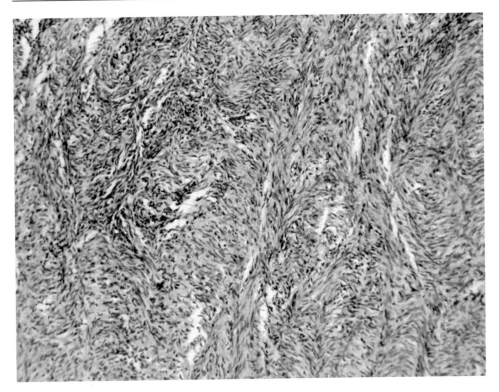

FIGURE 10-77
Fibroma. Cellular spindle-cell neoplasm resembling ovarian stroma is growing in fascicular and herringbone patterns. Neither cellular anaplasia nor mitotic activity is present.

MIXED SEX CORD-STROMAL TUMORS

These tumors comprise two or more identifiable types of sex cord-stromal tumors.

CLINICAL FEATURES

Mixed sex cord-stromal tumors occur in children and adults. The presenting feature is unilateral testicular enlargement. Gynecomastia may be present. Mortality may be related to the predominant histologic pattern and any foci of histologically atypical features.

PATHOLOGICAL FEATURES

GROSS FINDINGS

Tumors may be solid or cystic and grossly may resemble their various components.

MICROSCOPIC FINDINGS

Tumors may demonstrate characteristic granulosa, Leydig, or Sertoli cell elements in varying amounts. Features that are suggestive of malignancy are large tumor size, vascular and extratesticular invasion, nuclear anaplasia, increased mitotic activity, and necrosis.

ANCILLARY STUDIES

IMMUNOHISTOCHEMISTRY

The elements in a mixed sex cord-stromal tumor stain in the same manner as the individual pure tumors.

PROGNOSIS AND TREATMENT

The primary therapy is orchiectomy.

UNCLASSIFIED SEX CORD-STROMAL TUMORS

These tumors are also characterized as incompletely differentiated sex cord-stromal tumors. They are tumors with histologic features suggesting testicular, ovarian, and sex cord-stromal elements, but they lack the definitive features of a particular tumor.

CLINICAL FEATURES

Unclassified sex cord-stromal tumors are rare tumors that manifest as painless testicular masses in children and adults. Patients may have gynecomastia. Tumors are almost always benign in children, but as many as 25% are malignant in adults.

PATHOLOGIC FEATURES

GROSS FINDINGS

Tumors vary in shape and may replace testicular parenchyma or extend into extratesticular tissues. Tumors are yellow to white, mainly solid, and may be partly cystic.

MICROSCOPIC FINDINGS

Tumors have combinations of epithelial cells growing in solid and cystic patterns with tubule and cord formation. Cells may resemble Sertoli and Leydig cells. Spindle cells may be cellular and sarcomatoid. Both epithelial and stromal elements do not exactly resemble patterns of pure sex cord-stromal tumors. Features suggestive of malignancy are the same as in mixed sex cord-stromal tumors.

ANCILLARY STUDIES

IMMUNOHISTOCHEMISTRY

Spindle cell areas are positive for smooth muscle actin and S-100 protein and may be focally positive for cytokeratin.

DIFFERENTIAL DIAGNOSIS

The most important aspect of the differential diagnosis of the unclassified sex cord-stromal tumors is to make certain that the neoplasm is in the sex cord-stromal category and not a sarcoma of testicular or paratesticular origin. In this regard, gross examination of the tumor should make certain that the tumor is, in fact, of testicular origin. In largely spindled tumors, the pathologist should search for epithelial areas that would place the tumor in the sex cord-stromal category.

PROGNOSIS AND TREATMENT

These tumors are almost always benign in children, but about 25% are malignant in adults. Primary therapy is orchiectomy. Staging should be done, and in those patients with retroperitoneal lymph node involvement, an RPLND may be performed. Most of the reported

tumors have not been subjected to central pathology review by one or a group of pathologists, so there may be some variation in classification, particularly between mixed and unclassified sex cord-stromal tumors.

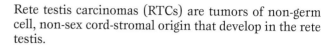

RETE TESTIS CARCINOMA

Rete testis carcinomas (RTCs) are tumors of non-germ cell, non-sex cord-stromal origin that develop in the rete testis.

CLINICAL FEATURES

RTCs are rare, with 42 tumors recorded through 1995. The tumor develops in the hilus of the testis and may involve the epididymis. According to reports in the

---

RETE TESTIS CARCINOMA—FACT SHEET

Definition
▶ Adenocarcinoma developing primarily in the rete testis and straight ducts of the testis

Incidence and Location
▶ Rare; 43 cases reported through 1995
▶ Develops in the hilus of the testis and may involve the epididymis

Morbidity and Mortality
▶ In a review of the literature, 33% of patients died of RTC, 75% of those within 1 year after diagnosis

Age Distribution
▶ Usually occurs in men older than 30 years of age, mostly from the fourth through the eighth decade

Clinical Features
▶ Usually painful, unilateral scrotal mass
▶ Onset may be brief or may extend for longer than 1 year
▶ May have associated back pain
▶ May have associated hydrocele, fistulas, sinus, or epididymitis
▶ Recurrent nodules may develop in scrotal and perineal skin

Radiologic Features
▶ Ultrasound may indicate the testicular hilar location

Prognosis and Treatment
▶ Primary treatment is orchiectomy
▶ Staging for distant disease should be done
▶ RPLND has produced long-term complete remission in a patient with micrometastatic neoplasm

literature, 33% of the patients have died of RTC, 75% of those within 1 year after diagnosis. RTC occurs in men older than 30 years of age, most in their fourth through eighth decades. The tumor onset may be brief or longer than 1 year. The presentation is usually with a painful unilateral testicular mass. There may be associated back pain, hydrocele, scrotal fistula, sinuses, and/or epididymitis. Recurrent nodules may develop in scrotal or perineal skin.

RADIOLOGIC FEATURES

Ultrasonography may demonstrate the hilar location of the tumor.

RETE TESTIS CARCINOMA—PATHOLOGIC FEATURES

Gross Findings
- ▶ Poorly circumscribed gray nodules at testicular hilus
- ▶ Mostly a single mass, but may be multiple
- ▶ Size ranges from 1 to 15 cm
- ▶ There may be gross spermatic cord involvement

Microscopic Findings
- ▶ Criteria for diagnosis are (1) absence of a histologically similar extratesticular tumor, (2) hilar location, (3) absence of primary testicular tumor of germ cell or non-germ cell origin, (4) transition from benign rete testis to RTC, and (5) a solid growth pattern
- ▶ Predominant growth pattern is papillary, with solid, spindled, and cystic areas less common
- ▶ Tumor cells are columnar to cuboidal with acidophilic to amphophilic cytoplasm
- ▶ Nuclei are enlarged, pleomorphic, and round to oval, with coarsely granular chromatin and sometimes prominent nucleoli
- ▶ Mitoses may be frequent

Immunohistochemical Features
- ▶ Tumor cells are positive for EMA, vimentin, keratin, and occasionally CEA
- ▶ Tumor cells are negative for AFP, hCG, and PSA

Differential Diagnosis
- ▶ Embryonal carcinoma
- ▶ Sertoli cell tumor
- ▶ Metastatic carcinoma
- ▶ Tumors of ovarian-type epithelium
- ▶ Malignant mesothelioma

PATHOLOGIC FEATURES

GROSS FINDINGS

RTC consists of one or multiple poorly circumscribed, gray nodules located at the hilus of the testis. Tumors range from 1 to 15 cm in diameter. There may be gross spermatic cord involvement.

MICROSCOPIC FINDINGS

Criteria for diagnosis have been stated to be absence of a histologically similar extratesticular tumor, hilar location, absence of a primary testicular tumor of germ cell or non-germ cell origin, histologic transition from benign rete testis epithelium to RTC, and a solid growth pattern. It may not be possible to demonstrate histologic transition, and a solid pattern may not be present, but the diagnosis of RTC can be made if the other criteria are satisfied. The predominant growth patterns are tubular and papillary adenocarcinoma, with solid, spindled, and cystic areas less common (Fig. 10-78). Tumor cells are cuboidal to columnar, with oxyphilic to amphophilic cytoplasm. Nuclei are enlarged, round to oval, and pleomorphic, with coarsely granular chromatin and sometimes with prominent nucleoli. Mitoses may be frequent.

ANCILLARY STUDIES

IMMUNOHISTOCHEMISTRY

Tumor cells are positive for EMA, vimentin, cytokeratin, and occasionally carcinoembryonic antigen (CEA). Tumor cells are negative for AFP, hCG, and PSA.

DIFFERENTIAL DIAGNOSIS

EC may have solid, papillary, or cystic formations, but EC is not generally centered on the testicular hilus; EC nuclei are larger and overlapping, and the cell borders are indistinct. IGCNU usually is present at the periphery of EC. SCT NOS often has tubular formations but is not generally centered on the hilus. Cells of SCT NOS are more regular and lack the atypia of RTC. The possibility of metastatic adenocarcinoma must be considered and ruled out. The presence of multifocality and extensive vascular invasion would cause further suspicion of metastatic adenocarcinoma. Papillary formations in the tumor raise the differential diagnosis of a tumor of ovarian epithelial origin or malignant mesothelioma. The former should resemble corresponding ovarian tumors, and the latter usually manifests predominantly on the mesothelial surfaces of the testis, often within a hydrocele sac. Each has characteristic histologic and immunohistochemical findings.

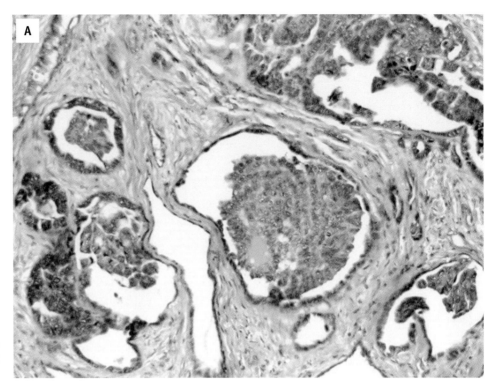

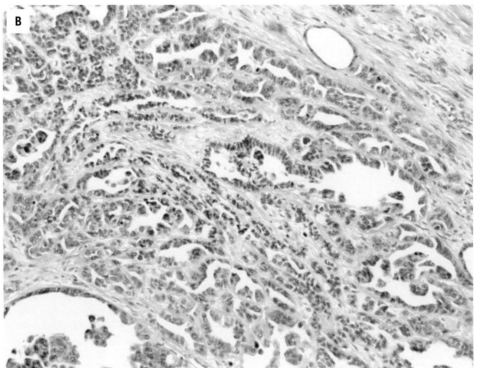

FIGURE 10-78

Rete testis carcinoma. **A**, Papillary formations composed of neoplastic cells with vesicular nuclei and prominent nucleoli project into lumina of the rete testis. Residual benign epithelium is present. **B**, Papillary and glandular formations infiltrate connective tissue.

MALIGNANT MESOTHELIOMA

CLINICAL FEATURES

These are tumors of mesothelial origin of the tunica vaginalis sac. By 1995, 81 cases of malignant mesothe-

lioma had been reported. The age range was 6 to 91 years, with a mean of 54 years. Forty-one percent of the patients who were asked reported occupational asbestos exposure. The majority of patients presented with persistent or recurrent hydrocele. In some, there were masses that involved spermatic cord, paratesticular structures, or testes. Malignant mesotheliomas are usually unsuspected and discovered in a hydrocele sac.

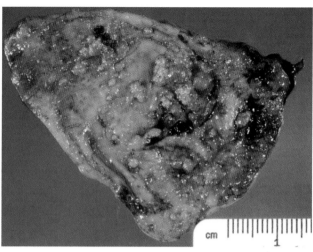

FIGURE 10-79

Malignant mesothelioma of tunica vaginalis. Raised yellow tumor foci ranging from less than 1 mm to 1.5 cm in diameter project from the gray mesothelial surface of a hydrocele specimen.

RADIOLOGIC FINDINGS

Imaging studies may suggest the diagnosis of malignant mesothelioma.

PATHOLOGIC FINDINGS

GROSS FINDINGS

Malignant mesothelioma usually occurs with a background of hematocele or hydrocele. The surgical hydrocele specimen consists of a thickened tunica vaginalis studded with often-friable papillary masses of variable size, ranging from less than 1 mm to several centimeters in diameter (Fig. 10-79). In cases where the testis is resected, papillary excrescences may be observed on the tunica albuginea. White or tan masses may invade spermatic cord, testis, or epididymis.

MICROSCOPIC FINDINGS

In a study by Jones and colleagues, the majority of malignant mesotheliomas were epithelial, and approximately 25% were biphasic. Epithelial tumors grow in papillary and/or tubular patterns (Fig. 10-80). Cellular

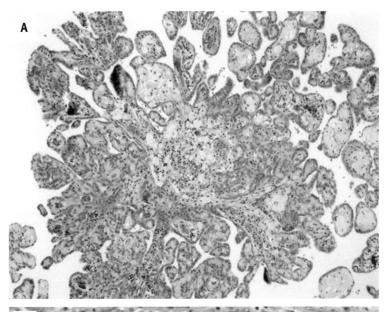

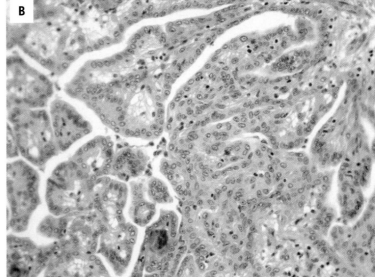

FIGURE 10-80

Malignant mesothelioma. **A,** A single layer of mesothelial cells lines complex papillary structures. Macrophages are present within some stalks. (Low-power magnification.) **B,** In the same specimen as in **A,** papillary formations are lined by columnar cells with vesicular nuclei and nucleoli. Unequivocal invasion is not identified. **C,** An invasive focus of malignant mesothelioma similar to that in the hydrocele specimen (**A** and **B**) shows a solid growth pattern and tubule formation. A foreign-body giant cell reaction to suture is present in the center. This image, from the orchiectomy specimen, demonstrates persistent tumor.

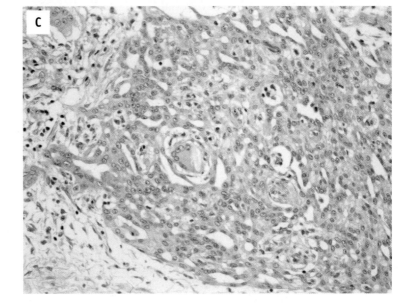

anaplasia varies from absent to marked. Most tumors grow on fibrous papillary stalks. The more anaplastic cells contain eosinophilic cytoplasm and hyperchromatic nuclei with prominent nucleoli and frequent mitoses. Solid sheets and complex papillary formations may be present. There is usually invasion of connective tissue. Mitoses may be numerous. The sarcomatous component of biphasic tumors grows in fascicular and storiform patterns and sometimes has numerous mitoses. Occasional psammoma bodies are present. Tumors may metastasize to inguinal and retroperitoneal lymph nodes; they may be present in surgical scars, skin, or spermatic cord; and they may metastasize to lungs, mediastinum, bone, or brain.

ANCILLARY STUDIES

IMMUNOHISTOCHEMISTRY

The cells, including spindle and epithelioid cells of malignant mesothelioma are positive for calretinin, cytokeratin 5 (CK5), CK6, and AE1-AE3. EMA and vimentin are usually positive. Malignant mesothelioma cells are negative for B72.3, LeuM1, Ber-Ep4, and CEA.

DIFFERENTIAL DIAGNOSIS

It is important to distinguish malignant mesothelioma from reactive mesothelial hyperplasia. The latter tends to occur in hernia sacs rather than in hydroceles, and often in young boys. Reactive mesothelial hyperplasia is quite cellular but noninvasive. Malignant mesothelioma must be distinguished from metastatic adenocarcinoma, serous tumors of borderline malignancy, and RTC. Serous borderline tumors often have papillae with stratified epithelial cells having a more columnar appearance. Tumors of ovarian-type epithelium (TOTEs) will generally stain positively for one or more of CEA, Ber-Ep4, LeuM1, and B72.3 and negatively for calretinin, in contrast to malignant mesotheliomas. The diagnosis of RTC should be considered and all or most of the criteria satisfied before rendering a definitive diagnosis. RTC is negative for calretinin.

PROGNOSIS AND TREATMENT

The diagnosis of malignant mesothelioma is usually not suspected preoperatively. If the initial presentation is a scrotal mass, orchiectomy should be performed with en bloc excision of involved adjacent structures. If the tumor is discovered during a transscrotal procedure, frozen sectioning should be performed, and, if the

diagnosis is made, an inguinal orchiectomy should be performed after consultation with the patient. Staging should be done after final pathologic evaluation. There is little experience to address further surveillance, treatment, or therapy. Consultation should be obtained with oncologists who treat malignant mesothelioma in other parts of the body. Follow-up of patients with malignant mesothelioma should be long-term, because these patients may develop mesothelioma in peritoneum or pleura at a later time.

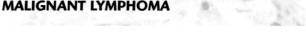

MALIGNANT LYMPHOMA

CLINICAL FEATURES

Malignant lymphomas of the testis may occur in prepubertal boys or adults, but the large majority are in men older than 50 years of age. Approximately 2% to 5% of testicular tumors are malignant lymphomas, and more than 50% of testis tumors in men older than 65 years of age are malignant lymphomas. In 20% to 38% of tumors, malignant lymphoma is bilateral and usually asynchronous. Survival is generally poor. Recent studies have recorded survival rates of 37% to 48% at 5 years and 19% to 27% at 10 years. Median survival times in two recent studies were 32 and 58 months. Malignant lymphomas usually manifest as painless testicular masses. Occasionally, bilateral testicular malignant lymphomas are initially present. Testicular malignant lymphoma usually is not associated with systemic disease at presentation.

PATHOLOGIC FEATURES

GROSS FINDINGS

Most malignant lymphomas involve the testis but often extend into epididymis and/or spermatic cord. In general, the testis is extensively replaced by an ill-defined, unencapsulated, tan-gray mass (Fig. 10-81).

MICROSCOPIC FINDINGS

Any type of non-Hodgkin's malignant lymphoma may occur in the testis.

Tumor cells infiltrate the interstitium, separating and infiltrating seminiferous tubular tunica propria and blood vessel walls (Fig. 10-82). In many areas, testicular architecture is totally obliterated. Tumor cells may extend into surrounding organs and soft tissues. The histologic appearance of the individual malignant lymphoma cells is similar to that in lymph nodes.

MALIGNANT LYMPHOMA—FACT SHEET

Definition

▶ A group of neoplasms composed of malignant lymphoid cells

Incidence and Location

▶ Most malignant lymphomas involving the testis are primary
▶ Intrascrotal malignant lymphoma predominantly involves the testis but may involve epididymis and spermatic cord
▶ Approximately 2% to 5% of testis tumors are malignant lymphomas
▶ Malignant lymphomas are bilateral in 20% to 38% of cases, usually asynchronous

Morbidity and Mortality

▶ Survival is generally poor
▶ Lymphoma grade and stage are related to survival
▶ 5- and 10-year survival rates are 37% to 48% and 19% to 27%, respectively

Race and Age Distribution

▶ Usually occur in men older than 50 years of age
▶ Most frequent testicular tumor in men older than 65 years of age
▶ May occur in prepubertal boys
▶ No racial predisposition

Clinical Features

▶ Usually manifest as painless testicular masses
▶ Usually unassociated with systemic lymphoma at presentation

Radiologic Features

▶ Ultrasound demonstrates the presence of a mass and may indicate extratesticular involvement
▶ Ultrasound may demonstrate multifocal bilateral tumors
▶ Ultrasonic appearance is not diagnostic of malignant lymphoma

Prognosis and Treatment

▶ Prognosis and treatment depend on cell type and tumor stage
▶ Most malignant lymphomas are stage IE
▶ Primary treatment is orchiectomy
▶ Additional treatment is chemotherapy and/or radiation
▶ Stage I unilateral tumors with microscopic sclerosis and follicular B cell lymphomas in prepubertal boys have a better prognosis
▶ Median survival times in two recent studies were 32 and 58 months
▶ Relapse from testicular malignant lymphoma occurs in extranodal sites, notably bone, central nervous system, skin, orbit, paranasal sinuses, stomach, nose, thyroid, and larynx

ANCILLARY STUDIES

IMMUNOHISTOCHEMISTRY

Because most patients with malignant lymphoma of the testis do not have a prior diagnosis of lymphoma, it is important to perform lymphoid marker studies. CD20 for B cell, CD3 for T cell, and CD45RB for leukocyte common antigen studies can be done on paraffin-embedded tissue.

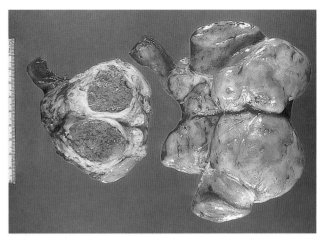

FIGURE 10-81
Malignant lymphoma in a bilateral orchiectomy specimen. Tan, homogeneous tumor massively obliterates one testis and focally involves the testis and paratesticular tissue of the other.

A small number of malignant lymphomas do not stain for these markers, and gene rearrangement studies for B-cell or T-cell receptor rearrangements may be helpful. Gene rearrangement study may be done on formalin-fixed, paraffin-embedded tissue by PCR. If a frozen section has been done and malignant lymphoma is suspected, if sufficient tissue is available, flow cytometry studies may allow detailed phenotyping.

MALIGNANT LYMPHOMA—PATHOLOGIC FEATURES

Gross Findings

▶ Mostly involves testis, but often extends into epididymis or spermatic cord
▶ Testis is extensively replaced by an ill-defined, tan-gray mass

Microscopic Findings

▶ Any type of non-Hodgkin's lymphoma can occur
▶ Tumor cells infiltrate the interstitium, separating and infiltrating seminiferous tubules and blood vessel walls
▶ May obliterate much testicular parenchyma
▶ Tumor cells may extend into rete testis, epididymis, tunica albuginea, or paratesticular soft tissue

Immunohistochemical Features

▶ Malignant lymphomas stain in the same way as those involving lymph nodes
▶ Malignant lymphomas are generally of large B cell type

Differential Diagnosis

▶ Seminoma
▶ Nonspecific granulomatous orchitis
▶ Specific (infectious) granulomatous orchitis
▶ Malakoplakia

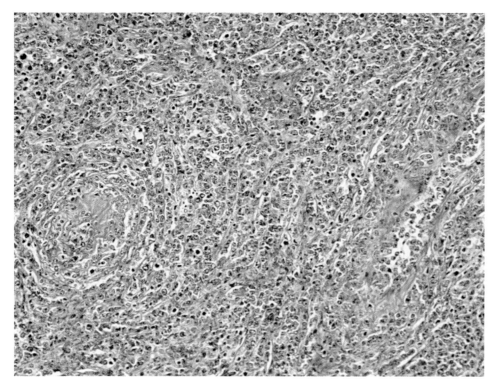

FIGURE 10-82
Massive infiltration of testicular parenchyma by malignant lymphoma, diffuse large B cell type. No residual testicular architecture is present.

DIFFERENTIAL DIAGNOSIS

The most important distinction is between a primary seminoma and malignant lymphoma. This usually is not a problem, and the diagnosis can be confirmed by using immunohistochemical lymphoma markers and PLAP and/or CD117, both of which mark seminoma cells. Rarely, non-neoplastic conditions mimic malignant lymphoma. Nonspecific granulomatous orchitis has a marked cellularity with lymphoid cells and may involve seminiferous tubular walls. The cell population of nonspecific granulomatous orchitis is variable, often comprising histiocytes and plasma cells. Lymphoma markers show monoclonality in malignant lymphoma and polyclonality in nonspecific granulomatous orchitis. A cellular population of histiocytes characterizes malakoplakia, which can be diagnosed by the demonstration of Michaelis-Gutmann bodies.

PROGNOSIS AND TREATMENT

The initial treatment of malignant lymphoma of the testis is orchiectomy. Prognosis and treatment are dependent on cell type and tumor stage. Most tumors are staged 1E. Further treatment consists of chemotherapy and/or irradiation. Most favorable malignant lymphomas are unilateral with microscopic sclerosis. Follicular B-cell lymphoma in prepubertal boys also has

a better prognosis. Relapse from primary testicular malignant lymphomas occurs in extranodal sites, including bone, central nervous system, skin, orbit, contralateral testis, paranasal sinuses, stomach, thyroid, and larynx. Tumors recurring in the testis (secondary malignant lymphomas) usually are primary in extranodal sites.

PLASMACYTOMA

Plasmacytoma is a malignant neoplasm, composed of plasma cells in any stage of differentiation, that may involve testicular and paratesticular structures.

CLINICAL FEATURES

Testicular plasmacytoma is a rare tumor, with 42 reported cases by 2001. Most patients either had known multiple myeloma or developed multiple myeloma after discovery of testicular plasmacytoma. Most patients die within 2 years after orchiectomy, although occasional long survival times, up to 26 years, have been reported. Most patients who have survived without evidence of disease after orchiectomy have had only a very short follow-up. The age range at the time of diagnosis is 2

Definition

▶ A tumor composed of malignant plasmocytes at any stage of differentiation

Incidence and Location

▶ Rare; 42 cases reported by 2001
▶ Primarily present in testis, but may be present in paratesticular tissue

Morbidity and Mortality

▶ Most patients develop plasma cell myeloma and die within 1 to 2 years.
▶ Long survival times have been reported rarely

Race and Age Distribution

▶ Age at discovery ranges from 26 to 89 years, with a mean of 55 years

Clinical Features

▶ The majority of patients have prior or subsequent multiple myeloma
▶ Most plasmacytomas develop a unilateral, painless intrascrotal mass
▶ 20% of patients develop asynchronous involvement of opposite testis
▶ Most have plasmacytoma at other sites at the time of diagnosis
▶ Most reported cases without clinical multiple myeloma have short follow-up

Radiologic Features

▶ Ultrasound demonstrates the presence of a mass
▶ There may be extratesticular lytic bone lesions in patients with multiple myeloma

Prognosis and Treatment

▶ Primary treatment is orchiectomy
▶ Prognosis is generally poor, because most patients have multiple myeloma
▶ Further therapy after orchiectomy depends on the diagnosis of multiple myeloma, which is treated with chemotherapy

to 89 years, with a mean of 55 years. Initially, tumors manifest as painless masses. At the time of diagnosis, most patients have plasmacytoma at other locations. Twenty percent of patients develop asynchronous involvement of the opposite testis.

RADIOLOGIC FEATURES

Ultrasonography demonstrates the presence of a mass. Radiologic studies of the skeleton may demonstrate lytic foci of multiple myeloma.

PATHOLOGIC FEATURES

GROSS FINDINGS

Tumors are solid, nonencapsulated, and tan to white masses that infiltrate and may replace testicular parenchyma. Plasmacytoma may extend into epididymis and/or spermatic cord and may be present exclusively or predominantly in an extratesticular location.

MICROSCOPIC FINDINGS

The growth pattern of plasmacytoma is similar to that of malignant lymphoma, although the cytology of tumor cells differs. Tumor cells extensively involve the interstitium and compress and invade the tunica propria of seminiferous tubules and the walls of blood vessels. Plasma cells may obliterate testicular architecture. Some cells have typical plasma cell morphology, with eccentric nuclei and perinuclear hofs, whereas

Gross Findings

▶ Plasmacytomas are solid, nonencapsulated, tan-white masses that infiltrate and may replace testicular parenchyma
▶ Plasmacytomas may extend into the epididymis and/or the spermatic cord

Microscopic Findings

▶ Tumor cells extensively involve the interstitium, compress and invade seminiferous tubules, and may obliterate testicular parenchyma
▶ Plasmacytomas are composed of masses of plasma cells in varying stages of differentiation
▶ Tumor cells may have typical plasma cell morphology with eccentric nuclei and perinuclear hofs, or they may be quite atypical with multinucleated cells
▶ The growth pattern of plasmacytoma is similar to that of malignant lymphoma, although the cytology of the tumor cells differs

Immunohistochemical Features

▶ Plasmacytoma cells express cytoplasmic immunoglobulin A (IgA) or IgM
▶ Plasmacytoma is positive for CD138
▶ Plasmacytoma cells may be weakly positive for CD45RB, and CD20
▶ Tumor cells may stain for EMA
▶ Tumor cells are negative for PLAP

Differential Diagnosis

▶ Malignant lymphoma
▶ Seminoma
▶ Spermatocytic seminoma
▶ LCT
▶ Granulocytic sarcoma
▶ Acute and chronic leukemias
▶ Malignant melanoma

others are quite atypical, with large multinucleated hyperchromatic cells.

ANCILLARY STUDIES

FLOW CYTOMETRY

Flow cytometry can be done on fresh tissue after notification of the laboratory that the case is possibly a plasmacytoma. The presence of κ or λ light chains can be identified.

IMMUNOHISTOCHEMISTRY

Plasmacytoma is strongly positive for CD138 and for κ or λ light chains.

DIFFERENTIAL DIAGNOSIS

A number of entities have somewhat similar features to plasmacytoma. Malignant lymphoma, large B cell type, may be difficult to distinguish from plasmacytoma. Large B cell lymphoma should be positive for CD20, weak or negative for κ or λ light chains, and variable for CD138. Plasmacytoma is negative or weakly positive for CD20 and CD45RB, positive for κ or λ light chains, and positive for CD138. Plasmacytoma may be mistaken for seminoma, but it lacks the distinctive cytologic appearance of seminoma cells and the associated granulomatous and lymphocytic foci. Immunohistochemical markers, CD117 and PLAP, should resolve diagnostic problems with seminoma. Spermatocytic seminoma occurs in similarly aged patients and is a very cellular neoplasm, but it has a characteristic triphasic appearance. Granulocytic sarcoma and leukemia have an intratesticular cellular distribution similar to that of plasmacytoma but are composed of different cell populations. Myeloperoxidase stains should confirm the presence of a granulocytic sarcoma or leukemia. Almost invariably, there is a history of leukemia. Metastatic cellular neoplasms such as malignant melanoma may present a diagnostic problem that can be solved with immunohistochemical markers. There should be a prior history of malignant melanoma, and the cells should be positive for HMB45 and S-100 protein. LCT is a potential differential diagnostic problem, but Leydig cells have more abundant eosinophilic, usually granular, cytoplasm, as well as a central nucleus and nucleolus. LCTs should stain prominently for inhibin.

LEUKEMIA

Acute and chronic leukemias may have testicular involvement.

CLINICAL FEATURES

Clinical involvement of the testis in leukemia is rare, affecting only about 5% of clinical cases, but may occur in both children and adults. However, approximately 63% of males with acute leukemia and 22% of those with chronic leukemia have testicular involvement at autopsy. In children with acute lymphoblastic leukemia, recurrence after remission may initially manifest in the testis. Testicular involvement is usually asymptomatic.

RADIOLOGIC FEATURES

Ultrasonography should demonstrate the presence of a gross mass, but it may be insensitive to small foci of recurrence.

PATHOLOGIC FINDINGS

GROSS FINDINGS

The leukemic involvement of testes mimics malignant lymphoma. Granulocytic sarcomas in other parts of the body may be green and have been called chloromas. Microscopic foci of leukemia are not identifiable grossly. Massive tumors are nonencapsulated, gray-white, and may obliterate testicular architecture and invade paratesticular tissues.

MICROSCOPIC FINDINGS

The growth pattern of leukemia mimics that of malignant lymphoma. Cellular morphology depends on the leukemic cell type and the degree of cellular differentiation. Cells may be immature myeloid or lymphoid types. The identification of eosinophilic myelocytes is suggestive of the diagnosis of granulocytic sarcoma. The recognition that the tumor is composed of immature cells of hematopoietic or lymphoid type points the way to further immunohistochemical and enzyme histochemical stains to obtain the correct diagnosis.

ANCILLARY STUDIES

HISTOCHEMISTRY

Enzyme histochemistry for lysozyme and acetyl chloresterase should be diagnostic of granulocytic leukemia.

IMMUNOHISTOCHEMISTRY

Lymphocytic markers can confirm the nature of a lymphocytic leukemia and can be used to investigate changes in tumor phenotype.

FLOW CYTOMETRY

Flow cytometry can be used on fresh tissue to obtain the phenotype.

DIFFERENTIAL DIAGNOSIS

The growth patterns of malignant lymphoma, plasmacytoma, and the leukemias are similar. The methods of distinguishing the types of neoplasm have been described earlier. In addition, orchitis enters the differential diagnosis from a histologic point of view. In mumps orchitis, there may be a massive intratubular and interstitial inflammation that raises the differential diagnosis of leukemia. The classic clinical history and the absence of immature cells should indicate the diagnosis of an inflammatory process. In cases of chronic orchitis of various causes, the absence of a monoclonal lymphoid population points to an inflammatory etiology.

PROGNOSIS AND TREATMENT

Only rarely does a testicular mass precede diagnosis of leukemia. In such cases, orchiectomy serves as a diagnostic procedure. Treatment of leukemia is with chemotherapy.

TUMORS OF OVARIAN-TYPE EPITHELIUM

The TOTEs resemble similarly named tumors of ovarian epithelial origin.

CLINICAL FEATURES

These tumors are quite rare, with approximately 22 cases reported by 1995. They are probably slightly more common than that, because TOTEs may have been misdiagnosed as other tumors. TOTEs occur in and around the testis and may extend beyond the tunica vaginalis. The age of patients with TOTEs reportedly ranges from 1 to 68 years, with a median age of 47 years. The median age in a series of six serous tumors on one study was 31 years. There may be an associated hydrocele.

RADIOLOGIC FEATURES

Ultrasonography should indicate the cystic and solid nature of the tumor and may suggest an intratesticular or extratesticular location.

TUMORS OF OVARIAN-TYPE EPITHELIUM—FACT SHEET

Definition
► Tumors which are histologically identical to tumors in the female that are derived from ovarian-type epithelium.

Incidence and Location
► Rare; approximately 22 cases were reported by 1995
► Serous tumors of borderline malignancy are most frequent
► TOTE may be underreported because of incorrect diagnosis
► Tumors occur in and around the testis and may extend beyond the tunica vaginalis

Morbidity and Mortality
► Most borderline serous tumors and Brenner tumors behave in a benign fashion if completely excised
► At least three tumors have been malignant, with at least one death
► At least one serous borderline tumor has metastasized

Age Distribution
► Age range is 11 to 68 years, with a median age of 47 years
► Median age of a series of serous carcinomas was 31 years

Clinical Features
► Tumors manifest as a testicular or paratesticular mass
► There may be an associated hydrocele
► Tumor recurrence may be preceded by or associated with elevated levels of serum CA-125

Radiologic Features
► Ultrasound should indicate the cystic and/or solid nature of the tumor and may suggest intratesticular or extratesticular location

Prognosis and Treatment
► Orchiectomy with complete excision of tumor is primary therapy
► Most borderline papillary serous tumors do not recur if completely excised, but one tumor with minimal invasion metastasized after 7 years
► Tumor should be diagnosed and staged accurately, using criteria for similar ovarian tumors
► Treatments should probably follow consultation with a gynecologic oncologist

TUMORS OF OVARIAN-TYPE EPITHELIUM—PATHOLOGIC FEATURES

Gross Findings

▶ Tumors are solid and cystic and may principally involve testicular or paratesticular tissue

▶ Serous tumors of borderline malignancy are cystic with papillary excrescences

▶ Serous carcinomas are solid and may be gritty

▶ Brenner tumors may be solid and/or cystic

▶ Mucinous tumors are predominantly cystic

Microscopic Findings

▶ By definition, the histology of the ovarian tumors resembles that of identically named tumors of the ovary

▶ Tumors thus far reported have been serous tumor of borderline malignancy, serous carcinoma, mucinous cystic tumor of borderline malignancy, mucinous cystadenocarcinoma, clear cell adenocarcinoma, endometrioid carcinoma, and endometrioid adenoacanthoma

▶ Careful gross and microscopic evaluation should be made of the location of the tumor

Immunohistochemical Features

▶ Serous tumors are usually positive for EMA, LeuM1, B72.3, and BerEp4 and negative for calretinin

Differential Diagnosis

▶ Teratoma with mucinous glandular areas vs. mucinous cystadenoma or mucinous cystadenocarcinoma of ovarian-type epithelium

▶ Malignant mesothelioma vs. serous borderline tumor and serous carcinoma

▶ Papillary serous adenoma and clear cell carcinoma of the epididymis vs. clear cell carcinoma of ovarian epithelial origin

PATHOLOGIC FEATURES

GROSS FINDINGS

Tumors are solid or cystic and may involve testis and/or paratesticular tissue. Serous tumors of borderline malignancy are cystic with papillary excrescences. Serous carcinomas are solid and may be gritty. Brenner tumors may be solid or cystic or both. Mucinous tumors are predominantly cystic.

MICROSCOPIC FINDINGS

By definition, the histology of TOTEs resembles that of similarly named tumors of the ovary. Tumors in the testis or paratesticular tissue reported thus far have been serous tumors of borderline malignancy, serous carcinoma, mucinous cystic tumor of borderline malignancy, mucinous cystadenocarcinoma, clear cell adenocarcinoma, endometrioid carcinoma, and Brenner tumor. Careful gross and microscopic evaluation should be made to ascertain the location of the tumor, and an attempt should be made to ascertain whether the tumor develops in the appendix testis, in the testicular-

epididymal groove, or from the mesothelium, or whether the tumor is completely intratesticular.

ANCILLARY STUDIES

IMMUNOHISTOCHEMISTRY

Serous tumors are usually positive for EMA and at least one of LeuM1, B72.3, CEA, and Ber-Ep4; they are negative for calretinin.

DIFFERENTIAL DIAGNOSIS

As in all testis tumors, it is necessary to rule out a primary GCT. Teratoma with mucinous glandular areas might mimic a mucinous cystadenoma or mucinous cystadenocarcinoma of ovarian-type epithelium. However, the latter tumor would have no IGCNU or nonmucinous teratomatous elements. Malignant mesothelioma with papillary formations enters the differential diagnosis of serous borderline malignant tumor and serous carcinoma, but mesothelioma usually has a single layer of cells covering papillary surfaces, in contrast to serous neoplasms. Mesothelioma is positive for calretinin, in contrast to TOTEs. Metastatic carcinoma should always be excluded, and a complete medical history should be obtained. Papillary cystadenoma and clear cell carcinoma of the epididymis might mimic a clear cell carcinoma of ovarian epithelial origin. Papillary cystadenomas of the epididymis are restricted to the epididymis, are often bilateral, and are usually associated with von Hippel-Lindau syndrome. Clear cell carcinomas of the epididymis are extremely rare, have a tubulopapillary growth pattern, and are histologically malignant.

PROGNOSIS AND TREATMENT

The primary treatment of TOTEs is orchiectomy. The pathologist should indicate whether the tumor appears to be completely excised or is at the margin of excision. Because of the rarity of the tumor, the urologist should probably consult with a gynecologic oncologist regarding possible further therapy.

METASTATIC TUMORS

In an autopsy population, metastatic carcinoma in the testis is identified from time to time. However, in clinical situations, metastatic tumors involving testis and paratesticular areas are quite rare.

CLINICAL FEATURES

The incidence of metastatic tumors is less than 1% of testicular tumors. These tumors are mostly carcinomas, may involve testis and paratesticular tissues, and occur mostly in men older than 50 years of age. The tumors usually manifest as a painless mass and are bilateral in 15% to 20% of cases. The origins of these neoplasms in clinical cases, in order of descending frequency, are prostate, renal cell carcinoma, malignant melanoma, lung, and carcinoid. The origins of neoplasms in autopsy studies, in descending order of frequency, are lung, malignant melanoma, prostate, and pancreas. In clinical situations, adenocarcinoma of the prostate is far more frequent than other carcinomas. In the past, this situation resulted from pathologic evaluations of testes in patients who had bilateral orchiectomy for palliation of hormone-resistant advanced prostatic adenocarcinoma. These metastatic prostatic adenocarcinomas in the testis were not symptomatic and usually not clinically palpable. Metastatic tumors in the testis usually occur in patients with known primary tumors; rarely, metastatic carcinoma involving the testis is the presenting finding.

RADIOLOGIC FEATURES

Ultrasonography should demonstrate tumors. Multifocality and bilaterality should raise the possibility of a metastatic tumor.

PATHOLOGIC FEATURES

GROSS FINDINGS

The neoplasm may have one or multiple masses or be vaguely nodular (Fig. 10-83). The size of the tumors is variable. Metastasis may cause replacement of the testis. Multiple nodules may occur in extratesticular locations.

MICROSCOPIC FINDINGS

The morphology of the tumor depends on the origin of the neoplasm. Neoplastic foci are usually multifocal in the intertubular areas, including intravascular spaces (Fig. 10-84). Neoplasm may be present in extratesticular tissue.

ANCILLARY STUDIES

IMMUNOHISTOCHEMISTRY

These studies are very important in regard to pinpointing the origin of the tumor. In cases where the

---

METASTATIC TUMORS—FACT SHEET

Definition
▶ Malignant neoplasms of extratesticular origin involving the testis

Incidence and Location
▶ Extremely rare, comprising fewer than 1% of testicular tumors
▶ May also involve paratesticular structures
▶ The large majority of metastatic neoplasms are discovered at autopsy
▶ Origins of neoplasms in clinical cases, in order of descending incidence, are prostate, renal cell carcinoma, malignant melanoma, lung, and carcinoid
▶ Origins of neoplasms in tumors at autopsy, in descending order of incidence, are lung, malignant melanoma, prostate, and pancreas

Morbidity and Mortality
▶ All tumors are malignant by definition

Race and Age Distribution
▶ Occur mostly (two thirds of cases) in men older than 50 years of age

Clinical Features
▶ Usually manifests as a painless mass
▶ Bilateral in 15% to 20%
▶ Usually occurs in a patient with a known primary tumor

Prognosis and Treatment
▶ In clinical situations, because the patient presents with a testicular mass, orchiectomy is the primary therapy. Further therapy depends on the nature of the primary tumor.
▶ Prognosis is usually poor

METASTATIC TUMORS—PATHOLOGIC FEATURES

Gross Findings
▶ Multiple or solitary masses in the testis and paratesticular tissue.
▶ Size can vary from barely visible to total replacement

Microscopic Findings
▶ Morphology of the tumor depends on the organ and tissue of origin
▶ Neoplasm is usually multifocal in intratubular areas and intravascular spaces
▶ Tumor may be present in extratesticular tissues
▶ Most metastatic tumors are carcinomas or malignant melanomas

Immunohistochemical Features
▶ Findings are characteristic of the primary tumor

Differential Diagnosis
▶ Primary testicular GCT
▶ Primary testicular LCT or SCT
▶ RTC
▶ Malignant lymphoma
▶ Plasmacytoma
▶ TOTE

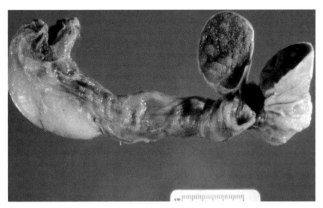

FIGURE 10-83

Metastatic small cell carcinoma of lung. Vaguely nodular formations are visible on the surface of the bivalved testis.

primary is known and the morphology of the testis tumor is similar to the primary, immunohistochemistry probably is not necessary.

DIFFERENTIAL DIAGNOSIS

The most important tumor in the differential diagnosis is a primary testicular GCT, because these tumors can be treated with specific and efficacious chemotherapy. LCT should be considered in the differential diagnosis of metastatic clear cell carcinoma of the kidney or adrenocortical carcinoma. SCT NOS enters the differential diagnosis of metastatic prostatic carcinoma and carcinoid. Testicular teratoma and mucinous cystadenocarcinomas of ovarian epithelial origin are in the differential diagnosis of metastatic intestinal carcinoma. Scattered small metastases from adenocarcinoma of the colon in the spermatic cord may raise the differential diagnosis of vasitis nodosum. In this situation, it is important to make certain that the patient did not have a prior vasectomy. The pathologist should attempt to verify the presence of intracytoplasmic or intraluminal mucin, which would be suggestive of a metastatic colonic tumor. Malignant lymphoma and plasmacytoma are in the differential diagnosis of metastatic cellular neoplasms. RTC is in the differential diagnosis of metastatic adenocarcinoma.

The pathologist should always be aware of the patient's previous medical history. Most primary tumors are known by the time a metastasis occurs in the testis. However, I have seen metastatic adenocarcinoma of the right colon that metastasized to paratesticular tissues and a small cell carcinoma of the lung that metastasized to the testis before discovery of the respective primary tumors. Clues to the site of origin of the colon cancer were the presence of stainable mucin and nuclear atypia. Multifocality and intravascular spread raised the suspicion of metastatic small cell carcinoma of the lung in the second case.

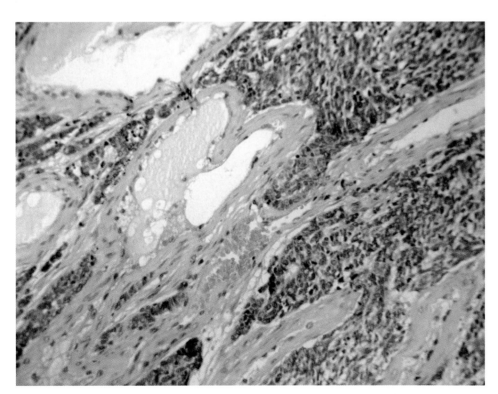

FIGURE 10-84

Metastatic small cell carcinoma of lung: microscopic findings. From the same case as Figure 10-83; multiple aggregates of metastatic undifferentiated small cell carcinoma are present in the interstitium.

PROGNOSIS AND TREATMENT

The therapy for a malignant testis mass is orchiectomy. However, there is nothing curative in the procedure for a patient with metastatic carcinoma. Metastasis in the testis indicates advanced disease and, hence, a poor prognosis. The correct diagnosis allows administration of appropriate chemotherapy and the assignment of an accurate prognosis.

Paratesticular Tumors

There are numerous tumors involving paratesticular structures that have identical features with those tumors elsewhere in the body. A few tumors that stand out because of their clinical importance or unique morphology are discussed here.

ADENOMATOID TUMOR

CLINICAL FEATURES

Adenomatoid tumors can occur in young children or older adults, but most occur in the third through fifth decades. There is no racial predominance. Similar tumors occur elsewhere in the body, such as the adrenal, retroperitoneum, or omentum. Adenomatoid tumor is the most frequent benign paratesticular neoplasm. It occurs in the epididymis, spermatic cord, and tunica albuginea. Adenomatoid tumors may have been present for months to years before discovery, and they may be first identified on a routine physical examination.

RADIOLOGIC FEATURES

Adenomatoid tumors are recognizable as a mass on ultrasound examination. The extratesticular location and diameter less than 5 cm should suggest the correct diagnosis.

PATHOLOGIC FEATURES

GROSS FINDINGS

Adenomatoid tumors are solid, resilient, firm, gray-white masses (Fig. 10-85). They are usually less than 3 cm and rarely greater than 5 cm in diameter. They are not associated with hemorrhage or necrosis.

ADENOMATOID TUMOR—FACT SHEET

Definition
▶ Benign tumor of mesothelial origin composed of structures often resembling glands

Incidence and Location
▶ The most frequent benign paratesticular neoplasm
▶ Occurs in epididymis, spermatic cord, and tunica albuginea
▶ Occurs most frequently in adults from the third to the fourth decades, and occasionally in children
▶ Similar tumors occur in other locations, including adrenal, peritoneum, and omentum

Morbidity and Mortality
▶ Benign

Gender, Race, and Age Distribution
▶ There is no racial predisposition
▶ Similar tumors appear in females, in proximity to the uterus and fallopian tubes

Clinical Features
▶ Usually discovered by the patient or by an examining doctor as a solitary, painless mass
▶ Rarely associated with pain
▶ May have been present for a long time

Radiologic Features
▶ Ultrasound demonstrates extratesticular location

Prognosis and Treatment
▶ Therapy is local excision, sparing the testis
▶ Location and tumor size should suggest the diagnosis

MICROSCOPIC FINDINGS

The tumors are predominantly extratesticular, may involve the tunica albuginea, and may infiltrate testicular parenchyma (Fig. 10-86). Adenomatoid tumors have an infiltrating growth pattern within fibrous tissue and smooth muscle. Tubular structures are comprised of epithelioid to endothelioid cells and may be plexiform, tubular, or canalicular (Fig. 10-87). Individual cells are often present and may have a signet-ring cell appearance. Vacuolated cells lining tubular structures may form spider web-like configurations, so-called threadlike bridging strands. The individual cells may have abundant eosinophilic cytoplasm or a flattened, attenuated appearance. Nuclei are usually small with small nucleoli. Lymphoid or plasma cell aggregates may be present. Rarely, adenomatoid tumors may infarct, produce pain, and have necrosis and reactive changes associated with them that may confound the diagnosis. Viable adenomatoid tumor, present in cases with infarction, should help to make the diagnosis.

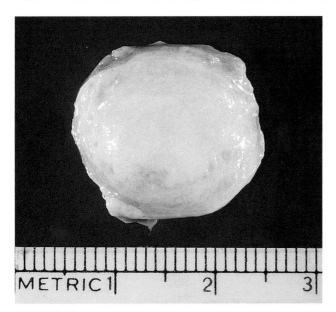

FIGURE 10-85
Adenomatoid tumor of epididymis. Resilient ,1.5-cm, white nodule.

ANCILLARY STUDIES

HISTOCHEMISTRY

The vacuoles and lumens contain acid mucin, which may be demonstrated by Hale's colloidal iron stain and Alcian blue stain at pH 2.5.

ELECTRON MICROSCOPY

Adenomatoid tumors have mesothelial features characterized by long, thin, nonbranched microvilli without a glycocalyx coating over much of the free surface. Microvilli project into intracellular lumina. The tumor cells contain tonofilaments. Junctional complexes are present between tumor cells. Spider webs are formed by juxtaposition of the plasma membrane of two apposed vacuolated mesothelial cells.

IMMUNOHISTOCHEMISTRY

Adenomatoid tumors stain positively for cytokeratin, EMA, and calretinin.

DIFFERENTIAL DIAGNOSIS

If it is recognized that the tumor is extratesticular, then the correct diagnosis is usually evident. If, however, the tumor involves testicular parenchyma, or if it is not recognized that the tissue of origin is extratesticular, then possible differential diagnoses include LCT, LCCSCT, YST, and histiocytoid hemangioma. LCTs tend to grow in sheets and aggregates and may have

---

ADENOMATOID TUMOR—PATHOLOGIC FEATURES

Gross Findings

► Solid, resilient to firm, gray-white, extratesticular mass less than 6 cm and usually less than 2 cm in diameter

Microscopic Findings

► Infiltrating growth pattern within fibrous and smooth muscle tissue
► Tubular structures comprise cells with an epithelioid to endothelioid appearance
► Individual cells may have abundant eosinophilic cytoplasm or a flattened, attenuated appearance
► Cells may be vacuolated with a "spider web" appearance
► There may be a lymphocytic or plasmacytic reaction

Ultrastructural Findings

► The mesothelial origin of the cell is demonstrated by long, nonbranched microvilli of the cell surface, which project into intracellular lumina

Immunohistochemical Features

► Tumor cells are positive for AE1-AE3, EMA, and calretinin
► Tumor cells are negative for endothelial markers, Ber-Ep4, CEA, B72.3, and LeuM1

Histochemical Features

► Hale's colloidal iron and Alcian blue stain at pH 2.5 demonstrate the presence of intracellular acid mucin

Differential Diagnosis

► YST
► Metastatic adenocarcinoma including signet-ring cell adenocarcinoma
► Malignant mesothelioma
► Histiocytoid hemangioma
► LCT

---

diagnostic intracytoplasmic Reinke's crystals. A cellular adenomatoid tumor might resemble the "tumor" of CAH, but cells of the latter lack vacuoles and grow more in a sheet-like or nodular pattern. In addition, the clinical history of a patient with CAH is characteristic. LCCSCT comprises large eosinophilic cells, but these are multifocal in the testis, may be present within seminiferous tubules, and are associated with laminated calcifications. Histiocytoid hemangioma may have a similar histologic appearance to adenomatoid tumor. The cells of histiocytoid hemangioma may contain intracytoplasmic vacuoles. However, blood may be recognized within lumina, the tumor may have a lobular configuration, and the cells should be positive for immunohistochemical markers for endothelial cells. The glandular pattern of YST could be confused with adenomatoid tumor. YST occurs within the parenchyma of the testis. However, on frozen section, the pathologist may not be able to determine the tissue of origin. In this case, it is mandatory to recognize that the tumor

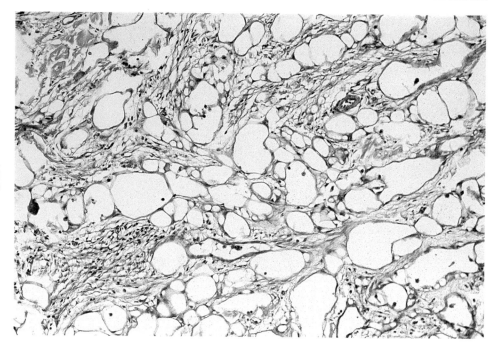

FIGURE 10-86

Adenomatoid tumor of epididymis. Infiltrating tubular structures lined by attenuated cells. Note numerous "spider webs."

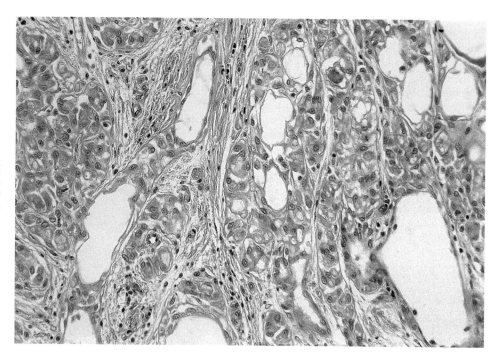

FIGURE 10-87

Extratesticular adenomatoid tumor. Cells with abundant cytoplasm, and others that are attenuated, line tubular structures. Some cells are vacuolated. Rare "spider webs" are present.

has originated in extratesticular tissue. On permanent section, characteristic patterns of YST should be present and some cells should be positive for AFP.

PROGNOSIS AND TREATMENT

All adenomatoid tumors are uniformly benign. The therapy is local excision, sparing the testes.

SARCOMA

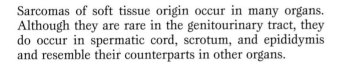

Sarcomas of soft tissue origin occur in many organs. Although they are rare in the genitourinary tract, they do occur in spermatic cord, scrotum, and epididymis and resemble their counterparts in other organs.

CLINICAL FEATURES

Sarcomas usually manifest as painless intrascrotal masses. Most childhood sarcomas are rhabdomyosarcomas, which have peak incidences at 4 to 6 years and in adolescence. Rhabdomyosarcomas occur with less frequency into the mid-30s. In adults, by far the most frequent sarcoma is liposarcoma, with a median age of 58 years. Other sarcomas that occur with some frequency are leiomyosarcoma and malignant fibrous histiocytoma. Mortality and morbidity depend on histologic tumor type, tumor stage, and the presence of sarcoma at the surgical margin of the specimen. There is no known racial predisposition. In patients with childhood rhabdomyosarcoma, there is a worsened prognosis for patients who are older than 10 years of age and have tumors greater than 5 cm in diameter.

RADIOLOGIC FEATURES

Sarcomas and their location should be identified with ultrasonography.

PATHOLOGIC FEATURES

GROSS FINDINGS

Embryonal rhabdomyosarcoma tends to be lobulated and soft, with focal hemorrhage and necrosis. Well-differentiated liposarcomas are usually large and yellow and resemble lipomas. Other types of liposarcomas may be fleshy, firm, myxoid, and gray-white. Leiomyosarco-

---

PARATESTICULAR SARCOMAS—FACT SHEET

Definition
- ▶ Malignant tumors of mesenchymal origin that almost always occur in a paratesticular location and are histologically similar to sarcomas elsewhere in the body

Incidence and Location
- ▶ Sarcomas of the genitourinary tract account for fewer than 5% of sarcomas in all parts of the body
- ▶ Spermatic cord tumors are 30% of genitourinary sarcomas and number approximately 100 cases per year in the United States

Morbidity and Mortality
- ▶ Morbidity and mortality depend on histologic type, tumor stage, and the presence of tumor at the surgical margin of resection
- ▶ Morbidity consists of local recurrence and distant metastasis

Race and Age Distribution
- ▶ There is no known racial predisposition
- ▶ Pediatric sarcoma in boys younger than 16 years of age are almost invariably rhabdomyosarcoma
- ▶ Childhood rhabdomyosarcoma has peak incidences at age 4 to 6 years and again in adolescence
- ▶ Adult sarcoma (16 years of age and older) may be of any type
- ▶ The median age of adult sarcoma is 58 years

Clinical Features
- ▶ Palpable mass in the scrotum or inguinal region
- ▶ Liposarcomas are often discovered at the time of inguinal hernia repair

Radiologic Features
- ▶ Ultrasound detects the presence of an intrascrotal or inguinal mass. Additional radiologic studies should detect retroperitoneal or pulmonary involvement

Prognosis and Treatment
- ▶ Prognosis depends on histologic type, tumor stage, and complete excision
- ▶ Poor prognosis relates to histologic type of rhabdomyosarcoma. The small number of cases makes it difficult to assess the affect of tumor grade in other types of sarcoma
- ▶ Primary treatment consists of wide local excision, with re-excision and orchiectomy, if needed, to ensure negative margins
- ▶ RPLND is used for some cases of rhabdomyosarcoma and for other sarcomas with proven lymphatic invasion
- ▶ Liposarcoma rarely metastasizes but can recur
- ▶ Chemotherapy and radiation therapy are used to treat rhabdomyosarcoma and have been used to treat other types of sarcoma

---

mas occur mostly in the spermatic cord and may be gray-white and whorled. High-grade sarcomas tend to be hemorrhagic and necrotic. It is important to identify the location of sarcomas. Primary sarcomas of the testis are rare, including those that occur in association with GCTs.

MICROSCOPIC FINDINGS

The majority of rhabdomyosarcomas are embryonal rhabdomyosarcoma, including a spindle cell variant. Rarely, alveolar and mixed alveolar/embryonal types occur in a pediatric population. Pleomorphic rhabdomyosarcoma is rare and tends to occur in older patients. The histology of rhabdomyosarcoma is similar to that in other parts of the body, with the exception of the spindle cell variant. This variant is comprised of medium-sized spindle cells in a storiform and whorled pattern. The cells have ovoid nuclei and prominent nucleoli. The non-spindle cell embryonal rhabdomyosarcoma is composed of malignant small cells with little eosinophilic cytoplasm. Small foci of elongate cells with abundant cytoplasm may be present. The small cells infiltrate structures of the spermatic cord, epididymis, or tunica albuginea, surrounding and compressing any ducts in the area (Fig. 10-88). Liposarcomas in paratesticular locations resemble those elsewhere. The surgeon and the pathologist should ascertain whether these tumors are present in paratesticular structures alone or have extended from or to the retroperitoneum. The majority of liposarcomas are well differentiated and may be lipoma-like or sclerosing. The second most frequent type of sarcoma is the dedifferentiated liposarcoma of high or low grade. Rare myxoid/round cell liposarcomas may occur.

ANCILLARY STUDIES

ELECTRON MICROSCOPY

Electron microscopy may be used to identify rhabdomyosarcoma by identifying thick and thin filaments and Z-bands. Electron microscopy rarely may be useful to distinguish rhabdomyosarcoma from other malignant small cell tumors.

IMMUNOHISTOCHEMISTRY

Rhabdomyosarcoma cells are positive for muscle-specific actin, desmin, and vimentin, and they are less frequently positive for myoglobin and troponin T.

DIFFERENTIAL DIAGNOSIS

The paratesticular location should be carefully ascertained, and sarcoma should be distinguished from sarcomas of testicular, scrotal, or retroperitoneal locations. Rhabdomyosarcomas should be distinguished from other small cell tumors, including melanotic neuroectodermal tumor (retinal anlage tumor) and desmoplastic small round cell tumor (DSRCT). Melanotic neuroectodermal tumors occur in infants and young boys, usually in the epididymis, and consist of nests of melanin-containing epithelioid cells, gland-like structures, and small round cells resembling neuroblasts. These tumors, which also occur in the orbit, generally have a benign behavior but rarely metastasize. DSRCT is a tumor of adolescents and young adults that occurs in the scrotum as well as the peritoneum. This tumor contains nests of numerous small cells growing within a desmoplastic stroma. The tumor cells are small, round to spindled, with scant cytoplasm, small hyperchromatic nuclei, and small nucleoli. Mitoses are frequent. Tumor cells are positive for cytokeratin, EMA, neuron-specific enolase, desmin, and WT1. DSRCTs are more aggressive than rhabdomyosarcomas in the paratesticular region.

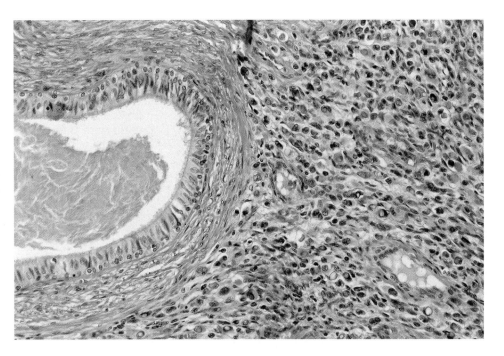

FIGURE 10-88

Infiltrating embryonal rhabdomyoblasts at the edge of the epididymal duct.

Well-differentiated liposarcoma must be distinguished from lipoma. Identifying lipoblasts or atypical cells within dense collagenous tissue confirms the diagnosis of liposarcoma.

PROGNOSIS AND TREATMENT

In patients with rhabdomyosarcoma, prognosis relates to tumor histology and surgical-pathologic staging. The latter is based on the Intergroup Rhabdomyosarcoma Study Group (IRSG) staging system and relates to the extent of the tumor, its complete or incomplete excision, and the presence or absence of metastases. Of the tumor types, embryonal rhabdomyosarcoma, particularly the spindle cell variant, has the best clinical prognosis. In the two most recent IRSG studies, the 3-year failure-free survival rates were 95% and 81% for embryonal rhabdomyosarcoma. In the two most recent Malignant Mesenchymal Tumor studies of the International Society of Pediatric Oncology, overall the 5-year survival rate was 92%, with an event-free survival rate of 82%. In this study, boys younger than 10 years of age with a tumor less than 5 cm in diameter had a better prognosis. Patients with alveolar rhabdomyosarcoma fare worse than those with embryonal rhabdomyosarcoma and are treated more intensively. Alveolar rhabdomyosarcoma in the paratesticular region has a better prognosis than does alveolar rhabdomyosarcoma in other parts of the body. The treatment of localized rhabdomyosarcoma consists of surgery and chemotherapy. Retroperitoneal lymph node biopsy is not done routinely but only if there is radiologic suspicion of retroperitoneal tumor in boys younger than 10 years of age. Staging ipsilateral RPLND is done for boys older than 10 years. Liposarcomas are treated by complete excision. Well-differentiated liposarcomas tend to recur over many years, but they do not metastasize. There are no large studies of liposarcomas with adequate follow-up, but myxoid/round cell and dedifferentiated liposarcomas may persist, recur, or metastasize.

PAPILLARY CYSTADENOMA OF THE EPIDIDYMIS

Papillary cystadenoma of the epididymis (PCE) is a unique lesion of the head of the epididymis that consists of papillary formations and cysts.

CLINICAL FEATURES

More than 50 cases of PCE have been reported, approximately 60% of which have been associated with von Hippel-Lindau disease. Approximately 17% of patients with von Hippel-Lindau syndrome have PCE, which in most cases is bilateral. Rare cases have occurred in the spermatic cord. The tumors manifest as intrascrotal masses with or without pain. Some patients present with infertility. It is possible that the papillary formations within the epididymis obstruct the egress of spermatozoa. There is no racial predisposition. PCEs have been reported in patients aged 16 to 81 years.

PATHOLOGIC FEATURES

GROSS FINDINGS

PCEs may be solid or multicystic and can measure up to 6 cm in diameter. They occur in the head of the epididymis near the efferent ducts. Cystic tumors may contain fluid.

PAPILLARY CYSTADENOMA OF THE EPIDIDYMIS—FACT SHEET

Definition

▶ A benign epithelial tumor of the epididymis growing in a tubulopapillary pattern

Incidence and Location

▶ Rare; more than 50 cases reported
▶ Occurs in the head of the epididymis
▶ Rare cases have occurred in the spermatic cord

Morbidity and Mortality

▶ Benign
▶ If the patient has von Hippel-Lindau disease, mortality and morbidity relate to the other manifestations of the disease
▶ May be associated with infertility

Race and Age Distribution

▶ No racial predisposition
▶ Age ranges from 16 to 81 years

Clinical Features

▶ Intrascrotal mass with or without pain
▶ Some men present with infertility
▶ Usually bilateral in patients with von Hippel-Lindau disease
▶ Approximately 60% of cases are associated with von Hippel-Lindau disease, and approximately 17% of patients with the disease have papillary cystadenoma of the epididymis

Prognosis and Treatment

▶ Treatment is local excision; results are excellent results in men without von Hippel-Lindau disease
▶ Prognosis in patients with von Hippel-Lindau disease relates to other manifestations of the disease

MICROSCOPIC FINDINGS

The tumor is composed of intraductal or intracystic papillary formations, ectatic ducts, microcysts, and intervening fibrous stroma (Fig. 10-89). Epithelial cells lining cysts and papillae are cuboidal to columnar, often with cleared cytoplasm, and contain glycogen and secretory droplets. Cysts may contain eosinophilic material.

ANCILLARY STUDIES

IMMUNOHISTOCHEMISTRY

Epithelial cells are positive for keratin (AE1-AE3 and CAM5.2) and EMA.

DIFFERENTIAL DIAGNOSIS

Although PCE has a distinct appearance, there is possible confusion with metastatic renal cell carcinoma and adenocarcinoma of the epididymis. Patients with von Hippel-Lindau disease often have multifocal bilateral renal cell carcinomas of clear cell type. These may have low-grade nuclei, but renal cell carcinoma, clear cell type, may also show more nuclear variability. The likelihood of a renal cell carcinoma metastasizing to the epididymis is small. Only a few primary adenocarcinomas of the epididymis have been reported. Although the latter have comprised tubulopapillary formations

FIGURE 10-89
Papillary cystadenoma of the epididymis. **A,** Solid and tubular structures are composed of cells with clear cytoplasm, round nuclei, and small nucleoli.

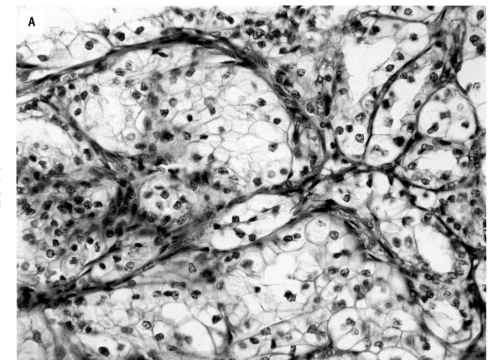

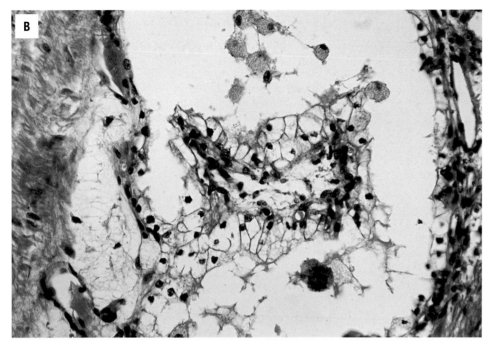

FIGURE 10-89, CONT'D

B, In the same tumor, a papillary structure is observed within a small cyst lined by clear cells.

PAPILLARY CYSTADENOMA OF THE EPIDIDYMIS—PATHOLOGIC FEATURES

Gross Findings

▶ Solid and cystic or multicystic masses up to 6 cm in diameter in the head of the epididymis near the efferent ducts

Microscopic Findings

▶ Intraductal or intracystic papillary formations, ectatic ducts, microcysts, and fibrous stroma
▶ Epithelial cells lining cysts and papillae are cuboidal to columnar and contain glycogen and secretory droplets
▶ Cysts may contain eosinophilic material

Immunohistochemical Features

▶ Epithelial cells are positive for keratin (AE1-AE3 and CAM5.2) and EMA

Differential Diagnosis

▶ Metastatic renal cell carcinoma
▶ Adenocarcinoma of the epididymis

---

and clear cells as well as tubular formations, adenocarcinomas have an infiltrating growth pattern and the capability to metastasize. There has been no known association between primary epididymal adenocarcinoma and von Hippel-Lindau disease. Other carcinomas may metastasize to the epididymis, but they should demonstrate features unlike those of PCE.

SUGGESTED READINGS

Germ Cell Tumors

Tumours of the urinary system and male genital organs: WHO histological classification of testis tumors. In Eble JN, Sauter G, Epstein J, Sesterhenn I (eds.): World Health Organization Classification of Tumours: Pathology and Genetics. Lyon, France, IARC Press, 2004, pp 218–219.

Ulbright T: Testicular and paratesticular neoplasms. In Sternberg SS (ed.): Diagnostic Surgical Pathology, 4th ed. Philadelphia, Lippincott Williams & Wilkins, 2004, pp 2168–2171.

Ulbright T, Amin M, Young R: Tumors of the testis, adnexa, spermatic cord and scrotum: Classification of testicular and paratesticular tumors and tumor like lesions. In Rosai J, Sobin L (eds.): AFIP Atlas of Tumor Pathology, 3rd series, Fascicle 25. Washington, DC, Armed Forces Institute of Pathology, 1999, pp 16–17.

Intratubular Germ Cell Neoplasia Unspecified

Berthelesen JG, Skakkebaek NE, Mogensen P, Sorensen BL: Incidence of carcinoma in situ of germ cells in contralateral testis of men with testicular tumors. Br Med J 1979;2:363–364.

de Jong B, Oosterhuis W, Castedo S, et al: Pathogenesis of adult testicular germ cell tumors: A cytogenetic model. Cancer Genet Cytogenet 1990;48:143–167.

Fowler JE, Whitmore WF Jr: Intratesticular germ cell tumors: Observations on the effect of chemotherapy. J Urol 1981;126:412–414.

Grigor KM, Wylie CC: The origin and biology of CIS cells: general discussion. APMIS 1998;106:221–224.

Jorgensen MN, Muller J, Giwercman A, Skakkebaek NE: Clinical and biological significance of carcinoma in situ of the testis. Cancer Surveys 1990;9:287–302.

Jorgensen N, Rajpert-De Meyts E, Graem N, et al: Expression of immunohistochemical markers for testicular carcinoma in situ by normal human fetal germ cells. Lab Invest 1996;180:206–213.

Krabbe S, Berthelesen JG, Volsted P, et al: High incidence of undetected neoplasia in maldescended testes. Cancer 1979;44:1357–1362.

Müller J, Skakkebaek NE: Testicular carcinoma in situ in children with the androgen insensitivity (testicular feminization) syndrome. Br Med J 1984;288:1419–1420.

Skakkebaek NE: Carcinoma in situ of testis in testicular feminization syndrome. Acta Pathol Microbiol Scand 1979;87A:87–89.

Skakkebaek NE: Carcinoma in situ of the testis: Frequency and relationship to invasive germ cell tumors in infertile men. Histopathology 1978;2:157–170.

Van Echten J, van Gurp RJ, Stoepker M, et al: Cytogenetic evidence that carcinoma in situ is the precursor lesion for invasive testicular germ cell tumors. Cancer Genet Cytogenet 1995;85:133–137.

Von der Maase H, Rorth M, Walbom-Jorgenson S, et al: Carcinoma in situ of contralateral testis in patients with testicular germ cell cancer: Study of 27 cases in 500 patients. Br Med J 1986;293:1938–1401.

Seminoma

Daugaard G, Petersen PM , Rorth M: Surveillance in stage I testicular cancer. APMIS 2003;111:76–85.

Hori K, Uematsu K, Yasoshima H, et al: Testicular seminoma with human chorionic gonadotrophin production. Pathol Int 1997;47:592–599.

McGlynn RA, Devesa SS, Sigurdson AJ, et al: Trends in the incidence of testicular germ cell tumors in the United States. Cancer 2003;97:63–70, 203.

Nazeer T, Ro JY, Amato RJ, et al: Histologically pure seminoma with elevated alpha-fetoprotein: A clinicopathologic study of ten cases. Oncol Rep 1998;5:1425–1429.

Rhagavan D, Sullivan AL, Peckham MJ, Neville AM. Elevated serum alpha-fetoprotein and seminoma. Cancer 1982;50:982–989.

Warde P, Specht L, Horwich A, et al: Prognostic factors for relapse in stage I seminoma managed by surveillance: A pooled analysis. J Clin Oncol 2002;20:4448–4452.

Yuasa T, Yoshiki T, Ogawa O, et al: Detection of alpha-fetoprotein mRNA in seminoma. J Andrology 1999;20:336–340.

Zuckman MH, Williams G, Levin HS: Mitosis counting in seminoma: An exercise of questionable significance. Hum Pathol 1988;19:329–335.

Spermatocytic Seminoma

Eble JN: Spermatocytic seminoma. Hum Pathol 1994;25:1035–1042.

Floyd C, Ayala AG, Logothetis CJ, Silva EG: Spermatocytic seminoma with associated sarcoma of the testis. Cancer 1988;61:409–414.

True LD, Otis CN, Delprado W, et al: Spermatocytic seminoma of testis with sarcomatous transformation: A report of five cases. Am J Surg Pathol 1988;12:75–82.

True LD, Scully RE, Delprado W: Spermatocytic seminoma of testis with sarcomatous transformation [letter to the editor]. Am J Surg Pathol 1988;12:806.

Ulbright TM: Neoplasms of the testis: Spermatocytic seminoma. In Bostwick DG, Eble JN (eds): Urologic Surgical Pathology. St Louis, Mosby, 1997, pp 585–587.

Embryonal Carcinoma

Ulbright T, Amin M, Young R: Tumors of the testis, adnexa, spermatic cord and scrotum: Embryonal carcinoma. In Rosai J, Sobin L (eds.): AFIP Atlas of Tumor Pathology, 3rd series, Fascicle 25. Washington, DC, Armed Forces Institute of Pathology, 1999, pp 103–118.

Woodward P, Heidenreich A, Looijenga L, et al: Tumors of the urinary system and male genital organs: Embryonal carcinoma. In Eble J, Sauter G, Epstein J, Sesterhenn I (eds): WHO Classification of Tumours: Pathology and Genetics. Lyon, France, IARC Press, 2004, pp 236–237.

Yolk Sac Tumor

Czaja JT, Ulbright TM: Evidence for the transformation of seminoma to yolk sac tumor, with histogenetic considerations. Am J Clin Pathol 1992;97:468–477.

Grady R, Ross J, Kay R: Patterns of metastatic spread in prepubertal yolk sac tumors. J Urol 1995;153:1259–1261.

Hu LM, Philipson J, Barsky SH: Intratubular germ cell neoplasia in infantile yolk sac tumor: Verification by tandem repeat sequence in-situ hybridization. Diagn Mol Pathol 1992;1:118–128.

Klepp O, Olsson A, Henrickson H, et al: Prognostic factors in clinical stage I nonseminomatous germ cell tumors of the testis: Multivariate

analysis of a prospective multicenter study. J Clin Oncol 1990;8:509–518.

Levy D, Kay R, Elder J: Neonatal testis tumors: A review of the Prepubertal Testis Tumor Registry. J Urol 1994;151:715–717.

Logothetis C, Samuels M, Trindade A, et al: The prognostic significance of endodermal sinus tumor histology among patients treated for stage III nonseminomatous germ cell tumors of the testis. Cancer 1984;53:122–128.

Palmer HE, Safaii H, Wolfe HF: Alpha-1-antitrypsin and alpha-fetoprotein: Protein markers in endodermal sinus (yolk sac) tumors. Am J Clin Pathol 1976;65:575–582.

Perlman E, Hu J, Ho D, et al: Genetic analysis of childhood endodermal sinus tumors by comparative genomic hybridization. J Pediatr Hematol Oncol 2000;22:100–105.

Talerman A: Endodermal sinus (yolk sac) tumor elements in testicular germ cell tumors in adults: Comparison of prospective and retrospective studies. Cancer 1980;46:1213–1217.

Talerman A: The incidence of yolk sac tumor (endodermal sinus tumor) elements in germ cell tumors of the testis in adults. Cancer 1975;36:211–215.

Teilum G: Special Tumors of Ovary and Testis: Histological Identification. Philadelphia, JB Lippincott, 1976, pp 146–147.

Ulbright T, Roth L, Broadhecker C: Yolk sac differentiation in germ cell tumors: A morphologic study of 50 cases with emphasis on hepatic, enteric and parietal yolk sac features. Am J Surg Pathol 1986;10:151–164.

Teratoma

Baniel J, Perez J, Foster R: Benign testicular tumor associated with Klinefelter's syndrome. J Urol 1994;151:157–158.

Berdjis C, Mostofi FK: Carcinoid tumors of the testis. J Urol 1977;118:777–782.

Fishleder A, Tubbs R, Levin H: An immunoperoxidase technique to aid in the differential diagnosis of prostatic carcinoma. Cleve Clin Q 1981;48:331–335.

Heidenreich A, Engelmann U, Vietsch H, Derschum W: Organ-preserving surgery in testicular epidermoid cysts. J Urol 1995;153:1147–1150.

Hosking D, Bowman D, McMorris S, Ramsey E: Primary carcinoid of the testis with metastases. J Urol 1981;125:255–256.

Jalota A, Middleton R, McDivitt R: Epidermoid cyst of the testis in Gardner's syndrome. Cancer 1974;34:464–467.

Michael H, Hull M, Ulbright T, et al: Primitive neuroectodermal tumors arising in testicular germ cell neoplasms. Am J Surg Pathol 1997;21:896–904.

Michael H, Lucia J, Foster R, Ulbright T: The pathology of late recurrence of testicular tumors. Am J Surg Pathol 2000;24:247.

Price EB Jr: Epidermoid cysts of the testis: A clinical and pathologic analysis of 69 cases from the testicular tumor registry. J Urol 1969;102:708–731.

Ross J, Kay R, Elder J: Testis-sparing surgery for pediatric epidermoid cysts of the testis. J Urol 1993;149:353–356.

Strahlberg M, Brown J: Concomitant bilateral epidermoid cysts of the testis. J Urol 1973;109:343–435.

Ulbright T: Testicular and paratesticular neoplasms: Teratomas. In Sternberg SS (ed): Diagnostic Surgical Pathology, 4th ed. Philadelphia, Lippincott Williams & Wilkins, 2004, pp 2188–2191.

Ulbright T, Amin M, Young R: Tumors of the testis, adnexa, spermatic cord and scrotum: Teratoma. In Rosai J, Sobin L (eds.): AFIP Atlas of Tumor Pathology, 3rd series, Fascicle 25. Washington, DC, Armed Forces Institute of Pathology, 1999, pp 147–164.

Ulbright T, Loehrer P, Roth J, et al: The development of non-germ cell malignancies within germ cell tumors: A clinicopathologic study of 11 cases. Cancer 1984;54:1824.

Unger P, Cohen P, Talerman A: Mixed germ cell tumor of the testis: A unique combination of seminoma and teratoma composed predominantly of prostatic tissue. J Urol Pathol 1998;9:257.

Woodward P, Heidenreich A, Looijenga L: Tumors of the urinary system and male genital organs: Teratoma. In Eble J, Sauter G, Epstein J, Sesterhenn I (eds): WHO Classification of Tumours: Pathology and Genetics. Lyon, France, IARC Press, 2004, pp 243–246.

Zavala-Pompa A, Ro J, el-Naggar A, et al: Primary carcinoid tumor of testis: Immunohistochemical, ultrastructural and DNA flow cytometric study of three cases with review of the literature. Cancer 1993;72:1726–1732.

Choriocarcinoma

Brigden M, Sullivan L, Comisarow RH: Stage C pure choriocarcinoma of the testis: A potentially curable lesion. Cancer J Clin 1982;32:82–84.

Ulbright T, Amin M, Young R: Tumors of the testis, adnexa, spermatic cord and scrotum: Choriocarcinoma and other rare forms of trophoblastic neoplasia. In Rosai J, Sobin L (eds.): AFIP Atlas of Tumor Pathology, 3rd series, Fascicle 25. Washington, DC, Armed Forces Institute of Pathology, 1999, pp 138–147.

Ulbright T, Young R, Scully R: Trophoblastic tumors of the testis other than classic choriocarcinoma: "Monophasic" choriocarcinoma and placental site trophoblastic tumor. A report of two cases. Am J Surg Pathol 1997;21:282–288.

Woodward P, Heidenreich A, Looijenga L: Tumors of the urinary system and male genital organs: Trophoblastic tumors. In Eble J, Sauter G, Epstein J, Sesterhenn I (eds): WHO Classification of Tumours: Pathology and Genetics. Lyon, France, IARC Press, 2004, pp 240–243.

Mixed Germ Cell Tumors

Greene FL, Page DL, Fleming ID, Balch CM (eds): AJCC Cancer Staging Manual, 6th ed. New York, Springer, 2002, pp 317–322.

Mostofi FK, Sesterhenn I, Davis CJ: Immunopathology of germ cell tumors of the testis. Semin Diagn Pathol 1987;4:320–341.

Ulbright T, Amin M, Young R: Tumors of the testis, adnexa, spermatic cord and scrotum: Mixed germ cell tumors. In Rosai J, Sobin L (eds.): AFIP Atlas of Tumor Pathology, 3rd series, Fascicle 25. Washington, DC, Armed Forces Institute of Pathology, 1999, pp 175–181.

Woodward P, Heidenreich A, Looijenga L, et al: Tumors of the urinary system and male genital organs: Tumours of more than one histological type (mixed forms). In Eble J, Sauter G, Epstein J, Sesterhenn I (eds): WHO Classification of Tumours: Pathology and Genetics. Lyon, France, IARC Press, 2004, pp 246–249.

Leydig Cell Tumor

Billings S, Roth L, Ulbright T: Microcystic Leydig cell tumor mimicking yolk sac tumor: A report of four cases. Am J Surg Pathol 1999;23:546.

Canto P, Soderlund D, Ramon G, et al: Mutational analysis of leuteinizing hormone receptor gene in two individuals with Leydig cell tumors. Am J Med Genet 2002;108:148–152.

Collins D, Cameron K: Interstitial-cell tumor. Br J Urol Suppl 1964;36:62–69.

Dieckmann K, Loy V: Metachronous germ cell and Leydig cell tumors of the testis: Do testicular germ cell tumors and Leydig cell tumors share common etiologic factors? Cancer 1993;72:1305–1307.

Gabrilove J, Nicolis G, Mitty H, Sohval A: Feminizing interstitial cell tumor of the testis: Personal observations and a review of the literature. Cancer 1975;35:1184–1202.

Gittes R, Smith G, Conn C, Smith F: Local androgenic effect of interstitial cell tumor of the testis. J Urol 1970;104:774–777.

Jockenhovel J, Rutgers J, Mason J, et al: Leydig cell neoplasia in a patient with Reifenstein syndrome. Exp Clin Endocrinol 1993;101:365–370.

Kim F, Young R, Scully R: Leydig cell tumors of the testis: A clinicopathologic analysis of 40 cases and review of the literature. Am J Surg Pathol 1985;9:177.

Moul J, Schanne R, Thompson I, et al: Testicular cancer in blacks: A multicenter experience. Cancer 1994;73:388–393.

Palazzo J, Peterson R, Young R, Scully R: Deoxyribonucleic acid flow cytometry of testicular Leydig cell tumors. J Urol 1994;152:415–417.

Poster R, Katz D: Leydig cell tumor of the testis in Klinefelter syndrome: MR detection. J Comput Assist Tomogr 1993;17:480–481.

Sesterhenn I, Cheville J, Woodward P: Tumors of the urinary system and male genital organs: Leydig cell tumour. In Eble J, Sauter G, Epstein J, Sesterhenn I (eds): WHO Classification of Tumours: Pathology and Genetics. Lyon, France, IARC Press, 2004, pp 250–251.

Sohval A, Churg J, Gabrilove J: Ultrastructure of feminizing testicular Leydig cell tumors. Ultrastruct Pathol 1982;3:335–345.

Ulbright T: Testicular and paratesticular neoplasms: Leydig cell tumor. In Sternberg S (ed): Diagnostic Surgical Pathology, 4th ed. Philadelphia, Lippincott Williams & Wilkins, 2004, pp 2198–2200.

Ulbright T, Amin M, Young R: Tumors of the testis, adnexa, spermatic

cord and scrotum: Leydig cell tumor. In Rosai J, Sobin L (eds.): AFIP Atlas of Tumor Pathology, 3rd series, Fascicle 25. Washington, DC, Armed Forces Institute of Pathology, 1999, pp 210–218.

Ulbright T, Srigley J, Hatzianastassiou D, Young R: Leydig cell tumors of the testis with unusual features: Adipose differentiation, calcification with ossification, and spindle shaped tumor cells. Am J Surg Pathol 2002;26:1424–1433.

Sertoli Cell Tumor

Amin M, Young R, Scully R: Immunohistochemical profile of Sertoli and Leydig cell tumors of the testis. Mod Pathol 1998;11:76A.

Henley J, Young R, Ulbright T: Malignant Sertoli cell tumor of the testis: A study of 13 examples of a neoplasm frequently misinterpreted as seminoma. Am J Surg Pathol 2002;26:541–550.

Sesterhenn I, Cheville J, Woodward P, et al: Tumors of the urinary system and male genital organs: Sertoli cell tumour. In Eble J, Sauter G, Epstein J, Sesterhenn I (eds): WHO Classification of Tumours: Pathology and Genetics. Lyon, France, IARC Press, 2004, pp 252–255.

Ulbright T, Amin M, Young R: Tumors of the testis, adnexa, spermatic cord and scrotum: Sertli cell tumors. In Rosai J, Sobin L (eds.): AFIP Atlas of Tumor Pathology, 3rd series, Fascicle 25. Washington, DC, Armed Forces Institute of Pathology, 1999, pp 193–202.

Young R, Koelliker D, Scully R: Sertoli cell tumors of the testis, not otherwise specified: A clinicopathologic analysis of 60 cases. Am J Surg Pathol 1998;22:709–721.

Zukerberg L, Young R, Scully R: Sclerosing Sertoli cell tumor of the testis: A report of 10 cases. Am J Surg Pathol 1991;15:829–834.

Large Cell Calcifying Sertoli Cell Tumor

Dryer L, Jacyk WK, du Plessis DJ: Bilateral large cell calcifying Sertoli cell tumor of the testes with Peutz-Jeghers syndrome: A case report. Pediatr Dermatol 1994;11:335–337.

Kratzer SS, Ulbright TM, Talerman A, et al: Large cell calcifying Sertoli cell tumor of the testis: Contrasting features of six malignant and six benign tumors and a review of the literature. Am J Surg Pathol 1997;21:1271–1280.

Nara M, Ray R, Bergada I, et al: Sertoli cell proliferation of the infantile testis: An intratubular form of Sertoli cell tumor. Am J Surg Pathol 2001;25:1237–1244.

Nogales F, Andujar M, Zuluaga A, Garcia-Puche J: Malignant large cell calcifying Sertoli cell tumor of the testis. J Urol 1995;153:1935–1937.

Proppe K, Scully R: Large-cell calcifying Sertoli cell tumor of the testis. Am J Clin Pathol 1980;74:607–619.

Tetu B, Ro J, Ayala A: Large cell calcifying Sertoli cell tumor of the testis: A clinicopathologic, immunohistochemical and ultrastructural study of two cases. Am J Clin Pathol 1991;96:717–722.

Ulbright T, Amin M, Young R: Tumors of the testis, adnexa, spermatic cord and scrotum: Large cell calcifying Sertoli cell tumor. In Rosai J, Sobin L (eds.): AFIP Atlas of Tumor Pathology, 3rd series, Fascicle 25. Washington, DC, Armed Forces Institute of Pathology, 1999, pp 202–210.

Granulosa Cell Tumors

Chan J, Chan V, Mak K: Congenital juvenile granulosa cell tumor of the testis: Report of a case showing extensive degenerative changes. Histopathology 1990;17:75–80.

Lawrence W, Young R, Scully R: Juvenile granulosa cell tumor of the infantile testis: A report of 14 cases. Am J Surg Pathol 1985;9:87–94.

Raju U, Fine G, Rajasekharan W, et al: Congenital testicular juvenile granulosa cell tumor in a neonate with X/XY mosaicism. Am J Surg Pathol 1986;10:577–583.

Ranaka Y, Sasaki Y, Tachibana K, et al: Testicular juvenile granulosa cell tumor in infant with X/XY mosaicism clinically diagnosed as true hermaphroditism. Am J Surg Pathol 1994;18:316–322.

Sesterhenn I, Cheville J Woodward PJ, et al: Tumors of the urinary system and male genital organs: Granulosa cell tumour group. In Eble J, Sauter G, Epstein J, Sesterhenn I (eds): WHO Classification of Tumours: Pathology and Genetics. Lyon, France, IARC Press, 2004, pp 256–257.

Shukla A, Huff D, Canning, et al: Juvenile granulosa cell tumor of the testis: Contemporary clinical management and pathologic diagnosis. J Urol 2004;171:1900–1902.

Fibroma-Thecoma

Sesterhenn I, Cheville J, Woodward PJ, et al: Tumors of the urinary system and male genital organs: Tumours of the thecoma/fibroma group. In Eble J, Sauter G, Epstein J, Sesterhenn I (eds): WHO Classification of Tumours: Pathology and Genetics. Lyon, France, IARC Press, 2004, p 257.

Ulbright T, Amin M, Young R: Tumors of the testis, adnexa, spermatic cord and scrotum: Tumors in the fibroma/thecoma group. In Rosai J, Sobin L (eds.): AFIP Atlas of Tumor Pathology, 3rd series, Fascicle 25. Washington, DC, Armed Forces Institute of Pathology, 1999, pp 226–227.

Mixed Sex Cord-Stromal Tumors

Jorgensen N, Müller J, Jaubert F, et al: Heterogeneity of gonadoblastoma germ cells: Similarities with immature germ cells, spermatogonia and testicular carcinoma in situ cells. Histopathology 1997;30:177–186.

Scully RE: Gonadoblastoma: A review of 74 cases. Cancer 1970;25:1340–1356.

Sesterhenn I, Cheville J, Woodward P, et al: Tumors of the urinary system and male genital organs: Tumours containing both germ cell and sex cord/gonadal stromal elements. In Eble J, Sauter G, Epstein J, Sesterhenn I (eds): WHO Classification of Tumours: Pathology and Genetics. Lyon, France, IARC Press, 2004, pp 259–260.

Talerman A, Delemarre JFM: Gonadoblastoma associated with embryonal carcinoma in an anatomically normal male. J Urol 1975;113:355–359.

Ulbright T: Mixed sex cord-gonadal stromal tumors: Testicular and paratesticular neoplasms. In Sternberg S (ed): Diagnostic Surgical Pathology, 4th ed. Philadelphia, Lippincott Williams & Wilkins, 2004, pp 2205–2206.

Ulbright T, Amin M, Young R: Tumors of the testis, adnexa, spermatic cord and scrotum: Gonadoblastoma. In Rosai J, Sobin L (eds.): AFIP Atlas of Tumor Pathology, 3rd series, Fascicle 25. Washington, DC, Armed Forces Institute of Pathology, 1999, pp 185–191.

Unclassified Sex Cord Tumors

Sesterhenn I, Cheville J, Woodward PJ, et al: Tumors of the urinary system and male genital organs. Sex cord/gonadal stromal tumors: Incompletely differentiated. In Eble J, Sauter G, Epstein J, Sesterhenn I (eds): WHO Classification of Tumours: Pathology and Genetics. Lyon, France, IARC Press, 2004, p 257.

Sesterhenn I, Cheville J, Woodward P, et al: Tumors of the urinary system and male genital organs. Sex cord/gonadal stromal tumors: Mixed forms. In Eble J, Sauter G, Epstein J, Sesterhenn I (eds): WHO Classification of Tumours: Pathology and Genetics. Lyon, France, IARC Press, 2004, pp 257–258.

Ulbright T, Amin M, Young R: Tumors of the testis, adnexa, spermatic cord and scrotum: Sex cord-stromal tumors, mixed and unclassified. In Rosai J, Sobin L (eds.): AFIP Atlas of Tumor Pathology, 3rd series, Fascicle 25. Washington, DC, Armed Forces Institute of Pathology, 1999, pp 227–229.

Rete Testis Carcinoma

Nochomovitz L: Tumors of the urinary system and male genital organs: Tumors of collecting ducts and rete. In Eble J, Sauter G, Epstein J, Sesterhenn I (eds): WHO Classification of Tumours: Pathology and Genetics. Lyon, France, IARC Press, 2004, pp 265–266.

Orozco R, Murphy W: Carcinoma of the rete testis: Case report and review of the literature. J Urol 1993;150:974–977.

Stein J, Freeman J, Esrig D, et al: Papillary adenocarcinoma of the rete testis: A case report and review of the literature. Urology 1994;44:588–594.

Ulbright T, Amin M, Young R: Tumors of the testis, adnexa, spermatic cord and scrotum: Carcinoma of the rete testis. In Rosai J, Sobin L (eds.): AFIP Atlas of Tumor Pathology, 3rd series, Fascicle 25. Washington, DC, Armed Forces Institute of Pathology, 1999, pp 240–243.

Malignant Mesothelioma

Davis C, Woodward P, Dehner L, et al: Tumors of the urinary system and male genital organs: Malignant mesothelioma. In Eble J, Sauter G, Epstein J, Sesterhenn I (eds): WHO Classification of Tumours: Pathology and Genetics. Lyon, France, IARC Press, 2004, pp 267–270.

Jones M, Young R, Scully R: Malignant mesothelioma of the tunica vaginalis: A clinicopathologic analysis of 11 cases with review of the literature. Am J Surg Pathol 1995;19:815–825.

Plas E, Riedl C, Pfluger H: Malignant mesothelioma of the tunica vaginalis testis: Review of the literature and assessment of prognostic parameters. Cancer 1998;83:2437–2446.

Ulbright T, Amin M, Young R: Tumors of the testis, adnexa, spermatic cord and scrotum: Malignant mesothelioma. In Rosai J, Sobin L (eds.): AFIP Atlas of Tumor Pathology, 3rd series, Fascicle 25. Washington, DC, Armed Forces Institute of Pathology, 1999, pp 247–253.

Malignant Lymphoma

Ferry J, Harris N, Young R, et al: Malignant lymphoma of the testis, epididymis, and spermatic cord: A clinicopathologic study of 69 cases with immunophenotypic analysis. Am J Surg Pathol 1994;18:376–390.

Finn L, Viswanatha D, Belasco J, et al: Primary follicular lymphoma of the testis in childhood. Cancer 1999;85:1626.

LaGrange J, Ramaioli A, Theodore C, et al: Non Hodgkin's lymphoma of the testis: A retrospective study of 84 patients treated in the French Anticancer Centers. Ann Oncol 2001;12:1313–1319.

Marks A, Woodward P: Tumors of the urinary system and male genital organs: Lymphoma and plasmacytoma of the testis and paratesticular tissues. In Eble J, Sauter G, Epstein J, Sesterhenn I (eds): WHO Classification of Tumours: Pathology and Genetics. Lyon, France, IARC Press, 2004, pp 263–264.

Ulbright T, Amin M, Young R: Tumors of the testis, adnexa, spermatic cord and scrotum: Malignant lymphoma. In Rosai J, Sobin L (eds.): AFIP Atlas of Tumor Pathology, 3rd series, Fascicle 25. Washington, DC, Armed Forces Institute of Pathology, 1999, pp 272–277.

Zietman AL, Coen JJ, Ferry JA, et al: The management of outcome of stage IAE non Hodgkin's lymphoma of the testis. J Urol 1996;155:43–46.

Zucca E, Conconi A, Mughal T, et al: Patterns of outcome and prognostic factors in primary large cell lymphoma of the testis in a survey by the International Extragonadal Lymphoma Study Group. J Clin Oncol 2003;21:20–27.

Plasmacytoma

Levin H, Mostofi FK: Symptomatic plasmacytoma of the testis. Cancer 1970;25:1193–1203.

Marx A, Woodward P: Tumors of the urinary system and male genital organs: Lymphoma and plasmacytoma of the testis and paratesticular tissues. In Eble J, Sauter G, Epstein J, Sesterhenn I (eds): WHO Classification of Tumours: Pathology and Genetics. Lyon, France, IARC Press, 2004, pp 263–264.

Oppenheim PI, Cohen S, Anders KH: Testicular plasmacytoma: A case report with immunohistochemical studies and literature [review]. Arch Pathol Lab Med 1991;115:629–632.

Ulbright T, Amin M, Young R: Tumors of the testis, adnexa, spermatic cord and scrotum: Multiple myeloma and plasmacytoma. In Rosai J, Sobin L (eds.): AFIP Atlas of Tumor Pathology, 3rd series, Fascicle 25. Washington, DC, Armed Forces Institute of Pathology, 1999, pp 277–279.

Leukemia

Buchanan G, Boyett J, Pollock B, et al: Improved treatment results in boys with overt testicular relapse during or shortly after initial therapy for acute lymphoblastic leukemia: A Pediatric Oncology Group study. Cancer 1991;68:48–55.

Ulbright T, Amin M, Young R: Tumors of the testis, adnexa, spermatic cord and scrotum: Leukemia including granuocytic sarcoma. In Rosai J, Sobin L (eds.): AFIP Atlas of Tumor Pathology, 3rd series, Fascicle 25. Washington, DC, Armed Forces Institute of Pathology, 1999, pp 279–281.

Tumors of Ovarian-Type Epithelium

De Nictolis M, Tommasoni S, Fabris G, Prat J: Intratesticular serous cystadenoma of borderline malignancy: A pathological histochemical and DNA contents study of a case with long term follow-up. Virchows Archiv A Pathol Anat 1993;423:221–225.

Jones M, Young R, Srigley J, Scully R: Paratesticular serous papillary carcinoma: A report of 6 cases. Am J Surg Pathol 1995;19:1359–1365.

Ulbright T, Amin M, Young R: Tumors of the testis, adnexa, spermatic cord and scrotum: Ovarian-type epithelial tumors. In Rosai J, Sobin L (eds.): AFIP Atlas of Tumor Pathology, 3rd series, Fascicle 25. Washington, DC, Armed Forces Institute of Pathology, 1999, pp 235–239.

Young R, Scully E: Testicular and paratesticular tumors and tumor-like lesions of ovarian common epithelial and Müllerian types. Am J Clin Pathol 1986;86:146–152.

Metastatic Tumors

Davis C. Tumors of the urinary system and male genital organs: Secondary tumors. In Eble J, Sauter G, Epstein J, Sesterhenn I (eds): WHO Classification of Tumours: Pathology and Genetics. Lyon, France, IARC Press, 2004, pp 277–278.

Haupt H, Mann R, Trump DL, et al: Metastatic carcinoma involving the testis: Clinical and pathological distinction from primary testicular neoplasms. Cancer 1984;54:709–714.

Price EB Jr, Mostofi FK: Secondary carcinoma of the testis. Cancer 1957;10:592–595.

Tiltman A: Metastatic tumors of the testis. Histopathology 1979;3:31–37.

Ulbright T, Amin M, Young R: Tumors of the testis, adnexa, spermatic cord and scrotum: Secondary tumors. In Rosai J, Sobin L (eds.): AFIP Atlas of Tumor Pathology, 3rd series, Fascicle 25. Washington, DC, Armed Forces Institute of Pathology, 1999, pp 281–285.

Adenomatoid Tumor

Davis C, Woodward P: Tumors of the urinary system and male genital organs: Adenomatoid tumour. In Eble J, Sauter G, Epstein J, Sesterhenn I (eds): WHO Classification of Tumours: Pathology and Genetics. Lyon, France, IARC Press, 2004, p 267.

Hes O, Peres-Montiel D, Alvarado-Cabrero I, et al: Thread-like bridging strands: A morphologic feature present in all adenomatoid tumors. Ann Diagn Pathol 2003;7:273–277.

Schwartz E, Longacre T: Adenomatoid tumors of the female and male genital tracts express WT1. Intl Gynecol Pathol 2004;23:123–128.

Skinnider B, Young R: Infarcted adenomatoid tumor: A report of five cases of a benign neoplasm that may cause diagnostic difficulty. Am J Surg Pathol 2004;28:77–83.

Ulbright T, Amin M, Young R: Tumors of the testis, adnexa, spermatic cord and scrotum: Adenomatoid tumor. In Rosai J, Sobin L (eds.): AFIP Atlas of Tumor Pathology, 3rd series, Fascicle 25. Washington, DC, Armed Forces Institute of Pathology, 1999, pp 243–246.

Sarcoma

Coleman J, Brennan M, Alektiar K, et al: Adult spermatic cord sarcomas: Management and results. Ann Surg Oncol 2003;10:669–675.

Crist W, Anderson J, Meza L, et al. Intergroup rabdomyosarcoma study IV: Results for patients with nonmetastatic disease. J Clin Oncol 2001;19:3091–3102.

Davis C, Woodward P: Tumors of the urinary system and male genital organs: Desmoplastic small round cell tumour. In Eble J, Sauter G, Epstein J, Sesterhenn I (eds): WHO Classification of Tumours: Pathology and Genetics. Lyon, France, IARC Press, 2004, pp 272–273.

Davis C, Woodward P: Tumors of the urinary system and male genital organs: Melanotic neuroectodermal tumour. In Eble J, Sauter G, Epstein J, Sesterhenn I (eds): WHO Classification of Tumours: Pathology and Genetics. Lyon, France, IARC Press, 2004, pp 271–272.

Davis C, Woodward P: Tumors of the urinary system and male genital organs: Mesenchymal tumours of the scrotum, spermatic cord, and testicular adnexa. In Eble J, Sauter G, Epstein J, Sesterhenn I (eds): WHO Classification of Tumours: Pathology and Genetics. Lyon, France, IARC Press, 2004, pp 273–276.

Leuschner I, Newton WA, Schmidt D, et al: Spindle cell variants of embryonal rhabdomyosarcoma in the paratesticular region: A report of the Intergroup Rhabdomyosarcoma Study. Am J Surg Pathol 1993;17: pp 221–230.

Montgomery E, Fisher C: Paratesticular liposarcoma: A clinicopathologic study. Am J Surg Pathol 2003;271:40–47.

Raney B, Anderson J, Barr F, et al.: Rhabdomyosarcoma and undifferentiated sarcoma in the first two decades of life: A selective review of Intergroup Rhabdomyosarcoma Study Group experience and rationale for Intergroup Rhabdomyosarcoma Study V. J Pediatr Hematol Oncol 2001;23:215–220.

Stewart R, Martelli H, Oberlin O, et al: Treatment of children with nonmetastatic paratesticular rhabdomyosarcoma: Results of the Malignant Mesenchymal Tumors studies (MMT 84 and MMT 89) of the International Society of Pediatric Oncology. J Clin Oncol 2003; 21:793–78.

Ulbright T, Amin M, Young R: Tumors of the testis, adnexa, spermatic cord and scrotum: Desmoplastic small round cell tumor. In Rosai J, Sobin L (eds.): AFIP Atlas of Tumor Pathology, 3rd series, Fascicle 25. Washington, DC, Armed Forces Institute of Pathology, 1999, pp 253–254.

Ulbright T, Amin M, Young R: Tumors of the testis, adnexa, spermatic cord and scrotum: Retinal anlage tumor. In Rosai J, Sobin L (eds.): AFIP Atlas of Tumor Pathology, 3rd series, Fascicle 25. Washington, DC, Armed Forces Institute of Pathology, 1999, pp 256–259.

Ulbright T, Amin M, Young R: Tumors of the testis, adnexa, spermatic cord and scrotum: Sarcoma. In Rosai J, Sobin L (eds.): AFIP Atlas of Tumor Pathology, 3rd series, Fascicle 25. Washington, DC, Armed Forces Institute of Pathology, 1999, pp 265–271.

Papillary Cystadenoma of the Epididmyis

Davis C, Woodward P: Tumors of the urinary system and male genital organs: Papillary cystadenoma of epididymis. In Eble J, Sauter G, Epstein J, Sesterhenn I (eds): WHO Classification of Tumours: Pathology and Genetics. Lyon, France, IARC Press, 2004, pp 270–271.

Jones E, Murray M, Young R: Cysts and epithelial proliferations of the testicular collecting system (including rete testis). Semin Diagn Pathol 2000;17:270–293.

Leung S, Chan A, Wong M, et al. Expression of vascular endothelial growth factor in von Hippel-Lindau syndrome-associated papillary cystadenoma of the epididymis. Hum Pathol 1998;29:1322–1324.

Price EB Jr: Papillary cystadenoma of the epididymis: A clinicopathologic analysis of 20 cases. Arch Pathol 1971;91:456–470.

Ulbright T, Amin M, Young R: Tumors of the testis, adnexa, spermatic cord and scrotum: Papillary cystadenoma of the epididymis. In Rosai J, Sobin L (eds.): AFIP Atlas of Tumor Pathology, 3rd series, Fascicle 25. Washington, DC, Armed Forces Institute of Pathology, 1999, pp 254–255.

Index

Genitourinary Pathology

Genitourinary Pathology

A Volume in the Series
Foundations in Diagnostic Pathology

Edited by

Ming Zhou, MD, PhD
Staff Pathologist
Anatomic Pathology, Urology and Cancer Biology
Cleveland Clinic
Cleveland, Ohio

Cristina Magi-Galluzzi, MD, PhD
Director, Genitourinary Pathology
Department of Anatomic Pathology
Cancer Biology and Glickman Urologic Institute
Cleveland Clinic
Cleveland, Ohio

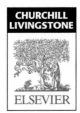

CHURCHILL
LIVINGSTONE

ELSEVIER

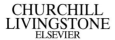

1600 John F. Kennedy Blvd.
Ste 1800
Philadelphia, PA 19103-2899

GENITOURINARY PATHOLOGY (A VOLUME IN THE   ISBN-13:   978-0-443-06677-1
FOUNDATIONS IN DIAGNOSTIC PATHOLOGY SERIES,   ISBN-10:   0-443-06677-9
Series Edited by John R. Goldblum)

Notice

Knowledge and best practice in this field are constantly changing. As new research and experience broaden our knowledge, changes in practice, treatment and drug therapy may become necessary or appropriate. Readers are advised to check the most current information provided (i) on procedures featured or (ii) by the manufacturer of each product to be administered, to verify the recommended dose or formula, the method and duration of administration, and contraindications. It is the responsibility of the practitioner, relying on their own experience and knowledge of the patient, to make diagnoses, to determine dosages and the best treatment for each individual patient, and to take all appropriate safety precautions. To the fullest extent of the law, neither the Publisher nor the Authors assume any liability for any injury and/or damage to persons or property arising out or related to any use of the material contained in this book.

The Publisher

Library of Congress Cataloging-in-Publication Data

Genitourinary pathology / Ming Zhou, Cristina Magi-Galluzzi, [editors];
series editor, John R. Goldblum.
    p. cm. — (Foundations in diagnostic pathology)
    ISBN 0-443-06677-9
    ISBN-13: 978-0-443-06677-1
    1. Genitourinary organs—Diseases. I. Zhou, Ming, MD, PhD II. Magi-
Galluzzi, Cristina. III. Series.
    RC871.G455 2007
    616.6—dc22

                     2006040173

Acquisitions Editor: Belinda Kuhn
Developmental Editor: Heather Krehling
Project Manager: David Saltzberg
Design Direction: Louis Forgione

Printed in China

Last digit is the print number: 9   8   7   6   5   4   3   2

To my wife, Lan
To my daughters, Grace and Rebecca
To my parents, Yinhai Zhou and Xiudi Guo
Ming Zhou

To the memory of my mother, Federica Bizzarri
To my father, Orfeo Magi Galluzzi
Cristina Magi-Galluzzi

Contributors

Mahul B. Amin, MD
Chairman
Department of Pathology and Laboratory Medicine
Cedars-Sinai Medical Center
Los Angeles, California
Diseases of the Penis, Urethra, and Scrotum

Lois J. Arend, MD, PhD
Associate Professor
Director, Renal Pathology and Electron Microscopy Services
Pathology and Laboratory Medicine
University of Cincinnati Medical Center
Cincinnati, Ohio
Introduction to Renal Biopsy

Laura Barisoni, MD
Assistant Professor
Department of Pathology
Renal Pathology Laboratory
New York University Medical Center
New York, New York
Introduction to Renal Biopsy

Stephen M. Bonsib, MD
Director
Surgical Pathology Professor
Department of Pathology
Indiana University School of Medicine
Indianapolis, Indiana
Non-neoplastic Diseases of the Kidney

Liang Cheng, MD
Associate Professor
Department of Pathology
Indiana University School of Medicine
Indianapolis, Indiana
Neoplasms of the Kidney

John N. Eble, MD, MBA, FRCPA
Nordschow Professor and Chairman
Department of Pathology and Laboratory Medicine
Van Nuys Medical Science Building
Indianapolis, Indiana
Neoplasms of the Kidney

Jonathan I. Epstein, MD
The Reinhard Professor of Urologic Pathology
Departments of Pathology, Urology, and Oncology
Director of Surgical Pathology and Anatomic Pathology
The Johns Hopkins Hospital
Baltimore, Maryland
Non-neoplastic Diseases of the Prostate
Neoplasms of the Prostate and Seminal Vesicles
Non-neoplastic Diseases of the Urinary Bladder
Neoplasms of the Urinary Bladder

Eyas M. Hattab
Assistant Professor
Department of Pathology
Indiana University School of Medicine
Indianapolis, Indiana
Neoplasms of the Kidney

Howard S. Levin, MD
Staff Pathologist Emeritus
Department of Anatomic Pathology
Cleveland Clinic
Cleveland, Ohio
Non-neoplastic Diseases of the Testis
Neoplasms of the Testis

Cristina Magi-Galluzzi, MD, PhD
Director, Genitourinary Pathology
Departments of Anatomic Pathology,
  Cancer Biology, and Urology
Cleveland Clinic
Cleveland, Ohio
Non-neoplastic Diseases of the Prostate
Neoplasms of the Prostate and Seminal Vesicles
Non-neoplastic Diseases of the Urinary Bladder
Neoplasms of the Urinary Bladder

Shane Meehan, MD
Assistant Professor
Pathology Department
University of Chicago
Chicago, Illinois
Introduction to Renal Biopsy

Rajal B. Shah, MD
Associate Professor of Pathology and Urology
Chief, Section of Urologic Pathology
University of Michigan Medical School
Ann Arbor, Michigan
Diseases of the Penis, Urethra, and Scrotum

Ming Zhou, MD, PhD
Staff Pathologist
Departments of Anatomic Pathology,
  Urology, and Cancer Biology
Cleveland Clinic
Cleveland, Ohio
Non-neoplastic Diseases of the Prostate
Neoplasms of the Prostate and Seminal Vesicles
Non-neoplastic Diseases of the Urinary Bladder
Neoplasms of the Urinary Bladder

Foreword

The study and practice of anatomic pathology are both exciting and overwhelming. Surgical pathology, with all of the subspecialties it encompasses, and cytopathology have become increasingly complex and sophisticated, and it is not possible for any individual to master the skills and knowledge required to perform all of these tasks at the highest level. Simply being able to make a correct diagnosis is challenging enough, but the standard of care has far surpassed merely providing a diagnosis. Pathologists are now asked to provide large amounts of ancillary information, both diagnostic and prognostic, often on small amounts of tissue, a task that can be daunting even to the most experienced pathologist.

Although large general surgical pathology textbooks are useful resources, they, by necessity, could not possibly cover many of the aspects the pathologist needs to know and include in their reports. As such, the concept behind *Foundations in Diagnostic Pathology* was born. This series is designed to cover the major areas of surgical and cytopathology, and each edition is focused on one major topic. The goal of every book in this series is to provide the essential information that any pathologist, whether general or subspecialized, in training or in practice, would find useful in the evaluation of virtually any type of specimen encountered.

My colleagues at The Cleveland Clinic, Drs. Cristina Magi-Galluzzi and Ming Zhou, both superb genitourinary pathologists, have edited what I believe to be an outstanding, state-of-the-art book on the essentials of genitourinary pathology. The list of contributors is impressive and includes renowned pathologists from across the United States, all of whom have built a national and international reputation in this field. The content in each chapter is extremely practical, well-organized, and concisely written, focusing on the thorough evaluation of both needle biopsy and resection specimens. Since virtually all practicing pathologists encounter these specimens with some regularity, the information provided by these experts will contribute to resolving problems encountered at the microscope on virtually any sign-out day.

This edition is organized into ten chapters covering the full spectrum of genitourinary disorders. Drs. Magi-Galluzzi, Zhou, and Epstein provide separate chapters on non-neoplastic and neoplastic diseases of the prostate and urinary bladder. Dr. Bonsib provides a straight-forward and practical review of non-neoplastic diseases of the kidney, followed by a cutting-edge discussion of renal neoplasms by Drs. Hattab, Cheng, and Eble. A unique chapter by Drs. Barisoni, Meehan, and Arend discusses an approach to the renal biopsy. Diseases of the penis, urethra, and scrotum are reviewed by Drs. Shah and Amin, followed by chapters on non-neoplastic and neoplastic diseases of the testis by my colleague and longtime mentor, Dr. Howard Levin.

I wish to extend my sincerest gratitude to Drs. Magi-Galluzzi and Zhou for pouring their heart and soul into this edition of the *Foundations in Diagnostic Pathology* series. I also would like to extend my appreciation to the authors who took time from their busy schedules to contribute their knowledge and expertise. I sincerely hope you enjoy this volume of *Foundations in Diagnostic Pathology*.

JOHN R. GOLDBLUM, M.D.

Preface

We have more than a dozen textbooks on genitourinary pathology in our possession. This book, *Genitourinary Pathology, A Volume in the Foundations in Diagnostic Pathology Series*, of which we are privileged to be the editors, however, has several distinct features that set it apart from other books.

First, this book has "Disease fact" and "Pathologic feature" tables for each major disease entity of the genitourinary tract, so that the essential clinical and pathological features of each entity can be easily digested and comprehended, and as such can serve as a quick reference during daily sign-out.

Second, succinct clinical features of each disease that are most relevant to the pathological diagnosis and prognosis are discussed in well-defined categories that include epidemiology, clinical symptomatology, prognosis, and management. Such knowledge is important to practicing pathologists as it will not only help us formulate diagnoses and understand the impact of our diagnoses on patient care, but also drive us to modify our practice to meet the demand of the ever-changing medical practice in general.

Third, this book includes a chapter on medical kidney diseases, an important topic, yet rarely covered by other genitourinary pathology textbooks. End-stage kidneys removed for a variety of medical conditions are not infrequently encountered in pathology laboratories. An understanding of the basic clinical and pathological features will greatly facilitate our handling and interpretation of these specimens.

This book is primarily intended to be a comprehensive genitourinary pathology textbook, providing up-to-date information on the surgical pathology of the wide array of neoplastic and non-neoplastic diseases of the genitourinary tract, and emphasizing the practical diagnostic aspects. These are addressed with more than 1000 high-quality, full color illustrations, as well as numerous boxes and tables to enhance and facilitate the presentation of information. Thus, it is a book with substantial content that one expects from a major genitourinary pathology textbook, but with a novel format that allows easy use and learning.

We are very fortunate to have many world renowned genitourinary pathologists contribute to this book. To all, we are immensely grateful.

MING ZHOU, MD, PhD
CRISTINA MAGI-GALLUZZI, MD, PhD

Our thanks go to Dr. John Goldblum, our colleague and the editor of this book series, and to Dr. Jonathan Epstein, both for their support and mentorship. We would also like to thank Heather Krehling, Belinda Kuhn, and the staff at Elsevier, who have lent us all the support and resources necessary to finish this project. Finally, we would like to acknowledge the superb secretarial support of Debbie Mitchell and Kelly Uterhark.

Ming Zhou, MD, PhD
Cristina Magi-Galluzzi, MD, PhD

Contents

1

Non-neoplastic Diseases of the Prostate

Cristina Magi–Galluzzi • Ming Zhou • Jonathan I. Epstein

THE PROSTATE GLAND

ANATOMY AND HISTOLOGY

In an adult man without prominent prostatic hyperplasia, the average weight of the prostate gland is approximately 30 to 40 g. The shape of the gland is that of an inverted cone, with the base located approximately at the bladder neck and the apex distally at the urogenital diaphragm (Fig. 1-1A). The prostatic urethra runs through the center of the gland, with a 35-degree anterior bend at the verumontanum. Posteriorly, Denonvillier's fascia, a thin layer of connective tissue, separates the prostate and seminal vesicles from the rectum.

Anatomically, the prostate is divided into inner and outer regions. The inner region is affected predominantly by benign prostatic hyperplasia (BPH), and the outer region shows predilection for carcinoma, although some prostatic cancer occurs centrally and BPH nodules may be seen peripherally. The prostate gland is divided into four zones: (1) anterior fibromuscular stroma; (2) central zone (CZ); (3) peripheral zone (PZ); and (4) preprostatic regions that comprise the periurethral ducts and the larger transition zone (TZ) (Figs. 1-1 and Fig. 1-2).

The anterior fibromuscular stroma occupies approximately one third of the prostate, contains very few glands, and consists of smooth muscle and dense fibrous tissue. The CZ forms a cone-shaped area surrounding the ejaculatory ducts, with the apex at the verumontanum, and the base at the bladder neck. The PZ is the prominent area distal to the CZ; it corresponds to a horseshoe-shaped structure extending posteriorly, posterolaterally, laterally and anteriorly around the inner aspect of the prostate.

The outer aspect of the prostate gland is divided into CZ and PZ based on histologic differences affecting these two areas. From a diagnostic standpoint, the CZ histology may mimic high-grade prostatic intraepithelial neoplasia (PIN). The PZ is frequently affected by carcinoma; the CZ is an uncommon site for origin of carcinoma, although it may be secondarily invaded by large PZ tumors.

The prostate consists of epithelial and stromal cells. The epithelial cells are arranged in tubuloalveolar glands consisting of ducts that branch out from the urethra and terminate into acini (Fig. 1-3A). The acini are characterized by papillary infoldings (Fig. 1-3B).

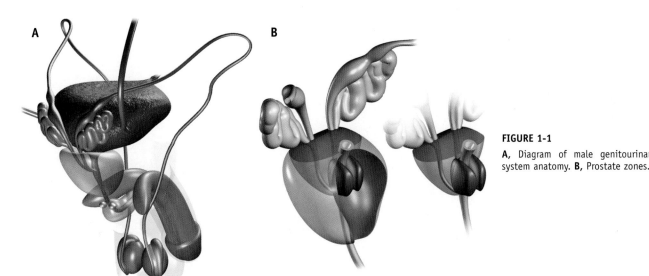

A **B**

FIGURE 1-1

A, Diagram of male genitourinary system anatomy. **B,** Prostate zones.

1

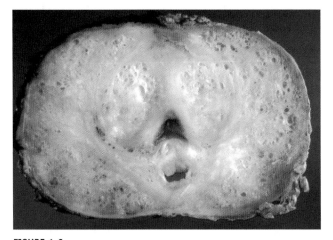

FIGURE 1-2

Cross-section of the prostate of an adult man at the level of the utricle. The nodular periurethral area represents the transition zone. The white-gray fibrous tissue surrounding the utricle divides the TZ from the peripheral zone.

Epithelial cells in the prostate are secretory cells, basal cells (Fig. 1-3B), transitional (urothelial) cells, and neuroendocrine cells. The proximal portion of the prostatic ducts is lined by urothelium, similar to the urethra. The distal portion of the prostatic ducts, as well as some prostatic acini, may show cuboidal and columnar epithelium mixed with urothelium (Fig. 1-3C). The urothelium or transitional epithelium is composed of spindle-shaped epithelial cells with occasional nuclear grooves, which are often oriented with their long axis perpendicular to the basement membrane. The columnar secretory epithelial cells are tall, with pale to clear cytoplasm (Fig. 1-3D). These cells are terminally differentiated and stain positively with prostate-specific antigen (PSA) and prostate-specific acid phosphatase (PSAP). Secretory cells lack immuno-reactivity with antibodies to high-molecular-weight cytokeratin (HMWCK) and p63. Basal cells lie beneath the secretory cells. The nuclei are cigar shaped or

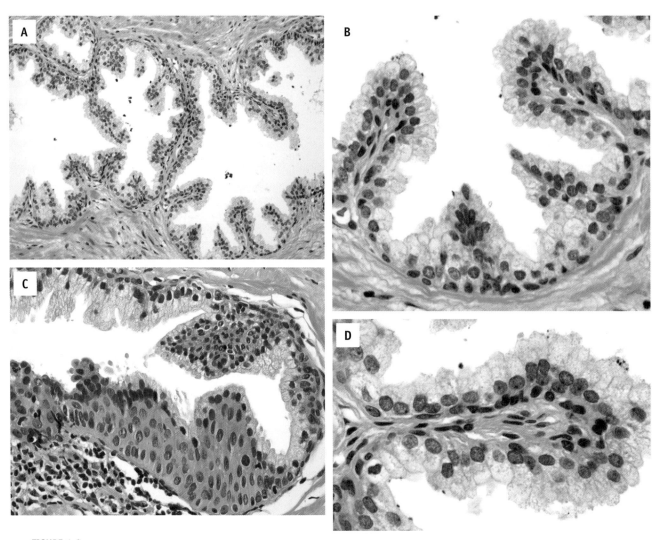

FIGURE 1-3

A, The epithelial cells are arranged in tubuloalveolar glands consisting of ducts branching out from the urethra and terminating into acini. **B,** The acini are characterized by papillary infoldings lined by secretory and basal cells. **C,** Some prostatic acini show cuboidal and columnar epithelium mixed with urothelium. **D,** The columnar secretory epithelial cells are tall with pale to clear cytoplasm. The basal cells lie beneath the secretory cells; the nuclei are cigar shaped and oriented parallel to the basement membrane.

resemble those associated with fibroblasts and are oriented parallel to the basement membrane (Fig. 1-3D). Frequently, basal cells are inconspicuous in benign glands and are difficult to distinguish from surrounding fibroblasts. It is important to differentiate basal cells from fibroblasts, because basal cells are absent in adenocarcinoma of the prostate (PCa) and may be identified in conditions that mimic prostate cancer. Occasionally, basal cells show prominent nucleoli, mimicking high-grade PIN. They may be identified by their immunoreactivity with antibodies to HMWCK or p63 or both. Basal cells are almost devoid of secretory products such as PSA and PSAP. Basal cells are not myoepithelial cells and do not react with antibodies to muscle-specific actin (MSA) or S-100. The prostate contains the largest number of endocrine-paracrine cells of any genitourinary organ.

The stroma comprises skeletal and smooth muscle cells, fibroblasts, nerve cells, and endothelial cells. The most apical portion of the prostate gland is characterized by skeletal muscle of the urogenital diaphragm extending into the prostate. Although mostly exterior to the prostate gland, skeletal muscle fibers not uncommonly extend into the peripheral portion of the prostate gland, especially apically and anteriorly. In a normal prostate, one can also find small nerve bundles. Occasionally, ganglion cells and paraganglia may be seen in the prostate, but they also are more commonly identified exterior to the gland. Cowper's glands may occasionally be seen in needle biopsy. Corpora amylacea are seen in approximately 25% of prostate glands in men age 20 to 40 years, whereas they are rare in adenocarcinomas. Corpora amylacea are round, laminated, hyaline eosinophilic structures that may become calcified. Lipofuscin is seen in approximately 60% of cases of benign prostate glands in sections stained with hematoxylin and eosin (H&E) and in almost all cases stained with Fontana-Masson.

BENIGN PROSTATIC HYPERPLASIA

BPH is a common urologic condition that is defined as a benign enlargement of the prostate gland, caused by increase in cell number, which commonly occurs in older men and is often accompanied by lower urinary tract symptoms. In the United States, approximately 14 million men have BPH, and the estimated annual cost of treatment is $4 billion. Prevalence increases with age, with only a few percent of men younger than 40 years of age, but 88% of men older than 80 years, having histologic BPH. The prevalence of histologic BPH at autopsy has been reported to be the same in various countries around the world; however, more recent studies have shown significantly less histologic BPH and significantly less volume of histologic BPH in Southeast Asian men compared with North American men. Little is known about the natural history of BPH. Besides older age, other risk factors are normal androgenic function and positive family history.

BENIGN PROSTATIC HYPERPLASIA—FACT SHEET

Definition
▶ Benign enlargement of the prostate gland due to increase in cell number, often accompanied by lower urinary tract symptoms

Incidence and Location
▶ Commonly occurs in older men
▶ Most common in transition zone and periurethral area; rarely in peripheral zone

Morbidity and Mortality
▶ 14 million men affected
▶ Estimated annual cost of treatment is $4 billion

Gender, Race, and Age Distribution
▶ Incidence seems to be higher among Caucasians than Asians
▶ Incidence increases with age

Clinical Features
▶ Firm enlargement of the prostate associated with urinary tract obstructive symptoms
▶ Increased PSA

Prognosis and Treatment
▶ Medical therapy: α-blocker, 5-α-reductase inhibitor
▶ Surgical therapy: open prostatectomy, TURP
▶ Minimally invasive surgical treatment: balloon dilatation, transurethral needle ablation, transurethral microwave thermotherapy, interstitial laser coagulation, and laser vaporization

---

CLINICAL FEATURES

BPH results in a smooth, firm enlargement of the prostate associated with urinary tract obstructive and irritative symptoms. However, the size of the gland does not correlate closely with the degree of obstruction or with clinical symptoms. Early symptoms of obstruction include decrease in the caliber and force of the urinary stream, hesitancy in initiating urination, inability to abruptly terminate micturition without dribbling, sensations of incomplete emptying of the bladder, and, occasionally, urinary retention. When symptoms progress, bladder compliance decreases and bladder instability develops, with frequency, urgency, and incontinence. BPH alone can elevate the serum PSA, and, indeed, BPH is the most common cause of elevated PSA.

Clinically, hyperplasia is classified into lateral, middle lobe, and posterior lobe enlargement. Typical hyperplastic tissue lateral to the urethra (TZ) is designated as lateral lobe enlargement. Middle lobe enlargement refers to a nodule arising at the bladder neck, which may then project into the bladder, creating a ball-valve obstruction (Fig. 1-4A). In posterior lobe hyperplasia, a bar of tissue, termed the median bar, arises posterior to the urethra.

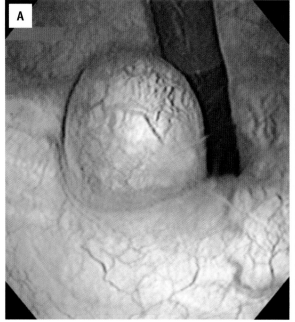

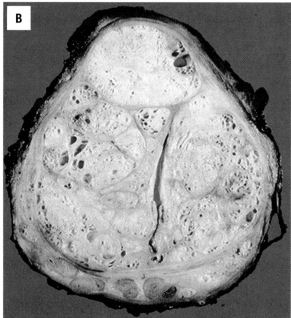

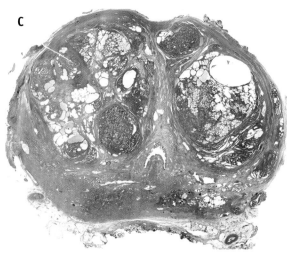

FIGURE 1-4

A, Intravesical endoscopic appearance of enlarged middle lobe of the prostate that arises at the bladder neck and projects into the bladder. (Courtesy of Dr. Stephen Jones, Cleveland, OH). **B,** Cross-section of the prostate from an adult man showing marked enlargement of the transition zone (TZ) by benign prostatic hyperplasia (BPH) with compression of the urethra and peripheral zone. **C,** Whole-mount cross-section of the prostate of an elderly man at the level of the verumontanum, showing massive enlargement of the TZ by BPH, with a compressed, horseshoe-shaped peripheral zone (PZ).

PATHOLOGY FEATURES

GROSS FINDINGS

Nodule formation is the hallmark of prostatic hyperplasia. BPH affects primarily the TZ of the prostate, consisting of bilateral nodules immediately external to the smooth muscle sphincter that surrounds the urethra (Fig. 1-4B,C). Hyperplastic nodules occasionally occur in the PZ. Only the histologic identification of nodules is diagnostic for BPH. By definition, specimens obtained through transurethral resection of the prostate (TURP) may be diagnosed as hyperplasia, because surgery has been performed for urinary obstructive symptoms. Many needle biopsy specimens do not sample the TZ, and the histologic findings do not correlate with the size of the prostate or with symptoms of urinary obstruction. Therefore, benign needle biopsies should be diagnosed as "benign prostate tissue" rather than BPH.

MICROSCOPIC FINDINGS

Prostatic hyperplasia is a proliferation of either pure stromal cells or both epithelial and stromal cells (Fig. 1-5). Franks described five histologic subtypes of BPH based on epithelial and stromal components. The smallest nodules, located in the periurethral submucosa, are predominantly stromal (Fig. 1-5A) and are composed of loose mesenchyme containing prominent small, round vessels (Fig. 1-5B). Occasionally, stromal nodules composed almost entirely of smooth muscle can be seen and may account for some of the reports of leiomyoma of the prostate. The glandular component of BPH is made up of small and large acini, some showing papillary infolding and projections (Fig. 1-5C,D). The luminal secretory epithelium consists of tall columnar cells with pale-staining granular cytoplasm. Basal cells are variably seen, ranging from difficult-to-detect to hyperplastic. The stroma consists of smooth muscle and fibrous tissue, which can occasionally display nuclear palisading mimicking a neural tumor. Lymphocytes and plasma cells are often present around the hyperplastic glands.

ANCILLARY STUDIES

IMMUNOHISTOCHEMISTRY

Immunohistochemically, the pattern of staining of BPH is similar to that of normal prostatic glands. The basal cells stain positively for HMWCK, p63, and cytokeratin CK5/6 (Fig. 1-6). The secretory cells are PSA and PSAP positive.

DIFFERENTIAL DIAGNOSIS

The presence of hyperplastic nodules in the PZ, although rare, can mimic carcinoma on digital rectal examination and on ultrasound studies. The main histologic differential diagnosis of stromal BPH is with a stromal neoplasm of the prostate. The diagnosis of prostatic leiomyoma should be restricted to large, symptomatic masses of small muscle. Epithelial hyperplasia should be distinguished from low-grade PIN, adenosis,

and well-differentiated carcinoma. Nucleomegaly and anisocytosis are features of low-grade PIN but not of BPH. Adenosis has a higher density of small, closely packed glands; a fragmented rather than complete basal cell layer; and often intraluminal crystalloids. BPH glands are typically not as crowded and lack the luminal cell nuclear atypia that are characteristic of pseudohyperplastic PCa.

PROGNOSIS AND THERAPY

The most common initial medical therapy is the use of α-adrenergic blockers, which relax the prostatic smooth muscle tone. If this therapy is not effective, α-blockers can be combined with a 5-α-reductase inhibitor. Many new, minimally invasive surgical treatments can be performed for BPH recalcitrant to medical therapy, but TURP remains the most effective treatment for BPH in terms of reducing symptoms. The more recent techniques used to treat BPH include balloon dilatation of the prostate, transurethral needle ablation, transurethral microwave thermotherapy, interstitial laser coagulation, and laser vaporization. Enucleation of the gland (open prostatectomy) is performed for very large prostate glands.

INFLAMMATORY AND INFLAMMATORY-LIKE LESIONS OF THE PROSTATE

Inflammation of the prostate (prostatitis) and infection of the gland are common clinical problems. The prostatitis syndrome is one of the most common entities encountered in urologic practice and accounts for more than 25% of male office visits for genitourinary complaints. It has been estimated that 9% to 11% of adult men have symptoms of prostatitis at any given time. Compared to prostate cancer and BPH, prostatitis is more likely to affect younger men, 18 to 50 years of age. The classification of prostatitis syndrome includes acute bacterial prostatitis (ABP); chronic bacterial prostatitis (CBP); chronic pelvic pain syndrome (CPPS) or, synonymously, chronic nonbacterial prostatitis; and asymptomatic inflammatory prostatitis (AIP). CPPS is divided in two subgroups, inflammatory and noninflammatory CPPS. Nonbacterial prostatitis is an inflammatory condition of unknown origin; it is the most common cause of prostatitis symptoms. Clinically, nonbacterial prostatitis is similar to CBP, except that both bacteriologic cultures and history of urinary tract infections are negative.

Patchy acute and chronic inflammation is present in the prostate of most adult men without symptoms. Histologically, symptomatic CBP cannot be distinguished from chronic inflammation commonly seen in specimens removed from patients with BPH. Therefore, it is preferable to diagnose inflamed prostate specimens

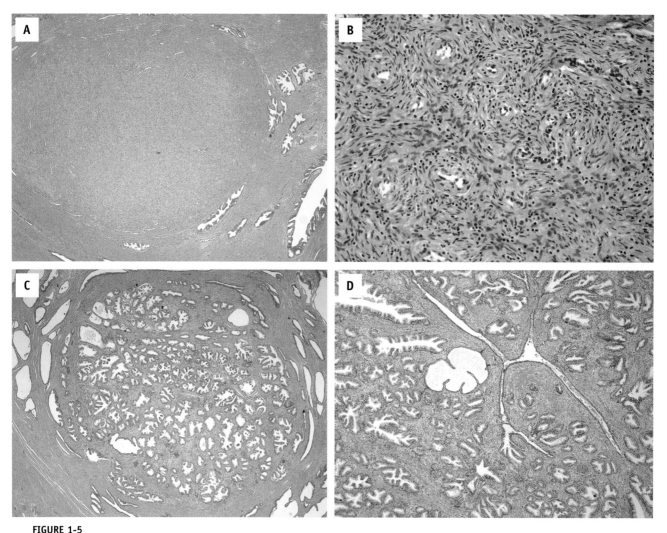

FIGURE 1-5

A, At low power, a periurethral stromal nodule *(left)* is present in the transition zone (TZ), in proximity to the prostatic urethra *(right)*. **B,** At high power, the stromal nodule is composed of cellular mesenchyme containing prominent small, round vessels. **C,** Low-power view of a well circumscribed, predominantly epithelial nodule within the TZ. **D,** Intermediate-power view of mixed epithelial-stromal nodule.

as showing acute or chronic inflammation, rather than acute or chronic prostatitis.

Bacterial prostatitis is associated with urinary tract infections, increased number of inflammatory cells in prostatic secretions, and growth of bacterial organisms from prostatic secretions. The organisms causing bacterial prostatitis are similar in type and incidence to those resulting in urinary tract infections.

NONSPECIFIC GRANULOMATOUS PROSTATITIS

Granulomatous prostatitis is a distinctive form of prostatitis that can be mistaken for carcinoma. It is subclassified into infectious granulomas, nonspecific granulomatous prostatitis (NSGP), postbiopsy granulomas, and systemic granulomatous prostatitis (also referred as allergic granulomatous prostatitis). NSGP

is an inflammatory response of foreign body type to extravasated prostatic fluid. NSGP is a rare disorder, but it is the most common granulomatous prostatitis seen on needle biopsy. The incidence is less than 3.4% in unselected series of patients. Systemic granulomatous inflammation encompasses cases with tissue eosinophilia, such as Churg-Strauss syndrome, as well as those without eosinophilia, such as Wegener's granulomatous prostatitis.

CLINICAL FEATURES

Most patients with NSGP are 54 to 65 years of age. Most have a history of urinary tract infection and may present with dysuria, frequency, acute urinary retention, and high-grade fever. Patients frequently have associated BPH with persistent obstructive symptoms

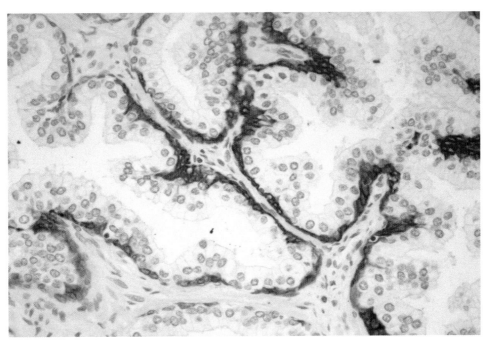

FIGURE 1-6

Immunohistochemically, the pattern of staining of benign prostatic hyperplasia (BPH) is similar to that of normal prostatic glands. The basal cells stain positively for high-molecular-weight cytokeratin (HMWCK).

NONSPECIFIC GRANULOMATOUS PROSTATITIS—FACT SHEET

Definition
► Focal or diffuse histiocytic inflammatory response to extravasated prostatic fluid

Incidence and Location
► Relatively rare disorder
► Incidence less than 3.4% in unselected series of patients

Morbidity and Mortality
► Painful, fixed, and nodular enlargement of the prostate
► Persistent obstructive symptoms and significant residual urine

Gender, Race, and Age Distribution
► Mean age is 54-65 years

Clinical Features
► History of urinary tract infection
► Patients may present with dysuria, frequency, acute urinary retention, high-grade fever
► Prostate gland is often hard, fixed, and nodular on DRE

Prognosis and Treatment
► Preferred treatment is either conservative or surgical
► Prognosis is excellent
► Combination therapy with an antimicrobial agent and hydrocortisone
► Steroids resolve clinical symptoms and lead to marked histopathologic improvement

---

and significant residual urine. The prostate gland is often hard, fixed, nodular, and closely mimics cancer clinically.

PATHOLOGIC FEATURES

GROSS FINDINGS

NSGP appears as small, firm, yellow granular nodules.

MICROSCOPIC FINDINGS

NSGP is characterized by a noncaseating, lobular, dense infiltrate of lymphocytes, plasma cells, eosinophils, epithelioid histiocytes, and scattered neutrophils (Fig. 1-7A). Many of the histiocytes have a foamy appearance, and some are multinucleated. These dense nodules tend to obscure and efface ductal and acinar elements. The epithelium is destroyed, and cellular debris, prostatic secretions, and corpora amylacea are common findings. The earliest lesion of NSGP consists of dilated ducts and acini filled with neutrophils, debris, and desquamated epithelial cells. Focal rupture of those ducts and acini results in a localized granulomatous and chronic inflammatory reaction (Fig. 1-7B). Older lesions of NSGP show a more prominent fibrous component.

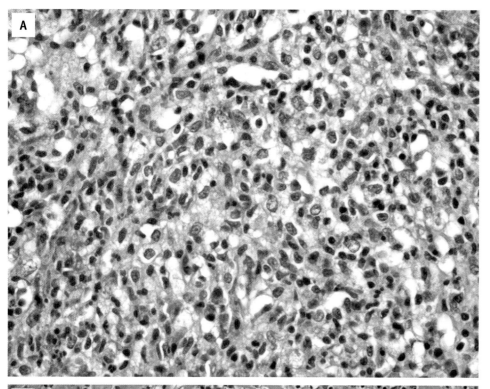

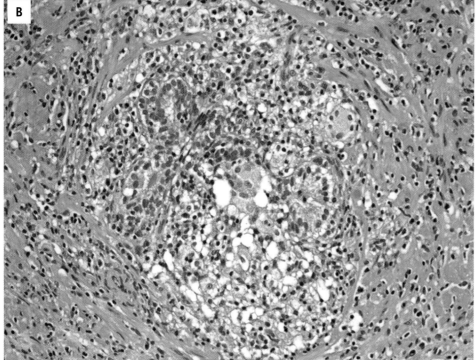

FIGURE 1-7

A, In nonspecific granulomatous prostatitis (NSGP), the lesion is characterized by a noncaseating, lobular, dense infiltrate of lymphocytes, plasma cells, eosinophils, and epithelioid histiocytes. Some of the histiocytes have a foamy appearance. **B,** In the earliest lesion of NSGP, focal rupture of ducts and acini results in a localized granulomatous and chronic inflammatory reaction.

ANCILLARY STUDIES

FINE-NEEDLE ASPIRATION BIOPSY

Fine-needle aspiration is a reliable procedure for the morphologic diagnosis of granulomatous prostatitis, which can clinically mimic prostatic carcinoma when it presents as a diffuse or nodular prostate enlargement with increased consistency. The findings in the typical cases are distinctive, with epithelioid and multinucleated histiocytes easily recognized.

IMMUNOHISTOCHEMISTRY

The epithelioid histiocytes are negative for cytokeratin (AE1-AE3), PSA, and PSAP and positive for histiocytic markers such as KP-1 and CD68.

NONSPECIFIC GRANULOMATOUS PROSTATITIS— PATHOLOGIC FEATURES

Gross Findings
- ▶ Small, firm, yellow granular nodules

Microscopic Findings
- ▶ Nodular granulomatous inflammation centered on ducts and acini
- ▶ Lobular, dense infiltrate of lymphocytes, plasma cells, eosinophils, epithelioid histiocytes and scattered neutrophils
- ▶ Earliest lesion: dilated ducts and acini filled with neutrophils, debris, and desquamated epithelial cells
- ▶ Older lesions: more prominent fibrous component
- ▶ Caseous necrosis absent

Fine-Needle Aspiration Biopsy Findings
- ▶ Epithelioid and multinucleated histiocytes are easily recognized

Immunohistochemical Features
- ▶ Negative for cytokeratin (AE1-AE3), PSA, and PSAP
- ▶ Positive for histiocytic markers (KP-1 and CD68)

Differential Diagnosis
- ▶ High-grade prostate adenocarcinoma
- ▶ Infectious granulomatous prostatitis
- ▶ Allergic granulomatous prostatitis

DIFFERENTIAL DIAGNOSIS

NSGP may simulate carcinoma both clinically and microscopically. Concurrent NSGP and PCa is rare. On needle biopsy, NSGP can be confused with high-grade prostate cancer, particularly in cases with prominent epithelioid histiocytes. The key feature to avoid a misdiagnosis of cancer is the recognition of a mixed inflammatory infiltrate. The presence of multinucleated giant cells may also aid in the diagnosis of NSGP. If difficulty persists, immunohistochemical stains for histiocytic and epithelial markers can differentiate the two entities.

In most cases, there is little histologic similarity between NSGP and infectious granulomatous inflammation of the prostate. Although discrete small granulomas can be seen with NSGP, they are always seen in the early lesion surrounding ruptured dilated ducts or acini. Allergic granulomatous prostatitis consists of multiple small, ovoid, necrobiotic granulomas surrounded by numerous eosinophils.

PROGNOSIS AND THERAPY

Irrespective of the choice of treatment (conservative or surgical), the prognosis of NSGP is excellent. NSGP responds favorably to combination therapy with an antimicrobial agent and hydrocortisone. Steroid therapy can promptly resolve clinical symptoms and provide marked histopathologic improvement.

ACUTE AND CHRONIC PROSTATITIS

Most cases of ABP are caused by gram-negative organisms, including *Escherichia coli* (80% of infections); other Enterobacteriaceae, such as *Pseudomonas, Serratia,* and *Klebsiella* (10% to 15%); and Enterococci (5% to 10%). Although prostatitis due to *Neisseria gonorrhoeae* was common in the preantibiotic era, it is rare today. CBP is characterized by recurrent urinary tract infections caused by the same pathogens. Patients with human immunodeficiency virus (HIV) infection or acquired immunodeficiency syndrome (AIDS) have an increased incidence of bacterial prostatitis. The association of infection or inflammation of the prostate with prostate cancer has been suggested but is not established.

CLINICAL FEATURES

The most common presentation of ABP is sudden onset of fever, chills, irritative and obstructive voiding symptoms, and pain in the lower back, rectum, and perineum. The prostate is swollen, tender, and warm and may be partially or totally indurated. Diagnosis is based on the finding yielded by the urine culture and expressed prostatic secretions, and biopsy is contraindicated because of the potential for sepsis. Abscess is a potential but rare complication of ABP. Clinical prostatitis may give rise to elevated serum PSA.

PATHOLOGIC FEATURES

GROSS FINDINGS

Examination of the specimen is uncommon.

MICROSCOPIC FINDINGS

ABP consists of sheets of neutrophils within and around acini, intraductal desquamated cellular debris, stromal edema, and hyperemia (Fig. 1-8A,B). The stroma is edematous and hemorrhagic, and microabscesses may be present. The presence of acute inflammation by itself without the clinical history of acute prostatitis should be diagnosed as "acute inflammation" not "acute prostatitis." Histologically, symptomatic CBP cannot be distinguished from chronic inflammation commonly seen in specimens removed for BPH; a histologic diagnosis of "chronic prostatitis" should not be made, and merely "chronic inflammation" should be noted. Chronic inflammation typically has a periglandular distribution and contains an admixture of lymphocytes

---

ACUTE AND CHRONIC PROSTATITIS—FACT SHEET

Definition
▶ Inflammatory condition clinically manifesting with urethral and prostatic symptoms and sexual dysfunction

Incidence and Location
▶ Common entity
▶ Accounts for more than 25% of male office visits for genitourinary complaints
▶ 9-11% of the adult male population has symptoms of prostatitis at any given time

Morbidity and Mortality
▶ Recurrent urinary tract infections and pain

Gender, Race, and Age Distribution
▶ Affects men 18-50 years of age

Clinical Features
▶ Sudden onset of fever, chills, and irritative and obstructive voiding symptoms
▶ Lower back, rectum, and perineum pain
▶ Elevated serum PSA

Prognosis and Treatment
▶ Antimicrobial therapy and α-blocker therapy
▶ May respond favorably to oral fluoroquinolone therapy
▶ TURP is an alternative surgical management
▶ Surgical or percutaneous drainage is required for prostatic abscess
▶ Biopsy is contraindicated for ABP because of the potential for sepsis

---

ACUTE AND CHRONIC PROSTATITIS—PATHOLOGIC FEATURES

Gross Findings
▶ Examination of the specimen is uncommon

Microscopic Findings
Acute
▶ Sheets of neutrophils within and around acini
▶ Intraductal desquamated cellular debris
▶ Stromal edema and hyperemia
▶ Microabscesses may be present
Chronic
▶ Periglandular distribution of a mixture of lymphocytes and plasma cells
▶ Occasional large nucleoli are not uncommon in both acute and chronic inflammation

Immunohistochemical Features
▶ Epithelial component positive for high-molecular-weight cytokeratins and PSA
▶ Inflammatory component positive for leukocyte common antigen (LCA)

Differential Diagnosis
▶ Prostatic adenocarcinoma
▶ Atrophy
▶ Urothelial metaplasia

---

and plasma cells (Fig. 1-8B,C). Occasional large nucleoli are not uncommon in areas of both acute and chronic inflammation.

DIFFERENTIAL DIAGNOSIS

Acute or chronic inflammation within the prostate can cause both architectural and cytologic abnormalities that may be confused with carcinoma. The glands frequently have an atrophic appearance. There may be streaming of basophilic epithelium resembling urothelial metaplasia.

PROGNOSIS AND THERAPY

Antimicrobial therapy and α-blocker therapy is effective in the majority of men with ABP or CBP. The minority of patients continues to respond favorably to oral fluoroquinolone therapy. TURP is an alternative for surgical

management of bacterial prostatitis. Surgical or percutaneous drainage is usually required in presence of prostatic abscess.

Although there is cumulative evidence demonstrating that chronic inflammation may play a role in prostate carcinogenesis, more studies are needed to prove its etiologic role in prostate cancer.

POSTBIOPSY GRANULOMA

Postbiopsy granuloma is a reaction to altered epithelium and stroma from previous cautery involving predominantly the periurethral zone tissue. It is the second most common subtype of granulomatous prostatitis (21% to 24% of TURP cases) after NSGP, and it accounts for approximately 7% of all cases of prostatitis.

CLINICAL FEATURES

Patients are 51 to 87 years of age. Granulomas may be seen in the prostate from 7 days to 52 months after TURP. Although is it more common to have a granulomatous reaction after TURP, similar linear granulomas

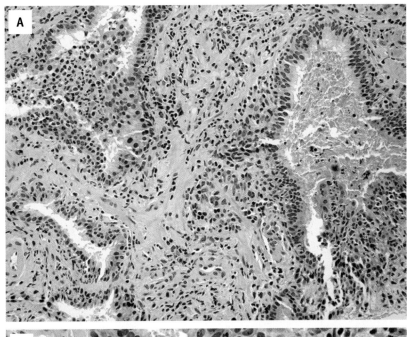

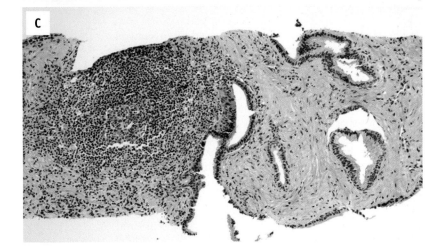

FIGURE 1-8

A, At low power, acute bacterial prostatitis consists of neutrophils within and around acini. A stromal chronic inflammatory infiltrate is also frequently present. **B,** At high power, the neutrophils are present within the columnar epithelium and inside ducts and acini filled with desquamated cellular debris. **C,** Chronic inflammation typically has a periglandular distribution and contains an admixture of lymphocytes and plasma cells.

POSTBIOPSY GRANULOMA—FACT SHEET

Definition
► Subtype of granulomatous prostatitis
► Reaction to altered epithelium and stroma from the previous cautery

Incidence and Location
► Second most common form of granulomatous prostatitis (21-24% of TURP cases)
► 7% of all cases of prostatitis
► Involves periurethral transition zone tissue

Morbidity and Mortality
► Seen in the prostate from 7 days to 52 months after TURP

Gender, Race, and Age Distribution
► Patients are 51-87 years of age

Clinical Features
► Persistent prostatism
► Urinary obstruction or retention
► Hematuria

Prognosis and Treatment
► Asymptomatic incidental finding requiring no treatment

may rarely develop after needle biopsy. Patients present with persistent prostatism, urinary obstruction or retention, and hematuria.

PATHOLOGIC FEATURES

GROSS FINDINGS

The gross findings are non-specific.

MICROSCOPIC FINDINGS

Postbiopsy granulomas are composed of a central region of fibrinoid necrosis surrounded by palisading epithelioid histiocytes (Fig. 1-9). Multinucleated giant cells are frequently present. Those lesions can assume a multitude of shapes, including wedge-shaped, ovoid, and elongated dissecting through the tissue. After TURP, nonspecific foreign body giant cell granulomas are frequently seen in addition to the characteristic necrobiotic granulomas. Abundant eosinophils may be identified if the TURP occurred within 1 month. In cases with a long interval since the prior TURP, the inflammatory infiltrate surrounding postbiopsy granulomas is usually minimal, consisting predominantly of lymphocytes and plasma cells with scattered eosinophils.

ANCILLARY STUDIES

IMMUNOHISTOCHEMISTRY

The lesion is so characteristic and distinct from infectious granuloma that stains for organism usually are not necessary.

DIFFERENTIAL DIAGNOSIS

This entity is often mistaken for other conditions such as rheumatoid nodule, tuberculous granulomatous prostatitis, and allergic granulomatous prostatitis. In contrast to infectious granulomas, the necrosis in postbiopsy granulomas often contains ghost-like structures of vessels, acini, and stroma. The irregular shape of the postbiopsy granulomas also distinguishes them from infectious granulomas. In contrast to allergic granulomatous prostatitis, the eosinophils are localized around postbiopsy granulomas, rather than diffusely infiltrating the stroma.

PROGNOSIS AND THERAPY

Postbiopsy granulomas are asymptomatic, incidental findings requiring no treatment.

POSTBIOPSY GRANULOMA—PATHOLOGIC FEATURES

Gross Findings
► Nonspecific

Microscopic Findings
► Granulomas with central region of fibrinoid necrosis surrounded by palisading epithelioid histiocytes
► Multinucleated giant cells are frequently present
► Elongated granulomas dissecting through the tissue are the most common shape
► Abundant eosinophils identified if TURP occurred within 1 month
► Lymphocytes and plasma cells predominate in cases with a long interval since TURP

Immunohistochemical Features
► Stains for organism are negative

Differential Diagnosis
► Rheumatoid nodule
► Tuberculous granulomatous prostatitis
► Allergic granulomatous prostatitis

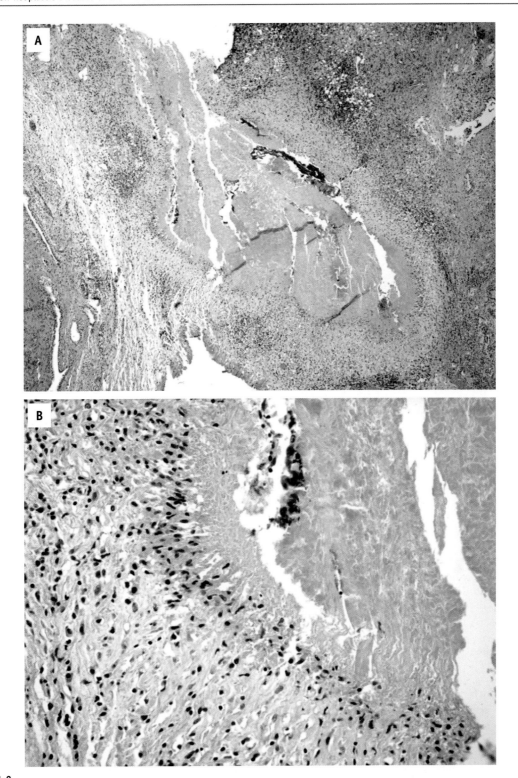

FIGURE 1-9

A, At low power, postbiopsy granulomas are composed of a central region of fibrinoid necrosis surrounded by palisading epithelioid histiocytes. The inflammatory infiltrate surrounding the granulomas is variable and consists predominantly of lymphocytes. **B,** High-power view of palisading histiocytes surrounding fibrinoid necrosis.

XANTHOMA

Xanthoma is a rare form of idiopathic granulomatous prostatitis that is characterized by a localized collection of cholesterol-laden histiocytes. It may be also seen in patients with hyperlipidemia.

CLINICAL FEATURES

Xanthoma occurs in older men and is usually an incidental finding in patients undergoing TURP or needle biopsy, although it can appear as a palpable nodule. In cases where xanthoma is associated with typical granulomatous prostatitis, it is appropriate to use the term *xanthogranulomatous prostatitis*. It is more commonly seen in the PZ, yet can also be present in the TZ.

PATHOLOGIC FEATURES

MICROSCOPIC FINDINGS

Xanthoma is a localized, circumscribed cluster of loosely cohesive histiocytes. The cells have a clear to foamy, vacuolated cytoplasm and benign-appearing nuclei without prominent nucleoli (Fig. 1-10).

XANTHOMA—FACT SHEET

Definition
► Collection of lipid-laden histiocytes

Incidence and Location
► Rare entity
► Incidental finding in patients undergoing TURP or needle biopsy
► Rarely may be seen in patients with hyperlipidemia
► Involves peripheral or transition zone

Morbidity and Mortality
► Benign condition

Gender, Race, and Age Distribution
► Occurs in older men

Clinical Features
► When associated with typical granulomatous prostatitis, it is appropriate to use the term xanthogranulomatous prostatitis

Prognosis and Treatment
► Clinically irrelevant in most of the cases

XANTHOMA—PATHOLOGIC FEATURES

Gross Findings
► Usually an incidental histologic finding

Microscopic Findings
► Circumscribed cluster of uniform cells
► Clear to foamy vacuolated cytoplasm
► Benign-appearing nuclei without prominent nucleoli
► Lack of gland formation

Immunohistochemical Features
► Positive for CD68
► Negative for cytokeratin, PSA, and PSAP

Differential Diagnosis
► Foamy gland prostatic adenocarcinoma

ANCILLARY STUDIES

IMMUNOHISTOCHEMISTRY

Xanthoma cells are positive for KP-1, a lysosomal marker, and CD68, a macrophage marker; they are negative for cytokeratin (AE1-AE3), PSA, and PSAP.

DIFFERENTIAL DIAGNOSIS

Prostatic xanthoma, particularly on needle biopsy, may resemble foamy gland PCa. Features that aid in the recognition of xanthoma include circumscription, lack of glandular formation, and bland cytologic features. Immunohistochemistry may assist in the differential diagnosis.

PROGNOSIS AND THERAPY

Xanthoma is a benign condition of inflammatory origin related to granulomatous prostatitis; it is clinically irrelevant in most cases.

MALAKOPLAKIA

Malakoplakia is a specific variant of granulomatous prostatitis that occurs rarely in the prostate. Because of its association with urinary tract infection, it could be categorized as an infectious type of inflammation. Malakoplakia is associated with a defective intracellular lysosomal digestion of bacteria.

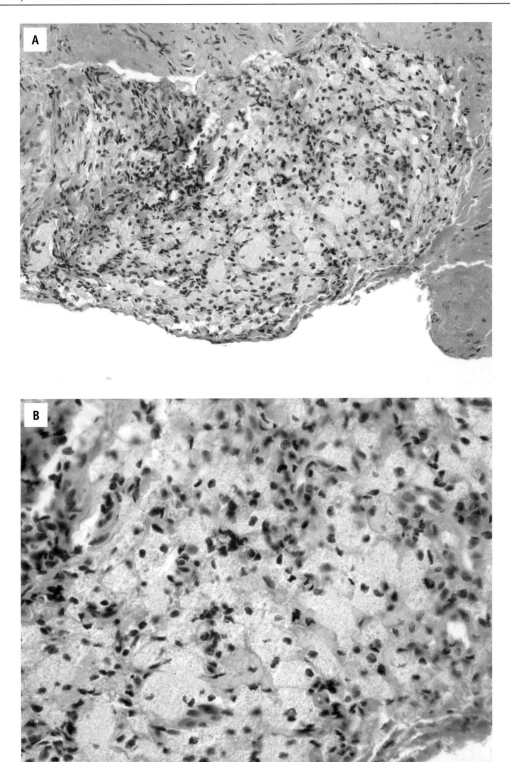

FIGURE 1-10
A, At low power, xanthoma consists of a localized, circumscribed cluster of loosely cohesive histiocytes. **B,** At high power, the cells have a clear to foamy, vacuolated cytoplasm and benign-appearing nuclei without prominent nucleoli.

CLINICAL FEATURES

The urinary tract infection is most frequently due to *E. coli,* which is commonly isolated from urine cultures. Patients with prostatic malakoplakia usually are in their 60s (range, 49 to 85 years) and present with symptoms and physical findings similar to those of prostatism. In half of the patients the differential diagnosis includes malignancy, mainly because of the presence of a hard nodule on digital rectal examination. Additionally, cases of malakoplakia can show hypoechoic lesions on transrectal ultrasound, mimicking adenocarcinoma. Occasionally malakoplakia occurs in combination with prostate carcinoma, and it can be associated with immunosuppression.

PATHOLOGIC FEATURES

GROSS FINDINGS

The prostate is diffusely hard, a finding suggestive of prostatic carcinoma. On the urothelial surface, *malakoplakia* ("soft plaque" in Greek) appears as a soft, yellowish nodule.

MALAKOPLAKIA—FACT SHEET

Definition
▶ Variant of granulomatous prostatitis associated with defective intracellular lysosomal digestion of bacteria

Incidence and Location
▶ Rare (about 30 cases reported to date)
▶ Prostate primarily involved in 10% of all cases

Morbidity and Mortality
▶ Can be associated with immunosuppression

Gender, Race, and Age Distribution
▶ Patient age range is 49-85 years

Clinical Features
▶ Associated with urinary tract infections
▶ Symptoms similar to prostatism: dysuria, frequency, urinary retention
▶ Enlarged firm to hard prostate by digital rectal examination
▶ Urine culture positive for *E. coli*

Prognosis and Treatment
▶ Prognosis is related to extent of renal and urinary tract involvement
▶ Antibiotic treatment to control urinary tract infection

MALAKOPLAKIA—PATHOLOGIC FEATURES

Gross Findings
▶ Soft, yellowish nodule (urothelial surface)
▶ Diffusely hard prostate

Microscopic Findings
▶ Infiltrative lesion
▶ Diffuse sheets of macrophages admixed with lymphocytes and plasma cells
▶ Intracellular and extracellular Michaelis-Gutmann bodies

Immunohistochemical Features
▶ Michaelis-Gutmann bodies are positive for von Kossa and PAS-D and generally negative for Perls Prussian blue stain
▶ Negative for PSA, PSAP, cytokeratins
▶ Positive for CD68

Differential Diagnosis
▶ Poorly differentiated prostatic carcinoma
▶ Granulomatous prostatitis

MICROSCOPIC FINDINGS

Malakoplakia is an infiltrative lesion characterized by diffuse sheets of macrophages admixed with lymphocytes, plasma cells, and neutrophils (Fig. 1-11). The macrophages contain intracytoplasmic, sharply demarcated, often concentrically laminated, spherical, basophilic inclusions, measuring 2 to 10 μm in diameter. These are the characteristic Michaelis-Gutmann bodies, which represent calcified bacterial debris. Michaelis-Gutmann bodies can also be extracellular.

ANCILLARY STUDIES

HISTOCHEMISTRY AND IMMUNOHISTOCHEMISTRY

Michaelis-Gutmann bodies contain calcium phosphate, and special histochemical stains can be used to better visualize these structures. They are typically periodic acid-Schiff-positive after diastase digestion (PAS-D) (Fig. 1-12A), von Kossa stain (for calcium) (Fig. 1-12B) positive, and weak to negative with Perl's Prussian blue stain (for iron). The absence of cytokeratins, PSA, and PSAP, together with positive staining for CD68, may be a helpful diagnostic tool.

DIFFERENTIAL DIAGNOSIS

Malakoplakia may mimic poorly differentiated PCa clinically, ultrasonographically, and histologically. The

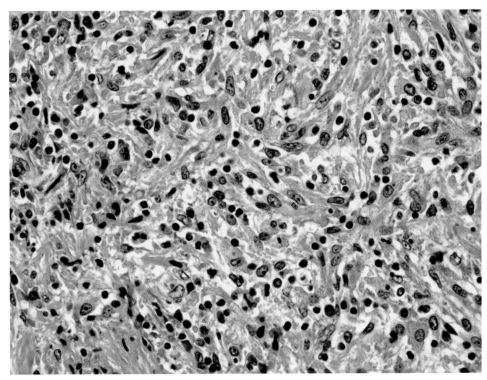

FIGURE 1-11
Malakoplakia is an infiltrative lesion characterized by diffuse sheets of macrophages admixed with lymphocytes, plasma cells, and occasional neutrophils. The macrophages contain intracytoplasmic, sharply demarcated, spherical, basophilic inclusions called Michaelis-Gutmann bodies.

finding of Michaelis-Gutmann bodies excludes a diagnosis of high-grade carcinoma and also distinguishes malakoplakia from other types of granulomatous prostatitis.

PROGNOSIS AND THERAPY

The prognosis is related to the extent of the renal and urinary tract involvement. Biopsy of the prostate should be performed. The symptoms disappear after prolonged antibiotic treatment to control the urinary tract infection.

MIMICKERS OF PROSTATE ADENOCARCINOMA

The diagnosis of PCa, especially when present in small amounts, is often challenging. Before making the diagnosis of prostate carcinoma, the pathologist should consider the various benign lesions that may mimic PCa. Most of those mimickers are easily recognized, but they may represent a challenge when dealing with

limited sampling in thin-core needle biopsies. Most tumor-like lesions mimicking PCa are small gland proliferations, the most common of which are atrophy, partial atrophy, atypical adenomatous hyperplasia or adenosis, basal cell hyperplasia (BCH), and seminal vesicle tissue. Sclerosing adenosis and cribriform clear cell hyperplasia are benign mimickers of high-grade PCa.

ATROPHY

Atrophy of the prostate is a common process that is typically, but not exclusively, found in older patients. Four main subtypes of atrophy are recognized: simple atrophy (previously known as lobular atrophy), cystic atrophy, postatrophic hyperplasia (PAH), and partial atrophy. Combined patterns (mixed type) are common. Glandular atrophy is commonly associated with chronic inflammation, which may have an active component characterized by intraglandular neutrophils. Inflammatory infiltrates are often found in and around foci of atrophy characterized by an increased proliferative index. These foci, called proliferative inflammatory atrophy (PIA), share some molecular traits with PIN and prostate cancer; they may be precursors of early prostate cancer, or they may indicate an intraprostatic environment favorable to cancer development.

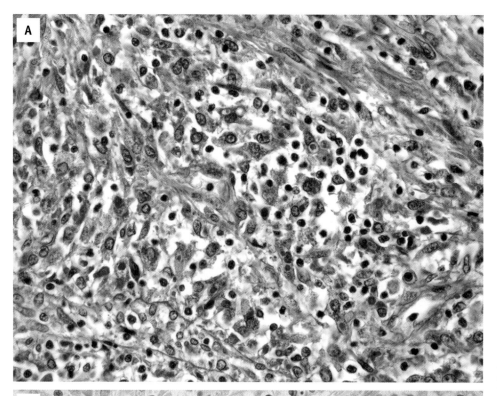

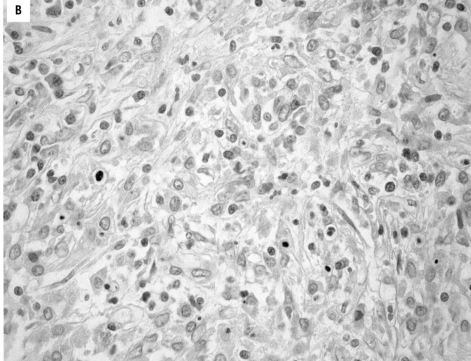

FIGURE 1-12

A, Michaelis-Gutmann bodies contain calcium phosphate and are typically periodic acid-Schiff-positive after diastase digestion (PAS-D). **B,** von Kossa stain (for calcium) is also positive.

CLINICAL FEATURES

Atrophy is typically considered to be a process affecting the elderly; however, it is present in at least 70% of men between 19 and 29 years of age. Its frequency and extension increase with advancing age. The prostate may be firm at digital rectal examination and may show hypoechoic lesions on transrectal ultrasound. Although atrophy is common in the PZ, it may also be seen in the CZ and in the TZ. Its pathogenesis is still unknown, although inflammation and chronic ischemic disease seem to be potential factors. Atrophy can be the result of treatment with antiandrogens and radiation.

PATHOLOGIC FEATURES

GROSS FINDINGS

Atrophy is grossly visible only when there is cyst formation.

MICROSCOPIC FINDINGS

All forms of atrophy are characterized by the presence of well-formed glands that exhibit a reduction in cytoplasmic volume of luminal epithelial cells. At low magnification, atrophy may be confused with prostate carcinoma because of the prominent acinar architectural distortion and the basophilic quality caused by scant cytoplasm and crowded nuclei. Although the glands may appear infiltrative, they appear circumscribed as a group, without infiltration of individual glands between benign glands. Stromal alterations, such as fibrosis and sclerosis, are also present.

Simple atrophy is the most common type of atrophy. It is characterized by isolated, not particularly crowded, atrophic glands of the same size as adjacent nonatrophic glands (Fig. 1-13).

In cystic atrophy, a varying degree of acinar dilatation is seen. Usually, other areas of more typical, simple atrophy are adjacent to the cystic areas. The term *cystic atrophy* is applied restrictively only to glands that have a sharp luminal border without infolding (Fig. 1-14).

PAH consists of a crowded cluster of small, atrophic acini with distorted contours, often arranged around a larger dilated duct (Fig. 1-15A,B). The small acini appear to abut the dilated duct, when it is present, imparting a lobular appearance to the lesion. The acini are lined by cuboidal secretory cells that have mildly enlarged nuclei and an increased nucleus-to-cytoplasm ratio when compared with adjacent benign epithelial cells (Fig. 1-15C). The stroma surrounding PAH may be sclerotic (Fig. 1-15D).

Partial atrophy is another variant of atrophy that may be confused with carcinoma. It may still retain the lobular pattern of atrophy, or it may have a more disorganized and diffuse appearance (Fig. 1-16A). It lacks

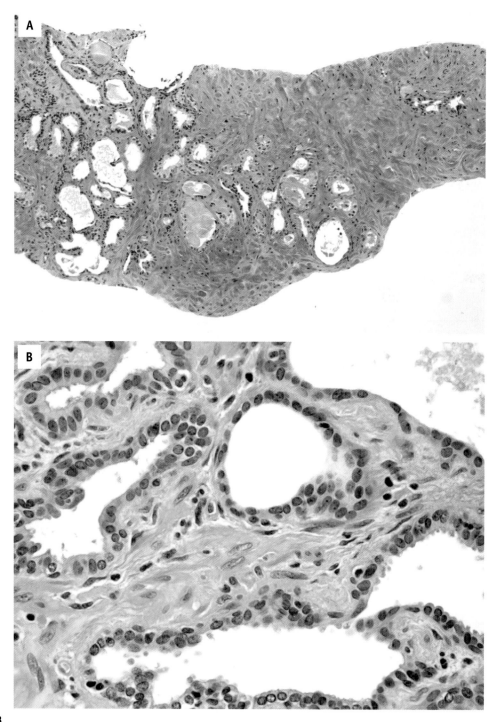

FIGURE 1-13

A, At low power, simple atrophy is characterized by crowded glands with acinar architectural distortion, as well as a basophilic quality resulting from scant cytoplasm and crowded nuclei. **B,** At high power, a characteristic reduction in cytoplasmic volume of the luminal epithelial cells and relatively benign-appearing nuclei are noted.

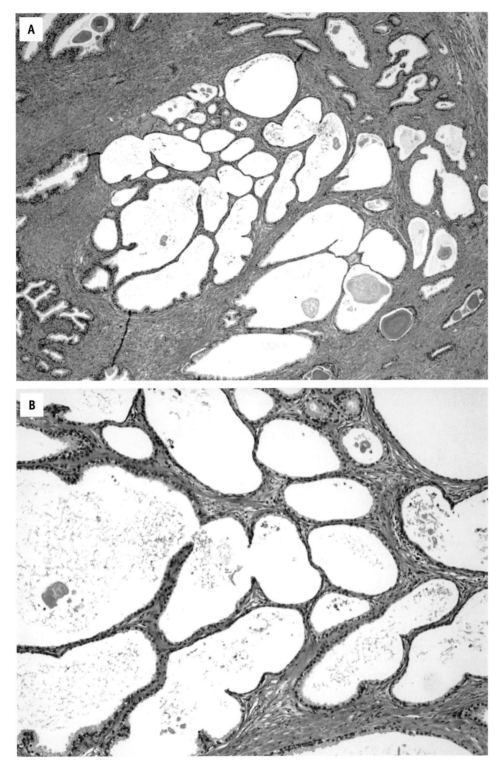

FIGURE 1-14
A, At low power, a varying degree of acinar dilatation is seen in cystic atrophy. **B,** The glands have sharp luminal borders without infolding.

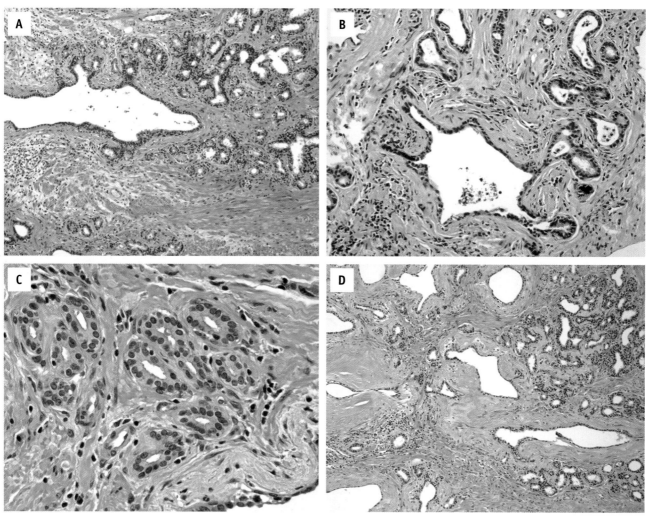

FIGURE 1-15

A and **B,** At low power, postatrophic hyperplasia (PAH) is characterized by clusters of small atrophic acini with distorted contours arranged around a larger dilated duct. The small acini appear to bud off the dilated duct, imparting a lobular appearance to the lesion. **C,** At high power the acini are lined by cuboidal secretory cells with mildly enlarged nuclei and an increased nucleus-to-cytoplasm ratio. **D,** The stroma surrounding PAH may be sclerotic.

the basophilic appearance of fully developed atrophy, because the nuclei are more spaced apart and in areas reach the full height of the cell (Fig. 1-16A,B). Benign features include pale-clear cytoplasm, relatively bland nuclear features without prominent nucleoli, and an undulating luminal surface with papillary infolding (Fig. 1-16C).

ANCILLARY STUDIES

IMMUNOHISTOCHEMISTRY

Double layering of cells is often seen in atrophic lesions, but in some instances it may be difficult to appreciate because of marked atrophy of the secretory cells. In such cases, stains for high-molecular-weight cytokeratin (34BetaE12 or HMWCK) or p63 may be employed to highlight the basal cell compartment to confirm the benign nature of the process. Whereas PAH tends to have complete staining with basal cell antibodies, partial atrophy often shows patchy immunoreactivity, in which not all glands in a focus are positive; among those that are positive, staining is often incomplete, with only one or two immunoreactive basal cells per gland (Fig. 1-17). Immunohistochemistry for α-methylacyl-coenzyme A racemase (AMACR) also shows positivity in some cases of partial atrophy, further mimicking prostate cancer.

DIFFERENTIAL DIAGNOSIS

PAH is at the extreme end of a morphologic continuum of acinar atrophy and most closely mimics PCa. PAH

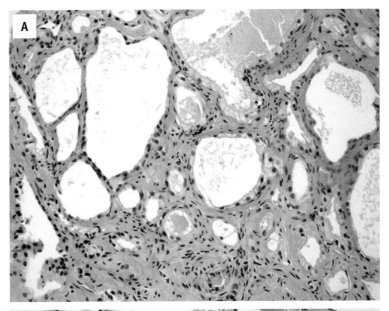

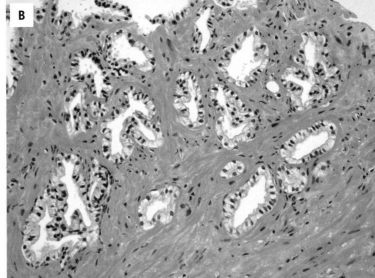

FIGURE 1-16

A and **B,** At low power, partial atrophy may retain the lobular pattern of atrophy. The lesion lacks the basophilic appearance of atrophy, because the nuclei are more spaced apart. **C,** At high power, the cells have pale-clear cytoplasm, relatively bland nuclear features without prominent nucleoli, and an undulating luminal surface with papillary infolding.

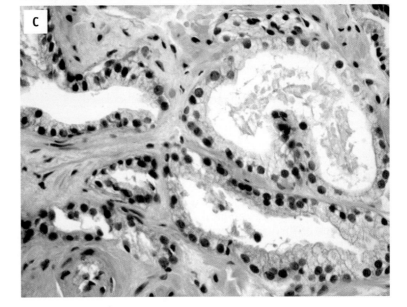

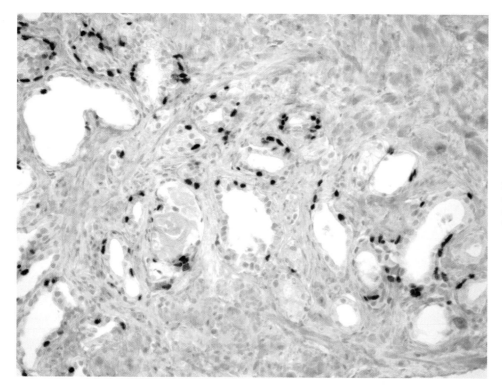

FIGURE 1-17
Immunoreactivity for p63, a basal cell marker, is often patchy in partial atrophy, with only few reactive basal cells per gland.

is distinguished from carcinoma by its characteristic lobular architecture with stromal fibrosis, intact or fragmented basal cell layer, and, at most, occasional mildly enlarged nucleoli. Atrophy with visible nucleoli can also be confused with the flat type of high-grade PIN. However, in flat PIN, the glands tend to be larger and the nucleoli more prominent.

PROGNOSIS AND THERAPY

Atrophy is a benign lesion, and patients should be monitored conservatively. Although atrophy mimics adenocarcinoma of the prostate and has been detected adjacent to cancer, there is no conclusive evidence suggesting that patients with atrophy have an increased risk of harboring or developing PCa.

ADENOSIS (ATYPICAL ADENOMATOUS HYPERPLASIA)

Adenosis, also known as atypical adenomatous hyperplasia, is one of the most common lesions that may be confused with PCa. It is characterized by a localized proliferation of small, closely-spaced glands within the prostate, arranged in a circumscribed cluster or nodule. Adenosis is an incidental histologic finding.

CLINICAL FEATURES

Adenosis has a predilection for the TZ, periurethral area, and apex of the prostate. It has been identified more frequently on TURP (1.5% to 19.6%) than on needle biopsy (approximately 0.8%), and it is present in up to 33% of radical prostatectomy specimens. The mean age of patients diagnosed with adenosis is 64 to 70 years. The volume and number of foci of adenosis increase with age. The biologic significance of adenosis is still unclear. The lesion morphologically simulates low-grade PCa of the TZ. Examples of small acinar carcinoma arising in relationship to adenosis have been reported. The biologic significance of the expression of AMACR, a protein highly expressed in PCa, in a small subset of adenosis cases remains to be determined.

PATHOLOGIC FEATURES

GROSS FINDINGS

Adenosis is not recognizable grossly because is a minute proliferation.

MICROSCOPIC FINDINGS

At scanning magnification, adenosis is characterized by a lobular proliferation of small glands with minimal

---

ADENOSIS (ATYPICAL ADENOMATOUS HYPERPLASIA)—FACT SHEET

Definition
▶ Localized proliferation of small, closely-spaced glands within the prostate, arranged in a circumscribed cluster or nodule

Incidence and Location
▶ 1.5-19.6% of TURP, 0.8% of needle biopsy, and 33% of radical prostatectomy specimens
▶ Predilection for transition zone, periurethral area and apex

Morbidity and Mortality
▶ Benign lesion

Gender, Race, and Age Distribution
▶ Occurs in men usually 5-10 years younger than those with adenocarcinoma
▶ Mean age: 64-70 years

Clinical Features
▶ Incidental finding

Prognosis and Treatment
▶ No treatment needed
▶ No established guidelines available

ADENOSIS (ATYPICAL ADENOMATOUS HYPERPLASIA)—PATHOLOGIC FEATURES

Gross Findings
▶ Nonrecognizable

Microscopic Findings
▶ Lobular proliferation of small glands
▶ Minimal infiltration into the surrounding stroma
▶ Cytoplasm is abundant, pale to clear
▶ Bland-appearing nuclei with inconspicuous to small nucleoli
▶ Fragmented basal cell layer

Immunohistochemical Features
▶ Some positivity for PSA and PSAP
▶ Discontinuous basal pattern with HMWCK and/or p63

Differential Diagnosis
▶ Well-differentiated prostatic adenocarcinoma

---

infiltration into the surrounding stroma (Fig. 1-18A). Within a nodule of adenosis, there are elongated, larger, more obviously benign glands with papillary infoldings and branching lumina admixed with small glands that, out of context, could be confused with cancer (Fig. 1-18B). The cells have abundant pale to clear cytoplasm and bland-appearing nuclei with inconspicuous to small nucleoli (Fig. 1-18C). The small, tubular glands have a fragmented basal layer.

ANCILLARY STUDIES

IMMUNOHISTOCHEMISTRY

By immunohistochemistry, the glands of adenosis exhibit some positivity for PSA and PSAP and typically a discontinuous basal pattern with HMWCK and/or p63 (Fig. 1-19).

DIFFERENTIAL DIAGNOSIS

Adenosis may be misdiagnosed as PCa. In contrast to adenosis, adenocarcinoma has a haphazard, irregular, infiltrative pattern of growth. The most important features separating adenosis from PCa are (1) significantly enlarged nuclei are lacking; (2) very large nucleoli are absent; (3) small, crowded glands mimicking cancer share cytoplasmic and nuclear features with adjacent, more recognizably benign glands within the nodule; and (4) a fragmented basal cell layer is present. Corpora amylacea are commonly seen in adenosis and are rare in carcinoma.

PROGNOSIS AND THERAPY

Although adenosis mimics adenocarcinoma of the prostate, there is no conclusive evidence suggesting that patients with adenosis have an increased risk of harboring or developing prostatic carcinoma. Adenosis should be considered as a benign lesion and treated conservatively.

SCLEROSING ADENOSIS

Sclerosing adenosis of the prostate consists of a benign, circumscribed proliferation of small acini set in a dense spindle-cell stroma. Sclerosing adenosis is an uncommon lesion found in men in their 60s and 70s and in less than 2% of transurethral resections performed for urinary obstructive symptoms associated with BPH. It is largely restricted to the TZ.

CLINICAL FEATURES

Sclerosing adenosis is rarely seen in needle biopsies. Rare cases are associated with elevated serum PSA levels. Usually, the lesion is solitary and microscopic, however, it may be multifocal and extensive.

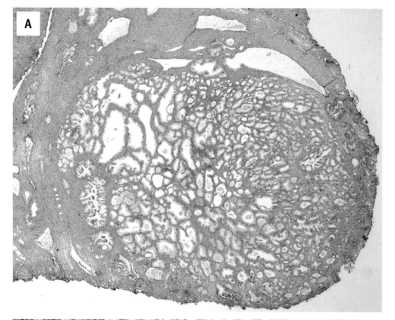

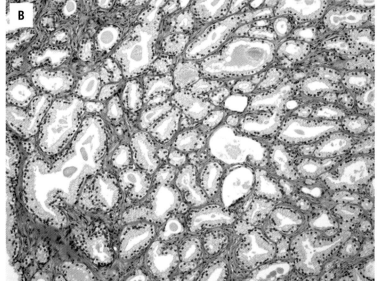

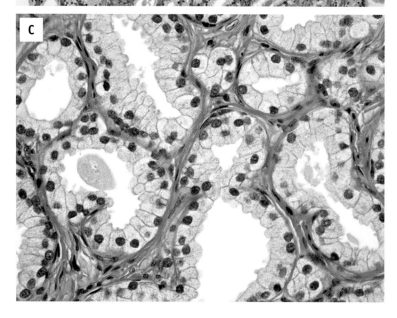

FIGURE 1-18

A, At scanning magnification, adenosis is characterized by a well-circumscribed nodule of small glands with minimal infiltration into the surrounding stroma. **B,** Within the nodule, elongated, larger, more obviously benign glands with papillary infolding are admixed with smaller glands. **C,** At high power, the columnar cells have abundant pale to clear cytoplasm and bland-appearing nuclei with inconspicuous to small nucleoli. Basal cells are focally identifiable.

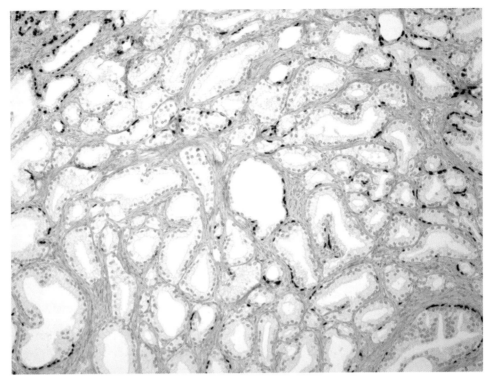

FIGURE 1-19
Adenosis (atypical adenomatous hyperplasia), showing discontinuous basal pattern of staining with p63.

SCLEROSING ADENOSIS—FACT SHEET

Definition
► Benign, circumscribed proliferation of small acini set in a dense spindle-cell stroma

Incidence and Location
► Uncommon lesion
► Incidental microscopic finding found in <2% of TURP specimens for BPH
► Largely restricted to transition zone

Morbidity and Mortality
► Metaplastic proliferation arising from basal cells

Gender, Race, and Age Distribution
► Men in their 60s and 70s

Clinical Features
► Detected in specimens from TURP performed for urinary obstructive symptoms associated with BPH
► Rarely associated with elevated serum PSA levels

Prognosis and Treatment
► No known malignant potential
► Benign course

PATHOLOGIC FEATURES

GROSS FINDINGS

Sclerosing adenosis is not recognizable grossly.

MICROSCOPIC FINDINGS

Sclerosing adenosis is characterized by a more or less circumscribed proliferation of well-formed, small- to medium-sized acini, as well as more poorly formed glands and even single cells embedded in a cellular and often edematous stroma (Fig. 1-20A). The proportion of stroma and glands varies in different lesions. The cells lining the acini display a moderate amount of clear-to-eosinophilic cytoplasm, often with distinct cell margins. The basal cell layer may be focally prominent and hyperplastic, particularly in acini rimmed by pauci-cellular hyalinized stroma (Fig. 1-20B). There is usually no significant cytologic atypia of epithelial cells or stroma cells, but some cases may show moderate atypia. Glandular lumen may contain crystalloids or occasional acid mucin. Characteristic features are the presence of a thick eosinophilic basement membrane around at least some glands and the presence of myoepithelial cells within the basal cell lining of the glands and in the spindle-cell population of the stroma.

SCLEROSING ADENOSIS—PATHOLOGIC FEATURES

Gross Findings
▶ Nonrecognizable

Microscopic Findings
▶ Relatively localized proliferation of well-formed, small- to medium-sized glands and individual cells embedded in a cellular and often edematous stroma
▶ Cells lining the acini display clear-to-eosinophilic cytoplasm, with distinct cell margins
▶ Basal cells may be focally prominent and hyperplastic
▶ Usually there is no significant cytologic atypia of glandular epithelial or stroma cells, although single cells may have prominent nucleoli
▶ Glandular lumen may contain crystalloids or occasional acid mucin
▶ Thick eosinophilic basement membrane around some glands
▶ Myoepithelial cells within basal cell lining of the glands and stromal spindle-cell population

Ultrastructural Features
▶ Basal cells show abundant microfilaments with prominent dense bodies

Immunohistochemical Features
▶ Basal cells coexpress HMWCK, MSA, and S-100 protein
▶ The acinar cells are PSA and PSAP positive

Differential Diagnosis
▶ Prostatic adenocarcinoma

ANCILLARY STUDIES

ULTRASTRUCTURAL EXAMINATION

Basal cells in sclerosing adenosis show abundant microfilaments with prominent dense bodies, in keeping with myoepithelium.

IMMUNOHISTOCHEMISTRY

Sclerosing adenosis is unique in that the basal cells undergo myoepithelial metaplasia and show coexpression of both HMWCK and muscle-specific actin (MSA) (Fig. 1-21A,B). S-100 protein is also positive in these cells. The acinar cells are PSA and PSAP positive.

DIFFERENTIAL DIAGNOSIS

The key feature in distinguishing sclerosing adenosis from PCa is the distinctive cellular stroma seen within sclerosing adenosis. Immunohistochemistry for HMWCK and MSA can be used in problematic cases.

PROGNOSIS AND THERAPY

Sclerosing adenosis is currently viewed as a metaplastic proliferation arising from basal cells, with no known malignant potential. Follow-up has revealed a benign course.

CRIBRIFORM CLEAR CELL HYPERPLASIA

Clear cell cribriform hyperplasia is an unusual form of BPH that is seen in 8% of untreated prostate glands. It occurs in the central region of the prostate, within the TZ. It is mostly seen in TURP specimens removed for urinary obstructive symptoms and is rarely seen on needle biopsy. Cribriform hyperplasia is a completely benign entity and is not a risk factor for subsequent development of neoplasia.

CLINICAL FEATURES

Patients with cribriform hyperplasia have a mean age of 64 to 72 years and usually present with a clinical diagnosis of BPH.

CRIBRIFORM CLEAR CELL HYPERPLASIA—FACT SHEET

Definition
▶ Unusual form of benign prostatic hyperplasia

Incidence and Location
▶ Seen in 8% of untreated prostate glands
▶ Predominantly involves the central region of the prostate, within the transition zone

Morbidity and Mortality
▶ Benign entity; not a risk factor for subsequent development of neoplasia

Gender, Race, and Age Distribution
▶ Mean age: 64-72 years

Clinical Features
▶ Patients present with a clinical diagnosis of BPH
▶ Can be seen after androgen deprivation therapy

Prognosis and Treatment
▶ Benign entity
▶ No treatment required

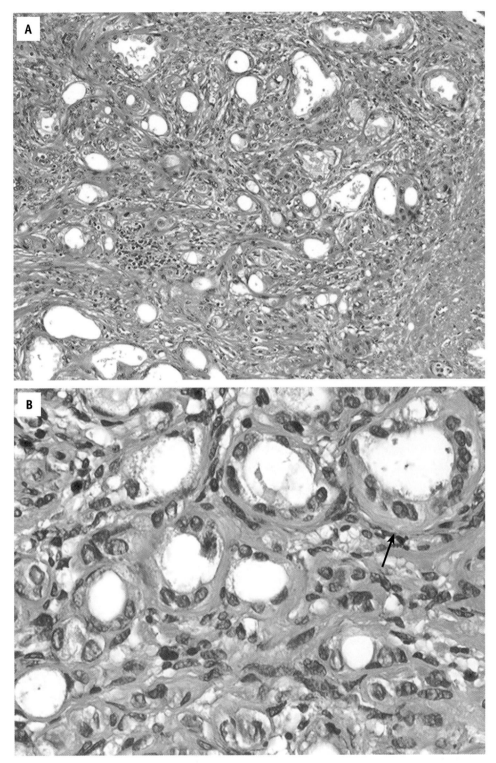

FIGURE 1-20

A, Sclerosing adenosis, showing proliferation of well-formed, small- to medium-sized acini, poorly formed glands, and even single cells embedded in a cellular and often edematous stroma. **B,** The cells lining the acini display a moderate amount of clear-to-eosinophilic cytoplasm, with distinct cell margins. The basal cell layer may be prominent in acini rimmed by paucicellular hyalinized stroma *(arrow)*.

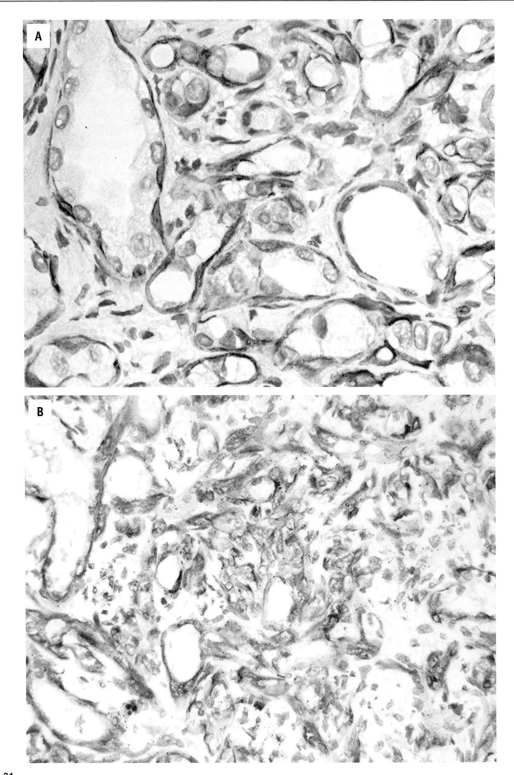

FIGURE 1-21
The lesion of sclerosing adenosis is unique in that the basal cells undergo myoepithelial metaplasia and show co-expression of both high-molecular-weight cytokeratin (HMWCK) (**A**) and muscle-specific actin (MSA) (**B**).